潮汕文库·文献系列

汕头福音医院年度报告编译（1866—1948）

（上卷）

[英] 吴威凛（William Gauld）等著

朱文平 编译

暨南大学出版社
JINAN UNIVERSITY PRESS

中国·广州

图书在版编目（CIP）数据

汕头福音医院年度报告编译（1866—1948）（上卷）/［英］吴威凛（William Gauld）等著；朱文平编译. —广州：暨南大学出版社，2016.8
（潮汕文库. 文献系列）
ISBN 978-7-5668-1665-8

Ⅰ. ①汕… Ⅱ. ①吴…②朱… Ⅲ. ①医院—史料—汕头市—近代 Ⅳ. ①R199.2

中国版本图书馆 CIP 数据核字（2015）第 263203 号

汕头福音医院年度报告编译（1866—1948）
SHANTOU FUYIN YIYUAN NIANDU BAOGAO BIANYI（1866—1948）
［英］吴威凛（William Gauld）等 **著** 朱文平 **编译**

出 版 人：徐义雄
项目统筹：黄圣英
责任编辑：颜 彦 杨柳婷 龙 欣
责任校对：王嘉涵 姚晓莉
责任印制：汤慧君 王雅琪

出版发行：暨南大学出版社（510630）
电　　话：总编室（8620）85221601
营销部（8620）85225284 85228291 85228292（邮购）
传　　真：（8620）85221583（办公室） 85223774（营销部）
网　　址：http：//www.jnupress.com http：//press.jnu.edu.cn
排　　版：广州市天河星辰文化发展部照排中心
印　　刷：广东信源彩色印务有限公司
开　　本：787mm×1092mm 1/16
印　　张：50.75
字　　数：1215 千
版　　次：2016 年 8 月第 1 版
印　　次：2016 年 8 月第 1 次
定　　价：160.00 元（上下卷）

（暨大版图书如有印装质量问题，请与出版社总编室联系调换）

总 序

潮汕文化历千年久远，底蕴渊深，泱泱广袤，又伴随着潮人的迁播而兼收并蓄，独树一帜，是中华文明中的重要一脉。

秦汉之前，潮汕囿于海角一隅，与中原殆少来往；自韩愈治潮，兴学重教，风气日开，人文渐著。宋朝文教兴盛，前七贤垂范乡邦；明朝人才辈出，后八贤称显于时。明清以来，粤东地区借毗邻大海的地理优势，与域外商贸频仍，以陶朱端木之业，成中西交汇之势，造就多元开放的文化格局。饶宗颐等学界巨匠引领风骚，李嘉诚等商海翘楚造福民生，俊采星驰，郁郁称盛。

而今国家稳步发展，蓬勃兴盛，潮汕地区凭借深厚的历史积淀，务实进取，努力发展传统文化及其产业，如潮剧、潮乐、潮菜、工夫茶、陶瓷、木雕、刺绣等，保持并革新精巧特色，在世界各地广泛传播，备受青睐。更有海外潮人遍布全球，为经济文化交流引桥导路，探索共赢模式，拓宽发展空间。

为促进潮汕文化的传承与创新，进一步推动潮汕文化“走出去”，在广东省委宣传部的大力支持下，海内外学者编写《潮汕文库》大型丛书。本丛书包括文献系列和研究系列，涉及历史、文学、方言、民俗、曲艺、建筑、工艺美术等多方面，囊括影印、笺注、点校、碑铭、图文集、口述史等多种形式，始终秉承整理、抢救传统文化的原则，尊重潮汕地区的家学渊源和治学传统。以一腔丹心，在历史沿袭中为文化存证，修旧如旧，求新而不媚俗于新；以一笔质朴，在字斟句酌中为品质立言，就事论事，求全而不迷失于全；以一纸恳切，在纷扰喧嚣中为细节加冕，群策群力，求深而不盲目于深。惟愿以此丛书，提升潮汕文化品位，凝聚海内外潮人，齐心发展，助力腾飞。

在成书过程中，广东省委宣传部高度重视，协调汕头、潮州、揭阳、汕尾市委宣传部，委托潮汕历史文化研究中心、韩山师范学院、暨南大学出版社组织编写与出版。海内外潮学研究专家倾注笔墨，潮汕历史文献收藏机构及热心人士鼎力襄助，更蒙粤东籍一批著名艺术家慷慨捐赠宝贵书画作品助力出版，在此一并致谢！

《潮汕文库》大型丛书编委会

2016 年 7 月

目 录

REPORT

OF THE

MEDICAL MISSIONARY HOSPITAL

SWATOW,

UNDER THE CARE OF

WILLIAM GAULD, M.D.

For 1866.

HONGKONG:
PRINTED BY DE SOUZA & Co.
1867.

REPORT.

THE present Report extends over a period of 15 months, from 20th September 1865 to 31st December 1866. During this interval, however, the dispensary and hospital work was, from various causes, suspended for nearly 3 months; so that the actual working period embraced is little more than a year.

The plan of operation has been the same as that detailed in last Report. At Swatow, the dispensing days for the people generally are twice a week, on Tuesday and Friday, while hospital patients are received at any time, and attended to daily.

During the year, dispensaries have been opened in *Ampow* and *Tathanpow*, two populous towns lying in opposite directions from Swatow, each about 9 miles distant by water. Wednesday is set apart for Ampow, and Saturday for Tathanpow. The visits to these places are made as regularly as circumstances permit. The result of our experiment is such as to encourage a continuance of this kind of work, and, if possible, an extension of it to other towns within a convenient distance. Visits have also been made to other parts of the country.

In addition to this, regular supplies of the more important and easily used medicines are sent to the various Mission Stations in the country, the demand for them being usually greater than we can fully meet.

The Chinese assistant is now of considerable service. He has been with us for three years, and, though at first wholly inexperienced, he has gradually become acquainted with the various drugs we use, can compound many of them himself, and has some skill in using them. In the opening of abscesses, and the other minor details of surgical practice, he is very much at home, and can perform some of the more simple eye operations successfully.

It will be seen, from the following statistics, that the Medical Mission work has, on the whole, been making progress during the past year.

Total number of patients for year ending 31st December, 1866	2,738
Number of *Female* patients included in above, ...	465
„ of *Hospital* patients do., do.	515
Total attendances, ...	10,854
Average on stated dispensing days at Swatow, ...	46
Greatest number treated on any one day, ...	96

In the register there are the names of over 400 places from which patients have come for treatment. These embrace towns and villages in every district of Tiechew, as well as some within the borders of the Fokien Province.

The number of *hospital patients* has greatly increased. Considering that they form in every respect, both for medical and missionary purposes, the most hopeful class, this increase is a matter for thankfulness and encouragement. These in-patients provide their own food and bedding, pecuniary help being but occasionally given when it seems advisable.

The *daily attendance* is nearly a third above last year's, and is noteworthy as indicating the average number of times each patient has been seen. If the number of patients and the number of daily attendances are nearly equal, it is manifest that, to a great proportion of the patients, a single visit could have brought little benefit. On this account it is, that a purely dispensary practice among the Chinese is comparatively so unsatisfactory.

An increased confidence on the part of the Chinese seems to manifest itself by a greater willingness to submit to the treatment prescribed.

To one who is acquainted with the habits of the Chinese it will not appear strange that the males among the patients should so far outnumber the females. It is difficult for women to leave their homes if at all distant from Swatow.

The following is a rough classification of the diseases, medical and surgical, treated during the year :—

Diseases of digestive organs, and general debility,	376
Do. of respiratory organs,	180
Rheumatic affections,	206
Scrofula (enlarged lymphatic glands, &c.)	23
Ague,	52
Fever,	42
Dropsy, and Œdema of limbs,	35
Paralysis,	28
Epilepsy,	6
Insanity,	3
Heart disease,	10
Leprosy,	112
Opium Smokers,	26
Diseases of eye,	626
„ of ear and nose,	22
„ of bone,	26
„ of joints,	67
„ of skin,	231
„ of genitals,	62
Wounds, ulcers, and abscesses,	453
Tumours,	40
Hernia,	14
Fistula in ano,	8
Hæmorrhoids,	4
Harelip,	1

Curvature of spine,	5
Burns,	5
Dislocations,	2
Fractures,	2
Cancer,	11
Dog bites,	4
Gangrene (dry,)	1

Of medical diseases, those affecting the *digestive system* are at once the most numerous and the most difficult to manage. They consist chiefly of cases of indigestion and debility among the poor. Usually of long standing, they are on this account naturally obstinate. Induced, as they are, by the bad quality or insufficiency of their food, the very causes which produced the disease are very often at work while the patients are under treatment. Moreover, if the patient has come to stay for a time, he not unfrequently puts himself on even a more meagre diet than at home; that he may be able to maintain himself longer in the hospital. Thus the drugs have not a fair field for their operation, and to be effectual would have to be backed up by food of a nourishing kind. This however the limited state of the funds at our disposal forbids except in a very few cases. Other diseases in this group, such as dysentery and diarrhœa, are more amenable to treatment, and produce more satisfactory results.

In diseases of the *respiratory organs*, phthisis, or pulmonary consumption, holds a conspicuous place. It is interesting to observe that, both in the frigid and torrid zones, in the Arctic regions and in the Tropics, this disease seems to prevail. It is perhaps, proportionally, as common among the natives of the South of China as among the Esquimaux of Greenland.

From the foregoing table it might be judged that *heart disease* was comparatively rare among the Chinese. Besides the cases noted, however, many of the patients treated for other maladies were afflicted with disease of the heart more or less advanced.

Of 100 cases of *leprosy*, made the subject of special observation and inquiry, those who had no known relatives affected with the disease numbered 78, or more than three-fourths of the whole; 14 of the lepers had some one or more relatives also leprous; 7 formerly had syphilitic disease; and one could give no other explanation of the origin of his trouble than that he lived with a leper. The ages of these patients ranged from 11 to 67 years. One case, that of a lad of 17, began after inoculation. Another, 15 years of age, was born a leper of a leprous mother; the patient aged 67 had been a leper for 10 years. The variety more frequently seen was the tubercular. The predisposing cause of leprosy is yet unknown, the exciting cause being, probably, whatever produces debility of the system.

Between 40,000 and 50,000 pills for the cure of *Opium smoking* have been used during the year. Among other instances of the benefit derived from them is the following:—The patient, a middle aged man, had been an Opium smoker for 10 years, and was using two drachms weight of the prepared extract of Opium daily. Determined at length to break off the habit, he began by taking 10 pills a day. At the end of 50 days, during which time he gradually diminished the number, he was taking only 2 pills a day, and about to give up even these. His case seemed a hopeful one.

A case of cystitis, or inflammation of the bladder, occurring in an Opium smoker, may be noticed as singular from the rapidity with which symptoms, apparently severe, subsided. The patient was suddenly affected with bloody urine a thick ropy (mucus) being abundantly discharged with it. There was little pain. He was ordered Castor Oil, the hot bath, Dover's powder, and rest. In a day or two he was quite well, somewhat to our surprise for the case looked serious.

Of surgical cases, by far the most numerous, are those affecting the *eye*. The operations on the eye have been as follows :--

For entropium and trichiasis,	64
Tumours removed from conjunctiva,	5
Pterygiums removed,	17
Tapping anterior chamber of eye,	13
Division of Iritic adhesions,	2
Iridectomy (for artificial pupil,)	6
Cataract (hard) extraction,	11
Operation for soft cataract,	1
Removal of Staphyloma,	1
Slitting up lacrymal canal,	1

The tumours removed from the conjunctiva, or lining of the eyelid and eyeball, are usually small, and derive any interest they may have from the importance of the organ whose functions they interrupt. One may be noted. It was attached to the conjunctiva covering the eyeball above the margin of the cornea, and extended to the angle formed by the reflexion of the conjunctiva on the lid. Of the size of a large hazel nut, it was round and smooth like a clot of blood, but of a blackish colour, and apparently cancerous in its nature. It had been growing for four months. There was no difficulty in removing it with the knife.

A number of people have been coming lately from the Southern District of the Fokien Province, affected with large unhealthy *ulcers* on the lower limbs. These are accompanied in many cases with greatly enlarged spleens, and a debilitated state of the system generally. They thought the disease was induced by the Taipings having polluted the water with dead bodies. If the rebels were responsible for this, it was more likely on account of their wasting the fields around, and thus causing a scarcity of food, which would press most heavily on these poor people, already living on the barest allowance.

A woman, troubled with a very large *abscess* of the loin, gave a curious account of it. It had been gathering in various parts of the body and had been driven from place to place by the application of chopped grass poultices. Such was the story. She was at once relieved by having the abscess opened.

Of *skin diseases*, perhaps the most interesting were several cases of *Kelis*. Uniformly the disease was found to be spreading, and attended with a hot itching pain. One was that of a woman aged 20, who came to me when in the country. The disease was confined to one spot over the breast bone. It was a raised patch of a dull, reddish colour, about the size of a large bean, and quite moveable. It began to appear 2 or 3 years ago, and was gradually enlarging. I cut it out along with some healthy skin around it, and stitched the wound, but was obliged to leave for Swatow before it had quite healed. Probably little care was afterwards taken to heal the sore, and ere long I heard the disease had returned. Another case was that of a boy of 16 years. He showed me a button-like tumour on his breast which he wished removed. On examination I found the trunk and limbs studded with tubercles of different sizes, round and oval, of the same nature as that on the breast. To cut was out of the question, and medicine was given, the efficacy of which there was no opportunity of testing as the lad soon after left. Kelis in some respects resembles cancer, though by no means such a formidable disease.

The general surgical operations have not been of any special importance. Excluding the opening of abscesses and such like, they number about 50 and embrace the removal of various kinds of tumours, removal of polypi, hæmorrhoids, and diseased bone, evulsion of the toe nails, amputation of the thumb, operations for harelip and fistula in ano, cutting out of bullets, &c.

A case of *distortion* resulting from a burn was operated on. The patient, a strong healthy looking man from the country, came with the fourth and fifth toes of one foot drawn up at right angles to the back of the foot by the cicatrix of a burn. He could not wear a shoe, and on that account wished to have the deformity removed. I cut across the thick raised belt of cicatrix and then dissected along to the roots of the toes. After forcibly straightening these, a splint was applied to the sole, and the toes were tightly bandaged to it. A pretty large ulcer was the result, which however gradually healed, the two toes being all the while kept level with the others by means of the splint. The foot got well.

A commencement has been made in *Vaccination.* Over 60 children were vaccinated in latter part of the year. The prejudices against our performing this little operation are very strong among the Chinese here, but having once made a beginning there is every prospect of so palpable a benefit being gradually more and more appreciated and sought for.

Through the liberality of the English Presbyterian Missionary Society, aided largely by the foreign community in Swatow and elsewhere, we have been enabled to erect a *new Hospital* far more suitable and commodious than any place we have hitherto occupied. It is a large two storied building, with easy accommodation for over 50 people. On the ground floor is a meeting room for the patients, where religious services are regularly conducted. Above this are a dispensary and spare room for the Missionary. The whole building, including cost of site, has been completed for about $4,000. The names of the contributors will be found at the end of the Report, and we would here return our sincere and hearty thanks for the ready and generous way in which our appeal for assistance has been met. The Chinese subscriptions have been obtained through the Seen-Hing Hong, and in connection with this we gladly acknowledge the kind services of Captain Morrison before his leaving for England.

Our desire and prayer is, that the new hospital may, every successive year, be a means of increasing blessing both to the bodies and to the souls of multitudes from every part of Tiechew. May they within its walls obtain the end for which they come, in health restored or improved, and pain exchanged for the comfort of ease. But not this only. May they, in addition, through the glad tidings of salvation daily brought within their hearing, be led to seek Him who is the only, but ever efficacious Physician of souls, the Lord Jesus Christ. This is the great object of our work, and according to our success in this are we glad. We have reason to believe that the past year has not been without fruit of this kind, and many of the patients have returned to their homes, in different part of the Department, with such knowledge of the "way of life" as needs but the Spirit of God to kindle into a saving faith.

SUBSCRIPTIONS FOR NEW HOSPITAL.

E. Vincent, Esq.,	$100
Rev. Wm. C. Burns, Peking,	100
H. D. Williams, Esq.,	50
H. A. Dircks, Esq.,	50
C. W. Bradley, Esq.,	50
Dr. Scott,	50
Rev. C. Douglas, Amoy,	36
Wm. M. Cooper, Esq.,	25
R. J. Lent, Esq.,	25
Captain Morrison,	25
Captain Locke, "*Belted Will,*"	25
E. Saltzkorn, Esq.,	20
Jas. Goodrich, Esq.,	20
Messrs. Fischer & Co.,	15
R. J. Abbott, Esq.	10
J. H. May, Esq.,	10
James M. Beatty, Esq.,	5
Thomas Stewart, Esq.,	5
Captain Newton, "*Roscote of Spool,*"	5
Captain Lister, "*Britain's Pride,*"	5
Captain Lyall, "*Memento,*"	5
B. Evan Hove, Esq.,	5
Swatow Eng. Presb. Missionaries,	300

CHINESE SUBSCRIPTIONS.

Chun-a-Lien, Swatow,	$100
Deputy Yu, Swatow Customs,	10
Ho-a-Low, "	10
Koo-Sung-Chow, "	10
Seen-Hing Hong, Swatow,	10
Foong-Sow-Sun, "	10
Chim-a-Fook, of Kwong-Chun Hong,	10
Kwok-a-Lun, Swatow,	40
Soon-Wo Hong, Swatow,	5
Tak-Foong Hong, "	6
Kwong-Tak-Seng, "	10
Hip-Mow Hong, "	6
Lee-Teen Kee, "	5

Hoy-Yuon-Chan, Swatow,	$	8
Yung-Yue-Hing, „		5
Yung-Chit-Soon, „		10
Ming-Foong Hong, „		10
Hop-Yue Shop, „		6
Seng-Hop „ „		5
Yuen-Mow Hong, „		8
Yeong, Military Officer of Chinghae,		10
Chun, Officer for Treasury, „		4
Yung-Yu-Foong, Swatow,		5
Fei-Tai Hong, „		6
Lu-Lin Hong, (Dircks & Co.),		6
Leong Hing, Swatow,		5
Kai Hing, „		5
Kwong Hing, Customs Bank,		5
Him-Seng, Swatow,		5
Kwong Hop, „		3

The following *Subscriptions* have been used to help in defraying the current local expenses of the dispensary during the past two or three years, having been contributed in 1864 and 1865 :

Dr. Scott,	$	50
Shipping in harbour,		53
Captain of "*Robert and Alexander*,"		10
Captain Howieson and crew, "*Spec*,"		22
Captain Murray and crew, "*Finella*,"		26.50
Messrs. Drown & Co.,		25
Mr. Botefuhr,		25
Shipmasters pr. Messrs. Drown & Co.,		10
Mr. and Mrs. Fischer, and Shipmasters pr. Mr. Fischer		92
Captain Grigs "*British Banner*,"		5
Captain Reid, "*Capiolani*,"		4

REPORT

OF THE

MEDICAL MISSIONARY HOSPITAL

AT

SWATOW.

IN CONNECTION WITH THE

ENGLISH PRESBYTERIAN MISSIONARY SOCIETY

UNDER THE CARE OF

WILLIAM GAULD, A.M., M.D., C.M.

For 1868-1869.

Printed by DE SOUZA & Co.,
HONGKONG.
1870.

REPORT.

Two years have elapsed since we published the last Report of our Medical work in connection with the English Presbyterian Mission to the Chinese of the Swatow region, and we have now, as then, the pleasure of recording steady progress in the number of *Hospital* patients. So much is this the case that the Hospital, which was built two years and a half ago, and then supposed to be sufficiently large for our purpose, is found to be much too small to accommodate the numbers which occasionally throng its wards. As stated in previous Reports, the in-patients are our chief care, and yield most satisfaction to us whether as physicians or missionaries. The number of these has been larger this last year than in any Hospital in China, so far as I am aware. The out-patient or dispensary practice here, however, is exceedingly small, but as the other is sufficient to occupy our time and strength we do not regret this.

The two *Dispensaries* in the country, at Ampow and Tathaupow, are still in operation, and visited weekly, for the most part by the native medical assistants, in company with one or other of the preaching missionaries.

The plan of dispensing on two days a-week at Swatow is still adhered to, and the course of procedure is on the whole the same as noted in previous Reports.

At Chow-chow-foo, the chief city of this department, a public dispensary was started by the Chinese in 1868. I have little doubt our Swatow work was in a great measure the *stimulus* to this. Supported by public contributions, which at first came in freely, everything seemed to promise success, and crowds came to the two native physicians who alternately gave their attendance on nine days in the month. The patients received written prescriptions which they took to a native drug store, where they received the medicine *gratis*. Soon, however, the funds began to fail, and the people to become dissatisfied with the ability, or want of it, displayed by the medical men chosen. These had of course undergone no special training for their work, but, being able to read and having abundant leisure, had probably looked over some book of prescriptions, thereafter considering themselves qualified practitioners. The institution may now be said to be extinct, both in respect of any attendance of patients and any adequate supply of the necessary funds. This may be taken as the common history of such establishments in China. Only in countries where Christian principle more or less influences the character of the people can such benevolent schemes have permanence and stability; and from this, alas! China is still far distant. True philanthropy is a fruit of Christianity alone, for true love to men can never be dissociated from love to God.

The statistics given for 1869 are obtained by making a proportional estimate for the whole year of the number registered for about six months. During the latter half of the year, in which I was unfitted by sickness for full work and regular attendance, there were quite as many patients as in the ealier part. The work for the greater part of that time was almost entirely in the hands of the three native assistants, and it is gratifying to be able to report that they carried it on so as to give very general satisfaction. I believe the statistics for 1869 are within rather than above the mark.

	1868	1869
Total number of patients*	2,950	2,500
Hospital patients (included in above)	608	850
Female patients "	486	...
Average attendance on dispensing days at Swatow	52	63
Greatest " " "	91	128

A small ward of the Hospital is set apart for *women* and is usually full.

A Chinese house close at hand was rented last year for the use of *lepers*, and sometimes from 10 to 20 of these unfortunate people were living in it at one time. The treatment of leprosy is still as unsatisfactory as ever. Hearing of the fame of a Bombay physician in the treatment of this disease, I wrote to a medical friend there for information on the subject and was much disappointed to receive the following answer:—"I know him well and have seen some of his patients. It is my own decided opinion and that of nearly all the medical men in Bombay that the whole affair is quackery". There are Chinese doctors who undertake to cure this terrible malady, but I have had no satisfactory proof of a single complete cure,

* These numbers indicate only the *new* cases entered in the register. The *total attendance* of old and new cases together, represented by the 20,000 or 30,000 of some Medical Reports in China, may perhaps mislead when given as the *number of patients*. Thus 1 patient coming 6 times is by this system set down as 6 patients. Unless a distinct register of the *new* patients be kept, it is impossible to give their number.

or indeed, of anything beyond a partial and temporary improvement, and this our Swatow patients in many cases obtain. It is a most common ailment in this part of China, and though, so far as I have seen it, quite distinct from the leprosy described in Scripture, it is, I am convinced, as sure to lead, sooner or later, to a fatal issue. The Chinese give the most widely diverse and unconnected reasons for being the subjects of leprosy. The soil, the water, rain and sun-heat and night dew, measles and the small pox, and numberless other things are stated as a cause. While it is regarded by themselves as hereditary, yet the majority of the lepers who come to the hospital protest that they have no leprous progenitors and that their leprosy came not from family taint.

It is usual to give a table of the different diseases treated and the following list for 1868 may be interesting to medical friends and others :—

Diseases of Digestive Organs.

Toothache	15	
Indigestion	281	
Worms	19	
Colic	3	
Diarrhœa	12	
Dysentery	9	
		339

Diseases of Respiratory Organs.

Catarrh	50	
Laryngeal Affections	11	
Bronchitis	28	
Pneumonia	1	
Phthisis pulmonalis	37	
Hæmoptysis	16	
Asthma	47	
		190
Rheumatic affections		169
Heart disease		6
Scrofula		18
Fever, Remittent	25	
„ Intermittent (Ague)	56	
		81
Dropsy		10
Œdema of lower limbs		13
Paralysis, Partial or local	10	
„ Hemiplegia	1	
		11

Epilepsy	9
Insanity	2
Leprosy	134
Opium smokers (for cure)	3
Female diseases (Leucorrhœa, &c.)	9
Kidney disease	7
Diseases of Eye	426
,, of Ear	9
,, of Skin	150
,, of Joints	37
,, of Bones	15
,, of Genitals	34
Wounds, Ulcers, and Abscesses	302

Tumours.

Cancerous	14	
Fatty	5	
Fibrous	5	
Lardaceous	4	
Gelatinous	4	
Vascular or Nævous	3	
Nodes and Warts	9	
		44

Ranula	2
Harelip	17
Cleft palate (both hard and soft)	1
Inguinal Hernia (Rupture)	4
Fistula in Ano	13
Hæmorrhoids (Ext. 2 Int. 5)	7
Angular Curvature of Spine	5
Tetanus (with Emprosthotonos)	1
Fracture	1
Dog bites	5
Snake bite	1
Goitre	1
Gangrene from frost bite	2

A table of the diseases treated during the year 1869 would be little more than a repetition of the above, with slight difference as to numbers.

A glance at the table will show that the diseases of the Chinese are very much the same as are met with in the dispensary practice of a poor district in England. Take away leprosy, elephantiasis or œdema of limbs, and perhaps in some degree aguish fever, and the rest of the diseases named have nothing specially Chinese about them. Owing to the want of native medical skill, however, and the great poverty of many of the people, some diseases attain to a development here which we seldom witness at home. Ulcers, for example, are allowed to spread to a very dangerous as well as loathsome extent, and a similar remark holds true in regard to many skin and eye diseases.

Comparatively few cases of acute inflammatory diseases come under notice in the Hospital. The great majority are chronic cases of indigestion, debility, rheumatism, chest complaints, eye disease and ulcers. Many of the patients have been so long the subjects of disease that complete cure is hopeless and we are glad if they can be sent back relieved to any extent. Many however, receive benefit of such a marked kind as, on their return, to induce others in the same village or town to come for treatment, many of them at considerable expense and effort. We have heard of a man even selling one of his sons to get money to come to the Hospital,—having, moreover, to travel forty or fifty miles to reach it.

Now and again we come across curious specimens of Chinese practice. Take the following:—A man came to the dispensary suffering from some degree of enteritis or inflammation of the bowels. At first he had been troubled with constipation and colic, for which he applied to a Chinese doctor, who, to expel the supposed poison, gave him the following prescription!

Ten Spanish Flies,
Three Centipedes,
Ten Silk-worms,
Ten Scorpions,

to be rubbed up together and the whole taken at once. Inflammation was the result, as might have been expected; it was, however, soon relieved by poultices and opium.

Many of the diseases are of *Syphilitic* or *Scrofulous* origin, although ranked under other heads. Those marked *Scrofula* are cases in which the symptoms were purely scrofulous. *Lupus* in its various forms is very common, and Chinese may often be met with *minus* the nose, the organ having been eaten away by this destructive malady.

A remarkable case of *Chronic hydrocephalus*, or water in the head, was seen at the Ampow dispensary in a child two years old. The disease had lasted a year, and by that time his head was so large that he could not support it. His body in other respects was not out of proper development, and he seemed not wanting in intelligence. The circumference of the head across the brow measured 2 feet, and over the crown from the ear tips 1 foot 3 inches; the feeling of fluctuation, indicating the presence of fluid, was quite distinct; the parietal bones, forming the sides of the head, were far separated and could be felt only at the lower part of both sides.

The enormous head attached to such a puny body gave the child a very singular appearance. No treatment was attempted.

Very few of the Chinese come to the Hospital simply to be cured of *Opium-smoking*, but we still continue to dispose of quantities of pills at Swatow and the various mission stations in the country to those who apply for them. The following case which came under our observation here is interesting:—The patient was a man aged 35 years, suffering from asthma. Fifteen years ago he began to smoke opium for relief from this disease, but found it ineffectual. However the habit of opium-smoking had so grown upon him, that he reached the enormous consumption of about a Chinese ounce daily. Having determined at length to give up the vice, he had recourse to the pills. Of these he began by taking 32 a day, and when he came to the Hospital he had by a gradual reduction come to require only a single pill a day. He experienced no great difficulty in giving up the drug so long as he had the pills, but when these were intermitted he was attacked with dysentery. The evil effect of Opium-smoking on the body, mind, and morality of the Chinese have been recently detailed by several medical missionaries in the pages of the "Chinese Recorder" and with their statements generally we quite agree. Hitherto, however, all agitation of the subject has proved barren of practical results, and the victims of this vicious habit continue to increase through the length and breadth of China. Much as has been said of the physical and moral injury attendant on opium-smoking, no one who has seen the miserable specimen of humanity a confirmed opium-smoker presents, and who knows anything of the general effects of his vice not only on himself but on his family and all dependent on him, can say that the strongest statements are exaggerations. Rather would we say that words are inadequate to depict the fearful state of matters induced by the abuse of Opium. With regard to Christianity, every missionary knows in how many ways this evil comes between him and the success of his efforts to propagate the Gospel. The Chinese themselves feel the injury and wrong keenly, and none is more ready than the opium-smoker himself to deplore the sad state of things. More and more manifestly is it proving itself China's curse. All agree that opium-smoking is everywhere spreading through the Empire, and we have good authority for stating that even in Peking, and within the precints of the palace itself, the practice has spread to an alarming extent. Some will tell us other nations have their stimulants and sedatives, their intoxicating drinks and tobaccos, &c. True, we admit, to a greater or less extent. But China has not only its Opium, but its intoxicating drink and tobacco in addition; and most commonly we find the opium-smoker a tobacco smoker, and not unfrequently a Chinese-whiskey drinker as well. The Opium evil, however, so transcendently eclipses the others that, comparatively speaking, they sink out of notice.

Among *Surgical* cases, *eye* diseases still hold by far the first place. Not a few come who are totally blind and hopelessly incurable, but most receive benefit more or less marked, and in some cases the results are very gratifying. Take the following for instance:—A man came with the eyelids of one eye so closed in consequence of the healing up of a wound made by a bamboo, that only one fifth of his sight remained to him, or, to use the Chinese phrase, he could see only *two parts* out of *ten*. It was a marked case of *Anchyloblepharon*, and caused not only loss of sight, but no little deformity. The adhesion was cut open and the lids separated, the skin and the mucous membrane of the upper lid being stitched together to prevent the lids again adhering. The restoration of sight was perfect and the appearance of the face greatly improved. Another case of injury from a blow, resulting in complete destruction of the eye, came for treatment. The lens was partly separated from its capsule, and driven backwards into the posterior chamber of the eye, where it could be distinctly seen, quite opaque and cataractous. The other eye was being injured by sympathy, and the lens had to be removed, not to restore sight, which was impossible, but to get rid of what was a cause of irritation to both the blind eye and the sound one. In 1868 there were 142 operations performed on the eye, and in 1869 the number was 170. More than the half of these were for inversion of the lids (*Entropium*) and irregular growth of eyelashes (*Trichiasis*), injuring the eyeball by friction. The Chinese assistants often perform these operations, as well as operations for *Pterygium* which come next in frequency. *Squint* seems to be a comparatively rare deformity among the Chinese of this region, and though I have seen a few cases during the past six years, I have never had the opportunity of operating on one.

Mangling of the ears is a way of taking vengeance on an offender occasionally indulged in by the Chinese. A man came to us one day with the outer border (*Helix*) of both ears cut away. They had been clipped off with scissors by an angry creditor. A curious method of getting satisfaction from a debtor! Another man came not long ago with one ear cut and mangled all over. He had gone to demand field-rent from a tenant, and a fight followed, during which he was *bitten* on the ear in the savage manner stated. Sometimes girls come with the lobe of the ear slit open owing probably to the use of large ear-rings. This deformity is remedied by an operation similar to that for harelip.

Diseases of *bones* are frequent. In a case of *necrosis* of the lower jaw, nearly the half of the lower jaw bone was lying loose in the gums. With very little cutting, the dead bone was removed in two or three pieces, to the great satisfaction and comfort of the patient.

Elephantiasis, or enlargement of the lower limbs, is almost invariably accompanied with swelled glands in the groin over the large blood vessels of the thigh. The following case was so :—He was a man of 26 years of age and both legs began to swell 16 years ago. He then had aguish symptoms, rigors &c. When he came to the Hospital, the measurements of his legs were

round the calf of leg, 2 feet 7 inches in one leg and 2 feet $3\frac{1}{2}$ inches in the other,

round the ankle, 2 feet 7 inches in one and 2 feet 1 inch in other.

The skin and tissue under it hung in heavy folds over the feet. I lately saw a woman whose arm from the elbow downwards presented the same appearance as the leg in Elephantiasis does, and have no doubt the disease was identical. It is the only case of this kind I have seen in the upper limb. Elephantiasis of the legs does not, so far as I have seen it, usually extend above the knee,—the thigh being comparatively normal in size. Where the disease is slight, rest with elevation of the limb, bandaging, Iodine paint locally and Iodide of Potassium internally, give satisfactory results for the time at least; but where the swelling is great and the skin disorganized there is little hope of doing much good.

Tumours of various kinds, from the size of a pea to that of a person's head, are not at all uncommon. The manifest benefit of their removal, as well as, in most cases, the safety of the operation and rapid healing thereafter, all strike the Chinese most favorably and bring credit to Western surgical skill. All the more is this the case from the fact that in this department the Chinese doctors are, from the want of anatomical knowledge, comparatively helpless. The practice of dissecting dead bodies, now freely allowed among Western nations, can alone supply this deficiency in Chinese surgery. With the exception of an occasional *post mortem* examination in the Chinese Hospital at Shanghai, and a little dissection at Dr. Kerr's Hospital, Canton, I know of nothing of the kind in China. Chinese official *post mortem* examinations of those who have died by violence or under circumstances requiring investigation, need not be alluded to, as these are, I believe, conducted in a way completely at variance with our ideas on the subject, and not calculated to help forward a useful knowledge of anatomy.

Fatty tumours are the most common. One about the size of a small pumelo was hanging like a soft bag from the shoulder blade of a young man, who was in consequence unfitted to some extent for work. It was easily dissected off the muscles on which it rested, and the skin stitched together. A few days for the healing of the wound completed the cure. Another of the same kind, about as large as a boy's head, was hanging down over the back bone like a beggar's wallet. The patient was 31 years of age and the tumour had been growing from his birth. I marked the line of incision for the guidance of the Chinese assistants and then left them to operate, which they did in my absence. The operation was successful and the man soon got well.

Cancerous tumours among the Chinese are of the same varieties as among Europeans. *Hard* cancer of the breast (mamma) is more common in women than in men. We removed one, however, about the size of an oyster, from the breast of a male patient. The wound made in operating healed rapidly, as is usual in cancerous patients. A case of *soft* cancer of the side, growing over the ribs, came for operation. The surface of the tumour was ulcerated to the extent of about two inches, owing to the employment of caustics by the Chinese doctor. On cutting it, the cancer was found to consist of several distinct smaller tumours, bound together by fibrous meshes, which separated during the operation. After excising as cleanly as possible, the raw surface was well washed with Carbolic Acid and the skin stitched together. I cannot say whether the disease returned afterwards, as the patient, on leaving the hospital, returned to his home at a distance in the country, and has not since been heard of.

The largest tumours are not always the most dangerous. *Vascular* tumours, though usually small, are yet much to be dreaded from the tendency to bleed on slight interference. A boy aged five years had a tumour of this kind on his scalp. He came with it bleeding freely. This had happened several times before and now the child was quite blanched or anæmic and had a cough from debility. The tumour was scarcely the size of a chestnut and adhered to the head by a small root not much thicker than whipcord. Round this I tied a strong thread so as to strangle it, cutting away at the same time all the tumour except a little knob to keep the ligature from slipping. Several months afterwards I met with a case exactly similar in another part of the country which was cured in the same way. The child whose case has been above noted, would inevitably have died ere long from the constantly recurring hæmorrhages, and the very simple operation doubtless saved his life.

Fibrous tumours of the neck are frequently seen, and they sometimes attain a very large growth. One of these, nodulated and pendulous, which had been growing for 20 years, was removed from a man's neck and the patient cured in about 18 days.

An elderly gentleman from the Foo-city came with a large tumour under the tongue (*Ranula*) which prevented any distinct articulation, and projected so as to produce a large bulging under the chin. The tumour consisted of a thick bag of skin filled with a custardlike semifluid mass which flowed out when an opening was made. After emptying it, a piece of the bag was clipped away and the rest injected with Iodine Tincture. Ere the patient left, all deformity was removed and he could speak quite distinctly,—the cyst becoming obliterated. The removal of a piece of the cyst wall effectually prevented any refilling of the tumour. I heard afterwards that the cure was a permanent one.

We have had many *Harelip* operations, most of which have been performed by the Chinese assistants. They usually afford great satisfaction to the patients. A case presented itself which had previously been operated on by a Chinaman (a Hakka) for $2. The operation was fair, except that a large notch was still left in the lip which the man wished to have remedied. His desire was granted.

At Kway-tham, one of the mission stations about 60 miles S. W. of Swatow, a remarkable case of *Tetanus*, with *Emprosthotonos* or bending forward of the spine by spasms of the muscles, was seen in a boy aged 9 years, the subject of spinal disease. Owing to *lock-jaw*, he could not open his mouth and had to be fed with fluid food. He was pale and sickly and, when awake, perspired freely. His arms and legs were quite stiff. His trouble was complicated with dysentery and protrusion of the end of the bowel. He could not turn himself in bed and at times his agony was great. He was seen only once or twice and then I had to return to Swatow.

The Chinese very rarely submit to have an arm or leg removed, however painful and useless the limb may be from disease. A patient from Hai-mung, however, had suffered so much from extensive ulceration of the elbow and disease of that joint, his health being rapidly undermined from the constant irritation and discharge of matter, that he gladly consented to the *amputation* of his arm. Dr. Maxwell and Dr. Manson, both of Formosa, happened to be present, and gave their assistance. The greater part of the wound healed at once, and in a fortnight the patient was ready to leave the hospital. An artificial arm was ordered from home, but the poor man died of consumption about a year and a half after the operation. It is pleasant to be able to add that this patient forsook idolatry and embraced Christianity, his after life giving good evidence not only to us but to his family and friends at home that he really believed in Jesus Christ as his Saviour. "Disciple of Jesus" was engraved in Chinese characters on his tombstone by his heathen relatives at his own request when dying.

Amputation of half of one foot and the ends of the five toes of the other had to be performed on a middle aged Chinaman who was frost-bitten while serving on board ship at Newchwang. When he came to the Hospital, all the toes and part beyond of the left foot were black, the line between the living tissues and the dead being very distinct. The ends of the toes of the right foot had also mortified, and were as black as the others. It was a marked case of *dry gangrene.* Hey's operation was performed on the left foot, leaving the heel and ankle bones untouched,—thus preserving half the foot. Only the last joints of all the toes of the right were removed. After several weeks both feet healed perfectly, and the man is able to walk about without a staff, though with a considerable limp on one foot. He was an opium-smoker, but while in the Hospital gave up the practice. He afterwards desired to be baptized, and as he had acquired a very intelligent knowledge of the Truth and appeared sincerely anxious to follow it, his desire was complied with. He is at present acting as the Hospital door-keeper and gives satisfaction in that position.

Besides the above, operations for the removal of dead bone, of hæmorrhoids or piles, for fistula, hydrocele, fungus testis, extraction of teeth, extraction of bullets, with a large amount of abscess opening, &c., make up the sum of our surgical manipulations.

In 1868 about 160 children were *vaccinated*, chiefly in the country around. At present in many widely separated villages, mothers are anxious for a visit of the Medical Missionary to vaccinate their children.

The question of *Infanticide* has been lately discussed by some friends in the north and centre of China, and without much of agreement. It would be greatly for the benefit of all concerned, if those who write about China and its people would confine their remarks to what they *know* of their own region, and refrain from hasty conclusions regarding the whole Empire, in regard to which immensely extensive generalizations on very limited data are easy and tempting. Let each one speak for the district in which he resides and with which he is familiar. In this way we should be saved the contradictory statements which are constantly being made by residents in different parts of this large country. In this N. E. Department of the Canton Province, among a population of several millions, infanticide is, alas! very prevalent, and no one who travels much through the district can fail to have the fact brought disagreeably before him. In our journeys we have seen a dead child floating in the village pond, or drifting down the river, or stranded on the low bank with perhaps a crow perched on the little body, or in the early morning the father has been met going out with his newly born female child in a basket to cast it away. Sometimes again the child is strangled ere it leave the mother's side. Infanticide is so common that the guilty parties scarcely care to conceal the crime, and they are ever ready with excuses for it. It is said to be less prevalent in the cities than in the villages. In the former, the children are sometimes laid down in the streets, in the hope that they will be picked up by some benevolent individual, and perhaps be deposited in the Foundling Hospital. Foundling Institutions originally existed in each of the nine District cities, but they are now little more than a name, there being no funds regularly available for the necessary expenses. In the Foo-city Foundling Hospital, when flourishing, there maybe between 20 and 30 children. Each nurse has at the most two children, and gets $2 or $3 per month for her pay, the money being raised by public subscription. The children are occasionally taken from the Hospital to families in which they are brought up as wives for the sons. Infanticide is said to be less common among the Hakkas, owing to their custom of getting the daughters betrothed in infancy and brought up in the family of the future husband. Among them, too, the women are more valuable for field work, which may be another reason for their preservation. The pleas put forward for this unnatural crime are various. If a woman gives birth to a female child and rear it, she is not likely to have another for two or three years, whereas if she destroy it she has the chance of a male child much sooner. Again she objects to rearing it on the ground that it prevents her from working and earning a little to help in the feeding of the family, and that even if she do rear it, the daughter when grown up has to be given away to a husband and so all her labour is lost. This is their own reasoning. No doubt poverty has a great deal to do with the crime, but many who *could* feed all their offspring, are so influenced by the general feeling of the uselessness of female children that they *will not*. A graduate with whom I had some conversation on the subject estimated that about three *per cent* of the mothers are guilty of Infanticide, but I fear that almost any mother among the poorer classes who bears several female children will not scruple to destroy one or more of them. In any case the birth of a female is no matter of congratulation, but the opposite. So much so, that the Chinese who are acquainted with foreigners seldom think of congratulating them on the birth of a daughter, whereas, if a son is born the expressions of their pleasure are loud and profuse. They look to their sons as the support and stay of their declining years, and the parents who have many of these "arrows" in their "quiver" are considered greatly blessed.

In taking a retrospect of the Medical Mission work in Swatow during the last *six* years, we cannot sufficiently praise our gracious Lord and Master for all His goodness to us. It is through His blessing that many thousands of the Chinese of Tiechew have been relieved, to a greater or less extent, of the pains and sicknesses which brought them under our notice. Especially have we to praise Him for His mercy to not a few of the patients in shewing them His salvation. In one month of the year 1868; no fewer than *nine* persons were admitted into the Church by baptism who first heard the Truth in connection with the Medical work. In various Districts of this mission field, old patients are occupying important positions among the members of the native Church; while of one or two we have a good hope that they have already entered on the joys of heaven. Apart from cases of actual conversion in connection with the Hospital, we cannot but hope that the daily preaching of the Gospel to so many, who are at the same time experiencing in their own persons that "goodwill to men" which it proclaims, is acting as a leaven which, by God's blessing, is preparing for "greater things" than we have yet seen. The beneficial influence of the Institution on the people generally has radiated far in every direction, and gratifying testimony to this is again and again received from the missionary brothern. They find their way greatly facilitated by it in their journeyings through Tiechew among a people naturally jealous and suspicious of foreigners, and at times the good name of the Hospital has been helpful in circumstances of danger and embarrassment. The *religious services* have for some time been carried on entirely by Rev. Messrs. Smith and Mackenzie to whose assiduous cultivation of the field opened up to them by the Medical department of the work, is, under God, chiefly due the success which has accompanied it. When there is hearty co-operation of the preaching with the medical missionary, and the former is willing and ready to embrace the peculiar opportunities afforded by the work of the latter for making known the Gospel,—the work of both being done in faith,—we have no hesitation in declaring the Medical work a most valuable auxiliary to the missionary scheme.

Dr. Thomson, from Edinburgh, has opportunely arrived to carry on the medical mission in our absence.

We here gladly take occasion to tender our most grateful thanks to all, both Europeans and Chinese, who have helped us by their subscriptions. With a list of these we close our Report.

SUBSCRIPTIONS

FOR 1868.

J. C. A. Wingate, Esq., U. S. Consul...	$ 25
Captain Piersdorf, ...	50
Captain Willowby, ...	10
Ho-a-Low, ...	10
A friend, ...	10
Captain Thomas, ...	4
Rev. G. Smith, ...	100
Rev. H. L. Mackenzie, ...	100
W. Gauld, Esq., M. D., ...	100
	$409

FOR 1869.

Chaloner Alabaster, Esq., H. B. M's Act. Consul, ...	$ 25
J. C. A. Wingate, Esq., U. S. Consul,...	25
F. Kleinwächter, Esq., Commissr. of Customs, ...	50
do. (private)...	25
Messrs. Bradley & Co.,...	50
" Dircks & Co., ...	50
Dr. C. Scott,...	50
E. Vincent, Esq., ...	50
R. M. Hobson, Esq..	40
do.	25
R. J. Lent, Esq., ...	25
G. Glass Lowder, Esq., ...	25
Thos. P. Drown, Esq., ...	25
John Horne, Esq., Calcutta, ...	17.78
A. Huber, Esq., ...	15
Messrs. Meyer & Fehr., ...	15
B. C. George Scott, Esq., ...	10
C. B. Warner, Esq., ...	10
C. Grant, Esq., ...	10
O. Asverus, Esq., ...	10
A. L. Piersdorf, Esq.	10
Captain Owen, "Lammermuir"	10
Captain McRae, "Isabella Ridley"	10
M. Clausen, Esq., ...	5
A friend, ...	5
H. Johnson, Esq., ...	5
Rev. G. Smith, ...	100
Rev. H. L. Mackenzie, ...	100
W. Gauld, Esq., M. D.,...	100
	$897.78

CHINESE SUBSCRIPTIONS.

郭麟	$20	
謙盛	10	
中剪	5	
雲賓	10	
鍾劍卿	5	
何彬文	10	
協昌	10	
福和	10	
開源	10	
協茂	10	
永捷順	10	
乾裕	5	
源裕	10	
永源興	10	
榮源	5	
陳源盛	6	
陳德茂	6	
廣珍盛	6	
宏興	5	
容華隆	5	
永順美	5	
萬興	6	
佳興	5	
艮	6	
A friend	10—	$ 200.00
		$1,097.78

* Obtained through E. Vincent, Esq., and his shroff.

REPORT

OF THE

Medical Missionary Hospital

AT

SWATOW,

IN CONNECTION WITH THE

PRESBYTERIAN CHURCH OF ENGLAND.

UNDER THE CARE OF

William Gauld, M.A., M.D.

PRINTED BY

DE SOUZA & CO.

HONG-KONG.

1878.

REPORT.

May, 1878.

ALTHOUGH the usual routine of hospital and dispensary work has been carried on during the year without interruption, our time and attention have been largely taken up with the building of the *new hospitals*, to which allusion was made in last Report.

Through the kindness of the Taotai, a very suitable site for the *General Hospital* was obtained on the sea beach, immediately adjoining the mission compound on the West. In negotiating with the Chinese Mandarin for it, we were indebted to Mr. Forrest, H. B. M.'s Acting Consul, for his kind help. The ground has 120 feet of sea front to the South, and extends 180 feet backwards to the main road leading in to Swatow. It has a free exposure on all sides, and is somewhat sheltered from the East winds by the other mission buildings.

Having obtained the site, we proceeded to fill it up to the requisite level, and in September the foundations were laid. Through God's goodness to us, the building was finished in time for use before the beginning of the warm season, and on the 18th April it was dedicated as a Mission Hospital. On that occasion, the missionaries and native Christians in Swatow, including some of our friends of the American Baptist mission, met for prayer and praise in connection with the work. Interesting addresses were delivered by the missionary and native brethren, and for the new hospital was earnestly sought the blessing of Him in whose cause it has been built.

The hospital consists of three main double-storied buildings facing the South. The one in front is separated from the two behind by a space of twenty feet. Its lower floor is wholly occupied by the preaching hall or

Chapel (about 48 feet X 28 feet) which is capable of seating two hundred people. The upper floor has five rooms, (dispensing and operating rooms, with assistants' and private rooms.) The two blocks behind are entirely for the patients. They have, in all, eight wards (about 18 feet X 38 feet) each containing ten beds. The upper floors are connected with each other by a front verandah, and from it a cross passage goes to the dispensing room, &c. in the front building. On the one side of the latter is a single-storied building for women, and on the other side a similar building is divided into four small rooms for patients who may prefer to pay a little for the use of a separate room rather than go into a common ward. Along the enclosing walls on both sides are cook-houses, bath-rooms, &c. There is ample accommodation for a hundred patients, and, carrying out the principle of the "cottage" system, each ward is practically isolated from all the others.

The funds for building were obtained by the sale of the old hospital; by liberal contributions from the Swatow foreign community and from the Chinese, including a donation of 100 taels from the Taotai; by a contribution of £100 ($495) from the foreign mission Committee of the Presbyterian Church of England, and one of £50 ($250) collected in New Zealand by the Rev: George Smith.

While the General Hospital was being proceeded with, steps were also taken for the erection of a *Leper Hospital.* We felt impelled to this on account of the large numbers of lepers who come for treatment year by year, and whom we were unwilling to receive into the General Hospital. Could no relief be given to those afflicted with leprosy, we should not have thought of a leper hospital. But our experience is that in most cases where the desease has not advanced very far, improvement can be effected, while in some cases apparently complete cures have been obtained. Lately a patient left us after a prolonged course of treatment, free from all marks of leprosy, although when he came the disease was very marked. In some parts of India, in Trinidad and elsewhere, very encouraging results have been obtained in the treatment of this desease. So far as we have seen, it is different from the leprosy of Scripture, and seems less dangerous, although sooner or later, if unchecked, it leads to a fatal issue. The Chinese of this region do not isolate lepers from the rest of the family except in extreme cases, and their idea of its contagiousness, or of infection from it, may be judged from the following local proverb:

寧與癩痦人同床
勿與生疥人對門

"With a leper you may sleep in the same bed, but don't stay opposite the door of one who has itch."

A piece of ground was purchased outside the native town, and at some distance from any dwelling house, but within easy reach of the general hospital. On this a building was erected large enough to receive twenty patients, the chief expense of which was kindly defrayed by the Mission Committee in Edinburgh. The total cost of the General and Leper Hospitals will be seen in the statement of account at the end of the Report.

On arriving in 1863, we first began work in a small Chinese house in Swatow, which was rented for a year. We then removed to the old mission house, using part of it as a dispensary, while for in-patients we rented an adjoining house. The need for a larger hospital however soon became apparent. With considerable difficulty we obtained what was then considered a good airy site on the water side, and eleven years ago our first hospital was built. It seemed all we could desire, and we felt very thankful for the increased accommodation and convenience in working which it provided. By the rapid growth of the native town, however, it is now shut in on every side, and quite unsuitable for a hospital, while the increasing numbers of in-patients made a still larger building necessary. The leper patients also had too often been crowded together in a small Chinese building entirely unfit for our purpose. Now that we have a General Hospital with *four* times the amount of room for patients of the former one, and a Leper Hospital more comfortable than the ordinary run of Chinese houses we would record our thankfulness to the Giver of all good, and, under Him, to the kind friends in Swatow and elsewhere who have furnished the means with which to build these hospitals. We trust the increased facilities for work may stimulate us to do more for the physical and moral well-being of the Chinese. They will have the benefit at least of improvements in regard to healthiness of situation and extent of accommodation, which should render many of their ailments more easy of cure.

The attendance during the year was affected somewhat by an outbreak of cholera in Swatow in the end of summer, and partly too, I think, by the fact that so much time had to be transferred from the work of healing to the superintending of building operations. The native assistants, however, on whom much of the hospital work was thus thrown, performed it on the whole satisfactorily. During part of the year the in-patients were increasing so that I had to limit the number both in the general and leper hospitals, being afraid of evil results from overcrowding during the cholera outbreak. The numbers for 1877 are as follows:—

In-patients.

General Hospital	1,073	
Leper „	90	—1,163

Daily average number of In-patients.

In General Hospital	75	
Leper „	13	— 88

Out-patients.

General	1,104	
Leper	181	—1,285

Average attendance of Out-patients.

(On dispensing days twice a week)	— 35

Total number of new cases entered, 2,448.

Females included in above.

In-patients	115	
Out-patients	197—	312

The patients as heretofore are chiefly from the villages and towns of the extensive region accessible from Swatow, embracing the nine districts of the Tiechew or Chao Chow Department and parts of that of Hweichow and Kia Yung Chow, and also the southern border of Fokien. They are usually most numerous in the summer months, when the temperature is such that they can travel without much in the way of baggage. The following table shows the *daily average attendance* during the various months of the year:—

	In-patients.	*Out-patients (on Disp. days.)*
January	116	42
February	55	14
March	88	33
April	82	30
May	130	62
June	104	49
July	78	26
August	68	28
September	102	30
October	89	49
November	64	34
December	75	25

The nature of the diseases we have had under treatment may be understood from the subjoined table. It will be seen that diseases of the *eye* and *skin* make nearly a half of the entire practice:—

General Diseases.

Fever, Remittent	21	Scrofulous or Syphilitic	
Intermittent	49—70	Glandular Swellings.	15
Rheumatic Affections	145	General Debility	18
Leprosy	271	Opium smoking	3
Cancers	23	Dropsy, Anasarca	10
Anæmia	34	Ascites	5—15

Diseases of Nervous System.

Headaches	6	Epilepsy	3
Paralysis, Facial	4	Local Anæsthesia	1
Partial	3	Locomotor Ataxy	1
Hemiplegia	11—18	Muscular Atrophy	1

Diseases of Digestive System.

Throat Affections.........	2	Diarrhœa..................	9
Toothache and Carious Teeth....................	5	Dysentery................	14
Dental Fistula...........	1	Spleen Enlargement....	12
Tonsillitis.................	1	Jaundice.................	1
Dyspepsia..................	112	Stricture and Ulceration of Rectum...........	8
Hæmatemesis............	2	Prolapsus Ani...........	7
Enteralgia (Colic)........	5	Fistula in Ano...........	20
Worms, Lumbrici.......26 Ascarides	1—27	Hæmorrhoids, External 4 Internal 21	—25
Constipation..............	4		

Diseases of Respiratory System.

Aphonia....................	11	Hæmoptysis..............	4
Catarrh....................	29	Phthisis	46
Bronchitis.................	27	Pneumonia	2
Asthma.....................	24		

Diseases of Circulation.

Heart Disease.............	3	Aortic Aneurism.........	2

Diseases of Urinary and Generative Organs.

Kidney Disease...........	60	Ulceration of Penis......	6
Diabetes Mellitus.........	1	Cancer „ „	3
Dysuria....................	1	Orchitis.....................	1
Incontinence of Urine...	1	Enlarged Testicle........	3
Spermatorrhœa..........	6	Hydrocele.................	25
Gonorrhœa and Gleet...	4	Ulcered Scrotum.........	2
Bubo	1	Menorrhagia	1
Phymosis..................	4	Amenorrhœa.............	1
Inflamed Penis...........	1	Leucorrhœa..............	3

Diseases of Skin.

Eczema	16	Lupus Exedens	1
Impetigo...................	1	Elephantiasis, Leg......24 Scrotum. 8 Both	1—33
Trichosis Furfurans (Ringworm)..........	37		
Psoriasis Palmaris	13	Alopecia..................	1
Pityriasis..................	7	Horny Skin	1
Scabies.....................	14	Corns......................	1
Prurigo.....................	4	Boils.......................	8
Lichen......................	1	Carbuncles...............	3
Acne........................	3	Abscesses............... ..	27
Condylomata	2	Ulcers......................	242
Kelis	1		

Diseases of Eye.

Asthenopia	18	Corneitis	11
Hemeralopia	2	Ulcers of Cornea	53
Conjunctivitis	56	Opacity „	89
Chronic Chemosis of Conja	2	Conical	1
Granular Ophthalmia	39	Staphyloma	6
Entropium	98	Hypopyon	7
Trichiasis	25	Iritis	6
Hordeolum	1	Synechiæ	9
Tinea Tarsi	2	Cataract	16
Tarsal Tumour	2	Glaucoma	6
Mucocele	1	Sympathetic Ophthalmia	1
Pterygium	30	Amaurosis	4
Vascular Cornea	12	Cancer	2
Pannus	1	Incurable Blindness	39

Diseases of Ear.

Otorrhœa	3	Deafness	6

Diseases of Nose.

Inflammation	2	Epistaxis	1
Polypus	7	Foreign body in Nostril	1

Diseases of Bones.

Caries and Necrosis	31	Spinal Curvature	5

Diseases of Joints.

Inflammation	17	Anchylosis	1
Sprain	12		

Unclassified.

Tumours,—Fibrous	5	Wounds, Incised, &c.	33
Nævous	6	„ Gunshot	2
Fatty	5	Blows and Bruises	74
Lardy	3	Burns	3
Ganglionic	1	Dog Bites	5
Warty	1	Snake „	1
Vascular	3	Centipede Bites	1
Glandular	16	Slit Ear	10
Osseous	1	Harelip	45
Ovarian	1	Cleft Palate	3
Encysted	4	Deformity from Cicatrix	3
Windy	1—47	Talipes Varus	1
Dislocations	2		
Fractures	2		

The majority of the patients is, as in former years, from the peasantry and labouring class, but there are some from all grades of native society. The Taotai's son was under treatment while on a visit from Chaochowfoo to Swatow with his father. Before leaving they paid a visit to the mission compound, and among other things saw the Boys' Boarding School under Mr. Gibson's care, with the work done in which the Taotai seemed pleased.

In the beginning of October, Cholera was prevalent in Swatow and in some of the large towns and villages around. In Chaoyang a family of eight or nine persons was wholly swept away. In many cases death was preceded by pain and vomiting without purging. Out of six patients seized in the Hospital, two died, one almost immediately, the other from gradual exhaustion brought on by the after fever. These are the first deaths from cholera that have occurred in the hospital since its commencement. The epidemic was apparently much more severe elsewhere along the coast of China than in the Swatow region.

Last year I remarked on the infrequency of deaths in the wards. This year there have been more than usual. One of those who died, was the brother of a District Mandarin. He came to the hospital in a hopeless condition, but finding himself more comfortable than at home, he preferred to stay and die in it.

To "divide the inheritance" does not seem to be an easier matter in China than it once was in Judea. A young man came to the hospital with numerous large wounds on his head, face, and arms. These, he said, had been inflicted on him with a large knife by his elder brother, because he, the younger, had found fault with the mode of division of the family property after the death of their parents. The elder, fearing the consequences of his crime, fled to another District, leaving on his brother's person lifelong marks of his avarice, injustice, and cruelty. Curiously enough on the same day another young man came from a different part of the country, to be treated for a wound of the shin caused by a stab from his elder brother in a quarrel between them.

Hernia (Rupture) is common among the Chinese, but I have rarely seen it in an *irreducible* condition, and never *strangulated*. It is seen usually on the right side. The Chinese pay readily for a foreign made truss, although native articles of wood or iron are used. One man showed me an ingeniously contrived wooden truss of his own devising and manufacture. Though serving its purpose, it was clumsy and uncomfortable compared with the European article.

There were 299 *surgical operations* performed on the *eye* of which the chief were:—

For removal of *Entropium* (the eyelashes inverted and rubbing on the eyeball)................. 229

For removal of *Pterygium* (fleshy growth on eyeball).. 38

Iridectomy (for artificial pupil)................. 4

Removal of *Cataract*................................ 8

A girl came having a *nervous* tumour which covered nearly the whole of her upper eyelid to the lash border. It was ligatured, and though at first there seemed the prospect of an extensive eversion of the lid, owing to the loss of skin, it eventually healed up and left scarcely any deformity.

The *operations* on the *body generally* were the following:

Tumours removed		26
Dead Bone	,,	8
Bullets	,,	2
Hæmorrhoids (piles) removed		17
Fracture set		1
Harelip operations		40
Slit Ear	,,	9
Fistula in Ano operations		14
Phymosis	,,	3
Hydrocele	,,	25
Paracentesis Abdominis		1
Deformity from cicatrix removed		1—147.

Besides teeth extractions, opening of abscesses, &c.

On one day the native assistants performed no fewer than fourteen operations, eight on the eye, three for harelip, and three for hydrocele.

A series of *soft tumours* appeared on the body of a girl of twelve years of age. Though the skin was quite natural over them, they were exceedingly painful. On using the exploring needle only *serum* was found in one of the largest of them. With the exception of one or two in which suppuration occurred, they were gradually dissipated by Iodine paint locally, with the internal use of Iodide of Potassium and Cod Liver Oil. The girl got quite well.

An *open tumour* was removed from the back of the neck of an elderly man, which was found to be full of chalky masses, part of which adhered to the neck. The bleeding was very profuse, but was stopped by pressure, and the rest of the diseased substance was removed by escharotics. The wound healed in due course.

Last year we took notice of the number of *harelip* operations. This year they were still more numerous, and at one time there were no fewer than eight harelip patients in the hospital from various parts of the country. We operated on two brothers from the same village in which lived a father and son both formely cured of the same defect. Afterwards another father and son came for operation. From the beginning up to the present time, about 160 cases have been operated on.

A case of *deafness* presented itself in a woman who said it was caused by a native doctor piercing the drum of the ear to let out some supposed disease in the head. She had the choice given her of having her eyeball pierced instead! Another case of deafness on one ear resulted from a blow, which caused hæmorrhage both from the external ear and through the Eustachian tube into the mouth.

A man came with an *ulcer* of the leg which was the result of a *snake* bite five years ago. Another was bitten in the finger by a snake, and his arm above the elbow was tied so tightly by his doctor, that there was a firm cicatrix of considerable breadth all round the arm, the remains of extensive ulceration from the ligature. Below, the arm was much swelled from the obstruction to the venous circulation. Another patient, while cutting grass on the hill side, about five months previous to his coming to the hospital, was bitten at the root of the thumb by a large *centipede*. He afterward became feverish and at the end of ten days felt pain along the arm up to his elbow. After a further interval of ten or fifteen days, the pain had got as far as his head, and eventually it spread all over his body, like rheumatic pains. Such a result of a centipede bite is somewhat uncommon.

In the beginning of 1877, my chief assistant, who had been with me from the commencement of the medical mission here, left to begin practice on his own account in Swatow and the country around. He had proved himself an efficient helper, bold and skilful in surgical operations, and fertile in expedient. I was sorry to part with him. In his place, however, came another old assistant, who also had some years ago left for private practice in the neighbourhood of his own village. His success, financially, did not come up to his expectation, and he was glad to return to the hospital work. Although not equal to the other in energy and courage, he is very helpful both in the medical work and in conducting the religious services among the patients.

At the morning and evening meetings for worship, the patients have been daily instructed in Christian truth. As in past years, I have had the cordial help of my colleagues, of whom the Rev. Messrs. Mackenzie and Gibson are at present in the field. They now undertake for three mornings a week, the increased burden of general mission work in Swatow and in the country, preventing them from doing more. The native assistant shares with me in conducting the other meetings. On Sunday afternoon, a special service is held with the patients. The visible results have not materially differed from former experience. Many have been indifferent to what they heard, some have been so convinced of the truth of Christianity as to give up idolatry, and a few have cast in their lot with the Christians. Those who thus decide in favour of the gospel, are not long in discovering that it and heathenism are opposing forces. An elderly man from a village about twelve miles distant from Swatow, was recently baptized along with two other patients. After a time he went home, improved in health, and in possession, we trust, of eternal life through Christ Jesus. Subsequently he came back to the hospital with the news that his relatives, hearing he had become a worshipper of God, had ere his return home, greatly injured his house and destroyed its furniture. Those of them who were cultivating his fields refused to give him his due share of the produce. In this state of things he wished to sell his fields, but his relatives would neither allow any other to buy them, nor would they themselves pay him fair value for them. They also told him that as he had given up the worship of the idols and ancestors, they would not even allow him to live in the village. The old man was much distressed. He had once been in Singapore for some years, and had returned to his native land with a sum of $200. Of this he had spent about $80 in building his small dwelling house, the rest going mostly to buy the fields of which his relatives were dispossessing him. We advised him to return to his village and try in a peaceable way to come to some terms about his property. He did so, and afterwards came to tell us that he had got a few acres of ground out of his persecutors' hands, and had rented them out to a friend whom he thought he could trust. As his house was still unrepaired, we advised him to have it put right and to live in his village, with the hope that by a consistent life he might disarm the opposition of his relatives, and commend the cause of Christianity to them and to his fellow villagers generally. There are cases of persecution in other parts of the region more severe than his, in which the Christians have to endure reproach and loss of goods as best they can, through the sustaining power of God's grace. It is a mistake to suppose that a Chinaman necessarily profits in worldly circumstances by becoming a Christian, and that he only becomes one from hopes of wordly gain. Such cases there may be, but generally, in the first place, a profession of Christianity is followed by persecution and loss. In the country at least, away from the influence and help of foreigners, it is so. That many are found ready to bear all rather than forsake the truth, is a proof of its divine power over their hearts and lives.

We gladly record our obligation and thanks to the friends who have so liberally contributed of their means to help in the building of the new hospital; also to Mr. Schjöth for obtaining contributions from the native employees in the foreign and native customs; and to Chinese friends in the hongs of Messrs. Bradley & Co. and Messrs. E. Vincent & Co., for obtaining contributions from the Chinese merchants in Swatow. We have to thank some lady friends, also, for supplies of white cotton for surgical dressings, and for clothing and other things useful to the sick. Our old friend of the Tang Ngwan Seng Hong has again kindly given us 2,000 tickets for cash and rice to poor patients, value over $50. He is the purchaser of the old hospital on behalf of the members of a guild in a distant sea coast town. They have bought it for conversion into shops or storehouses, the yearly rent of which is to make a fund for the funeral expenses of sailors and others, who may be drowned along this part of the coast. Thus, though no longer used as a hospital, it is still apparently to serve a charitable purpose.

SUBSCRIPTIONS TOWARDS CURRENT EXPENSES.

"Offender," per R. J. Forrest, Esq., H. B. M. Consulate	$ 30.00
A Chinaman, per C. Hannen, Esq., Commissioner of Customs	100.00
Miss Fielde, for Hospital patient	5.00
Mr. Scott Chinese Customs, for patient	4.50
A young friend, per W. G.	25.00
A friend, proceeds of race prize	10.00
Captain Pitman	5.00
A friend	5.00
Rev. S. B. Partridge	10.00
Wm. M. Cooper, Esq, Shanghai	5.00
George Harrison, Esq., „	4.50
Consultation fees, per Dr. Gauld	85.00
	$289.00

SUBSCRIPTIONS TOWARDS BUILDING OF NEW HOSPITAL.

Drs. Scott and Scott	$ 200.00
T. W. Richardson, Esq	100 00
H. A. Dircks, Esq	100.00
Messrs. Herton Ebell & Co.	75.00
Rev. George Smith	55 00
William Gregory, Esq.	50.00
C. Hannen, Esq	50.00
Rev. J. C. Gibson	50.00
William Gauld, M D	50.00
Rev. H. L. Mackenzie	40.00
Rev. John Rutherfurd	30.00
Carried over	$800.00

Brought over	$800.00
W. Hülse, Esq.	30.00
C. Jeremiassen, Esq.	30.00
Rev. Dr. Ashmore	25.00
Rev. W. Duffus	25.00
R. H. Hill, Esq.	25.00
W. S. Fergusson, Esq.	25.00
G. D'Arnoux, Esq.	25.00
E. Vincent, Esq	25.00
C. C. Williams, Esq	25.00
P. Campbell, Esq	25.00
W. Laidlaw, Esq.	10.00
W. Rae, Esq.	10.00
J. W. P., Esq.	10.00
Otto Asverus, Esq	10.00
J. R. Bridgman, Esq	10.00
J. D. Meyer, Esq	10.00
E. Bois, Esq.	10 00
A. Crasemann, Esq	10.00
W. Watson, Esq.	5.00
W. Pollock, Esq.	5 00
P. H. King, Esq.	5.00
A. Witte, Esq	5.00
Chr. Nönchen, Esq	5.00
Samuel Paul, Esq	5.00
W. Harris, Esq	5.00
H. Ramsey, Esq.	5.00
F. W. Focken, Esq.	5.00
M. Jupiter, Esq	4 00
A. Norden, Esq	3.00
A. L. Piersdorf, Esq	3.00
J. Low, Esq	3 00
H. Schaumlöffel, Esq	3.00
P. Williams, Esq	2.00
J. Ecclestone, Esq	2.00
	$1,205.00

CHINESE SUBSCRIPTIONS TOWARDS BUILDING OF NEW HOSPITAL.

The Taotai ....100 taels=$144.00

現任潮州道憲張

Loo Leen Hong, Kueh Kee Yong 50.00

魯麟行司事郭繼榮

Chinese Customs' Deputy, Kui.............................. 30.00

督辦新關稅務委員貫

Tsan Thai Oon 20.00

曾泰運

Phok Hong Chiang.. 20.00

卜宏昌

Leem Khien Thai Hong.................................... 16.00

林泰乾行

China Merchants' S. N. Co.'s Hong.................... 12.00

輪船招商局

Chinese Customs' late Deputy, Ho 10.00

欽加同知銜前任文昌縣正堂何

Han Tsu Ngee 10.00

項子宜

Ho Teen Kwang.. 10.00

何鎮光

Ho Siu Iah, Gov. Bank.................................... 10.00

何守益官銀號

Carried over.......................... 332.00

Brought over	332.00
Hiap Moug Hong .... 協茂行	10.00
Kia Heng Hong .... 佳興行	10.00
Nam Chhiang Soon Hong .... 南昌順行	10.00
Kueh Khai Ngwan Hong .... 郭開源行	10.00
Tang Ngwan Seng Hong .... 陳源盛行	10.00
Khiam Seng Hong .... 謙盛行	10.00
Kwan Hwat Zoo Hong .... 光發裕行	10.00
Hok Chhiang Ie Hong .... 福昌洋行	10.00
Yong Seng Hwat Hong .... 永成發行	10.00
Lee Chhiou Chiu .... 李朝周	10.00
Kwang Tshoon Hong .... 廣春行	6.00
Hwa Soon Long Hong .... 和順隆行	6.00
Iah Seng Hong .... 益成行	6.00
Carried over	450.00

Brought over	450.00
Gek Lee Zoo Kee Hong 玉利裕記行	6.00
Iah Kee Hong 益記行	6.00
Tan Song Mong Hong 陳松茂行	6.00
Heng Seng Lee Hong 興盛利行	6.00
Lee Ngwan Hong 利源行	6.00
Ngee An Hong 義安行	6.00
Tong Hwa Khiam Kee Hong 中和謙記行	6.00
Chiap Heng Hong 洽興行	6.00
Tan Yong Heng Hong 陳永興行	6.00
Ko Kwan Heng, Gov. Bank 高廣恒官銀號	5.00
Lee Wang Ie 李汪洋	5.00
Beh Su Tee 麥士治	4.00
Ee Keet Hai Kee Hong 怡吉海記行	4.00
Carried over	522.00

Brought over	522.00
Siou Chiap Seng Hong 蕭捷盛行	4.00
Nie Loo Khee 梁汝頎	3.00
Kwang Joo Tung Joo 光裕堂俞	2.00
Lee Lee Teng 李麗亭	2.00
Ngeng Yien Tung, U 凝遠堂余	2.00
Phua Kiam Kok 潘謙谷	1.00
Gou Che Chiu 吳星洲	1.00
Ie Oo Cho 姚雨齋	1.00
Joo Tsu Ngiam 俞子嚴	1.00
Heng Noi Hwang 王蓮芳	1.00
Iap Hoon Lau 葉雲樓	1.00
Sia Tshau Tung 佘草堂	1.00
Siou Chiap Seng 蕭捷成	1.00
	$543.00

STATEMENT OF INCOME AND EXPENDITURE.

To wages of Assistants, Doorkeeper, Cook, &c., for 12 months to December 1877	......	$ 237.17
„ Current expenses, including medicines bought here	......	212.10
„ Printing Hospital Reports, &c.	......	27.80
„ Aid given to poor patients	......	20.00
„ Tickets for cash and rice to poor patients value	......	55.00
„ Medicines from London	......	340.00
„ Cost of new General Hospital :—		
Preparing site, stone bund, &c.	$ 553.16	
Building, painting, &c.	3,879.65	
Furniture, &c.	260.50	
		4,693.31
To Cost of Leper Hospital :—		
Purchase of site and filling	210.15	
Building, painting, &c.	718.35	
Furniture, &c.	23.00	
		951.50
Balance in hand to meet current expences for 1878	......	212.84
		$6,749.72

May, 1878.

Audited and found correct, by

H. L. MACKENZIE.

By Balance from 1876	$ 867.48
„ Contributions for current expenses as per list	289.00
„ Contributions for building New Hospital as per list	1,205.00
„ Chinese do., do., as per list	543.00
„ Cash and Rice tickets for poor patients, value.	55.00
„ Sale of Old Hospital	2,000.00
„ Grant from Foreign Missions Committee of Presbyterian Church of England, for General Hospital, £100	495.12
„ Grant from Mission Committee in Edinburgh, for Leper Hospital, £100	495.12
„ Contribution from New Zealand, per Rev. George Smith, £50 and Interest	253.03
„ Sundries	43.82
„ Sale of Medicines, trusses, &c.	131.31
„ „ of pills for Opium smokers	25.94
„ Medicines from London, paid by Mission Committee in Edinburgh	340.00
„ Contributions from patients, not included in above	5.90
	$6,749.72

WILLIAM GAULD

REPORT

OF THE

Medical Missionary Hospital

AT

SWATOW,

IN CONNECTION WITH THE

PRESBYTERIAN CHURCH OF ENGLAND.

UNDER THE CARE OF

William Gauld, M. A., M. D.

AND

Alexander Lyall, M. B., C. M.

FOR 1880.

PRINTED BY

DE SOUZA & CO.

HONG-KONG,

1881.

REPORT.

THE time has again come round when we are called upon to lay before the friends of the Swatow Mission Hospital a short statement of the work. The report for 1880 must be shorter and less complete than in former years. Dr. Gauld who has had the superintendence of the work, with only a short interval at home, for the last sixteen years, and who by his personal and professional accomplishments has been so instrumental in allaying suspicion and inspiring confidence in Western Medical Science, returned home in early spring for a season of well-earned rest. His interim successor's linguistic studies have to some extent limited his attention to the work.

The Hospital work in its twofold aspects,—Medical and Evangelistic—has, however, been kept going uninterruptedly throughout the year. Both in the Medical and Evangelistic work the native assistants, trained by Dr. Gauld, have taken an active part, and their conduct has given much satisfaction.

As in former years, two days of the week have been given specially to dispensary practice, and the other four days to hospital work and performing of operations, and the arrangement is found to be satisfactory both to patients and to those in charge.

In-patients.—The number of in-patients last year exceeds that of any previous year. There have been 2,403,—an increase of 375 over last year's numbers. Towards the end of summer and in the autumn months the wards of both the large and small hospitals were uncomfortably crowded, and it was difficult to overtake all the work. Although an attempt was made to keep down the numbers by making all living within an easy day's journey of Swatow dispensary patients, unless their diseases precluded satisfactory treatment as such, yet the daily attendance in September and October averaged 239, and in one week in the beginning of the latter month we had 304 patients under our care. This last number may be taken as the utmost limit of the accommodating powers of the two hospitals. From the fact that the largest proportion of our patients is drawn from the numerous towns and villages in the surrounding districts, to a distance of 60 or 80 miles, it is necessary, if we are to treat them at all, to receive them as in-patients irrespective of their diseases. This is by no means a disadvantage in ordinary times, as it allows us to treat their diseases in a more satisfactory manner, and it provides a fine field for missionary operations; but on occasions when sickness is rife, it hinders to some extent our control over the numbers, and compels us to take in more than we otherwise would do.

The difficulty of convincing a Chinaman who has come a distance of from 20 to 60 miles to Swatow for treatment, and who may have been saving his cash for weeks before to enable him to provide food for himself when there, that there is no room, needs only to be experienced to be appreciated. One day a party of six women came from Mi-ow, a large market town about 50 miles inland. They were suffering from entropium, and a small operation, with a few days after-treatment, would have been sufficient for a cure, as the disease was only beginning; but the hospital was full. They were told to go away, and return in another month. At sunset they were found spreading their mats under an outside stair, and the night being warm they intended to sleep there. In these circumstances it is best to give in; accommodation was found for them, and in a few days they returned home with their eyes cured. This is an example of what occurred pretty frequently during those two months.

The large influx of patients in autumn may have been partly due to the unhealthy summer. In spring and the beginning of summer there were unusually heavy and protracted rains, large tracts of land were flooded for a month or more, and the crops in many places entirely destroyed. The exposure and privation then endured by the inhabitants told badly on them as summer advanced; and after the planting of the winter rice crops was finished, we had numerous patients coming from the districts that had suffered from the floods.

The average length of stay in the hospital for each patient was 23 days.

Out-patients.—The number of out-patients treated at the dispensary in Swatow has been 1,346, an increase of 266 over last year's numbers. This branch of the work has almost entirely been conducted by the two senior assistants. It also shows a corresponding increase during September and October. These two months give an average of 66 for each dispensing day; and the largest number attending on any one day was 117. Several trips into the country have been taken, and 510 patients were seen and prescribed for, and a few small operations performed.

The following table giving the number of new patients registered in each month, and the other statistics, will give some idea of the amount of work done:—

	In-patients.	*Out-patients.*	*Total.*
January	129	55	
February	32	26	
March	202	106	
April	187	96	
May	279	88	
June	211	120	
July	207	86	
August	174	111	
September	267	134	
October	376	236	
November	129	132	
December	210	156	
	2,403	1,346 =	3,749
Patients seen in the country			510
			4,259

Daily average number of:—

In-patients from Jan. to July...... 124
" " July to Jan....... 183
Out-patients " Jan. to July...... 28
" " July to Jan....... 48

Females included in above:—

In-patients 465
Out-patients........................... 286=751

Many requests have been received for western medicines by sick people in the country, who, from various reasons, were unable to come to Swatow. Medicines for fevers, dysentery, diarrhœa, and debility were most sought after. Many of these requests were granted, care being taken to prevent any imposition.

The number of female in-patients this year is interesting from the fact that it is a certain indication of increasing confidence in the Hospital on the part of the people. There have been 465, an increase of 178 over last year, and amongst them were a considerable number of younger women. These came generally attended by an elderly female relative, who was frequently a patient herself. It has been found necessary to set apart another of the large wards, capable of holding 20 persons, for their accommodation, and even with the additional space their wards were often overcrowded. An intelligent elderly woman, a christian, has been appointed as matron over their part of the Hospital. She is expected to exercise a general supervision over the women and their wards, to help in dressing wounds and to do mission work in a quiet way. The patients have taken kindly to her, and she shows some tact in her dealings with them. She has only been at work for 10 weeks, but already she is found to be useful in various ways. The want of a few well trained natives to act as nurses has long been felt, and we hope that in her case a good beginning has been made to supply that want.

The class of patients varies little from that of former years. A few Mandarins of the smaller sort, and literary men of various ranks, have been treated as out-patients, but the great bulk of our patients are villagers,—tradesmen and farmers,—many of them very poor.—Tang Nguan Seng still continues to contribute liberally in rice and cash tickets for the assistance of the poorer patients. This year we have received ninety one dollars worth from him, and seven dollars worth from an anonymous donor. Several cases have received some assistance from the Hospital funds. Great care is taken in the distribution of the rice and cash tickets in order that they may not become an inducement for the recipient to stay longer in the Hospital than necessary.

A tabulated list of the diseases treated will be found appended. A short resume may be given for those readers who do not care to study it.

I.—MEDICAL.

Malarious Diseases.—41 cases of simple fever and 103 of intermittent fever have been under treatment: the tertian variety of ague being most prevalent. The majority of the fever patients were admitted during the summer months, and in many the disease was of long standing. Patients who had suffered more or less for six, eight, or ten months were not unfrequent; and then generally the disease was complicated with anæmia, local, and sometimes general œdema.

Of the **Sequelæ** of intermittent fever and Malaria we have had 10 cases of Hepatic (liver), and 33 of Splenic (spleen), enlargements; 165 cases of Anæmia; and a large number of ulceration of the extremities of malarious origin. In a few cases the Hepatic enlargement was very great, extending downwards to the brim of the pelvis, in others more or less of ascites was present. Amongst the anæmic cases is included a considerable number of examples of the disease called by the Chinese *pai sien*. There are doubts as to the nature of this disease. The symptoms are those of general debility with a marked increase of the normal solid ingredients of the urine. The Chinese dread it very much, and ascribe to it the origin of numerous other diseases. It is sometimes preceded by fever, but in other cases no history of fever can be made out. In many cases, at least, it seems to be an anæmia of malarious origin, with symptoms of nervous debility well marked. With regard to the results of the treatment of this class of diseases; the febricula and intermittent fevers were found in every case to yield quickly to quinine. The hepatic and splenic enlargements in some cases were rapidly reduced; in other cases, more especially in those complicated with anæmia and ascites, no benefit was received. The result in many of the anæmic cases was very unsatisfactory. This was mainly due to two reasons—(1) the long continuance of the disease, (2) the irritating effects of Iron on the gastro-intestinal mucous membrane, especially in the hot months. Not unfrequently diarrhœa, and even dysentery, has been produced by five minim doses of Tinct-Ferri perchloridi. The drug is more easily borne when given in pill.

Leprosy.—87 cases of this disease have applied for relief, but as no special provision for their treatment was made during the year—the small building which in former years was set apart for the accommodation of the lepers having been used throughout the year as a general hospital—there is not much to report in regard to them. A few attended the dispensary regularly for a time; but most of them, receiving or buying a quantity of medicine to last for one or two months, were sent home again. The anæsthetic variety has been more frequently seen than the tubercular, and the principal varieties of anæsthetic leprosy coming under our notice were as follows:—(1.) Small portions of skin most frequently over the ankle, knees, buttocks, or on the chest and arms, with impaired sensibility, but with no apparent alteration of structure. (2.) Similar patches, surrounded by a palish red line which sharply defines the healthy from the diseased skin. (3.) Reddish patches, slightly raised and thickened, with the edges ulcerated and the centre pale and anæsthetic. Between this and the former variety various intermediate stages are seen, some of which resemble common ringworm. (4.) Small deep circular ulcers—as if gouged out—on the sole of the foot, with the surrounding skin thickened and anæsthetic. (5.) Muscular atrophy causing contraction of fingers and toes. (6.) Ulceration around toes. (7.) Brown blotches of skin with loss of sensibility.

Blood Poisoning.—The eleven cases of blood poisoning were caused by eating the flesh of a buffalo that had died from disease. They all presented the same symptoms—gangrenous—looking pustules on legs and arms, in some accompanied by a considerable amount of fever. The fever quickly subsided—but recovery in some of the cases was prolonged.

Opium Smokers.—The wards of a large general hospital like ours are not suitable for the treatment of such cases, as more care and supervision are necessary than can be given with so many patients on hand. 20 cases applied for admittance to be cured of their evil habit, of these 12 submitted to the necessary restraint and left the hospital at least temporarily relieved of their craving. The plan adopted was to cut off the opium at once, and Quinine and aromatic stimulants were given in its place. Though the symptoms in some cases were severe, no return to the drug was found necessary. Of the other cases, one was in an advanced stage of Phthisis, and he was advised not to make the attempt. An emaciated wretched looking woman, who ate a large quantity of opium-refuse daily, was only half-hearted in her attempt to reform. She refused to stop the opium all at once, and, on the relief of some urgent disagreeable symptoms, left the hospital. Two men came who stated that they had been cured on a previous occasion, but had taken to the pipe again on their return to their homes. Their manner was somewhat suspicious, and, on demanding a guarantee of good faith, they left the hospital. Other two men made an attempt, but their resolution failed. After being five or six days in hospital and the usual symptoms connected with the cure not beginning to develope, occasion was made to visit their ward shortly before the time for closing the gates at night and they were found absent in Swatow "buying things." On suggesting to them that their visits to Swatow seemed to delay their cure, and that it would be better to hand their cash to the assistants, who would find a trustworthy man to do their shopping, they left. The daily consumption of the drug by the smokers who came to us varied from one to four drachms, and manifestly the chief motive for seeking a cure was the fear of starvation which threatened them if they continued the vicious habit. A mandarin, who was under treatment for another disease for some months consumed, with the assistance of his wife, one dollar's worth every day of the year.

Diseases of the Digestive System.—The most frequent disease in this group is dyspepsia. All the varieties were met with, but the one characterised by eructation of sour water and attacks of pain at intervals or periodically was most common. In many cases the general health was much impaired, and the treatment often exceedingly difficult. The chief causes seemed to be (1). The habit of taking too large quantities of rice at meals, (2), and more frequently, insufficiency of food both in quantity and quality. (3) in others, the cause seemed to be distinctly malarial. The treatment of the second class was most difficult, as the original cause was often still at work while the patient was in the hospital. Many of this class were the recipients of the rice and cash tickets, and their necessity could not be doubted.

Rheumatic Affections are as common in the hot as in the cold months. Muscular rheumatism is the commonest, but the chronic articular form is not infrequent. Only one case of acute rheumatism has come under observation.

Diseases of Respiratory Organs.—279 cases have been prescribed for. Chronic Bronchitis is the most frequent, and phthisis comes next on the list. This latter disease is by no means rare; it is seen in all its stages, and runs a very chronic course.

Enthetic Diseases are very common, and some of them, as well as some of the *lupus* cases, presented a very loathsome appearance.

Deaths.—There were five deaths in the hospital during the year. Two of these were not patients. One a young woman, a beggar, was found in a moribund state in the hospital grounds, having been placed there by her friends, and then deserted. She died two hours afterwards, and a decent burial was provided from the hospital funds. A young lad, a thief by profession, suffering from dysentery and anæmia, was brought in a semi-unconscious state to the dispensary by his friends, who quietly slipped away, leaving him in our hands. He lingered a few days, and in the meantime his friends were found out. Congestion of the liver, following acute dysentry, resulted fatally in the case of a middle aged man. A young lad, 16 years of age, an applicant for baptism, was treated for two months for anæmia. He had received considerable benefit, and was about to return home when he had an attack of dysentery. From this he also recovered; but two days afterwards, unknown to the assistants, he had gone out of the hospital for a walk, and in passing the refreshment stalls was tempted to buy a pine apple, of which he ate a considerable portion. Some hours afterwards he suddenly became unconscious and died. The last death was that of a travelling literary graduate from Kiangsi. He was a hard opium smoker and was suffering from an enlarged liver with ascites. His general condition did not admit of much hope of relief, but, pleading earnestly to be taken in if only to die, as he was starving, and the only other alternative for him was a speedy death in the streets, he was admitted.

II Diseases of Eye and Skin comprise fully a third of the cases treated. Of eye diseases alone we have had over 900 cases, and from their variety and numbers it is difficult to sum up briefly the year's work in such a Report as this. There have been about 70 cases where one or both eyes have been completely destroyed, generally from sloughing of the cornea, following *purulent* or *granular conjunctivitis*; and a number of cases of disease of the nervous apparatus of the eye; to whom no benefit could be given. Another class of cases where the disease was of old standing and of complicated nature, involving several of the parts of the eye has been more frequent. Many of these cases stayed with us a long time, and, as a general rule, the disease was checked, though more or less impairment of vision remained. However, in a large proportion of cases the disease was found in a form easily amenable to treatment.

III.—SURGICAL.

The following surgical operations have been performed during the year :—

On the Eye:

Operations for Entropium and Trichiasis	378	
„ Pterygium...........................	79	
„ Symphlepharon	2	
„ Anchyloblepharon	2	
„ Cataract	21	
Iridectomy	14	
Slitting up Canaliculi	4	
Tapping of anterior chamber	1	
Excision of eye ball................	3	
„ tumours (small)........................	3	
		507

On the Body generally:—

Operations for Fistula in Ano	32
„ Harelip	33
„ Slit Ear..................................	18
„ Closure of Nasal aperture	2
„ Contraction of Anus................	2
„ „ after burn.............	1
„ Tapping, &c., Hydrocele	31
Excision of Tumours	18
„ Elephantiasis Scroti....................	3
„ Epithelioma of Lip	2
„ Uterine Polypus	1
Plastic Operation of Lip..........................	1
Circumcision for Phymosis........................	5
Operation for Paraphymosis	2
Amputation of Finger	1
„ Penis	2
„ Hand	1
Extraction of Necrosed Bone	15
„ Teeth..	80
„ Bullets	3
„ Nasal Polypus	12
„ Foreign Bodies............................	2

Hæmorrhoids removed	45
Slitting up Sinuses	10
Operation for Anchylosis of Jaw	1
Fractures Set	4
Dislocation Reduced	5
Dilating Stricture of Urethra...............	3
	335
Total........................	842

The larger proportion of Entropium and Pterygium operations, and also a considerable number of the smaller operations on the body generally, have been performed by the two senior native assistants. Long and extensive experience has made them expert in such cases and the results were very satisfactory. Many of the Entropium cases were of old standing, and accompanied by inflammation and opacity of the cornea from the irritation of the inverted eyelashes. These opacities cleared up to some extent after the removal of the exciting cause, and frequently where there was only a glimmer of light before operative interference, 4 and 5 parts (normal-10) of vision would afterward be obtained;—a result much appreciated by the patients, who showed their feelings of gratitude in their own way by a plentiful presentation of cakes, &c.

Cataract.—There were 21 operations for the extraction or dispersion of cataract. Of these, 2 were failures, but the rest were successful and followed by more or less of vision.

Iridectomy.—These operations were performed for central corneal opacities, iritic adhesions, and glaucoma. In 5 cases no benefit accrued.

Harelip.—29 single and 4 double harelips have been cured by operation. Two cases of the above were complicated with cleft palate, and we expect them to return shortly to be cured of this also. Of the 33 cases, only 4 were females, a fact not so much due to any relative infrequency of this mal-development in the female sex, as to the indifference with which complaints of girls are regarded by Chinese parents.

Elephantiasis Scroti.—Three of these tumours have been removed during the year, and all made successful recoveries. The weights of the tumours were 112 oz., 166 oz., and 180 oz., respectively.

Polypus of uterus.—The patient was about 35 years of age and had suffered for a long time from hæmorrhagic discharges. A polypus about the size of a small pumelo was successfully removed by the ecraseur.

Amputation of hand.—A young man from a village near Swatow had his hand crushed between the revolving stones of a sugar mill. The tendons, vessels, and soft parts generally were much bruised and lacerated, and the bleeding had been restrained by tying a piece of bamboo fibre around the wrist. Amputation was performed; one of the flaps sloughed slightly, but the wound healed quickly by granulation.

Fish Bone in Foot.—A large piece of bone was removed from the sole of a man's foot where it had lain for five years, and had occasioned much suffering.

Tumours.—The most interesting of these cases were the tumours of the neck; 4 such of large size have been successfully removed. In one case the tumour, extending deeply in the parotid region, was found to involve the facial nerve, which had to be cut. Partial paralysis of the muscles followed on one side of the face. The patient was also an opium smoker, but being anxious for the removal of the tumour, he denied the fact. In the evening after the operation alarming symptoms began to manifest themselves, and the patient appeared as if he were going to sink. A large dose of opium was given with wonderful results. Finding on recovery that the paresis interfered with the comfort of his smoking, he gave up the habit.

There have been no deaths from any operation during the year. The Chinese make good surgical patients. They endure pain with stoical indifference, suffer little from shock, and the wounds heal kindly. It is difficult to understand why unfavourable results so seldom follow surgical interference. The conditions are often as unfavourable as they well could be; but, excepting a tendency to fever, which is easily prevented by a few days preliminary treatment with quinine and iron, little constitutional disturbance follows, and the wounds rarely take on an unhealthy action. There is a great readiness to submit to the knife, and operations on the eye, removal of tumours, &c., are often urgently entreated. They object, however, very strongly to amputations, no matter how urgent the case may be. A number of cases where amputation of the diseased part afforded the only, but good, chance of saving the life had to be sent home without anything being done. The following may be mentioned as instances. A man from the Island of Namoa, about 35 years of age, was admitted with caries of carpal and metacarpal bones. The hand had been diseased for 12 years, was entirely useless, and had to be supported on a wooden splint. For a good part of this time he had been unable to do any work and his general health was beginning to be shattered. A boy, 12 years of age, with ankle and foot disorganised, the bones being quite soft from caries, and the soft parts ulcerated was brought by his father to be cured. The foot had been diseased for 3 years and the boy was unable to walk. In neither case would the suggestion that the diseased parts be removed by amputation be listened to.

Gunshot Wounds.—Only one case was of recent occurrence, that of a young man, who, happening to get in front of an unshotted gun at the moment of firing, received its contents in his body. The injuries received were somewhat severe, consisting of large lacerated wounds in the lower part of the abdominal walls, in the groins, on the left shoulder, and hands. Extensive sloughing of the injured parts followed, and it was fully two months before he was able to leave the Hospital.

An old man was admitted who had received a shot in the left foot, 17 years ago. About half of the foot had been lost from the subsequent sloughing, and the stump was the seat of an unhealthy fungoid mass that bled on the slightest irritation. He objected to amputation ; and, other treatment failing to effect a cure, he returned home in a very weak condition.

Extraction of Bullets.—The position of the bullet in two patients showed what a narrow escape they had made. In one, the bullet had hit the clavicle, splintered it into two and lodged between the pieces. In the other case, it had entered the thigh on its anterior aspect, burrowed under the skin and lodged immediately over the inner surface of the great vessels of the leg. In both cases the bullet was easily extracted.

The work in the Hospital affords many glimpses into the social life and habits of the people, and these often reveal a state of matters far from pleasant. A man was admitted semi-unconscious from loss of blood and shock, with a scalp wound about 4 inches in length, and with one side of head and face much cut and bruised. His friends gave the following history: the patient was a cook on board one of the steamers engaged in the coolie trade, and had recently returned from a voyage to Singapore. On the way to his home in a fishing village a few miles from Swatow he was way laid, knocked on the head, and robbed of $30, the earnings of his last voyage. Assistance was given by us and others to the friends in their attempt to induce the Mandarin of the district to take the matter up, and if possible bring the perpetrators of the deed to justice. At one time it seemed as if an interesting medico-legal enquiry was about to commence, as a counter story was got up that the injuries were self-inflicted for the purpose of deceiving some person to whom patient was said to owe money. From the nature and extent of the wounds it would have required some credulity to believe the latter story, but it sufficed to satisfy the official ideas of justice. Illustrations were met with of some of the evils following the fashionable custom of binding the feet of the women, so common in this and other parts of China. A good looking, pleasant-mannered girl, 17 years of age, was admitted with gangrene of the great toes. A short time previous to her admittance, compression of her feet had been begun and the gangrenous condition was the result. Her mother, a hard-looking specimen of humanity, (who thought that, seeing she had other three daughters, great credit was due to her for not strangling this one at her birth) made some objections to the unbinding of the feet, but ultimately gave way. Great relief followed, a line of separation was forming between the healthy and the gangrenous parts, and the advisability of amputation was being considered. But the man to whom she had been betrothed in early life, and who had been averse to her coming to the Hospital, demanded the fulfilment of the engagement, and the girl was taken away. Six months afterwards, on inquiry, it was found that the toes were still sore, and that the compression of the feet was being persevered in.

Wounds, Bruises, &c.—The number of such cases admitted has been very considerable, and includes 5 dislocations and 4 fractures of recent occurrence, and a case of cerebral concussion. Most of the injuries, however, were slight. With regard to the Bruises, it is striking how many of them have been inflicted in village and family brawls. The chest, back, and legs are the favourite places for assault. These bruises are produced by blows from bamboo poles applied in a plunging method, the end of the pole striking the body. Although there is not much outside mark, yet the blow is followed by severe bruising of the muscles, which afterwards become the seat of pains of a Rheumatic character. These pains often continue to recur for years, and sometimes lead to the impairment of the general health. Hæmoptysis is a frequent result of beatings on the chest. Other cases have received their blows from friends and neighbours for conscience sake. The confession of Christianity in many of the Chinese villages is no easy matter, as the hospital work can testify. It is often rewarded with blows and maltreatment in various ways.

A few cases were the subjects of a disciplinary castigation for alleged misdemeanours. If these scourgings fail to produce law-abiding citizens, it is certainly not due to their want of severity. One case of stabbing was caused by a foreign seaman in a fit of drunken passion.

Evangelistic.—The religious services have been conducted in the same way as in former years. A morning service, prior to the commencement of the medical work, and worship in the evenings, have been maintained daily. On three days of the week the services have been conducted by the Rev. Messrs. Duffus and Gibson, and on the other occasions by the two senior assistants. Dr. Gauld in the beginning, and the Rev. Mr. Mackenzie in the end of the year have given assistance in this work. The women's wards have received occasional visits from the ladies of the mission, but other engagements and sickness have much interfered with their visits.

As to spiritual fruit, there have been numerous applicants for admission into the church, but in one case only has the request been granted. The others on leaving the hospital were urged to attend, for further instruction and examination, the chapel in the neighbourhood of their homes. Six of these applicants are known to have kept up their profession in their native village. One has given up his occupation as a sailor to keep the sabbath; another has endured a good deal of persecution. The latter, whose history is a very sad one, was a middle aged widow who had an operation on the eyes performed with a successful result in February. Her late husband's friends objected very strongly to her giving up the worship of idols, and, as she persisted in this, treated her very cruelly. Their unkind and cruel treatment caused her to have long fits of weeping, and about six months after her return home from the hospital an inflammatory affection of the eyes, excited by the fits of weeping, resulted in total blindness. She, however, maintains her constancy as a worshipper of God.

As many of the applicants were unable to read, a class in the afternoons was formed for their benefit, They were taught to read the hymn book, and had the meaning explained. The attendance at this class varied from 4 to 30. Two former patients were baptized at a station in the country, and we trust that many of last year's applicants will by-and-by be gathered in.

Financial—From the statement in the appendix it will be seen that the receipts for the year amount to $2013.13 and the expenditure to $1551.20 leaving a balance of $461.93 to tide over the earlier months of 1881. We beg to offer our hearty thanks to the community for their liberal contributions.

Dr. E. J. Scott has given assistance on many occasions throughout the year, and our thanks are due to him. We have also to express our deep obligations to the Rev. Messrs Duffus and Gibson for frequent assistance in interpreting and for help rendered in many ways.

Subscriptions for 1880

T. W. Richardson, Esq.	$50.00
William Gregory, Esq	50.00
A. Huber, Esq	50.00
Bernhard Schaar, Esq	50.00
W. Hälse, Esq	50.00
Messrs. Douglas Lapraik & Co. per G. D. Pitman, Esq	50.00
Rev. William Duffus	25.00
„ Dr. MacIver	25.00
G. D. Pitman, Esq.	25.00
P. Campbell, Esq.	25.00
William Gauld, Esq., M.D	25.00
Alexander Lyall, Esq.	25.00
Wm. Rae, Esq.	20.00
Otto Asverus, Esq	20.00
A Friend	20.00
London Med. Miss. Society—per—Ferguson, Esq.	26.09
Proceeds of Concert—per Captain Parker	13.00
J. R. Bridgman, Esq	10.00
W. S. Fergusson, Esq.	10.00
Fred. Schjöth, Esq.	10.00
T. H. Ewer, Esq.	10.00
Do.	5.44
H. Ramsay, Esq	10.00
J. D. Meyer, Esq	10.00
J. Eccleston, Esq	10.00
C. C. Williams, Esq.	10.00
A. Witte, Esq.	10.00
Captain Williams	10.00
A Patient per Miss. Fielde	10.00
Oct. Johnson, Esq.	5.00
W. N. Morehouse, Esq	5.00
W. Pollock, Esq	5.00
Do.	2.74
J. von Jezewski, Esq.	5.00
A. Gillanders Esq.	5.00
W. Watson, Esq.	5.00
Captain F. W. Focken	5.00
Captain A. L. Piersdorf	5.00
Captain Linklater	5.00
Miss Norwood	4.00
W. E. Moxham, Esq	3.00
Patient	1.00
	$720.27

STATEMENT OF INCOME AND EXPENDITURE.

To Wages of Assistants, &c.	$ 294.70
" Balance due Dr. Gauld for Medicines and Maps.	35.57
" Printing Hospital Report, Postage	29.91
" Medicines bought in China	161.31
" " from London for Sale	114.79
" " " " " Hospital	530.59
" Aid given to Poor Patients	14.95
" Repairs, Alteration of Drains, &c.	147.67
" Lards, Oils, Papers, &c.	47.04
" Cloth for Bandages	30.70
" Gin for Liniments and Tinctures	61.02
" Water	44.60
" Sundries	38.35
" Balance on Hand	461.93
	$2,013.13

By Balance from 1879	$ 264.03
" Contributions as per List	720.27
" Sales of Maps	3.60
" " of Trusses	27.48
" " Opium Pills	10.48
" " Medicines	385.85
" " Mils	37.33
" " Sundries	20.12
" Rent for small Ward	13.68
" Medicines from London paid by Missionary Committee in Edinburgh	530.59
	$2,013.13

List of Diseases Treated.

GENERAL DISEASES.

Chicken-pox 2
Febricula 41
Intermittent Fever :—
Quotidian 20
Tertian 74
Quartan 3
Irregular 6
Chronic Rheumatism 98
Pleurodynia 27
Lumbago 34
Sciatica 15
Chronic Articular Rheumatism and Rheumatic Arthritis 32
Syphilis 32
,, Congenital 5
Strumous & Syphilitic Glandular Enlargements 31
Lupus Excedens 13
Rodent Ulcer of Face 2
Anæmia 165

General Debility 34
Blood Poisoning 11
Opium Smokers 20
Tumours :—
Lardaceous 4
Fatty 8
Wens 2
Parotid 2
Submaxillary 3
Cervical 34
Osseous 2
Naevus 2
Epulis 1
Cysto Sarcoma 2
Scirrhus of Breast 2
Glandular ,, ... 3
64
Goitre 2
Ascites 14

Diseases of the Nervous System.

Locomotor Ataxia 4
Epilepsy 7
Paralysis-Facial 1
,, of Arm 1
Hemiplegia......... 6
Paraplegia 3

Sunstroke 1
Vertigo 13
Mania 1
Dementia 1
Neuralgia 5

Diseases of Respiratory System.

Asthma 39
Bronchites Acute & Chronic. 125
Phthisis Pulmonalis 69
Emphysema 11

Hæmoptysis 21
Pneumonia 2
Ulcer of Larynx 4

Diseases of Ear.

Otorrhœa 12
Inflammation 2
Eczema of Meatus 1

Tumours 2
Injury 1
Deafness 1

Diseases of Nose.

Ulceration of Mucous Membrane 8
Closure of Anterior Apertures 2
Epistaxis 1

Polypi-Mucous 14
,, Malignant 1
Foreign Body in 1

Diseases of Circulatory System.

Hypertrophy of Heart	1
Valvular Diseases	25
Varix	5

Diseases of Digestive System.

Ulceration of Lip	3
Epithelioma ,,	3
Harelip Single	32
,, Double	4
Gumboil	2
Aphthæ	5
Enlarged Papellae of Tongue.	3
Epithelioma ,,	3
Ulceration of Palate	3
,, Fauces	10
Tonsillitis	6
Stricture of Oesophagus	5
Dyspepsia	191
Colic	18
Dysentery	34
Diarrhœa	30
Vermes	25
Stricture of Rectum	9
Hæmorrhoids Internal	38
,, External	8
Fistula in Ano	39
Ulcer of Rectum	3
Prolapse ,,	3
Contraction of Anus	2
Condylomata	7
Cirrhosis of Liver	4
Enlargement ,,	10
Congestion ,,	3
Jaundice	3
Enlargement of Spleen	33
Hernia	33

Diseases of Eye.

Entropium & Trichiasis	216
Ophthalmia Tarsi	25
Adherent Lids	2
Symblepharon	4
Abscess of Lids	2
Hordeolum	3
Lardaceous Tumours of Lid.	3
Contraction of Lids	2
Suppuration of Lachrymal Sac	2
Fistula Lachrymalis	2
Sinus in Orbit	1
Obstruction of Puncta and Nasal Duct	25
Pterygium	57
Conjunctivitis Granular	117
,, Pustular	2
,, Purulent	8
,, Catarrhal	50
Opacity of Cornea	65
Ulcers ,,	85
Slough ,,	5
Destruction of one Eye	46
,, of both Eyes	28
Keratitis	16
,, Suppurative	3
Vascular Cornea	21
Anterior Staphyloma	8
Iritis	7
Iritic Adhesions	22
Hernia of Iris	29
Cataract Hard	42
,, Soft	6
Irido Choroiditis	2
Hypopion	5
Tremulous Iris	1
Glaucoma	7
Optic Neuritis	4
Atrophy of Optic Nerve	13
Amaurosis	3
Retinitis	3
Pigmentary Degeneration of Retina	1
Hemeralopia	2
Carcinoma of Eye	3
Orbital tumours	3
Injury Eye	2

Diseases of Genito Urinary System.

Hydrocele	39	Ulceration of Penis	10
„ of Cord	1	Rupture of Urethra	2
Scrotum Ulceration of	10	Fistula „	1
„ Sinuses	4	Stricture „	3
Orchitis	4	Incontinence of Urine	3
Tumours of Testicle	3	Cystitis	3
Lymph Scroti	4	Hæmaturia	1
Elephantiasis Scroti	19	Chronic Albuminuria	3
Spermatorrhœa	26	Leucorrhœa	16
Gonorrhœa	13	Amenorrhœa	4
Warts	3	Menorrhagia	2
Bubo	11	Metrorrhagia	3
Chancres	7	Dysmenorrhœa	1
Phymosis	5	Polypus of Uterus	1
Paraphymosis	2	Inflammation of Vulva	3
Epithelioma of Penis	3	Ovarian Tumours	2
Destruction „	2		

Diseases of Skin.

Elephantiasis of Limb	29	Ecthyma	5
„ Growths on Back.	1	Leucoderma	2
Eczema of Scalp	15	Keloid	1
Favus „	7	Melasma	3
Tinea Tonsurans	6	Frambœsia	4
„ Circinata	89	Osmidrosis	2
„ Mansonii	8	Zeroderma	2
Eczema	22	Onychia	1
Pityriasis Versicolor	2	Gangrene	1
Psoriasis	5	Whitlow	2
Scabies	25	Carbuncles and Boils	12
Achne	1	Ulcerations	260
Abscesses	19		

Dieases of Bones.

Caries and Necrosis	69	Spinal Curvature	14

Diseases of Joints.

Inflammation	33	Anchylosis	8
Sprains	14		

Unclassified.

Dislocation	8	Dog Bites	4
Fractures	7	Snake Bites	1
Contraction of Tendons and Cicatrices	9	Sinus in Cheek	2
Muscular Atrophy	3	Fish Bone in Foot	1
Deformity	2	Iron Splinter in Arm	1
Wounds, &c	33	Slit in Ear	18
Gunshot	4	Blows and Bruises	11
Bullets Lodged	3	Injury to Chest (from Burden-bearing and Beatings)	62
Burns and Scalds	7	Cerebral Concussion	1

REPORT

OF THE

Medical Missionary Hospital

AT

SWATOW,

IN CONNECTION WITH THE

PRESBYTERIAN CHURCH OF ENGLAND,

UNDER THE CARE OF

Alexander Lyall, M. B., C. M.

FOR 1882.

PRINTED BY

Kwai Fung,

PRINTER, BOOKBINDER & STATIONER,

SWATOW

1883.

REPORT

ABSENCE in the country on Medico-Evangelistic work for several weeks in the beginning of the year, and heavier work than usual during the Spring months, have hindered me from submitting earlier a short resume of the work that has been done in the Swatow Mission Hospital during the past year, for the information of friends who either contribute to the support of the Institution, or may desire to know what progress has been made.

There is perhaps little of general interest to report, but we have the satisfaction of feeling that we have been able to relieve, to a greater or less extent, the sufferings and ailments of many of the crowds of uncared for poor, and others who have resorted to us for treatment.

On two occasions I was compelled to leave my post for a few weeks owing to failure of strength, but the native assistants were able to carry on the work in my absence; on the latter occasion they had the benefit of the supervision of the Rev. Dr. Riddel of the Hakka branch of our Mission.

Our Staff of native assistants, exclusive of door-keeper, etc., consists of six men and one woman,—one of the former being a pupil and receiving no pay. On them necessarily devolves much of the routine work of the Hospital, and the carrying out of the after-treatment of Surgical patients, and this they do in a pleasant and satisfactory manner. The two senior assistants, however, can render even more valuable help, for, besides taking an active part in the Evangelistic work that is carried on in the Hospital, they can perform in a business-like fashion many of the minor surgical operations, and can treat satisfactorily the commoner diseases that come under notice. During the year two more of the assistants have been allowed to perform certain surgical operations, and they made a very creditable appearance in their first endeavours with the knife. Hence we have frequently had the pleasure of superintending four native youths operating at the same time.

Number of Patients.—Although during the year certain circumstances occurred that tended to keep down the number of patients—notably the prevalence of Cholera in Swatow during the month of October, yet the total number exceeds that of the previous year by 189. But for the occurrence of Cholera, and my absence for a time, both the number of patients and surgical operations performed would have been greater. There were a few cases of Cholera in our wards, but the fact did not seem to disconcert the patients in the least, as we experienced considerable difficulty in getting rid of a few of them in order that we might have an empty ward or two on hand. For a few weeks, however, we ceased to have patients coming from a distance, as they were afraid of travelling through the infected parts.

The numbers for 1882 are as follows:—

In-patients	2,738.
Out-patients	1,405.
Total	4,143.

Females included in above:—

In-patients	385.
Out-patients	238.
Total	623.

The daily average attendance of in- and out-patients during the year was as follows:—

	In-patients.	*Out-patients.*
January	174	26
February	97	22
March	115	25
April	141	32
May	233	45
June	248	47
July	232	44
August	181	42

	In-patients.		*Out-patients.*
September	233	......	59
October	212	......	57
November	122	......	35
December	162	......	29

The average length of stay in the Hospital for each in-patient was 16 days.

Out-patients are only seen on two days of the week—Tuesdays and Fridays, but we never refuse to prescribe for an urgent case if it should happen to come on any of the other days. The total number of visits made by them was 4,021, which gives nearly an average of three visits to each patient. A considerable number of them came from places at some distance from Swatow, but such were for the most part boatmen, and others who had come to Swatow in connection with business matters.

Several trips were made to preaching stations in the country, and a few hundreds of patients were seen and prescribed for, but an accurate record of their number has not been kept.

The native places of the patients are given in the following table, and, taken in connection with the table given in last year's report of the number of towns and villages represented by that year's patients, it may be of interest to those who value the Hospital as a missionary agency.

From the District of Ching-hai..................	571
,, ,, Chao-yang	996
,, ,, Kieh-yang	778
,, ,, Pu-ning	361
,, ,, Jao-ping	479
,, ,, Huei-lai	237
,, ,, Hai-yang	403
,, ,, Fung-shun	52
,, ,, Ta-pu	13
From the Island of Namoa	54
,, District of Lu-fung and Hai-fung	32
,, ,, of Kia-ying-chow	13
,, Province of Fokien	144
,, Other Provinces	10

In autumn a public dispensary was opened in Swatow by General Fang, and placed under the care of two native doctors from the Tung Wah Hospital in Hongkong. We understand that the native merchants have undertaken the support of the institution, and it is reported that a hospital for the accommodation of in-patients will by and bye be built. So far as we can learn, only native drugs and appliances are used; and it is interesting to know that the moral well-being of the patients has not been lost sight of. The "Sacred Edict," it is said, is read daily to the patients while they are being attended to by the physician and surgeon in charge. This feature looks rather like a set-off to the preaching of the Gospel in the establishment under our care. The presence of this dispensary, however, has tended to increase rather than decrease the number of our patients; at all events the work during the last two months of the year was heavier than in former years at the same time. This is not the first attempt of the kind that has been made, for in former years public dispensaries were opened in two of the large cities in this region, though only for a short time.

We are quite prepared to welcome any effort put forth by the Chinese themselves to alleviate the vast amount of disease and suffering for which so little is done, but we are afraid that the character and practices of the people will require to be materially changed before they will be able to carry on a true philanthropic work to any good purpose; and the Science and Art of Medicine as practised by the native faculty cannot be expected to make much impression on the diseases that are prevalent amongst the people.

We may also mention that another philanthropic work has been set agoing in Swatow, viz:—a poor-house for beggar women. It is simply a lodging house, however, as no food or money is given to the inmates. We have visited the place several times, and so far as we can see no objectionable feature has as yet appeared.

Evangelistic.—Morning and evening worship has been conducted daily with the patients either by my ordained Colleagues or by the senior native assistants. Miss Ricketts has frequently visited the female wards, and on several occasions has given instruction to a number of female patients who were applying for baptism. The services were well attended, and a very gratifying amount of interest in the Doctrine has been shown by a large number of the in-patients. During the year more than 140 men and women have given in their names as applicants for admission into the church. Special classes for the teaching of such have been held more or less regularly in the afternoons, and many have succeeded in acquiring a fair knowledge of the more essential doctrines of the Christian religion. On Sunday afternoons they were also assembled for an hour or so for examination, which was generally conducted by one of the Misssionaries, assisted by the native elders of the Swatow congregation. Of this large number of applicants only a few received baptism, as we generally require that they, before receiving the sacred rite, should go home, and show the sincerity of their profession by avowing and conducting themselves as Christians among their relatives and neighbours. On leaving the Hospital some of them go to places near which there is no chapel, and it is very difficult to follow them up; some, as might be expected, make no profession of Christianity at their homes; others however do, and hold on, often under pretty severe persecution.

It is to be expected that some of those who profess to be believers, while recipients of the benefits of the hospital, should relapse into their old ways on returning to their homes. Feelings of gratitude for bodily suffering relieved may lead a man to think favourably of the religion that we seek to propagate. But it requires something more substantial than gratitude to support a man in his religious profession in the face of a hostile community. And although such cases are disappointing, yet sometimes even through them others—heathen acquaintances or relatives—are brought to a knowledge of the truth. Two instances of this kind came under the notice of one of my colleagues. The first was that of a man who had been a patient of Dr.

Gauld's thirteen years ago. A hymn book was then given to him which he took home but laid aside as a book in which he felt no interest. Last year a brother of the patient came upon the book, read it, and becoming interested in the truths that it taught, went to the chapel at Kia-kng for further instruction. Now he and a friend have been baptized, and several men and women are interested, and meet nightly for worship in a room which they have rented for the purpose. One of these men, who is now a professing Christian, was rather notorious as a thief and gambler, and some of his fellow-villagers expressed their gratification at the great change that had come over him, saying they could now stay at home at nights instead of, as formerly, keeping watch in their fields against his thievish practices.

The other case was that of a man from a village near Kia-kng, who was an applicant for baptism when under treatment in the beginning of the year. He was twice visited at his native village, the first time shortly after leaving the Hospital, then six months afterwards when apparently he had drawn back from his profession; but two of his friends led partly by what our patient had told them of the doctrine, and partly by what they had heard on the occasion of the above mentioned visit to their village, had become interested, and were found to be very hopeful candidates for baptism.

Perhaps such incidents as the above may not be common; but we could relate many instances of others, who we trust have become sincere believers, being instrumental in bringing in relatives and neighbours. We give our notes of a few of these cases:—A Thiau, from the district of Huei-lai, baptized in 1881, has brought his mother and younger brother from their native village to Swatow, three days journey, in order to be under Christian instruction. The mother was seized with cholera a few days after arriving in Swatow, but recovered. Now both mother and brother are applicants for admission into the church. A Hien, from Hûa-phêng, a large village in the district of Chao-yang, baptized on the 1st of January, 1881, has influenced a number of friends in favour of the Gospel; and his brother, who came several times to Swatow to receive teaching, has been baptized. A Tsoi, a woman from the village of Sua-leng, also in the district of Chao-yang, baptized last year, has taught several neighbours what she herself knows of the truth, and lately has had to suffer persecution of a trying kind. A Chhim, a barber in Swatow, was admitted into the Hospital in order to undergo a surgical operation, and was under treatment for three weeks. He has attended Divine service regularly since, accompanied by two friends, and all of them are now candidates for baptism. As his associates in business objected to him not working on Sundays, he left them, and latterly has set up business in another part of the town with his two friends as partners.

Of the total number of adult baptisms (148) in connection with our Mission last year, some 17 or 18 heard for the first time, and accepted the Gospel, while under treatment in the Hospital.

We may also mention as a result of the Evangelistic work, that we frequently meet with former patients who have had their faith in idols undermined, and yet have not embraced the Christian religion. Every year a number of such cases come under our notice. On the other hand, others, who made no profession in the Hospital, are sometimes gathered in at preaching stations in the country, months, or even years, afterwards. The history of these cases is that they have secretly worshipped God since the time they were inmates of the Hospital.

We cite these facts to show that the Hospital is what it professes to be, a mission hospital. Medical missions, however, need no apologist, for they are abundantly useful both in relieving the sick and suffering, and in disseminating the Gospel. The medical art is naturally the handmaid of the Church, and we believe that Western Medical Science loses nothing but gains much in its introduction amongst a heathen people by being associated with the dissemination of true religion. At all events, it suffices some of us to know that the standing orders for the Christian soldier are, "Heal the sick, and say that the kingdom of God is at hand."

"The kingdom of God cometh not with observation:" thus, throughout the Swatow region Christianity is slowly, silently, but surely spreading amongst the people, brother telling brother of the good tidings, and friend passing the word to friend, and every now and again worshippers of the true God are discovered in villages where we thought there were none. We are humbly thankful that the Hospital under our care has helped, and is still helping forward the good cause.

A tabulated list of the diseases treated is appended. This list is as correct as it is possible for us to make it, but some diseases have been treated in greater numbers than we have indicated. Such skin diseases as ringworm, pityriasis, scabies might be numbered by hundreds.

MEDICAL.

Measles.—A mild epidemic of this affection occurred in April. It made its appearance amongst the boys in the Mission school, but in a mild form, and only ten of the boys were affected with the complaint. The Chinese are very careless in regard to this disease, children being allowed to run about as soon as the febrile symptoms have subsided.

Cholera.—During the month of October, Cholera was prevalent in Swatow and neighbourhood. It was imported from Manila viâ Amoy by returning emigrants. At first many fatal cases occurred, but fortunately the disease did not spread far into the country, and soon subsided. We had ten cases in the hospital, four of which died, the rest recovering. The first two cases occurred in the small hospital, and the probable source of infection was a small house, only a few yards distant, in which a large number of lepers reside. Four days before the appearance of Cholera in the hospital, an inmate of this house died from the disease, and his body was kept lying outside the building two days before being buried. Our two patients (husband and wife) recovered. There were no more cases in the small hospital, but about a week afterwards a young lad, under treatment in the large hospital for ulcer of the leg, was seized, and died in a few days. This patient had been under treatment for a long time, and, being strictly confined to bed, had not been out of the ward for three months at least. A few days afterwards other two patients were attacked and died. These cases happened during my absence in the north of China, and the day before my return another patient was seized, and was in the stage of collapse when I saw her. She, however, made a good recovery, as did three of the four others who were subsequently attacked with the disease.

There were about 240 in-patients at the time, but the disease showed no tendency to spread in the wards; only in two instances did we have two cases occurring in the same wards. Acute diarrhœa and dysentery were also very rife in the hospital, and in Swatow and villages around. By dismissing 30 or 40 of the patients, we were able to set apart two of the large wards for the purpose of isolating the cases of cholera and diarrhœa as they occurred. We also took the precaution to inspect all under treatment three times every day, so that every patient with relaxed bowels might be at once detected, isolated, and put under somewhat vigorous treatment.

Almost daily we had people from Swatow coming to the dispensary for medicine for friends who had been seized with cholera. Not unfrequently the request was for a medicine that would keep the patient alive till he could be removed to his native village in the country. This fact may throw some light on the question of the propagation of cholera. In a region thickly covered with overcrowded, filthy villages, it is surprising that there is not oftener an outbreak of cholera, and still more wonderful that the disease, when once introduced in an acute form, should not spread beyond 30 miles from the Port town. The Chinese do not adopt any preventative measures. They do indeed stick up lots of long bamboo poles, to which small red flags are suspended by day and lighted lanterns by night, to drive away the disease; but sanitary matters are left to be looked after by the pigs and dogs.

Opium Smokers.—128 men and one woman, desirous of breaking off the habit of opium smoking, came for treatment during the year. Of these, three who were hopelessly ill with pulmonary consumption, were sent home again; four came as out-patients, and were only seen once; the others (122) were under treatment as in-patients for a longer or shorter time. Below we give some statistics with reference to the quantity of the drug smoked, duration of habit, and age of the patients; the statistics are not quite complete.

AMOUNT USED PER DAY.

½ mace or less	15	3 mace	4
1 „ or more than ½ m.	29	5 „	1
1½ „ „ „ „ 1 m.	30	6 „	2
2 „	12	8 „	1
2½ „	6		

DURATION OF HABIT.

2 years or less	9	10 years	11
3 „	9	11 „	2
4 „	7	12 „	2
5 „	4	15-20 „	5
6 „	2	28 „	2
7 „	1	45 „	1
8 „	6		

The much larger proportion of the cases not included in the above table were smokers of less than ten years' standing.

AGE OF PATIENTS.

From 20—25 years	13	From 40—50 years	19
„ 25—30 „	26	„ 50—60 „	12
„ 30—35 „	23	„ 60—70 „	1
„ 35—40 „	22	„ 75 „	1

Foreign opium was used in every case. So far as we can learn, the poppy is not grown, and neither is the native drug used, in the districts of Chao-chow. One mace of prepared foreign opium costs the smokers 90 cash or 8 cents. Nearly all of these patients were in the habit of drinking a quantity of whiskey daily, and were also smokers of tobacco.

In the report for 1881 we estimated the number of opium smokers in hamlets and villages to be about 4 *per cent* of the population. This year the statistics obtained from a much more extensive series of inquiries give an average percentage of 3¼. Perhaps, therefore, it may not be wide of the mark to say that about 3 *per cent* of the population in rural districts are given to opium. In Swatow, with a population of about 20,000, there are, we understand, 73 opium shops. Opium smoking is more prevalent in places where facilities for smuggling abound.

Opium eating is very far from being unknown in this region. A number of our patients were *eaters* as well as *smokers* of the drug. Many opium smoking burden-bearers, chair-bearers, boatmen, while engaged in their usual occupation, are in the habit of quieting the appetite by swallowing at intervals a small pellet of opium; and the impecunious opium sot in order to satisfy his cravings takes to eating the ashes from the opium pipe. Notwithstanding the assertions of theorisers—professional and amateur—the effects of opium smoking and opium eating on the physical frame of man are just the same. They differ in degree no doubt, but we are inclined to believe from clinical observation that the difference in degree between them is not so great as is commonly supposed.

There is a variety of gangrene of the toes and fingers sometimes met with which apparently results from the constitutional effects of opium smoking. It is a form of dry or chronic gangrene, in which the toes and parts of the fingers are very slowly destroyed by sloughing. There is little constitutional disturbance accompanying the disease. Last year we had two cases of this malady under treatment for about eight or ten weeks. A few cases are seen every year, and in every instance of the disease that we have seen the patient was a confirmed opium smoker.

An old man, aged 75 years, stated that he had smoked opium for 45 years, and had consumed about an ounce daily for the last two or three years. He was in fairly good health, and was anxious to break off the habit, but he was taken away from the hospital by his friends on the third day after admission. Such cases are very exceptional. Amongst the labouring classes, at least, the effects of habitually smoking opium are undoubtedly injurious both to body and mind.

Another man resorted to the pipe to cure intermittent fever. He had smoked two years, but the disease was still unrelieved. His spleen was enormously enlarged, and he was deeply anaemic and debilitated. He left the hospital on the fourth day. During the last three years we have made many inquiries of patients, native doctors, and others concerning the supposed virtue of opium smoking in preventing *malarious fevers*, but without obtaining any definite evidence for or against the theory. It is not likely, however, that a lazy opium smoker spending, as he does, several hours every day indulging in the pipe, should be as liable to fever as another man, who perhaps works from day-light to dark in the fields, exposed to a fierce sun, and the vicissitudes of the weather.

In the treatment of opium smokers no opium or any of its alkaloids is given, and the patients have to provide their own food while with us. About one third of the cases ran away as soon the distressing symptoms in connection with the cure set in. The others were under treatment a longer or shorter time, and left relieved of their craving.

There have been under treatment 1,079 cases of **Eye Diseases** and 726 cases of **Skin Diseases** during the year.

SURGICAL.

The following surgical operations have been performed during the year :—

On the Eye:—

Operations for	Entropium and Trichiasis	...	361
,,	,, Pterygium	... ...	92
,,	,, Cataract	... ...	7
,,	,, Symblepharon	... ...	3

Operations for Hernia of Iris 5
" " Ptosis 1
" " Ectropium 3
Slitting up Canaliculus 12
Excision of Sarcomatous tumour of orbit ... 1
" Small tumours of Eyelid ... 2
" Eyeball 3
" Anterior Staphyloma 1
Puncture of Anterior Chamber 5
Iridectomy 31
Removal of Splinters from Cornea 3
Syndectomy ... ... 2=532

On the Body generally:—

Operation for Harelip 37
" " Fistula in Ano 53
" " Slit in Ear 31
" " Phymosis (Circumcision) ... 10
" " Sinuses 12
" " Ganglion 2
" " Webbed Fingers 1
" " Salivary Fistula 1
" " Fungus Testis 1
" " Cystic tumour of lower jaw ... 1
Excision of Tumours 35
" " Scirrhus of Breast 4
" " Wens 2
" " Elephantiasis of Labium ... 1
" " " of Scrotum ... 1
" " Lymph Scrotum 1
" " Tonsils 2
" " External Hæmorrhoids ... 7
" " Condylomata 1
" " Warts... 1
" " Callous Skin of Foot 7
" " Epulis 2
" " Keloid 1
" " Testicle 1
" " Epithelioma of Skin 4

Excision of Epithelioma of Lip	... ...	1
Extraction of Teeth	... ...	127
,, ,, Necrosed Bone	... ...	26
,, ,, Seed from Nostril	... ...	1
,, ,, bamboo splinters	... ...	2
,, ,, needle	... ...	1
,, ,, bullets	... ...	3
,, ,, Nasal polypi...	... ...	6
,, ,, Urethral calculus	... ...	1
Amputation of Thumb	... ...	1
,, ,, Fingers	... ...	5
,, ,, Toes	... ...	2
,, ,, Penis (epithelioma)	...	3
Lithotrity	... ...	1
Tapping Cystic Goitre	... ...	2
Do. and injecting Hydrocele	... ...	22
Tying Internal Haemorrhoids	... ...	25
Plastic operation for mutilated Ears	...	2
,, ,, slit in Nostril	...	1
Opening Abscesses, Whitlows, Carbuncles...		75
Cauterising	... ...	4
,, for Spermatorrhea	... ...	2
Dilating Stricture of Urethra	... ...	8
Reduction of Dislocations	... ...	5
Setting of Fractures	... ...	3=546
Total	... ...	1,078

There have been no deaths from any operation during the year.

Entropium and Trichiasis.—361 operations for the relief of these affections have been performed with satisfactory results. These very common conditions of the eyelids are caused by long continued granular conjunctivitis, and neglected muco-purulent inflammations of the conjunctiva. In many cases both of the upper eyelids were affected, and in a few cases the hair-lashes of all four eyelids were inverted. About 220 individual patients have been operated on. The palpebral aperture was also shortened in some of the more chronic cases, and this condition was remedied at the same time by slitting up the outer canthus.

Ectropium or evertion of the eyelid is not very common, and is much more difficult to treat than entropium. Three patients have been operated on for this affection. In two case the condition was caused by inflammatory thickening of the conjunctiva, and in the third case by the contraction of a cicatrix in the upper eyelid. In the latter case a plastic operation was necessary for a cure; and accordingly the cicatrix was excised, and a piece of healthy skin, cut from the forehead, was put in its place with a result that was gratifying both to patient and operator.

Iridectomy.—This operation was performed in 30 cases for corneal opacities, and only in three or four cases no benefit was obtained. Three patients, who were practically blind—there being only a bare perception of light in the eyes—before the operation, obtained such an amount of sight as to enable them to walk about without assistance. The same operation was also performed in one case for *glaucoma*, and resulted in the relief of the painful symptoms, and in a slight improvement of vision.

Excision of the Eyeball.—The Chinese object very strongly to the Excision of the Eyeball,—no matter how urgent the necessity for its removal may be. In three cases, however, we were allowed to excise a painful useless eye, where there was great danger of Sympathetic Ophthalmia being set up in the healthy eye.

Fistula in Ano is very common, and, as at home, there are cases met with where this condition is associated with disease of the lung. In the large majority of cases the disease results from an abscess in the cellular tissue surrounding the bowel. Many of this class of patients were farmers, and perhaps the fact of these men having to work for hours with their feet in water, when preparing their fields for the rice planting, may have something to do with the causation of these abcesses. The general health is also frequently below par in this disease. The treatment adopted is to lay the fistula open by means of the knife, and this has been done is 53 instances with satisfactory results.

Hydrocele is another very common disease. There were 22 cases treated last year, which is a smaller number than usual. The distended sac is tapped, and then a drachm and a half of strong tincture of iodine is injected into it. Occasionally this treatment is not sufficient to bring about a permanent cure.

Elephantiasis of Labium.—Two pedunculated growths, about the size of a pumelo, and resembling an Elephantiasis tumour in their structure, were successfully removed by the ecraseur from the labia minora of a woman aged 46 years.

Lymph Scrotum.—This peculiar disease is occasionally met with. The affected part is thickened, but soft and pliable to the touch, and the surface is roughened by the presence of numerous vesicles which discharge on pricking a quantity of thin clear fluid. This disease is closely allied to ELEPHANTIASIS. It is even maintained by some native doctors that it sometimes passes into elephantiasis. Four cases presented themselves during the year; one of whom was suffering from elephantiasis of the leg in addition to lymph scrotum. One patient only consented to have the disease excised. This was easily done, and a good recovery followed, the wound healing partly by first intention and partly by granulation.

Elephantiasis of Scrotum.—We operated on one case, that of a man aged 32, from the district of Huei-lai. He had been ill for more than a year, and the scrotal swelling was preceded by frequent attacks of ague, and by enlargement of the lymphatic glands in the groin. A tumour weighing 3 lbs. was removed, and recovery took place without a bad symptom.

Two patients with scrotal tumours of an enormous size came for treatment, but they would not consent to an operation being performed.

Urinary Calculi.—In one case the calculus was crushed four times, and more than an ounce of debris came away in the urine. There were still one or two small fragments to be removed when I was obliged to leave Swatow for a time, and the patient had left the hospital before my return.

Urethral Calculus.—One patient came to get a small calculus, which was lodged in the urethra near the triangular ligament, removed. One of the native assistants cut down on the calculus, and removed it. In a few days the wound was quite healed, and patient was dismissed cured.

Malignant Tumour of the Orbit.—This patient, a woman aged 42, had been ill for two years. She attributed the commencement of the disease to an injury which she received in the upper part of the orbit. The eye swelled, and irritant applications were used for a long time. A soft sarcomatous tumour as large as an orange projected from the orbit, pushing the eyeball upwards under the eyelid, which was stretched over the front of the mass.

As the patient was willing to submit to any operative interference that would afford relief from the disease even for a short time, she was put under chloroform, and the whole contents of the orbit were removed. The apex and floor of the cavity were also touched with the hot cautery, in order to destroy any remaining portions of the morbid growth. A part of the bony roof of the orbit was eroded, and on being touched with the finger crumbled into pieces. These fragments of bone were cautiously removed, and the outer membrane of the brain thereby exposed.

Patient made a good recovery, and left much pleased at getting rid of the unsightly and painful mass.

Scirrhus of the Female Breast.—Four such tumours were removed, and with one exception the wounds healed by first intention. In two of the cases a number of enlarged glands in the axilla were removed at the same time,—the operations being performed with strict antiseptic precautions.

Epithelioma.—A considerable number of patients have been operated on for this disease either by means of the knife, or by the thermo-cautery. The more interesting of these cases were :—(1) *Epithelioma of the angle of mouth,* involving to a small extent both lips, and extending a short distance into the cheek in line of the teeth. The gap remaining after the removal of the disease was filled up by flaps of healthy skin formed by making two incisions, one downwards into the submaxillary region, and the other upwards into the cheek. (2) *Epithelioma of the chin.*—In this case also a plastic operation was performed. (3) *Epithelioma of the penis.*—In three cases this organ was amputated for this disease in the usual way.

Plastic Operation for Mutilated Ear.—For certain offences against society, as adultery, the Chinese villagers are in the habit of taking the law into their own hands, and summarily inflicting on the offenders punishment of a somewhat savage kind. Occasionally patients, with the ears lopped off entirely or in part, or with the eyes completely destroyed by being pierced with some sharp instrument, will come hoping that the foreign Doctor will be able in some way or other to remedy their condition. It is not often we can help in such cases; but in one case, where the upper half of one ear only had been cut off leaving a good stump, we performed a plastic operation to the satisfaction of the patient, as it remedied to some extent the tell-tale condition of his ear. The operation was performed in two stages, first a flap of skin was dissected from behind the ear, and stitched to that part of the stump nearest it. Some weeks afterwards the attachment of this flap to the scalp was severed, and at the same time another flap was cut from the temple, and applied to the part of the stump that had not been covered by the first operation. A few weeks after the patient's return to his home, we had another man coming from the same neighbourhood, who had lost one ear entirely, and desiring to be treated as the former case had been.

Injuries, &c.—Most of the injuries, wound, &c.

were slight. In a few cases, however, they were so severe as to endanger the life of the patient. The most serious case treated was that of a ship coolie, aged 45, who fell from the top of a mast on to an awning. He fell on his face, and the lower jaw was fractured on the right side opposite the canine tooth, the nasal bones were smashed, the orbital margin of the superior maxilla was also fractured, and the skin of the face and forehead severely bruised. Patient smoked and ate opium ashes to the extent of two mace daily. After a long and lingering illness he ultimately recovered.

Dislocation of the Lower Jaw.—A man was twice treated for this condition at an interval of several months. On both occasions the dislocation was caused by opening the mouth too widely when yawning.

Financial.—From the statement in the appendix it will be seen that the receipts of the year amount to $2,237.23 and the expenditure to $1,903.80 leaving a balance of $333.43 in our hands.

The Tang Nguan Seng hong still continues to supply us with rice and cash tickets for the benefit of the poorer patients. These, to the value of about $120, have been received during the year.

In conclusion we have to acknowledge with hearty thanks the liberal contributions from the Swatow Foreign community and others; the kind assistance of Dr. Pollock in collecting a number of the contributions; the gift of a *Listers' Steam Spray*, for use in the antiseptic treatment of wounds, from the Rev. J. C. Gibson, M. A; and of a *Thermo-cautery* from my old teacher, Prof. Simpson, of the University of Edinburgh.

[We append a short report of the Hakka Medical work as the drugs used in the work were supplied by the Swatow Hospital.]

Report of the Hakka Medical Work for 1882.

The Rev. Dr. Riddel writes:—Medical work among the Hakkas has been carried on in a desultory manner since December, 1881. During visits to the preaching stations I had my basket of medicines always with me. The work done during these visits will not bear comparison with Hospital work for various reasons. The patients know that the doctor is to be there only a short time, and so there is often such a rush as makes it impossible to examine difficult cases satisfactorily. Then there is the limited pharmacopœia, and want of surgical appliances, and, moreover, seldom any opportunity of seeing the patients a second time to renew prescriptions.

In the early part of 1882, I stayed at Ng-yun-thung for periods of several weeks on end, and was thus able to give the patients much more attention, and secure, I hope, better results. In this region some 500 cases were treated. Afterwards during our stay at Ng-kang-phu we had more than 300 cases; and, during a visit to Ta-pu in August, more than 200 cases.

I find the total number of new cases from December 1881 to the end of 1882 to be over 1100, and of these more than 200 returned once or twice to have their medicines renewed.

With no place as yet purchased for dispensary, a few minor operations only, such as for entropium and slit ear, were all that it was thought wise to attempt.

SUBSCRIPTIONS FOR 1882.

Messrs. Bradley & Co.	$100.00
„ Dircks & Co.	100.00
„ Butterfield & Swire	50.00
„ Douglas Lapraik & Co.	50.00
Rev. W. Ashmore, D.D., *special*	50.00
Robert Craig, ...	50.00
Fred. H. Ewer, ...	50.00
W. Gregory, ...	50.00
Messrs. Campbell & Co.	30.00
Rev. D. MacIver, M.A.	30.00
W. Paton, ...	30.00
John Andrew, ...	25.00
Rev. J. A. B. Cook	25.00
„ W. Duffus	25.00
W. Gauld, M.A., M.D.	25.00
A. Huber, ...	25.00
Alexander Lyall, M.B., C.M.	25.00
Rev. H. L. Mackenzie, M.A.	25.00
G. D. Pitman, ...	25.00
"Shanghailander" per Dr. Pollock	25.00
Rev. G. Smith, M.A.	25.64
Messrs. Williams & Co.	25.00
Otto Asverus, ...	20.00
J. D. Meyer, ...	15.00
James Beaton, ...	10.00
J. R. Bridgman, ...	10.00
M. F. A. Fraser, ...	10.00
W. Krey, ...	10.00
Ed. Milne, ...	10.00

Capt. T. G. Pocock, s. s. *Thales*	10.00
H. Sage, ...	10.00
A. Montague Sowdon, ...	10.00
Capt. Whittle, per Dr. Pollock	10.00
Capt. P. Williams	10.00
D. W. Wright, ...	10.00
Rev. J. Rutherfurd, M.A., B.D.	6.74
J. K. W. Lange de la Camp, ...	5.00
C. C. Chamberlain, per Dr. Pollock	5.00
Capt. Clegg, Do.	5.00
Capt. F. W. Focken	5.00
J. C. Johnston, ...	5.00
J. Liddell, ...	5.00
T. N. Manners, ...	5.00
Capt. Peoples, per Dr. Pollock	5.00
J. Sjögren, ...	5.00
W. Lührss, ...	4.00
H. Haines, ...	3.00
Thos. W. Harrocks, ...	3.00
W. G. Tindall, ...	3.00
"Decision," per Mr H. Sage	2.00
J. Ferdes, ...	2.00
J. T. Manley, ...	2.00
E. Phair, ...	2.00
A. Smith, ...	2.00
Tsan Thai un	20.00
L. Wong	15.00
A Khiin Ia.	10.00
Ung Keang	5.00
Sam Tatling	5.00
Patients	2.79
Kwai Fung	2.00
Lin-su	2.00
Sim Kye Pang	2.00
Hau-ku	1.00
	$1,150.17

STATEMENT OF INCOME AND EXPENDITURE.

To	Wages of Assistants and Doorkeeper ...	$359.00
,,	Printing Hospital Reports, Postage	30.33
,,	Ground Rent, and Insurance on Building	25.00
,,	Repairing and White-washing Wards ...	55.48
,,	Lard and Oils	66.98
,,	Cloth for Bandages, Cotton Wool	57.91
,,	Gin and Rectified Spirits, for Liniments and Tinctures..........................	124.02
,,	Paper, Wax, Kerosine, Charcoal	11.50
,,	Sundries	61.70
,,	Water	44.45
,,	Aid to Poor Patients	162.71
,,	Foreign & Native Drugs bought in China	162.27
,,	Surgical Instruments	53.27
,,	Drugs, Surgical Dressings, Milk, from London, and Freight and Insurance...	129.18
,,	Drugs, &c. from London paid by Mission Committee in Edinburgh (about)......	500.00
,,	Rice and Cash Tickets (about)	120.00
,,	Balance on Hand	333.43
		$2,237.23

By	Balance from 1881	$ 293.89
,,	Contributions as per List	1,150.17
,,	Sale of Trusses	28.98
,,	,, Latrine Contents	29.18
,,	,, Sundries	4.13
,,	,, Drugs (profits of)	95.03
,,	Rent of Small Wards	15.85
,,	Rice and Cash Tickets (about)...........	120.00
,,	Drugs from London, paid by Mission Committee in Edinburgh (about)...	500.00
		$2,237.23

LIST OF DISEASES TREATED.

GENERAL DISEASES

Febricula	34
Intermittent Fever	131
Chronic Articular Rheumatism	43
Muscular Rheumatism	93
Lumbago	32
Pleurodynia	9
Rheumatic Arthritis	1
Gonorrhœal Rheumatism	2
Syphilis	30
,, Congenital	4
Syphilitic & Strumous Glandular Enlargement	30
Struma	5
Leprosy	150
Anæmia	139
Debility	69
Opium Smokers for cure	129
Goitre	7
Starvation	2
Tumours—Fatty	9
Lardaceous	8
Fibrous	10
Glandular	5
Malignant	17
Scirrhus of Breast	5
Cystic	6
Naevus	1
Wen	1
Ganglion	2
Unclassified	7
CancrumO ris	1
Measles	11
Cholera	10
Erysipelas	2
Gangrene	3
Blood Poisoning	1
Ascites	6
General Œdema	1
Local ,,	3

Diseases of the Digestive System.

Ulceration of Lip	6
Epithelioma of Lip	4
Harelip	41
Gumboil	2
Caries of Teeth	11
Epulis (Fibrous)	3
Enlarged Papillæ of Tongue	2
Salivary Fistula	1
Ulceration of Gums, Mouth or Fauces	21
Epithelioma of Tongue	1
Elongated Uvula	1
Tumours of Fauces	3
Tonsillitis	5
Cleft Palate	2
Stricture of Oesophagus	8
Dyspepsia	239
,, Alcoholic	2
Colic	28
Dysentery	25
Diarrhœa	27
Lumbrici	33
Hiccup (?)	1
Constipation	1
Stricture of Rectum	10
Internal Haemorrhoids	36
External ,,	14
Fistula in Ano	60
Ulcer or Fistula of Rectum	7
Prolapse of Rectum	2
Ulcer. of Anus (Sodomy)	17
Imperforate Anus	1
Hernia	34
Enlarged Spleen	33
,, Liver	5

Diseases of the Ear.

Deafness	8
Otorrhœa	7
Inflammation	1
Accumulation of War in Canal	1
Eczema	1
Injury of Ear	1
Fistula of Ear	1
Mutilation of Lobe	4
Wounds ,,	2
Closure of Orifice by Cicatricial Contraction	1

Diseases of the Circulatory System.

Valvular Disease of the Heart	7	Popliteal Aneurism	1
Varix	5		

Diseases of the Respiratory System.

Ulcer of Larynx	4	Phthisis Pulmonalis	72
Asthma	14	Emphysema	7
Bronchitis	133	Hæmoptysis	9
Pneumonia	2		

Diseases of the Nose.

Ulceration of Nose (Lupoid and Syphilitic)	23	Slit in Nose	2
Ulceration of the Mucous Membrane	6	Wound of Nose	1
		Polypus of Nose	11
		Malignant Polypus	1

Diseases of the Eye.

Entropium and Trichiasis	217	Slough of Cornea	18
Ectropium	6	Opacity „	86
Ptosis	1	Arcus Senilis	1
Hordeolum	2	Splinter in Cornea	2
Hypertrophy of Tarsal Cartilage	2	Injury of „	1
Tumours (small) of Eyelid	7	Iritis	14
Naevus of Eyelid	1	Iritic Adhesion	35
Ophthalmia—Granular	210	Hernia of Iris	16
„ Purulent	16	Hypopion	4
„ Catarrhal	63	Anterior Staphyloma	15
„ Pustular	2	Cataract	28
„ Gonorrhœal	1	Foreign Body in Lens	2
„ Tarsi	29	Glaucoma	9
Pterygium	74	Destruction of one or both Eyes	53
Obstruction of Punctum or Nasal Duct	15	Tremulous Iris	1
Lachrymal Abscess	5	Optic Neuritis	2
Symblepharon	3	Atrophy of Optic Nerve	3
Anchyloblepharon	3	Amaurosis	4
Keratitis	11	Night Blindness	3
Vascular Cornea	10	Extravasation of Blood into Retina	1
Ulcer of „	99	Malgnant Tumours of Orbit	4

Diseases of Joints.

Strumous disease of Hip joint	10	Bursitis	1
„ „ Knee „	4	Synovitis of Ankle Joint	15
„ „ Shoulder „	2	Anchylosis of Knee „	6
„ „ Elbow „	1	„ Ankle „	2
Synovitis (Acute & Chronic) of Knee joint	11	„ Elbow „	1
		„ Finger „	2

Diseases of the Nervous System.

Hemiplegia	5	Mania	2
Paraplegia	3	Dementia	3
Paralysis of Arm	4	Neuralgia	9
„ Facial	2	Sciatica	16
Epilepsy	9	Hysteria	1
Locomotor Ataxy	1	Vertigo	3
Local Anæsthesia	18	Spinal Disease	1

Diseases of the Skin.

Tinea Circinata	108	Herpes Zoster	1
„ Tonsurans	10	Ulticaria	1
„ Sycosis	14	Keloid	3
„ Favosa	4	Elephantiasis of Leg	35
Pityriasis	8	Corns	4
Scabies	20	Painful Cicatrix	2
Prurigo	5	Epithelioma	7
Eczema	32	Lupus	3
„ Capitis	5	Condylomata	8
Psoriasis	10	Warts	1
Pemphigus	2	Whitlows	12
Icthyosis	4	Carbuncles and Boils	6
Ecthyma	7	Inflammation	17
Alopeica	2	Abscesses	56
Leucoderma	2	Ulcerations	301
Acne	6	Sinuses	28
Lichen	1	Fissures and Cracks	9

Diseases of the Genito Urinary System.

Ulcer or Sinus of Scrotum	9	Fungus Testis	1
Eczema of Scrotum	7	Cystitis	1
Lymph Scrotum	4	Vesical Calculi	2
Elephantiasis of Scrotum	11	Chyluria	1
Epithelioma of Scrotum	1	Retention of Urine	1
Chancres and Ulcerations of Penis	16	Incompetence of Urine	2
Epithelioma of Penis	6	Impotence	1
Tumour (small) of Penis	1	Chronic Albuminuria	2
Phymosis	9	Maldevelopment of Genitals	1
Paraphymosis	1	Bubo	6
Gonorrhœa	20	Leucorrhœa	5
Stricture of Urethra	11	Menorrhagia	1
Injury of „	3	Irregular Menstruation	1
Urinary Fistula	2	Elephantiasis of Vulva	1
Calculus in Urethra	1	Uterine Fibroid	2
Spermatorrhœa	27	Carcinoma Uteri	1
Orchitis	1	Ovarian Tumours	2
Hydrocele	24	Tumours (not classified)	3

Diseases of Bones.

Caries and Necrosis	61	Spinal Curvature	10
Periostitis	1		

Wounds, Injuries, &c.

Dislocation of Lower Jaw ...	2	Gunshot Wounds	4
" Shoulder ...	3	Slit in Ear	27
" Elbow	1	Bruises and Injuries	53
" Finger	2	Injury to Chest (from burden-bearing and beating) ...	65
" Hip	5	Sprains	27
Fracture of Radius	4	Wounds	32
" Fibula	1	Burns and Scalds	14
" Lower Jaw, Nasal Bones, and Orbital process of Sup. Maxilla	1	Bamboo Splinter in hand ...	1
Compound Fracture of Humerus	1	" " in thigh ...	1
Compound Fracture of Great Toe	2	Needle in hand	1
		Bullets lodged	3
		Bites—Dog's	5
		Pig's	2

Unclassified.

Inflammation of Lymphatics of Leg	1	Enlarged Glands in Groin (Elephantiasoid)	7
Mal-development of Arm ...	1	Contraction of Tendons ...	4
Involuntary Muscular Twitchings	1	Supernumerary Thumb ...	1
		Opium Poisoning	1

REPORT

OF THE

Medical Missionary Hospital

AT

SWATOW,

IN CONNECTION WITH THE

PRESBYTERIAN CHURCH OF ENGLAND,

UNDER THE CARE OF

Alexander Lyall, M. B., C. M.

AND OF

MEDICAL MISSION WORK

IN THE

HAKKA COUNTRY,

UNDER THE CARE OF

Rev. Wm. Riddle, M. B., C. M.

FOR 1883.

PRINTED BY

Kwai Fung,

PRINTER, BOOKBINDER & STATIONER,

SWATOW,

1884.

REPORT.

THE past year has been to the native population of this region a rather unhealthy one. An unhealthy Spring season was followed by a long, hot, and unusually trying Summer, in the beginning of which a severe epidemic of cholera broke out in Swatow, and, spreading over the greater portion of the Department of Ch'ao-Chow, caused great havoc among the people; and as the year closes small-pox is very prevalent, and is being attended by a considerable mortality.

On the whole, therefore, the work in the Swatow Mission Hospital during the past year has been more than usually heavy and anxious.

During the cholera epidemic the native assistants worked well, and were always found willing, when called upon, to attend to cases outside. We are thankful to say that only one member of the Hospital Staff of assistants was knocked down with the disease, and that he made a good recovery from a pretty severe attack.

Number of Patients.—The total number of patients who have been under treatment is as follows:—

In-patients	2,838	
Out-patients	1,597	—4,435
Patients seen and prescribed for in the country,		1,150
Total		5,585

The total number of our patients when compared with the large number of out-patients at some other Hospitals in China may seem to be small; but, seeing that so large a proportion are in-patients, it indicates a pretty fair amount of work.

Perhaps the two following tables will give a better idea of the amount of work done.

(1) Table showing the number of new patients registered on their first visit only, during the various months of the year.

	In-patients.	*Out-patients,*
January	234	131
February	56	25
March	267	114
April	276	145
May	502	279
June	277	178
July	208	144
August	64	67
September	194	140
October	333	135
November	178	101
December	249	138
	2838	1597

(2) The daily average attendance of in- and out-patients during the year.

	In-patients.	*Out-patients.*
January	192	35
February	79	14
March	157	24
April	195	31
May	328	51
June	285	47
July	183	38
August	98	22
September	119	32
October	204	48
November	168	30
December	162	30

In-patients.—The medical institution under our care is, we believe, the only one in China where the number of in-patients is greater than the number of out-patients. We have had 2,835 in-patients, and of these 379 were women. Frequently during the year we have found the Hospital buildings too small to accommodate all who applied for admittance, and have had to send some away without their being properly attended to. In the month of May the daily average number amounted to 328.

Owing to the prevalence of cholera the in-patients diminished very much in numbers towards the end of Summer, so that in the month of August we had only a daily average of about 100. For some time we ceased to have patients coming from a distance, as they were afraid to travel through the infected parts.

During the whole Summer there was not a single case of cholera in the wards of the large Hospital although scores of people were dying from that disease only a few yards distant; but in the small Hospital we were not so fortunate. The assistant in charge, who was attending cases outside, was seized, and during the next fortnight or three weeks eight additional cases occurred. We then got rid of the other patients as soon as possible, and shut the building up for a time.

Towards the end of the year we had two cases of small-pox—one of them an assistant. They were isolated, and the disease did not spread further.

Last year more *deaths* than usual occurred in the Hospitals. In all eighteen persons died; but some of these were poor, friendless people who had been left on our hands. One a blind infant, about eighteen months old, was brought by her father for treatment. It was late in the afternoon when he arrived, and the assistants asked him to stay in the wards until next morning in order that he might see me; but during the night he decamped leaving the child on our hands. The child died some months after from dysentery. Another, a poor emaciated creature who was dying from starvation and dysentery, was found by some of the native Christians lying behind the Cantonese guild. At their request we took him in, but he died next day. He was, it is said, the son of a wealthy native merchant, who, getting into trouble with the mandarins, had to make a rapid flight to save his head. The lad being a broken down, dissipated youth had been left behind by his father. Two men, returning from abroad, were brought from the steamer in a moribund state, and died a few hours after admittance. In another case death was self-inflicted. This man came from the District of Lu-fung, and had been successfully treated for Granular Conjunctivitis. On being asked to return home, he poisoned himself. Three deaths were due to cholera.

Medical Missionaries differ in opinion as the best methods of carrying on medical mission work among the Chinese. Some prefer to give most of their time and strength to the out-patient department, and to have only a small hospital in which the graver cases of illness can be more carefully treated. This method certainly entails the least strain on one's strength, but the value of this kind of work may be questioned.

In a small place like Swatow, where the vast proportion of the patients come from the surrounding districts, to a distance of eighty or one hundred miles, it is necessary to take them into the hospital if they are to be treated at all; but apart even from our special circumstances we thoroughly believe in the superior value of the hospital *versus* the dispensary system. From some experience I am inclined to think that the work done in the dispensary is not satisfactory. A patient comes, gets medicine, and goes away again, and the probability of his following out the directions given is very small, as the Chinese way of taking medicine differs greatly from the Western method. The in-patient system, it is true, does not come up to what one could wish, still, having them under your care, the patients can be attended to once, twice or oftener, if necessary, every day, and the treatment can be altered or changed at will. This plan, of course, makes it necessary to admit cases that are, strictly speaking, not suitable hospital cases; but in a mission hospital this is not to be regretted, because evangelistic work is more easily, and perhaps more successfully also, carried on among patients who are not the subjects of severe or painful disease. A Medical Missionary can exert little influence over a person whom perhaps he only sees once in the out-patient department; but he can get much nearer to those who are living under his charge in his hospital. He gets to know them, or, what is perhaps more important in this part of the world, his patients get to know him. Consequently much more personal influence can be brought to bear on the patients in such circumstances.

We believe therefore that, for a medical missionary to accomplish really good work, medical or evangelistic, among the Chinese, he must have a good large building in which his patients can lodge, and where he can devote to them most of his time and strength.

We have no wish to see the number of our out-patients increased, but we would gladly welcome an addition to our hospital buildings.

The in-patients provide their own food while staying with us, but no charge is made for medicine or medical attendance.

Out-patients.—of the 1,597 out-patients 229 were women. They are seen only on two days of the week—Tuesday and Friday. During the year a considerable number of persons have been visited in their own houses in Swatow.

Visits to the Country.—About the time of the Chinese new year, in company with colleagues, I spent a month in visiting the more distant Hakka and Hoklo preaching stations in the West and South-west; and in autumn a fortnight was spent among the villages in the Chao-yang plain. During these trips about 1,150 persons were seen and prescribed for.

EVANGELISTIC.

The evangelistic work has been conducted as hitherto Before the work of the day begins the patients are assembled and have the word of God read and explained to them. About sunset they again meet together in the chapel, when a shorter service is held, generally by one of the native assistants. On several days of the week the morning service is conducted by the ordained missionaries and Mrs. Smith, Miss Ricketts and the Bible-women under her care have done good work among the women.

During the year twelve of the patients have been baptized, and many more have sought for admission into the Church. For these a special meeting has been regularly held on Sunday afternoon. Besides those who come forward as applicants for baptism, we find that many others get a clear mental knowledge of the Truth We are entitled to cherish the hope that from among these some will in days to come confess from the heart the Truth which they already in some measure know.

Through the liberality of the Scottish National Bible Society there is now a prospect of having a colporteur connected with the hospital. The above Society has kindly given a grant of £12 to pay the salary of an agent of this kind for one year; and one of the students, at present under instruction in Swatow, has been set apart for this work. He will enter upon his duties after the Chinese new year. He will be expected to visit old hospital applicants for baptism in their homes, and to take advantage of the opportunities that may arise for preaching and selling religious books and tracts.

In the evangelising of the Department of Ch'ao Chow the hospital has played a useful part. The opportunities it presents for making known the gospel are exceptionally favourable, for there is now a daily average during the year of nearly two hundred in-patients who come from all parts of the surrounding country. Moreover, the average length of stay in the hospital for each patient is about three weeks, and during this time he has the opportunity of receiving daily religious instruction.

Below we give a table showing the number of towns and villages in the different Districts from which patients have come; and also the number of persons from each District.

It will be seen that in all they came from 1439 towns and villages. This of itself will indicate the value of the Hospital as an Evangelistic Agency.

	No. of Villages.	*No. of Patients.*
Ch'ao-chow Department :—		
Ching-hai District	79	552
Chao-yang ,, ...	279	1139
Kieh-yang ,, ...	270	698
Hwei-lai ,, ...	88	232
Jao-ping ,, ...	200	629
Pu-ning ,, ...	168	361
Hai-yang ,, ...	157	380
Fung-shun ,, ...	34	91
Ta-pu ,, ...	12	27
Island of Namoa	12	65
District of Kia-ying-chow.........	19	31
,, of Lu-fung and Hai-fung	14	36
Province of Hokien	102	181
Other Districts or Provinces	5	13
	1439	4435

(7)

The following is a list of diseases, &c. which have beer under treatment :—

General Diseases.

Febricula	48	Congenital Syphilis	1
Intermittent Fever :—		Muscular Rheumatism	8
Quotidian	8	Lumbago	2
Tertian	23	Pleurodynia	2
Quartan	224	Syphilitic Rheumatism	1
Irregular	7	Rheumatic Arthritis	
Leprosy	218	Cholera	8
Anaemia	123	Small-pox	
General Debility	61	Typhus Fever	
Syphilitic & Strumous Glandular Enlargement	27	Erysipelas	
Syphilis	23	Diabetes	
Chronic Articular Rheumatism	41	Gangrene	
		Starvation	
		Opium Smoking (for cure)	11

Diseases of the Digestive System.

Harelip	27	Constipation	
Ulceration of Lip	3	Diarrhœa	2
Epithelioma of Lip	2	Dysentery	2
Gumboil	1	Haematemesis	
Dental Sinus	2	Enlarged Liver	
Caries of Tooth	2	„ „ with Jaundice	
Cleft Palate	3	Scirrhus of Liver	
Ulceration of Palate	1	Enlarged Spleen	4
Epithelioma of Palate	2	Stricture of Rectum	
Inflammation of Tongue	1	Fissure „ „	
Ulceration of Fauces	8	Polypus „ „	
Chronic Tonsillitis	16	Prolapse „ „	
Enlarged Papillæ of Fauces	1	Ulceration of Anus (Sodomy)	1
Stricture of Œsophagus	3	Wound of Rectum	
Dyspepsia	280	Fistula in Ano	5
Alcoholic Dyspepsia	1	Internal Haemorrhoids	4
Scirrhus of Stomach	1	External „	
Colic	47	Hernia	3
Gastro-intestinal Catarrh	1	Ascites	
Vermes	24	Fistula in Abdominalwall	

Diseases of the Lymphatic System.

Enlarged Glands in Groin with Fever	8	Lymph Scrotum	
Elephantiasis of Leg	42	Elephantiasis of Scrotum	1

Diseases of the Pulmonary System.

Congestion of Larynx	2	Asthma	1
Bronchitis	130	Haemoptysis	1
Phthisis Pulmonalis	92	Emphysema	

Diseases of the Eye.

Entropium and Trichiasis	204
Ectropium	1
Syphilitic Ulceration of Eyelid	2
Wound of Eyelid	1
Involuntary Twitching Eyelid	1
Abscess of Eyelid	1
Tumours (Small) Eyelid	4
„ (Malignant) Eyelid	2
Wart „ „	1
Thickening of Tarsal Cartilage	3
Tarsal Cyst	1
Ptosis	2
Hordeolum	2
Anchyloblepharon	6
Symblepharon	8
Ophthalmia—Tarsi	9
„ Catarrhal	71
„ Pustular	4
„ Purulent	6
„ Granular	349
„ Gonorrheal	4
Pterygium	58
Opacity of Cornea	66
Ulcer of „	47
Slough of „	14
Wound of „	3
Fibrous growth under Conjunctiva	2
Pannus	5
Keratitis	15
Irido-Keratitis	2
Anterior Staphyloma	23
Iritis	19
Hernia of Iris	8
Chronic Iritic Adhesion	37
Hypopion	7
Glaucoma	9
Atrophy of Optic Nerve	4
Amaurosis	10
Myopia	1
Night Blindness	2
Cataract	22
Wound of Cornea and Lens	2
Destruction of one or both Eyes	56
Malignant Tumour of Eyeball	2
„ „ of Orbit	5
Obstruction of Punctum or Nasal Duct	18
Blenorrhea	3
Fistula of Lachrymal Sac	3
Injury from Lime	1

Diseases of the Nose.

Polypus—Simple	10
„ Malignant	1
Ulceration of the Mucous Membrane	8
Ulceration of Nose and Lip	9
Disease of Nasal Bones	1
Epistaxis	2
Inflammation	2
Wound	1
Bruise	1
Closure of Nasal Orifice and of Mouth (partial)	1
Fruit Stone in Nose	1

Diseases of the Genito Urinary System.

Albuminuria	8
Vesical Calculus	3
Spermatorrhœa	31
Gonorrhœa	23
Stricture of Urethra	9
Extravasation of Urine	1
Urinary Fistula	2
Phymosis	13
Ulceration of Penis	25
Adherence of Prepuce to glans Penis	1
Epithelioma of Penis	6
Hypertrophy of Prepuce	1
Wound of Penis (dog's bite)	1
Ulceration of Scrotum	6
Eczema of Scrotum	3
Ringworm of Scrotum	4
Fungus Testis	2
Hydrocele	28
Scrotal Tumour	1
Impotence	1
Bubo	7
Uterine Tumour	1
Leucorrhœa	4
Amenorrhœa	2
Dysmenorrhœa	1
Pruritus of Vulvum	1
Tumours of „	2

Diseases of the Ear

Deafness	8	Malignant Tumour of Ear	2
Otorrhœa	8	Slit in Ear	19
Polypus in External Ear	1	Cyst in Lobe	1
Wax " " "	2	Earache	1

Diseases of the Skin.

Scabies	22	Icthyosis	4
Tinea Circinata	110	Ulcers	264
" Favosa	8	Epithelioma	8
" Tonsurans	8	Lupus	2
Eczema	40	Onychia	2
Psoriasis	9	Rupia	5
Pemphigus	1	Syphilitic Nodes	4
Acne	7	" Gumma	1
Pityriasis	6	Condylomata	2
Sudamina	1	Corns	9
Herpes Zoster	1	Carbuncles and Boils	12
Leucoderma	1	Warts	2
Keloid	1	Fissures	4
Prurigo	2	Sinuses	16
Ecthyma	8	Abscesses	48

Tumours.

Naevus	5	Glandular	7
Epulis	4	Malignant Tumours	15
Wen	1	" " of Jaw	5
Goitre	2	" " of female breast	3
Ranula	1	Cystic	7
Ganglion	3	" of lower jaw	2
Fatty	12	Unclassed	6
Fibrous	11		
Lardaceous	7		

Diseases of the Nervous System.

Epilepsy	9	Paralysis of Face	2
Sciatica	26	" Paraplegia	3
Neuralgia	11	" Hemiplegia	2
Local Anæsthesia	13	" Arm	2
Vertigo	7	Imbecility	1
Chronic Hydrocephalus	1	Dumb	1
Apoplexy	1	Disease of Spinal Cord (unclassed)	1
Locomotor Ataxy	3		

Diseases of the Vascular System.

Aneurism of Aorta	1	Enlarged Heart	1
Valvular Disease of Heart	7	Varix	7

Diseases of Bones.

Caries and Necrosis	61	Spinal Curvature	8
Periostitis	8		

Diseases of Joints.

Strumous disease of Hip joint	16
„ „ Knee „	5
„ „ Elbow „	1
„ „ Shoulder „	1
Synovitis of Knee Joint ...	7
„ of Ankle Joint ...	17
„ of Shoulder Joint...	1
„ of Wrist Joint ...	1
Synovitis of Metatarso-pharyngeal of little toe ...	1
Anchylosis of Ankle Joint...	1
„ of Knee „ ...	6
„ of Hip „ ...	2
„ of Elbow „ ...	2
Bursitis	1
Bruise of Joints	8
Knock Knee	1

Wounds, Injuries, &c.

Dislocation of Shoulder ...	2
„ Elbow	1
„ Ankle	1
„ Toe	1
Fracture of Tibia	2
„ Femur	1
„ Toe	1
„ Radius	1
Wounds	50
Bruises and Injuries	48
Injury to Chest (from burden bearing and beating) ...	45
Sprains	20
Burns and Scalds	5
Bites—Pig's	2
„ Cat's	1
„ Dog's	6
„ Woman's	1
Bullet lodged	1
Bamboo Splinter in Foot ...	1
Fish Bone in Oesophagus ...	1
Needle in Wrist	1
Piece of Glass in Foot	1

Unclassified.

Contraction after Burns and Ulceration	4
Muscular Twitchings	1
Midwifery	2
Cut Throat..........................	2
Stramonium Poisoning.........	1

Cholera.—This disease in an Epidemic form was prevalent to a fearful extent last Summer. It is stated by old residents to have been the most fatal Epidemic that has occurred since Swatow was made a treaty port. The origin of the Epidemic was currently reported to have been due to the opening of the coffins of two Chinese sailors who had died from the disease on board a steamer; but it is not likely that this was the cause. There was a good deal of Cholera in the Autumn of 1882, and I think that the disease was Endemic in Swatow during the Winter.

From the commencement of the hot weather acute Diarrhœa and Dysentery were very rife among the people; and a good many deaths especially among children occurred.

It was not, however, till near the end of June that Typical cases of Cholera began to appear, and once started, it spread rapidly all over the country. No reliable estimate of the mortality can be obtained, but it was very great. In Ch'ao-chow-foo alone, it is said that between 4,000 and 5,000 persons died.

Chinese friends reported to us many instances of the disease proving fatal in a few hours, and in many of these there was little or no purging or vomiting. We heard of many sad cases, for instance, a family living in the Foo city lost 9 out of 11 members.

The majority of the cases that came under our notice were fairly amenable to treatment, especially when the patient was seen at an early stage. An accurate list of the numbers treated was not kept, but of the 83 cases of which we have notes, fully three-fourths recovered.

Cholera mixtures were sent to many of the preaching stations connected with the Protestant Missions in Swatow; and some Chinamen bought large quantities of the same mixtures for distribution among poor people, or for selling over again. In these ways, as we afterwards heard, many cases were successfully treated.

Many different methods of treatment were tried, and on the whole we found that a mixture composed of equal parts of Tinctures of Opium, Capsicum, Rhubarb, and Spirits of Peppermint and Camphor was perhaps the most useful in the early stage of the disease. When the disease was fully developed the well known Indian "Cholera drops" was the best remedy tried. In the stage of collapse, or when the patient began to show symptoms of collapse, we gave Hypodermic injections of Ether or Brandy. Besides the medicinal treatment, hot bottles, Sinapisms &c. were applied to the patient, and hand friction was resorted to for relieve of Cramps. Diluted milk was cautiously given at short intervals in cases where the vomiting was not severe.

In one case a Hypodermic injection of Morphia at the beginning of the second stage had a marked beneficial result.

Three cases were reported to us as having been successfully treated with Carbolic Acid. A Chinese gentleman bought from the hospital a quantity of Carbolic Acid solution for disinfecting purposes; and he gave some of it to a family in which there was Cholera, to be used in disinfecting excreta &c. Misunderstanding his directions they used it as medicine, and drank some of it. In a short time after beginning to use it, the disease was checked, and they made a rapid recovery.

Malarial Diseases.—There has been a marked increase in the number of cases of Intermittent Fever as compared with former years, which is another indication of the unhealthiness of the season. During the year 282 cases of Intermittent and 48 cases of simple Fever have been treated, whereas in 1882 there were only 131 cases of the former and 34 of the latter. In addition to these, there have been about 280 cases of simple fever occurring among the patients in course of treatment for other diseases.

In treating Intermittent Fever we generally give both quinine and arsenic from the first. By this treatment a cure is more quickly obtained. Many of the cases are of long standing; and the Quartan variety of Intermittent Fever is by far the most common.

The only objection to quinine is its price; it is very expensive. We have tested the value of a considerable number of *Substitutes* for quinine, and of these *Cinchona Febrifuge*, largely used in India in treating ague among the poor, is perhaps one of the best. A little larger dose is required, and it is slightly more irritating to the stomach than quinine, but very good results can be obtained from its use. As it is much cheaper than quinine, we intend in future to use the Cinchona Febrifuge much more extensively. If India would send the *Cinchona Febrifuge* to China instead of *Opium*, it would be a great blessing to the Chinese people.

Opium Smokers.—We give a few statistics with reference to this class of patients for the information of those who take an interest in the subject of opium-smoking.

There were 111 opium-smokers admitted, but a few of them left the hospital after two or three days' attempt to break off the habit.

As formerly, no opium whatever was used in their treatment. In the course of the year we have come across a considerable number of our old patients, and of these we have reason to believe that most have not returned to the pipe. Two or three of this class have been admitted into the church.

AMOUNT USED PER DAY.

½ mace or less...	 15	2½ mace	... ...	5
1 „ or more than ½ m.	32	3 „	... ...	10
1½ „ or „ „ 1 m.	24	4 „	... ...	2
2 „	... 16	5 „	... ...	4

Duration of Habit.

1 year or less	6	12 years	3
2 ,,	9	13 ,,	1
3 ,,	7	14 ,,	2
4 ,,	10	16 ,,	1
5 ,,	5	17 ,,	2
6 ,,	5	18 ,,	1
7 ,,	2	20 ,,	6
8 ,,	2	25 ,,	2
9 ,,	1	30 ,,	2
10 ,,	17	34 ,,	1
11 ,,	1		

Age of Patient.

From 20—25 years	11	From 40—45 years	18
,, 25—30 ,,	15	,, 45—50 ,,	9
,, 30—35 ,,	24	,, 50—60 ,,	9
,, 35—40 ,,	21	,, 70	2

Eye Diseases.—More than 1,120 cases of Eye Diseases have passed through our hands.

SURGICAL.

The following Surgical operations have been performed during the year :—

On the Eye :—

Operations for Entropium and Trichiasis	326
,, ,, Pterygium	51
,, ,, Ectropium	1
,, ,, Anchyloblepharon	5
,, ,, Symblepharon	1
,, ,, Cataract	7
,, ,, Anterior Staphyloma	3
,, ,, Hernia of Iris	4
,, ,, Hypopion	4
Plastic operation for Slit of upper Eyelid	1
Iridectomy for Artificial Pupil	29
Excision of Eyeball	2
,, ,, Fibrous growths from Conjunctiva	3
,, ,, Tumours (small) from Eyelid	8
,, ,, ,, Malignant ,,	2
,, ,, Wart Eyelid	1
,, ,, Sarcomatous Tumour of Orbit	1
Opened Abscess of Eyelid	1=450

On the Body generally.—

Operations for Harelip	26
,, ,, Fistula in Ano	47
,, ,, Slit in Ear	21
,, ,, Phymosis (Circumcision) ...	14
,, ,, Ganglion	8
,, ,, Naevus	1
,, ,, Ulcer of Rectum	1
,, ,, Extravasation of Urine ...	1
,, ,, Caries of Bone	8
Excision of Tumours	46
,, ,, External Hæmorrhoids ...	14
,, ,, Shoulder Joint	1
,, ,, Elbow ,, ...	1
,, ,, Tonsils	2
,, ,, Epulis	4
,, ,, Scirrhus of Breast	2
,, ,, Portion of Lower Jaw	1
,, ,, Wen	1
,, ,, Epithelioma of Skin	2
,, ,, Hypertrophy of Prepuce ...	2
,, ,, Elephantiasis of Scrotum ...	3
,, ,, Elephantiasis of Clitoris and Labia Minora	1
,, ,, Corns	9
,, ,, Ranula	1
,, ,, Polypus of Rectum	1
Plastic operation for wound of Lip	1
,, ,, ,, deformity of Lip ...	1
,, ,, ,, closure of Nasal Orifice and Mouth (partial)	1
,, ,, ,, closure of outer canal of Ear	1
Lithotomy	1
Slitting open Sinuses	8
,, ,, Cystic Tumours in sub-maxillary region	2
Tapping and injecting Hydrocele	24
Slitting open Hydrocele	1
Tying Internal Hæmorrhoids	46
Amputation of Penis (Epithelioma) ...	4
Extraction of Necrosed Bone	27
,, ,, Teeth	67
,, ,, Polypus of Nose	16
,, ,, Bullet	1

Extraction of Seed from Nostril	...	...	1	
,, ,, Finger Nail ...	...	...	2	
,, ,, Bamboo Splinter	...	...	1	
,, ,, Piece of Glass	...	...	1	
,, ,, Needle ...	...	...	1	
Opening Whitlows, Abscesses, &c.		...	40	
Dilating Stricture of Urethra	...	...	5	
Reduction of Dislocations ...	...	...	2	=482
				932

There have been no deaths from any operation during the year.

Lithotomy.—This patient, a little boy about five years of age, had suffered more or less for two years from his complaint. He was in fairly good health. After a few days of preparatory treatment, Lithotomy by the lateral method was performed, and a calculus about the size of a small hen's egg was extracted. The little patient made an excellent recovery, and was able to leave the hospital about sixteen days after the operation.

Closure of Nasal Orifice and Contraction of Mouth.—The Nasal Orifices were entirely occluded, and the opening into the mouth was not more than half an inch in diameter. This condition of the parts was due to former Ulceration.

Two operations were performed; in the first an opening was made into each of the nostrils, and then silver tubes, which were connected in front by a narrow intermediate piece, were inserted into the nostrils in order to prevent them from filling up again. These tubes were kept in position by means of strings, one end of which was fastened to the tubes, and the other carried round the sides of the head and tied behind. At the same time, holes through the cheek were made on both sides of the mouth, and small bars of silver inserted, and tied in. Some weeks afterwards the second operation was performed, which consisted of cutting open the skin between the mouth and the holes which were now patent. The results were satisfactory.

Excision of part of Lower Jaw.—The patient, a young man, was suffering from a Cystic Tumour of the jaw, which was situated midway between the symphysis and the angle. In 1882 I opened the Tumour, cleared it out, and swabbed the cavity with a strong solution of Chloride of Zinc. The Tumour returned some months afterwards. This time the piece of jaw in which the Tumour was situated, was excised. The wound took rather a long time to heal, but the result was fairly good.

Elephantiasis Scroti.—Three cases were operated on, and the Tumours removed were 76 oz., 160 oz., and 100 oz. in weight respectively. The patients made good recoveries.

Elephantiasis of Labium.—Two Elephantiasis growths, one weighing 10 lbs., and the other 1 lb., were removed from the Clitoris and Labia Minora of a middle aged woman. An elastic band was tightly tied round the necks of the Tumours, and very little blood was lost during the operation. The patient made a good recovery.

Resection of Joint.—The shoulder joint of a young man, and the elbow joint of a boy were excised for caries of the bones, and disorganisation of the joints. In both cases the disease was of old standing, and the patient much reduced in health. It was necessary to remove a large piece of the bones, and the results were not very satisfactory.

Excision of Tumours.—A large number of Tumours of various kinds, have been removed from various parts of the body. Many of them were very interesting cases, but it is impossible to give an account of them in this report A few were of large size; one, a fatty Tumour removed from the buttocks weighed 81 ozs., an another, somewhat like an Elephantiasis growth, 2½ lbs. in weight, was removed from the iliac region.

FINANCIAL.

From the statement appended it will be seen that the receipts for the year amounted to $2,320.94, and the expenditure to $2,201.40, leaving a balance of $119.54 in our hand. A list of the Subscribers is also appended; and to them our hearty thanks are due for their liberal contributions. We trust that the medical institution under our care may still be deemed worthy of their support.

During the year Tan Nguan Seng has given rice and cash tickets to the value of $100 for distribution among the poorer patients. His generous help, now continued for some years, deserves grateful mention; it enables us to detain many poor patients until their cures are completed.

SUBSCRIPTIONS FOR 1883.

Messrs. Bradley & Co.	$100.00
„ Schaar & Co.	100.00
China Sugar Refining Company Limited and Messrs. Jardine, Matheson & Co. ...	100.00
Messrs. Butterfield & Swire	50.00
„ Douglas Lapraik & Co.	50.00
R. H. Hill for medical attendance	50.00
Rev. D. MacIver, M.A.	50.00
„ G. Smith, M.A.	35.00
Baron von Seckendorff	30.00
Children's Medical Mission Association, London, per Miss A. R. Butler	27.42
John Andrews	25.00
Rev. Wm. Duffus	25.00
Colin Jamieson	25.00
Alexander Lyall, M.B., C.M.	25.00
Rev. H. L. Mackenzie, M. A.	25.00
J. F. MacPhun, M.B., C.M.	25.00
Wm. Paton	25.00
Geo. D. Pitman	25.00
Otto Asverus	20.00
Presbyterian Church (native) Swatow	20.00
James Beaton	10.00
Rev. J. A. B. Cook	10.00
Ch. Lange de la Camp	10.00
L. Grunauer	10.00
W. F. Inglis	10.00
J. C. Johnston	10.00
A. Lay	10.00
T. N. Manners	10.00
Thomas Mitchell	10.00
J. F. Oiesen	10.00
G. Phillips	10.00
A. L. Piersdorf	10.00
D. W. Wright	10.00
P. Williams	10.00

"A grateful Patient"	$10.00
H. Sage	7.50
George Brown (for poor patients)	5.00
Capt. Clegg, S. S. *Keelung*, per Dr. Pollock ...	5.00
J. Dickie	5.00
F. W. Focken	5.00
Capt. Glasson, S. S. *Swatow*, per Dr. Pollock ...	5.00
H. Hyndman	5.00
W. Keeble	5.00
J. Liddell	5.00
M. Linklater	5.00
Capt. Lunt, S. S. *Meefoo*, per Dr. Pollock ...	5.00
Miss Norwood (for patient)	5.00
Clement Pape	5.00
Capt. Robinson, S. S. *Tientsin*, per Dr. Pollock	5.00
J. Sjögreen	5.00
Mrs. Smith	5.00
Capt. Whittle, S. S. *Changchow*, per Dr. Pollock ...	5.00
Capt. Wyles, S. S. *Tamsui*, per Dr. Pollock ...	5.00
W. Davidson	4.00
H. Haines	3.00
Capt. Macdonald	2.00
J. F. Manley	2.00
W. E. Southcott	2.00
Tsan Thai-un	20.00
L. Wong	15.00
Siou Hui-ngou	10.00
Siou Ek-keng	10.00
Wong Liu	3.00
Sim hut-tsho	2.00
S. Kye Pang	2.00
Ung Keang	2.00
Kwai Fung	2.00
Cliok Su	2.00
Han Tsu-ngi	2.00
U, Gou, Ie	3.00
Lam Tatting	2.90
Lu U-kheng	1.00
Kin-yung	1.00
Tan Hong-tng	1.00
Pho-ti	1.00
A patient.	2.00
Hospital Subscription box	10.84
	$1,179.76

STATEMENT OF INCOME AND EXPENDITURE.

To Wages of Assistants and Doorkeeper	$370.00
,, Printing Hospital Reports, Postage	30.50
,, Ground Rent, and Insurance on Building	25.60
,, White washing Wards, and Repairs and Painting	83.02
,, Lard, Oils, Paper, Wax, Charcoal	94.60
,, Cloth for Bandages, Cotton Wool	70.48
,, Gin and Rectified Spirits, for Liniments and Tinctures	130.19
,, Water	43.20
,, New Beds, Instrument Press and Sundries	130.10
,, Aid to Poor Patients	135.79
,, Drugs bought in China and Calcutta	170.63
,, Drugs and Surgical Dressings from London, Freight, Insurance and Landing Expenses	293.89
,, Drugs, &c. from London paid by Mission Committee in Edinburgh (about)	510.00
,, Rice and Cash Tickets (about)	100.00
,, Balance on Hand	119.54
	$2,320.94

By Balance from 1882	$333.23
,, Contributions as per List	1,179.76
,, Sale of Trusses	17.00
,, ,, Contents of Latrine	28.55
,, ,, Sundries	20.44
,, ,, Drugs	121.20
,, Rent of Small Wards	10.76
,, Drugs from London, paid by Mission Committee in Edinburgh (about)	510.(
,, Rice and Cash Tickets (about)	100.00
	$2,320.94

Report of the Medical Work in the Hakka Region for 1883.

In submiting a short account of my second year of Medical work among the Hakkas, I feel there is little to relate of much interest from a Medical point of view, although there is reason to believe that a good deal of suffering has been removed or alleviated, and some good done indirectly in thus commending the gospel by a practical exhibition of its spirit.

Since the beginning of the year I have carried on the work in conjunction with Dr. MacPhun, who meanwhile gives his chief attention to the language, but intends by and by to give his whole energy to Medical work. In addition to steady work at our centre at Ng-kang-phu for about 200 days when one or both of us were residing there, we made several visits to outstations taking a supply of medicines with us, the length of our visits varying from a few days to two or three weeks. Dr. MacPhun's visits were made in company with the Rev. D. Mac-Iver, and include an important visit to the Thai-pu region in the early part of the year.

Most work has been done at Ng-kang-phu and has been carried on in the chapel there. Towards the end of the year a house was mortgaged for a Hospital, but as it had to undergo extensive repairs, the new year found us still dispensing in the Chapel to the inconvenience both of doctors and preachers. Being so circumstanced, we have not this year professed to receive in-patients; but we found means from time to time of accommodating for some days a few urgent cases that we hoped to benefit.

Our Hospital, which is now all but ready, contains a pretty large ward for men, a ward for women, a surgery, a room for preaching, and two small ante-rooms which can be utilised in various ways. We shall be able to receive about 20 in-patients. We have already felt very much the need of such a place. Of the patients we advise to go to Swatow for better treatment very few ever go, the reason apparently being that most of them are too poor to undertake such a journey. With some it seems very difficult to make them understand the real state of the case. They seem to regard an advice to go elsewhere as a hint that they cannot be cured, or that we are for some reason unwilling to trouble ourselves with them. Some months ago two men came to us suffering from urinary calculus. We took pains to explain at length to them the nature of their disease, the uselessness of "eating medicine," and the benefit all but certain to be got by going to the Swatow Hospital. But their great reluctance to take our advice was evident.

The dangers attending the treatment of such diseases will make it unadvisable for us to attempt it here for some time to come; if indeed, it ever be considered worth while to raise the small Hospital at Ng-kang-phu to such a state of efficiency. Until such time at least there will always be cases that must be sent to Swatow. A great many of the less serious surgical cases, however, we hope soon to be able to treat with satisfactory results. We have already made a beginning, as the list of the surgical operations performed during the year will show; and such work we feel sure is worth doing. We have one native dispenser under training at Swatow, who will by and by dispense medicines for us, and dress wounds, work that has now to be done by ourselves, and entails a considerable loss of time.

Of the number of patients who came to us for treatment at Ng-kang-phu a pretty correct account has been kept. The total number of cases on record is 1,024. Not a few of these paid us two, three, or more visits, but an accurate account of these visits has not been kept. Of this number most were Hakkas, but a few scores were Hoklos, chiefly from near Miow. We have had patients coming to us from Sin-thyen in the South to Thong-hang in the North, and two or three came all the way from Chong-lok.

An approximate estimate of those seen during our visits to the out-lying country makes them about 576. If to these we add those treated by Dr. MacPhun in the Thai-pu region, at Thong-hang, Hopho, and other places, the number treated at outstations will be about 1,000: making the total number of cases for the year to be upwards of 2,000.

A fair proportion of our patients have from the first been females, seeking relief chiefly from eye diseases or such ordinary complaints as Dyspepsia, Rheumatism, Chronic Cough, etc. Of the 1,024 patients treated at Ng-kang-phu about 340, or *one-third* were females.

At Ng-kang-phu we fixed 11 to 1 as the time when patients could be seen. The average number of new cases daily was about five. Though our aim is to make medical skill the handmaid of the gospel, yet the small daily attendance, together with the want of in-patients with whom we might conduct worship at stated hours, has rendered it impossible for us to preach to our patients as regularly as we would wish to do. When at any time they have been coming in larger numbers we got one of our students to preach to them, at other times we have simply talked to them about the doctrine and invited them to come to the Chapel and hear more.

Our Medicines continue to be supplied by Dr. Lyall, and our thanks are due to the friends who by their contributions continue to aid the Swatow Hospital It is right that our friends should know that country work uses up a large quantity of drugs—more perhaps in proportion to the number of patients than is used in a Hospital. While Hospital work is largely *operating*, our chief work we may say, is *dispensing*. To make such work efficient we need to be well supplied with Medicine. Hitherto we have dispensed Medicines *gratis*, and have sold only to a few who have bought from us in quantity.

The appended list of cases seen by us at Ng-kang-phu will give some idea of the kind and frequency of the diseases we are called upon to treat. We close with some remarks on the Medical and Surgical cases.

MEDICAL CASES.

Dyspepsia, *Ague*, *Chronic Bronchitis*, and *Muscular Rheumatism*, are the most common cases of disease.

Ague seems most common with us after the Autumn rice harvest, when the rice fields are dried up. The benefit derived from quinine is well known everywhere here, and if we use any other drug we are liable to be reminded that the "white medicine" is the best. In milder cases one dose of quinine, two or three grains, followed by a course of iron and arsenic often suffices to cure it.

To *Malarial* influence is probably also due much of the *Anaemia* and *Debility* that we meet with, but it is only in some cases that we get a history of Ague. The same medicines as are useful in ague are indicated in these cases; *quinine* and *iron*, or iron and arsenic being followed by marked improvement.

Of Children's diseases we found it in many cases difficult to make a satisfactory diagnosis. Most were chronic cases badly cared for, and for the want of a better name we class these under the head of *Infantile debility.*

Some of these were simple cases of *Lumbrici.* Others were due to weakness after acute diseases aggravated by improper treatment, in cases perhaps originally of a strumous tendency. A few of these children were much emaciated, the hands and feet swelled, the eyes firmly closed and requiring some trouble to get them opened, when it would be discovered that both were hopelessly diseased, the cornea sloughed, and the iris protruding. The people of this quarter give to these infantile troubles the name of "Kam-tsit." Most but not all are cases of *Lumbrici,* and *Santonine* produces almost immediate and visible improvement. In some of the worst cases we could do nothing better than try the effect of condensed Swiss milk. We found this did much good. The art of *nursing the sick* is apparently unknown among these people. If a child takes its ordinary food, well and good, if not they have no idea of preparing anything more easily digested.

We have had many applications from *Opium-smokers* for "stop opium pills," which we uniformly refused, from the firm conviction that by giving them we should only mislead those who hoped to benefit by them, to say nothing about the probability that some of the applicants knew what a "stop opium pill" is composed of as well as we did. We always advise them to go to the Swatow Hospital, and break off the habit at once.

SURGICAL CASES.

Of *Eye diseases* the greatest number of cases have been of *Granular Conjunctivitis.* Some were cured by repeated visits to us, but others did not come often enough to secure the best results.

A good many came with their eyes watery and uneasy but without inflammation or development of granules, a state apparently produced by constant irritation from smoke or dust, and apt to run into fully developed granular disease. A weak solution of *Zinc sulphate* is our usual remedy, and is now in such repute that we find it difficult to persuade our patients that they must not use it for all diseases.

For the cure of Entropium we have operated with success on about 10 individuals, performing 15 operations in all.

Of the other Surgical cases we shall mention only the following :—

Fracture of Lower Jaw and Scalp Wound.—A boy of 11 had his head crushed between the beams of a sugar-cane mill. A large flap of the scalp about five inches long, as much indeed as covered the temporal fossa, was torn away down to the ear, which was almost severed from the head. The lower jaw was broken about an inch from the middle line of the chin, and the mouth was awry from the posterior fragment projecting inwards. The wound had been daubed all over with some vegetable preparation intended to stop the bleeding. But the parents allowed this to be removed, and the wound washed. Some bits likely to slough were removed with the scissors, and the flaps replaced and retained in position by a few stitches. The jaw was easily set, retained its position without any bandage, and there must have been almost immediate union as the boy seemed to use his jaw easily some days after. The wound suppurated, and a little of the flap sloughed, but in course of time, with daily attention, it healed very satisfactorily.

Harelip.—For this congenital deformity we have operated in four cases. The first was an aggravated case of *Double Harelip*, a boy of seven years old, whose parents are both members of the church. The operation was performed by Dr. Lyall when on a visit to Ng-kang-phu in the beginning of the year. As the lad was rather unmanageable, the silver wire sutures, the best we had at hand, were hardly sufficient to keep the parts at rest; but the case nevertheless did fairly well.

The other cases were operated on during a visit to the Basel Mission Stations in Chong-lok, in the month of August. One was a lad of eleven years, one four years, and the other nine months. All did well.

Removal of Tumour (Fibroma).—During the visit to Chong-lok, a patient came with a large Pendulous Tumour hanging by a broad pedicle from his ribs close below the axilla. The Tumour was removed by seizing the pedicle by a rough clamp of wood, improvised for the occasion, and cutting on it with the knife. The patient had many other Tumours on his back and chest, but none of them larger than a small egg, while the one removed was found to weigh fully two pounds.

The following is a pre[illegible] correct list of the operations performed during the year:—

Harelip	4
Entropium, upper 11, lower 4	15
Pterygium	3
Slit Ear	4
Cleft lower Lip	1
Dent. Extract	6
Fractures Set	5
Tumour (Fibroma) removed	1
Tapping Cystic Tumour of upper jaw ...	1
,, ,, ,, ,, lower ,, ...	1
Extraction of Nasal Polypus	1
Abscesses opened	5
Tying Internal Hæmorrhoids	1
Fistula in Ano	1
	49

Summary of the Diseases Treated:—

General Diseases	263
Diseases of the Digestive system ...	119
,, ,, Circulatory ,, ...	9
,, ,, Respiratory ,, ...	72
,, ,, Nervous ,, ...	22
,, ,, Genito-urinary ,, ...	6
,, ,, Ear and nose	9
,, ,, Eye	160
,, ,, Joints	4
,, ,, Bones	2
,, ,, Skin	115
Wounds, Injuries &c.	44
Unclassified	199
Total	1,024

REPORT

OF THE

MISSION HOSPITALS

AT

SWATOW AND UNG-KANG-PHU,

IN CONNECTION WITH THE

PRESBYTERIAN CHURCH OF ENGLAND,

UNDER THE CARE OF

P. B. COUSLAND, M. B., C. M.

AND

J. F. McPHUN, M. B., C. M.

For 1886.

PRINTED AT KWAI-FUNG'S PRESS, SWATOW.

1887.

REPORT

THE number of patients for 1886 is given below. The slight falling off as compared with the previous year is more than accounted for by the new regulations for opium-smokers, which have reduced the number of those applying for cure of the habit. The dearness of rice too, during the summer months, led to a considerable falling off in the attendance while it lasted.

Number of Individual Patients:—

In-patients	3592
Out-patients	1944
Total...	5536
Females included in the above ...	842

In addition a large number were treated by the senior assistants out of dispensary hours. They were chiefly trivial accidents and cases of slight illness among those more or less connected with the Mission.

Daily Averages.—The daily average number of In-patients, and attendance of Out-patients, during the various months is given below:—

	In-patients.	*Out-patients.*
January	172	27
February	66	18
March	169	41
April	162	32
May	263	46
June	196	63
July	184	43
August	201	46
September	263	58
October	278	63
November	164	41
December	170	40

The Dispensary has been open as usual on Tuesdays and Fridays for out-patients, but those desiring admittance to the wards are also seen on Mondays, Thursdays, and Saturdays. Operations are performed on Wednesdays and Saturdays.

Swatow is comparatively a small place, and wholly given up to business. Very few families reside in it. It is marvellously destitute of accommodation for travellers. There are only a few inns and they charge prohibitory prices. Patients from a distance therefore, unless they have some acquaintance in the town who can take them in, must enter the Hospital. This leads to over crowding at times, and the Chapel and verandahs are often occupied in the warm summer nights.

Twice during last summer a number of women had to be accommodated in part of the Chapel. They had been saving up their cash for some time, and looking forward to having their eyes cured or their dyspepsia alleviated, and it would have been hard to turn them away.

The Hospital buildings consist of 3 two-storied blocks, one being administrative, and the other two having each four large wards—two upstairs and two downstairs. In addition there are small wards for special cases, private wards, students' rooms, and the former leper hospital, the latter distant a few minutes walk. Altogether there is accommodation for 150 patients.

One ward is reserved for Opium Smokers. Formerly no charge was made for this class of patients, but as this proved unsatisfactory, a new rule was institu ed last year requiring them to pay $1 as a guarantee of good faith. This has had the effect of reducing the numbers coming by more than one half, but the treatment of those who did come was much more satisfactory.

I have to gratefully acknowledge receipt of a telephone to connect the medical man's house with the Hospital, the gift of Miss Ricketts. In many ways it will be a great help.

Distribution of the Patients.

	Patients.
In the Chao-chow department:—	
From Ching-hai district	655
Chao-yang ,, ...	1345
Kieh-yang ,, ...	979
Hai-yang ,, ...	686
Jao-ping ,, ...	554
Pu-ning ,, ...	492
Hwei-lai ,, ...	331
Fung-shun ,, ...	69
Ta-pu ,, ...	15
Island of Namoa	90
In the Hwei-chow department:—	
From Lu-fung district	34
Hai-fung ,, ...	6
From Kia-ying-chow	26
In the Fokien Province:—	
From Chau-an district	226
Elsewhere	12
From other Provinces etc.	16
	5,536

EDUCATIONAL.

A class of six students was under instruction during the year. The subjects taken up were Materia Medica, Anatomy, and Physiology; Drs. Kerr and Osgood's works being used as text books. In Anatomy an articulated skeleton was the chief aid, but through the kindness of Mr. J. T. Morton of London, the students this year will have the enormous advantage of revising their Anatomy on a "*Modèle d'homme complet du Dr. Auzoux.*"

At the half yearly examinations a very fair knowledge of the subjects was shown.

Evangelistic.—There has been no change in the Evangelistic methods. The daily morning and evening services, and the Sunday afternoon inquirers' meeting have been held as usual.

There is no evangelist attached to the Hospital. The two senior assistants conduct the services and my ministerial

colleagues give a morning each per week. The students of the Theological Seminary when in session have conducted evening worship in the small Hospital. All the patients meet in the large Hospital chapel in the morning. As in former years there has been no visible fruit among the out-patients, but the work among the large number of inpatients has not been barren of results, twenty of them, seven women and thirteen men, having been received into the Church. It was decided to baptise another man but he died before the rite was administered. Some of those admitted heard for the first time during the past year. Many have been applicants for a longer period. It is not until they have proved their sincerity by professing Christianity at their homes that they are baptised. This is very necessary, for there is no way of testing the truth of their profession while in the Hospital.

SURGICAL OPERATIONS.

On the Eye:—

Operation for Entropion and Trichiasis—		
On the upper lid ...	313	
,, ,, lower lid ...	188	—501
,, ,, Symblepharon	...	4
,, ,, Ankyloblepharon ...	...	1
,, ,, Pterygium	...	55
,, ,, Pinguecula	...	1
,, ,, Conjunctival Cysts ...	...	2
,, ,, ,, Hypertrophy	...	2
Peritomy	...	1
Iridectomy	...	11
Extraction of Lens (Cataract) ...	...	13
Laceration of Opaque Capsule ...	...	5
Puncture of Anterior Chamber ...	...	1
Operation for Hypopyon	...	11
,, ,, Repair of Split Eyelid...	...	1
Excision of Eyeball	...	3
		612

On the Body generally:—

Amputation of Leg	1
,, Fingers	2
,, Supernumerary Thumb ...	2
,, Penis (Epithelioma)	5
Excision of Non-Malignant Tumours ...	21
,, Malignant ,, ...	13
,, Cystic ,, ...	15
,, Vascular ,, ...	1
,, Part of Sup: Max: (Sarcoma) ...	2
,, Sebaceous Cysts	12
,, Aneurism	1
,, Encysted Bullet	1
,, Enlarged Tonsils (Guillotine) ...	2
Operation for Harelip	39
,, Cicatricial Closure of Nostrils	2
,, Epithelioma of Lower Lip ...	1
,, Ranula...	3
,, Repair of Split Ear Lobule ...	42
,, ,, Upper Lip	1
,, ,, Split Nose	1
,, ,, Torn Scrotum ...	1
,, Fistula in Ano...	52
,, External Haemorrhoids ...	26
,, Internal ,, (tying)	42
,, Phimosis (circumcision) ...	10
,, Elephantiasis of Scrotum ...	4
,, Adenoid Pharyngeal Growths	1
,, Empyema ... ...,	1
,, Congenital Absence of Rectum	1
,, Ganglion	5
,, Ununited Fracture of Femur...	1
,, to straighten Finger	1
Electrolysis of Keloid...	3
,, Naevus	3
Aspirating Bladder	1
,, Abscess of Liver	1
,, Empyema...	3
Needling for Sciatica...	1
Tapping and injecting Hydrocele	27
,, ,, Cystic Goitre... ...	8
Perinotomy (Ruptured Urethra)	1
Extracting Fruit Stone from nose	1
Fish Bones ,, Pharynx ...	3

Extracting Sequestra	... ...	20
„ Nasal Polypus	... ...	8
„ Aural „	... ...	1
Subcutaneous Ligature of Naevus	... ...	1
Ligature of Naevus	... ...	1
Avulsion of Toe Nail	... ...	2
Total Number of Operations,	... ...	1004
Extracting Teeth	... ...	115

Besides opening abscesses and fistulae, reducing dislocations, catheterisation, etc., not included in the preceding table.

Entropion and Trichiasis.—Perhaps the most distinctive feature in the Surgical work at Swatow is the large number of operations for Entropion and Trichiasis, amounting to 501 last year. Cases are seen in all gradations of severity, from slight Trichiasis, to complete Entropion, the lashes of both lids lying flat against the cornea along their whole length. Very many come too late. The cornea is a net work of vessels, ulcerated, nebulous, or there has been perforation and more or less extensive Iritic prolapse. It is curious how little suffering is sometimes caused by the incurvation, and how people can do their daily work as if there was no sheaf of lashes rubbing an ulcer in their cornea. Women seen to suffer from this disease in a larger proportion than men. Last year of the male patients 120 or 2½ p.c. had entropion, as compared with 119 or 14 p.c. of the female. With granular ophthalmia the numbers were—men 290 or 6 p.c., women 86 or 10 p.c.

Dr. MacPhun informs me that Trachoma and Entropion are rarely met with among the Hakkas, the great majority of cases coming under his notice at Ng-kang-phu being Hoklos. Even along the borderland where the two races mingle it is the Hoklos who are affected. Although there is a great difference in the case of the women—the Hakka women do not bind their feet, and consequently help the men in field work, there is none with the men. As regards smoke, glare, and dirt, there is little to choose between them. I know of no reason to account for the unenviable pre-eminence which Swatow has in this disease. I cannot think that there can be any such difference in the mode of life of the people here as compared with the Cantonese and the inhabitants of the Fokien Province, to account for the greater prevalence of this disease among the Hoklo population of this region.

Abdominal Fistula.—Patient, a girl 11 years old. Duration, 3 months. Situation, a little below and to the light of the Umbilicus. Result of injury from buffalo's horn. Faeces partly passing by fistula and partly per anum. An attempt to close it by reflecting and stitching together the mucous membrane and then the skin failed. It was then cauterised twice, and after the second time closed up satisfactorily.

Empyema.—Duration of illness, five months. Left side of thorax much enlarged, especially posteriorly. Heart displaced to the right. The patient, a young man, emaciated. I aspirated three times in one week, removing 210 ounces of fluid, of which one-fourth was pus. As the relief was only temporary, the cavity was opened and drained, an inch of the eighth rib being removed with Hey's saw and bone forceps. Local anesthesia was obtained by means of Cocaine. As owing to the effects of the climate on the india rubber tube of the aspirator some air had unfortunately been admitted at the last aspiration, the operation was not made a strictly antiseptic one. Diarrhoea pointing to waxy degeneration of the intestines began not long afterwards. At his own urgent request he went home two months after the operation, and as the diarrhoea continued, and the discharge of pus had not lessened, recovery is hopeless. Probably if he had presented himself a little sooner the result might have been different.

Repair of Upper Lip in a girl. More than half of the centre of the upper lip, the columella, and part of the septum nares had ulcerated away after an attack of small-pox. Three incisions were required on each side before the flaps could be adjusted, viz.: (1) Up by the side of the alae. (2) From the same starting point out into the cheeks parallel with the lip. (3) From the corners of the mouth horizonately outwards. The result was very satisfactory as far as the lip is concerned, but the nose is still susceptible of improvement.

Electrolysis of Keloid and Naevus.—The results, in the cases that can be traced, have so far been satisfactory.

Elephantiasis of the Scrotum.—Four cases. Weights $2\frac{1}{2}$, 2, 21, and 20 lbs. In the second case there was reason to suspect Epithelioma of the penis from the discharge, and the diagnosis being vindicated during the operation the diseased member was removed. The only death from operation during the year occurred in the case of a man from Hokien. The drained tumour weighed 20 lbs. after removal. Both legs were also much enlarged with Elephantiasis. Shock was the cause of death. In future I shall be extremely chary about operating in cases where the legs are much affected.

Aspirating Abscess of Liver.—I record this case as it is the first I have come across among the Chinese. Duration of illness two months. Liver extended 3 inches below the margin of the ribs in the nipple line. The aspiration was diagnostic and little more than an ounce of thick pus was removed. The patient could not stay in the Hospital for treatment and nothing further was done for him.

Native worm-gut—(the silk spinning apparatus of the caterpillar of the Atlas Moth) was used in a number of operations during the year. It was found very useful as a suture, but for ligaturing vessels it was too stiff and insoluble. It is extremely cheap.

List of some of the Diseases treated.

General Diseases.

Intermittent Fever:—	Leprosy 270
Quotidian 9	(Macular 90 p.c.)
Tertian... 12	Beri-beri 10
Quartan 189	Goître 6
Irregular 8	Opium Smokers for cure ...306
Enlarged Spleen (Malarial) 19	

Nervous System.

Dementia 4	Epilepsy 7
Puerperal Dementia ... 1	

Digestive System.

Malignant Stricture of Œsophagus 4	Inguinal Hernia ... ... 42 (R. Side 70p.c.)
Ulceration and Stricture of Rectum (Unnatural Crime) 31	

Circulatory System.

Valvular Disease of the Heart 16

Eye.

Granular Ophthalmia ...376	Entropion and Trichiasis ...239

Lymphatic System.

Elephantiasis of R. leg only 14	Elephantiasis of Scrotum only 18
" of L. leg only 10	Lymph Scrotum 10
" of R. leg & scrotum 2	Enlargement of Inguinal Glands only 3
" both legs & " 2	
" both legs only ... 1	
Side not recorded 10	

Genito Urinary System.

Vesical calculus 2

Midwifery 3

Beri-Beri.—There was an outbreak of the atrophic variety of this disease in the middle school for boys and the girls' school of this Mission at Swatow.

The boys' school reassembled after the new Year's holidays by the beginning of March. The girls' school did not break up at the Chinese new year. The first cases were noticed about the beginning of May, when several boys who had been under treatment for dyspeptic symptoms began to complain of numbness of the skin of the abdomen and legs, and a little enquiry elicited the usual symptoms. Before long seven boys were down with it, and as nothing had the least influence in checking the course of the disease, they were sent sixty miles inland to the highland Hakka country, and placed under Dr. McPhun's care at Ng-kang-phu. This was on the 26th of May. Three days afterwards as seven more boys and the native teacher were affected the school was broken up and the boys sent home.

On the 2nd of June one girl was attacked, on the 11th another, and on the 17th two others. As 5 or 6 more had slight prodromata, the summer holidays were anticipated and the school dismissed.

The symptoms in those attacked differed but slightly. There was first a rheumatic sensation in the affected parts, and in many cases evidences of gastric catarrh. Then followed numbness of the anterior tibial and femoral regions, and of the abdomen as far up as the umbilicus. At the same time the muscles of those regions became hard and painful. The pain was of a hot, crawling, and cramping description, and in some cases prevented sleep. This was followed in a few days by marked flabbiness of the affected muscles and loss of power. The accompanying paresis was brought home somewhat forcibly to some of the boys by their legs suddenly giving way under them. This compelled them to take to bed. There was also pain in the knee, aggravated by stretching the leg. In some cases the partial anesthesia eventually extended to the forearms, but in no case, with one doubtful exception, to the lips.

The areas of anesthesia were not the same in all cases. One boy had none of the femoral region. Others had the calves and back of the thighs affected as well as the front.

The ankle-clonus and knee jerk were absent: unfortunately I have not kept a note of the skin reflexes. In the boys last attacked pain in the knee and in the Tendo Achillis behind the ankle-joint were the most prominent symptoms. Dyspnoea was pretty marked among the worst cases in the boys' school. In only two cases was there any oedema. In one there was slight oedema about the ankles. He had a systolic murmur in the mitral area. The oedema disappeared in a few days on the administation of Digitalis. In the other case, where the face was slightly puffy, there was reduplication of the second sound in the aortic and pulmonary areas. The dyspnoea was most marked in these two cases. In the others auscultation revealed only a somewhat tumultuous cardiac action. In all the boys there was tenderness on percussion of a varying number of the upper Dorsal vertebrae. This could not be elicited in the girls.

The excretions were quite normal.

In the case of two of the girls the onset of pain in the legs was quite sudden—one was seized while in the classroom and had to be carried howling upstairs. On the whole the girls suffered less than the boys. Before the girls' school was broken up, those affected were all able to shuffle about a little. The disease did not go on steadily from bad to worse as it did in the other school. Five or six girls had slight premonitory symptoms for a number of days but they never came to anything.

Of the boys who were sent to Ng-kang-phu, four soon recovered so far as to be sent to their homes. The other three remained at Ng-kang-phu for a month and a half. One of these is still at home. The other two returned to school this winter, 1886-7, and have been under treatment for some degree of stiffness and atrophy of the muscles of the calf. The others who were sent directly home recovered completely in the course of two or three weeks. I should have noted that strong and weak, older and younger were attacked indiscriminately. Of the three worst cases two had previously enjoyed good health, while the other had been in bed for a month with chronic articular rheumatism.

No medicinal treatment was found of any value, but the curative effects of removal from the site of infection were most marked. For the sequelae, cod liver oil, strychnine, and Faradaism were of some service. Prohibiting rice to those affected produced no apparent benefit.

I did not diagnose Beri-beri until the boys' school had been dismissed. The descriptions in the text books are quite in applicable to the dry form. Fortunately I came across Dr. Simmon's article in the Customs' Medical Report for 1879-80 which removed all doubts as to the nature of the outbreak.

As to the cause of the outbreak it is difficult to arrive at a satisfactory conclusion.

In the same compound with the affected schools are the mission houses, and Theological Seminary, while the Hospital is close by, and yet nobody outside of the schools was attacked. The food suggests itself as a probable vehicle for the introduction of a specific poison, especially as it has been stated that the spores of the suspected Bacillus have been found adhering to rice, and a large quantity of rice was being imported from Mid-China, Japan, and Siam at this time. But in that case there should have been some cases among the other Chinese in the compound and in Swatow, in fact all over the country. As it was I could not hear of a single case, and besides it was found on inquiry that imported rice was not used in the schools. Why such an outbreak should have occurred in two well ordered, clean, airy schools, built somewhat recently like the rest of the mission buildings, on land reclaimed from the sea, and having no communication with each other, in a district where Beri-beri has hitherto been unknown, while among the Chinese all around not a case seems to have been known, is a problem that awaits solution. The season, it may be remarked, was an exceptionally dry one. I believe that in the summer of 1884 there was a solitary case in the boys' school of what must have been Beri-beri.

Since the outbreak above described ten cases of Beri-beri have been treated in the Hospital. Two of those came from the neighbouring district of Hai-yang, and I have but little doubt that they were examples of the dry form of Beri-beri. Of the others, seven came from Singapore and one from Penang. They were all of the dropsical variety. The sea-voyage had apparently a beneficial effect, for by the time they reached Swatow the anasarca had almost disappeared, even when, according to their own statements, it was quite marked on embarking. The muscular atrophy and anesthesia were in the same localities as in the dry cases. In addition there was dyspnoea, a systolic murmur over the pulmonary area, and constipation. The affected muscles regained strength very slowly.

Recent investigators in Malaysia have stated that Beri-beri cases can infect a locality. Might it not be that its occurrence in the schools has some connection with the constant importation of these cases from the Straits' settlements?

Midwifery.—The worst case was one of cross-birth. The woman had been in labour for three days. On the second day the midwife had pulled the presenting arm off. The foetus was so firmly jammed I could not turn until I had eviscerated. The head was hydrocephalic and on introducing my hand to remove the placenta I found the uterus extensively ruptured where the head had been. She died thirty hours afterwards.

SUBSCRIPTIONS For 1886.

Two Friends	$83.00
Messrs. Bradley & Co.	50.00
„ Jardine, Matheson & Co.	50.00
China Sugar Refining Company, Limited ...	50.00
Messrs. Butterfield & Swire...	50.00
A Silent Donor	50.00
Rev. G. Smith, M. A.	30.00
Wm. Paton	30.00
P. B. Cousland, M.B., C.M., ...	30.00
W. Gregory	25.00
Dr. Pollock	25.00
Rev. W. Duffus	25.00
A. Lyall, M.B., C.M., ...	25.00
E. McKean	20.00
J. Jaques	20.00
D. MacIver	20.00
Rev. J. C. Gibson	20.00
Do. for 1885.	20.00
Dr. Gauld	17.56
D. C. Byworth	15.00
W. Allum	10.00
H. Matchitt	10.00
J. D. Monro	10.00
L. Grunauer	10.00
O. Asverus	10.00
C. B. Quelch	10.00
Cl. Pape	10.00
P. Williams	10.00
Miss Fielde, special	10.00
H. Sage	7.00
R. L. Richardson	5.00
G. L. Hummel.	5.00
W. Pollock	5.00
J. Dickie	5.00
L. Leslie	5.00
A. Rosthorn	5.00
A. L. Piersdorf	5.00
W. F. K.	5.00
H. Brockdorf...	5.00
F. W. Focken	5.00
J. Manley	5.00
W. M. Keeble	4.00

J. L. T.	3.00
J. D. Smith	3.00
W. G. Tindall	3.00
I. H. M. Noodt	3.00
C. Kerr	3.00
R. Adam	3.00
W. Davidson	3.00
R. Hamilton	3.00
Miss N.	2.00
A. Smith	2.00
A. Sutherland	2.00
S. Kye Pang	2.00
Professional	10.00
	$853.56

CHINESE SUBSCRIPTIONS.

Chinese Presb: Church, Swatow	25.00
Tai-Won	20.00
Ah Kim	20.00
Ko, Buey Tso	20.00
S. Kye Pang from "Breconshire"	20.00
Ee Kee	10.00
Eg Keng	10.00
Liao, Foo-Sang	10.00
Yuen Ding Fat	10.00
A Patient	9.79
Patients' box	7.45
Ben	5.00
Hok-lim	5.00
Siau Tai Fan	5.00
A Chhim	5.00
A Sew-Tsai	5.00
A Patient	4.00
Phó-ti	2.00
Kwai fung	2.00
T. Lam	2.00
A Pin-wen	1.00
	$108.24

During 1885, Tan Nguan-seng continued his supplies of rice and cash tickets, the total amounting to 6,000 tickets worth $191.36, and thus furnishing 8,000 meals for destitute patients.

In addition Tsan A Hi contributed 200 tickets, their money value being $13.18, and another friend 106 tickets worth $6.26.

By means of these tickets I am enabled to keep many chronic cases until a cure is effected, who, but for them, would be unable to remain long enough.

STATEMENT OF INCOME AND EXPENDITURE.

By Subscriptions—European	$853.56
,, ,, Chinese	198.24
,, Sale of Medicines, Trusses etc.	634.01
,, ,, Milk to Patients	101.95
,, Receipts from Opium Smokers	138.84
,, Rent of Private Wards	21.32
,, Miscellaneous Receipts	58.97
,, Medicines supplied by Mission Committee in Edinburgh	681.10
	$2,777.99

To Balance	$36.58
,, Wages and Travelling Expenses	364.96
,, Publishing Hospital Reports	31.00
,, Fire Insurance Premium for 2 years	40.00
,, Milk from London	229.41
,, Medicines bought in Swatow	64.01
,, ,, & Spirit from Hongkong & India	353.00
,, ,, from England etc.	258.38
,, Lard	23.17
,, Repairs	54.75
,, Oil	104.03
,, Wool	48.57
,, Water	49.08
,, Washing	9.82
,, Aid to Poor Patients and Burial Expenses	44.46
,, Miscellaneous expenses—Cloth, Paper, etc.	96.88
,, Medicines supplied by Mission Committee in Edinburgh	681.10
,, Balance on hand	288.79
	$2,777.99.

REPORT of the Medical Mission Work at Ung-kang-phu in the Hakka Region in 1886.

The work in the Hospital and Dispensary has been carried on almost continuously through another year.

During the month of August it was closed for about two weeks. The number of patients attending show only a slight increase on last year, and their attendance varies inversely with the amount of work to be done in the fields.

The work in the Hospital in so far as it affects the Hakkas is mostly confined to the Ung-kang-phu region. This is partly due to the position and nature of this part of the Hakka field. The Hakkas live near the hills, and along the upper reaches of streams which flow down through the plains inhabited by the Hoklos.

The field is thus divided into little districts the inhabitants of which have more and easier communication with the Hoklos below than with their Hakka brethern in the adjoining districts. The want of easy water communication greatly limits the field that comes under the influence of the Hospital, as few patients will undertake a long land journey.

From our proximity to the Hoklos a number of them come for treatment, and of the in-patients nearly one half were Hoklos.

During the months of April and May the rice was very dear, and this no doubt kept many poor people at home who sadly needed their diseases attended to. The majority of the people are so poor that even a small increase in the price of rice means much distress among them. One of our preachers told me that in his native district comprising three hundred families, it was reckoned that only about twenty families had plenty to eat.

As will be seen from the subjoined list, the number of operations performed bears a rather small proportion to the number of patients seen, about one operation to every ten patients. The Hakkas are rather unwilling to undergo any operation that involves cutting, and often in case of Tumours or Abscesses wish some medicine to take or apply that will *dissolve* them.

Some are becoming acquainted with the beneficial effects of western drugs, and not a few come prescribing for themselves, asking for such medicines as Quinine, Santonine, and Iodine.

The number of cases under treatment during the year is as follows:—

New Out-patients	2225
In-patients	315
Females included in the above:—	
In-patients	40
Out-patients	451
Children under 12 years	350

Besides the above many patients were seen during journeys to the country.

During the year a part of the afternoon has been given to teaching the assistants the elements of Anatomy and Physiology.

Evangelistic Work.—Morning and evening worship was daily held in the Hospital. Besides the stated services the Evangelist endeavours to have conversation with individuals, which is very useful not so much in exposing the foolishness of Idol worship, which they usually freely admit, as in removing some of the many foolish ideas entertained regarding the worship of God. Those willing to be instructed are taught to read the ten commandments,

Lord's prayer, and hymn book, which forms the chief theological reading of many even of our church members. Very few can read the scriptures, so passages are selected to be committed to memory. There were a number of patients who seemed much interested while in the Hospital, and on leaving had a fair knowledge of the doctrine. Two or three of them we think had their hearts influenced to serve the True God.

During the year Dr. Riddel and I paid a number of visits to the country stations and also to new districts. On these journeys, which are chiefly evangelistic, we are accompanied by a native preacher, and find abundant opportunities of preaching the word. From a medical point of view this is not equal to Hospital work, yet it is most important in breaking down prejudice, and opening the way into new districts. In this way the Gospel has been proclaimed in many new villages, and we would earnestly request the prayers of God's people that the seed thus sown may be blessed.

Congenital Absence of Anus.—A child two days old was brought in this condition. After cutting in for over an inch and finding no bowel, I was unwilling to proceed further at the time. The father took the child home the same day saying he would come back in the morning but did not return.

Traumatic Gangrene.—The patient in this case was a boy who had fallen and fractured his radius at the neck. The arm was bandaged up by a native practitioner who bound it too tightly. When admitted about ten days after the whole forearm was dead, the line of demarcation far advanced, and much inflammation and infiltration in the upper arm. Temp. 103. The line of demarcation formed at the elbow joint, and in a few days was nearly complete leaving only the head of the ulna to be cut out. Owing to the unwillingness of his father to have any further operation, the stump was left to granulate and healed up all right.

LIST OF DISEASES TREATED.

General Diseases.

Ague	45	Leprosy	63
Anaemia	19	Opium Smokers (for cure)	53
" with large spleen	4	Scrofula	12
General Debility	62	Typhus	1
Infantile "	31	Syphilis	5
Erysipelas	3	Dropsy (General)	8
Febricula	13		

Diseases of the Nervous System.

Neuralgia	3	Hydrocephalus	1
Paralysis (Facial)	3	Wry Neck	1
Paresis (leg extensors)	3	Mania	2
Hemiplegia	1	Hysteria	3
Anaesthesia (Local)	5	Vertigo	14
Epilepsy	4	Cerebral Tumour	1
Convulsions (Infantile)	1	Unclassed	6
Sciatica	7		

Diseases of the Circulatory System.

Aneurism	1	Heart Disease (Valvular)	3
Naevus	1	" " (Irregular)	9
Varicose Veins	3		

Diseases of the Respiratory System.

Asthma	20	Bronchitis	80
Laryngitis	2	Phthisis	11
Coryza	15	Haemoptysis	2
Pleurisy	1		

Diseases of the Digestive System.

Harelip	1	Apthae	5
Ulceration of Mouth & Fauces	8	Parotitis	4
Hypertrophy of Gum	2	Vermes	4
Tonsillitis	2	Jaundice	7
Irregularity of Teeth	4	Lumbrici	25
Caries of Teeth	36	Constipation	2
Ulceration of Pharynx	2	Haematemisis	3
Dysphagia	1	Haemorrhoids—Internal	3
Stricture of Oesophagus	1	External	2
Dyspepsia	164	Fistula in Ano	14
Diarrhoea	28	Ulceration of Anus	5
Colic	6	Congenital Absence of Anus	1
Dysentery	3	Prolapse of Rectum	6
Ascites	3	Unclassed	7
Hernia (Inguinal)	5		

Diseases of the Cellular Tissue.

Abscesses and Sinuses	82	Inflammation	51
Boils and Carbuncles	31		

Diseases of the Genito Urinary System.

Phimosis	3	Spermatorrhoea	9
Paraphimosis	1	Retention of Urine	1
Balanitis	5	Haematuria	1
Urethitis	3	Amenorrhoea	1
Chancre	9	Leucorrhoea	3
Gonorrhoea	2	Menorrhagia	3
Stricture of Urethra	5	Cystitis	1
Urethral Calculus	2	Prolapse of Uterus	1
Hydrocele	1		

Diseases of the Skin.

Acne	1	Scabies	13
Eczema	96	Painful Cicatrices	3
Ringworm	115	Prurigo	5
Favus	1	Psoriasis	1
Warts	5	Impetigo	4
Pigment Spots	1	Rupia	1
Corns	3	Unclassed	5
Erythema	2	Ulcers	122
Lichen	5		

Diseases of the Organs of Locomotion.

Rheumatic Pains (Muscular and Arthritic)	115	Synovitis	10
Lumbago	8	Oedema of Legs	3
Caries and Necrosis	16	Elephantiasis of Leg	1
Periostitis	2	Morbus Coxae	3
Bursitis	1	Posterior Curvature of Spine	2
		Traumatic Gangrene (fore-arm)	1

Diseases of the Eye.

Ptosis	1	Ulceration of Cornea	9
Hordeolum	1	Nebulae	5
Hypertrophy of Lower Lid	1	Leucoma	14
Entropium and Trichiasis	41	Staphyloma	11
Catarrhal Ophthalmia	108	Iritis	8
Granular "	98	Cataract	7
Purulent "	12	Night Blindness	3
Phlyctenular "	9	Amaurosis	2
Blenorrhoea	5	Posterior Synechiae	4
Pinguecula	1	Dislocation of Lens	1
Pterygium	15	Eye disorganized (one or both)	9
Corneitis	11	Foreign body in Cornea	1
" with Hypopyon	4	Unclassed	5
Occlusion of Pupil	1		

Diseases of the Ear.

Otorrhoea	4	Eczema of External Meatus	4
Split Lobule	6	Unclassed	2

Diseases of the Nose.

Polypus	4	Ulceration of Mucous Membrane	5
Epistaxis	3		

Tumours.

Cystic	18	Malignant	6
Fatty	2	Ganglion	3
Fibrous	2	Unclassed	9

Injuries.

Bruises	30	Dog Bites	5
Sprains	19	Foreign bodies lodged	5
Wounds	38	Fractures	4
Burns	6	Dislocations	11

OPERATIONS

Operation for Entropium and Trichiasis	44
,, ,, Pterygium	8
Iridectomy (for artificial pupil etc.)	2
Operation for Harelip	1
,, ,, Fistula in Ano	1
Removal of Tumours	11
,, Nasal Polypus	1
Excision of Ext. Haemorrhoids	1
,, Warts	3
,, Corns	1
Extraction of Necrosed Bone	1
,, Urethral Calculi	2
,, Teeth	41
,, Foreign Bodies	5
Repairing Split Ear	5
Slitting Prepuce	4
Opening Abscesses	26
Excision of Granulation tissue from Gum	3
Slitting up Sinuses	10
Wounds Stitched	7
Tying Int. Haemorrhoids	1
Bursting Ganglion	3
Reducing Dislocation	1
Operation for Contraction of Urethral Orifice	2
,, Imperforate Anus	1
Division of Cicatrix (Contracted)	1
Tapping Cyst	1
Amputation of Toe	1
Cutting out head of Ulna in case of Traumatic Gangrene	1

REPORT

OF THE

MISSION HOSPITAL

AT

SWATOW

IN CONNECTION WITH THE

PRESBYTERIAN CHURCH OF ENGLAND

UNDER THE CARE OF

P. B. COUSLAND, M. B., C. M.

For 1887.

PRINTED BY KWAI-FUNG, SWATOW.

1888.

REPORT.

THE work in the Hospital has as usual been carried on during the past year without a single day's interruption, and with undiminished acceptance. The decrease in the total number of patients has been wholly due to the smaller number of opium smokers attending since they were required to pay for admission. The number of ordinary patients is larger than ever, the increase being especially marked among the women. The proportion of females has been increasing of late years notwithstanding that many of them come from some distance up country and have to travel by boat.

STATISTICS.

Number of Individual Patients:—

In-patients	3242
Out-patients	2130
Total	5372
Females included in above	933
Cases seen out of Dispensary hours, chiefly by Senior Assistants about	2000
Daily average number of In-patients ...	174
Average attendance of Out-patients on Dispensary days	53
Number of Operations	863

No change has been made in the methods. Out-patients were seen on Tuesdays and Fridays, Wednesdays and Saturdays being set apart for operations. The patient are expected to provide their own food and charcoal, and to cook it for themselves in the Hospital kitchens, but medicines are supplied free, the only class required to pay being opium smokers, who are charged $1.

Some Chinese merchants have helped very much by putting in my hands a supply of rice and cash tickets which can be converted at their shops, the one into rice and the other into twenty-five cash each, to buy meat and vegetables with. By means of these I can provide a generous dietary for such patients as seem most necessitous, and can keep many until a cure has been effected, who otherwise would have to go home not much better than when they came. Last year 6,900 meals were thus supplied. The chief donor of these tickets—the head of the Tan-nguan-seng hong, has this year shown further interest by paying the passages home of those patients who had stayed at the Hospital until their money was exhausted, and also by donating 700 glass bottles for those who were too poor to buy proper bottles for themselves. Such interest is as refreshing as it is rare, for the well-to-do Chinese are inclined to fight shy of a foreign institution.

A very large quantity of the Anglo-Swiss Co.'s condensed milk is consumed by the patients. They have no prejudices against it as they have against what they call "raw" milk, indeed they look upon the tinned kind as partly a medicine, and get very partial to its sweetness. As nourishing and easily digested food is usually as much needed as drugs, a supply of such milk is kept on hand, and the patients are encouraged to use it. It is scarcely necessary to say that they are expected to buy it, but a considerable quantity has to be given to those who are too poor to do that. In the preliminary and subsequent treatment of operation cases it is very useful, and as alcohol *per se* is almost never used as a remedy, the motto of the Hospital might well be *Lacte, non vino.*

In some Districts condensed milk, the Chinese say, is much used by the wealthier classes, and probably many infants are saved from blindness or death by having it added to their unsuitable rice diet; but at the same time it is a pity that recourse should be had to it, when the milk of their own buffalos and cows could be easily had.

One patient exhibited the results of a somewhat drastic cure for gambling. He must have been an inveterate haunter of the tables, for his wife, probably finding gentler measures fail, had cut the muscles in front of his leg across with a chopper, thus laming him for life. The same form of treatment had been applied by the authorities to the legs of a number of rowdies, who were brought in from the neighbouring District city, but as the wounds had been somewhat aimlessly inflicted, no permanent damage was done.

EDUCATIONAL.

Four afternoons in the week were devoted to teaching the junior assistants and students, seven in number. Three of these were bound to the Hospital for a period of three years, their parents guaranteeing all their expenses, a fourth was an ex-student whose three years had expired, and whom we supported for another year that he might finish his curriculum, and the rest were paid assistants, one being under training with a view to accompanying me to Ch'ao-chow-foo.

The subjects studied were the Practice of Medicine and Surgery, Skin and Eye diseases, together with ~~Chemical~~ Clinical instruction. At the end of the year two young men left who had been with us for six and four years respectively. They will be the means of relieving much suffering, and, if they use their opportunities well, can be a great help to the progress of the Gospel in the cities in which they have settled

The Rev. Wm. Duffus kindly conducted a Bible class with the students during a part of the year.

The *mannikin* was an object of very great interest to the Chinese, and many were the petitions to be allowed to see it. Their wonder and delight as it was taken to pieces bit by bit was most amusing, and it is some satisfaction to think that their ludicrous ideas of Anatomy and Physiology were somewhat upset.

EVANGELISTIC.

The results of Hospital work from a missionary point of view are not always very apparent, but we have never lacked encouragement in disseminating Christian truth among the patients. At the meeting for inquirers on Sunday afternoon there are always some who profess to have given up heathenism and accepted Christianity, and of these last year at least three men and three women were admitted into the church. In addition, it should be noted that among the whole number baptised by the missionaries during the year, there were several who were friends or relatives of converts who first heard in the Hospital, and whose conversion therefore was indirectly due to the Hospital. Most of the inquirers are lost sight of for the meantime, for we have no adequate means of following them up, but in all probability some will yet be gathered in at the various stations of the mission. The results are not to be judged by even the number applying for admission into the church, for it has frequently happened that our agents travelling through the country have come upon former patients, who, although they showed no sign of awakening while in the Hospital, have remembered what they heard there, and have sought to worship God in their heathen homes according to their light.

In addition to the recognised usefulness of the Hospital as a means of removing dislike and prejudice by an exhibition of Christian philanthropy, the preaching of the Gospel in it exercises a powerful influence for the overthrow of idolatry and other degrading superstitions of the Chinese, and few of the in-patients can leave without having their faith in them seriously shaken, and in many cases destroyed. This effect of our work *plus* the imparting of a knowledge of God's revelation, must be leavening the whole Swatow Region and preparing the way for the final triumph of Christ's cause in it, while we have the further comfort of believing that year by year some are being saved.

It is worthy of notice as showing the wide reaching influence of our work, that the number of villages, towns, etc. from which patients come is about 1800.

SURGICAL OPERATIONS.

On the Eye:—

Operation for Entropion and Trichiasis :—		
On the upper lid	281	
„ „ lower „	129—410	
Operation for Pterygium		46
„ „ Conjunctival Tumours		4
„ „ Chalazion		1
Iridectomy for Artificial Pupil		6
Extraction of Lens (Cataract)		11
Laceration of Opaque Capsule		6
Tapping Anterior Chamber		1
Operation for Hypopyon		2
Excision of Melanotic Tumour of Inner Canthus		1
		488

On the Body generally :—

Amputation at the Hip Joint (death from shock)	1
,, of Arm	1
,, ,, Foot (Syme's)	1
,, ,, ,, (Chopart's)	1
,, ,, Toes	3
,, ,, Fingers	4
,, ,, Penis (Epithelioma)	2
Excision of Fatty Tumours	5
,, ,, Symmetrical Fibrous Tumours of Elbows and Thighs ...	3
,, ,, Dermoid Cyst	1
,, ,, Tumours of Breast	5
,, ,, Sebaceous Cysts	11
,, ,, other Tumours	20
,, ,, Callosities	7
,, ,, Encysted Bullets	2
,, ,, Enlarged Tonsils	3
Operation for Harelip	32
,, ,, Cicatricial Closure of Nostrils ...	2
,, on Mouth (Cheiloplastic)	3
,, for Ranula	3
,, ,, Aural Cysts	2
,, ,, Repair of Split Lobule	41
,, ,, ,, ,, ,, Nose	1
,, ,, Cyst of Antrum	1
,, ,, Cicatrices	4
,, ,, Fistula in Ano	58
,, ,, External Haemorrhoids	19
,, ,, Internal ,, ...	38
,, ,, Phimosis (Circumcision)	13
,, ,, Elephantiasis of Scrotum	8
,, ,, ,, ,, Foreskin	1
,, ,, Stricture of Meatus Urinarius ...	1
,, ,, Unnatural Anus	1
,, ,, Ganglion	4
Electrolysis of Naevus	4
,, ,, Keloid	1
Ligature of Naevus	3
Aspirating Abdominal (Lumbar) Cyst	1
Needling for Sciatica	1
Laying open Lymphocele	1
Tapping and injecting Hydrocele	16
Extracting Fruit Stone from Nose	1

Laying open Sinuses	6
Exploratory Operations	3
Plugging Posterior Nares	1
Opening large Abscesses	6
" Retropharyngeal Abscess	1
Cauterising for Bone Disease	1
Operation for Sequestrum	5
" " Nasal Polypus	16
" " Aural "	2
Excision of Horns, Warts, etc.	5
Total number of Operations	863
Extracting Teeth	117

A considerable number of minor operations such as opening abscesses, extracting loose sequestra, catheterisation, setting fractures etc. are not included in the above total.

List of a few of the Diseases treated.

General Diseases.

Intermittent Fever:—		Enlarged Spleen	7
Quotidian...	12	Leprosy	244
Tertian	12	Beri-beri	9
Quartan	117	Goitre	5
Double Quartan	2	Syphilis	207
Four day Ague	1	Opium Smokers for cure ...	94

Eye.

Granular Ophthalmia	430	Other Eye Diseases	528
Entropion and Trichiasis	270		

Lymphatic System.

Elephantiasis of right Leg ...	13	Elephantiasis of both Legs ...	2
" " left "	11	Side not recorded	3
" " " " and Scrotum	1	Elephantiasis of Foreskin......	1
		" of Scrotum......	21
" of both Legs and Scrotum	2	Lymph Scrotum..................	2

Genito-Unrinary System.

Vesical Calculus	6	Penile Calculus...	1

Beri-beri.—Eight returned emigrants came with Beri-beri, got at Singapore. In three of these cases the disease was the dry form, and in the others the dropsy had disappeared during the voyage to Swatow. Curiously enough one of these patients had been home for eight years, and yet had a yearly recurrence of the affection, the first symptoms manifesting themselves in April or May, and disappearing in November. I do not know of a similar case, as return home seems to effect a cure in every case. As this young man's village was in a low lying district, I advised change to a more hilly locality. Beri-beri recurred in the girl's school in 1887 and it had to be closed in con sequence. Although there was a virulent outbreak of it in the boys' school the year before, yet last year, strangely enough, not one boy was affected.

Spirit Drinking.—Of 1709 adult males whose habits as to spirit drinking were ascertained, it was found that 57 per cent took it occasionally—when they could get it, some said—36 per cent denied taking it, and 7 per cent confessed to the daily use of it. The average daily quantity consumed by the last class was eleven ounces, the amount varying from two ounces to the liberal allowance of thirty-two ounces. The spirit used was generally the cheap rice whisky, and it seems to be the custom to take it in the evening. While it is an extremely rare thing to see a Chinaman the worse of liquor, and I have never met with a case of true chronic alcoholism, yet one is called upon every year to treat a number of patients whose complaint has been brought on by the habitual use of alcohol, or rather I should say of native spirit, for it is probably very impure stuff. Unfortunately I do not know whether it has ever been analysed, and with what result.

It might be urged that these statistics are misleading, for if the result of spirit drinking is injurious, there should be a larger proportion of those addicted to it among the patients than among a similar number of adult males taken at random from the general populace. I do not think it is so, and for this reason: a large number stated that formerly they used to take it, but since their present illness began they had given it up. This was especially the case in Eye troubles, where its use aggravated the inflammation. So that I believe the true estimate should be rather over than under what is here given.

I do not intend to make any remarks on these statistics, but simply present them as some definite information on a subject whose importance it behooves all those labouring for the good of the Chinese to be alive to.

Fourteen per cent of the adult male patients had been abroad, the great majority having been to Singapore, and the others to Penang, Siam, and Annam. The average duration of their stay there was five years. Unfortunately they are seldom benefited physically or morally by their visit to "foreign parts," the proportion suffering from Syphilis, and more or less complete blindness from Gonorrhœal Ophthalmia being very high.

P. B. C.

Note.—With reference to the balance of $590, it may be stated that all of this sum will be required in a few weeks for necessary repairs of the hospital buildings and for enlarging the administrative department.

Dr. Lyall having returned from his furlough home, now resumes charge of the Medical work in Swatow.

SUBSCRIPTIONS for 1887.

Messrs. Bradley & Co.	$50.00
" Jardine, Matheson & Co.	50.00
China Sugar Refining Company, Limited ...	50.00
Messrs. Butterfield & Swire	50.00
A Friend	60.00
A Silent Donor	50.00
Per Wm. Paton to help poor patients	40.00
Rev. G. Smith	30.00
E. McKean	30.00
Wm. Paton	25.00
H. Matchitt	25.00
C. B Quelch	25.00
Rev. Wm. Duffus	25.00
Dr. Pollock	25.00
Rev. J. C. Gibson...	25.00
Dr. Lyall	25.00
Dr. Cousland	25.00
A Friend	24.00
H. Budler	20.00
H. M.	20.00
D. C. Byworth	15.00
J. D. Monro	10.00
W. E. Allum	10.00
J. de la Touche	10.00
Otto Asverus	10.00
L. Grunauer	10.00
R. L. Mansfield	10.00

L. Haesloop	... ...	10.00
P. Williams	... ...	10.00
Miss Fielde for Cataract Spectacles	... ...	10.00
C. A. Coleman	... ...	5.00
R. L. Richardson	... ...	5.00
D. Anderson	... ...	5.00
S. Leslie	... ...	5.00
L. Hayllar	... ...	5.00
H. Wilzer	... ...	5.00
C. Palmer	... ...	5.00
W. H. Wilkinson	... ...	5.00
W. Pollock	... ...	5,00
G. Keeble	... ...	5.00
J. J. MacGrath	... ...	5.00
F. W. Focken	... ...	5.00
A. L. Piersdorf	... ...	5.00
W. F. Inglis	... ...	5.00
K. Young	... ...	5.00
Miss. Hess	... ...	5.00
P. Plage	... ...	3.00
C. Ecallaw	... ...	3.00
J. D. Smith	... ...	3.00
J. O'Neill	... ...	3.00
A. Sutherland	... ...	2.00
		$873.00
Chinese Subscriptions	... ...	$271.80

Rice and Cash Tickets.

Tan, Nguan-Seng 4000 tickets	... ...	$119.50
Hiap-li 200 tickets	... ...	11.09
Anonymous 100 tickets.	... ...	4.91

STATEMENT OF INCOME AND EXPENDITURE.

By Balance	$320.46	To Wages	$355.33
„ Subscriptions—European	873.00	„ General Expenses	163.56
„ „ Chinese	271.89	„ Aid to Poor Patients	33.32
„ Sale of Drugs to European & Chinese	552.80	„ Repairs	56.44
„ „ „ Milk to Do. Do.	202.46	„ Milk from London	274.18
„ „ „ Sundries	81.21	„ Medicines bought in Swatow	44.04
„ „ „ Trusses	61.50	„ „ „ „ Hongkong	150.84
„ Receipts from Opium Smokers	92.00	„ „ from England, &c.	477.45
„ Rent of Private Wards	11.00	„ „ from Home Committee	620.00
„ Grant from Home Committee	620.00	„ Burial Expenses	28.89
		„ Oil	95.45
		„ Lard	24.32
		„ Wool	63.09
		„ Water	46.87
		„ Cloth	43.40
		„ Paper	10.93
		„ Washing Wards	10.82
		„ Balance on hand	590.39
	$3,095.32		$3,095.32

REPORT

OF THE

MISSION HOSPITAL

SWATOW

IN CONNECTION WITH THE

PRESBYTERIAN CHURCH OF ENGLAND

UNDER THE CARE OF

ALEXANDER LYALL, M.B., C.M.,

For 1888.

PRINTED BY KWAI-FUNG, SWATOW.

1889.

REPORT

AT the close of another year, in accordance with established custom, we beg to submit a short summary of the year's work for the information of the friends and supporters of the Swatow Mission Hospital. It is unnecessary to enter into details, as the various branches of the work were carried on as usual with a fair amount of success both from the medical and the missionary point of view. A glance at the statistics given below, and at the list of diseases treated, will show that a good deal of hard work has been done during the year. Dr. Cousland, who had charge of the Hospital during my furlough home, continued to give his help for several months until he left to begin work in Chao-chow-foo. He attended to the out-patients on the usual Dispensary days, thus giving me more leisure for the Hospital work—a leisure which was very grateful. The lamented death of the Community Doctor in September made it necessary for us, with the consent of our colleagues, to undertake the various duties of the Medical Officer of the Port. These we continued to perform as long as it was necessary, without neglecting our own proper work.

STATISTICS.

NUMBER OF INDIVIDUAL PATIENTS:—

In-patients	2719
Out-patients	2397
Total	5116
Females included in above	807
Cases seen out of Dispensary hours, chiefly by Senior Native Assistants about ...	1500
Visits paid to Chinese patients in their own homes	137
Daily average numbers of In-patients ...	160
Average attendance of Out-patients on Dispensary days	45
Total number of visits of Out-patients to the Dispensary	7500
Number of Operations	853

In addition, we have the medical care of a large number of Chinese living in the Mission Compound, as pupils, assistants, and servants.

Last summer was an unhealthy one to the native population of Chao-Chow. The Spring rains were more abundant and continued longer than usual, and were followed by a long spell of hot and comparatively dry weather. In May, cases of Cholera began to appear in Swatow and several other towns, but as long as the wet weather continued it did not spread much. The warm dry weather set in about the beginning of July, and the disease soon became prevalent all over the country. The type of Cholera was not of the most virulent kind, yet the mortality was very great in several of the larger cities. The cases of the disease which came under our notice were fairly amenable to treatment, and about 75 per cent recovered. The town of Swatow suffered greatly, but the neighbouring large villages which were severely attacked in the Epidemic of 1883, escaped almost entirely. Curiously enough, neither in 1883 nor last year did it invade the mountainous Hakka country to the West. Dr. McPhun did not see or hear of a case in Ng-kang-phu or neighbourhood, though the disease was very prevalent in villages on the Kit-yang river only a few miles distant.

The presence of Cholera lessened very considerably the number of our patients during July and August. For some weeks patients almost ceased to come from a distance, as they were afraid to travel, through the infected parts. Persons travelling in districts in which Cholera is prevalent run great risk of infection. Many of the cases which occurred in the Hospital were patients recently admitted who had evidently caught the disease on their way to Swatow. In Swatow we attended quite a number of intending Emigrants who had come in from the country to get a steamer for "Foreign parts." No hospital assistant or attendant was attacked, and when cases occurred in the hospital, the disease showed no tendency to spread in the wards.

Beriberi again broke out in the mission schools in Spring, but none of the cases were severe, and all speedily recovered on being sent to their homes. This disease appears to be becoming more prevalent every year. Nothing like an Epidemic of Beriberi has yet occurred in Swatow, but we may expect one soon. Of the cases treated in the hospital, several had never been abroad. We have had no death from this disease yet, but several of the cases were very severe. One man was unable to walk, or even to stand without support, for more than two months. This man, a native of Chao-yang, was in hospital for the cure of Opium smoking in the end of 1887, and some months after returning home he was attacked with Beriberi.

In the *annus medicus* of Swatow there are two events which deserve a passing notice, though neither is directly connected with the work under review. In November Dr. Cousland opened a dispensary in the prefectural city of Chao-chow, thus beginning a work which we trust and believe will be greatly beneficial to the people of that city and its vicinity. Almost from the first week the number of patients coming for treatment has been so numerous that it was necessary to limit the number admitted each day. So far, the premises are very unsuitable for medical purposes, but doubtless a more convenient habitation will be forthcoming.

The next event is the proposal by the native merchants of Swatow, to erect a large hospital to be conducted according to native principles, and to be placed under the charge of Chinese physicians imported from Shanghai or Hongkong. The foundations have already been built on a site near the Mission Hospital. It is gratifying to find that the Chinese themselves are beginning to move in the direction of providing charitable and benevolent institutions for the relief of the sick poor. In such a populous region as Chao-chow there must be, however, a vast amount of suffering untouched by hospitals placed in Swatow; so we trust that the wealthy native merchants will not limit their benevolent endeavours to this town only, when the necessity for such is so much greater in many other cities of this Prefecture.

In the beginning of the year, having a balance of $500 on hand, I enlarged the two small front blocks of the large hospital, thereby gaining six additional small rooms. The overcrowding for many months of the year is, however, too great to be remedied by such a small addition to the accommodation. It has often been remarked in our annual Reports that a large proportion of our patients come from a distance, and that it is necessary for us to provide a lodging for them, if we are to attempt the treatment of their ailments. Swatow is badly provided with good lodging houses. The inns for emigrants are very expensive and beyond the means of many of the patients. For the women patients, there is really no place for them to put up in Swatow. It is my intention, when I can get sufficient funds for the purpose, to enlarge the small hospital [formerly the leper hospital], and turn it practically into a hostelry. This will enable me to limit strictly the number of patients in the large hospital which can easily accommodate at least 120 Chinese. An arrangement of this kind would relieve me from a good deal of trouble and worry, and would provide as fine a field for missionary operations as could be desired.

EVANGELISTIC.

It has been remarked that there is this difference between a Medical and a Ministerial Missionary, viz:—that the people themselves come to the former, whilst the latter himself has to go to the people with his message. The truth of this remark is exemplified by our experience in Swatow. Last year we had patients coming from 1663 different towns and villages in the Prefectures of Chao-chow, Hwei-chow, and Kia-ying-chow, and from the southern part of the Hokien province. There is one advantage—and it is by no means a small advantage from a missionary point of view—of having a large hospital in or near the Mission Compound, that all the Missionaries can take part in the Evangelistic work which is carried on among the patients. Much of the success of the Swatow Hospital is due to this fact.

Number of Villages.

Chao-chow department:—	
Ching-hai district	115
Chao-yang ,, ...	339
Kieh-yang ,, ...	289
Hwei-lai ,, ...	130
Jao-ping ,, ...	170
Pu-ning ,, ...	190
Hai-yang ,, ...	224
Fung-shun ,, ...	26
Ta-pu ,, ...	19
From Districts of Hwei-chow	15
,, ,, ,, Kia-ying-chow	47
,, Province of Hokien	80
,, Elsewhere	19
Total	1663

At my request, my wife has written an account of the Evangelistic work. The plan which she has organised of taking native Christian women and setting them to work among the women patients, is a valuable one, and much fruit may be expected from it in the future. Of the total additions to the Church by Baptism during the year, twenty-one had heard for the first time, and accepted the Gospel, while patients in the hospital. Many of these had been under treatment in former years. Mrs. Lyall writes as follows:—"As in the past, much effort has been made to give the patients a knowledge of Christian Doctrine. The daily morning and evening services and the special service for inquirers on Sunday afternoon, have been continued as heretofore, and have been conducted by the missionaries, students from the college, and the two senior native assistants. Special efforts have been made by the ladies of the Mission that no woman among the patients should leave the hospital without having obtained sufficient knowledge of the Truth to lead, sooner or later, to her becoming a Christian, should she ever have a desire for something better than can be found in idolatrous worship. Such efforts have not been confined to the missionary ladies. Six or more of the young Christian women, most of them former pupils in the girls' school, now married and living in Swatow, have expressed a willingness to set apart an hour each week for visiting the women's wards, to help the occupants to a clearer knowledge of the Gospel. In addition to the ordinary assistance given to such as wish to learn to read the character hymn book, a class has been started for such of the women, girls, and boys as wish to read the colloquial books, of which a considerable number have been prepared by the Mission. This class was begun quite as an experiment, as it was feared that the short time most of the patients stay, would prevent much practical good resulting from it. But the result has been far from discouraging. Out of twenty-eight who have been for a longer or shorter time members of the class, nine have learned to read fairly well—so well that with a little practice after leaving the hospital they can read any of our romanised books.

Thus in every way possible has it been sought to disseminate Christian Truth. It can not be doubted that much good must result from these efforts. This year more than one hundred of the patients entered their names as applicants for baptism, of whom only a few were received.

Concerning the most of those not yet baptized, we have no reason to doubt their sincerity, but it is contrary to our practice to receive any who have not yet returned to their villages, and tested their sincerity by a consistent Christian life in their own homes. While many from various reasons, principally from living in villages remote from any chapel, are never again heard from, yet there is scarcely a visit paid to any of the country stations when there is not some one asking for baptism who was formerly a hospital patient, and, perhaps, a hospital inquirer.

Among such cases may be mentioned that of Teng-hai sim. She first heard at the hospital eight years ago. By the time she returned to her home she had lost all faith in idols, but did not at once become a Christian. She was far, however, from forgetting what she had heard, and was greatly troubled because of her sins, and very unhappy over them. Two years ago she came again to the hospital, and was so helped by further instruction that when she went back to her home, she began to worship God in secret, not yet daring, through fear of her husband, to confess herself a Christian. But, by means of various excuses, she managed to keep herself free from participating in idolatrous customs. This year, finding she must come again for treatment, before leaving home she found courage to tell her husband that she was determined to become a Christian, and the first Sunday after her arrival found her among the applicants. As her village is not far from one of the country stations she was advised to apply there. This she did, and on a recent visit paid by Mr. Mackenzie to that station, she was baptized.

At one of the most distant stations there was baptized a man who had heard ten years ago at the hospital, and has been a worshipper of God ever since. As he lives about 30 miles from the nearest chapel it was very seldom that he could attend worship, but he kept the Sabbath in his own home, and now, after all these years, he has asked for and received admission to the Church.

Sun-ho, another patient who was baptized this year, came to the hospital two years ago on account of his son whom he brought for treatment. He was so impressed by what he then heard that upon his return home he not only became a warm hearted worshipper himself, but, with much zeal and earnestness, sought to give others a knowledge of the Gospel. This brought upon him bitter persecution. Before this he had been a man of some influence in his village, and was often appealed to for help to settle petty disputes, but now he was everywhere reviled and made sport of, and even suffered the indignity of being beaten by his wife who was violently opposed to his new faith. But he has borne all this patiently, and now his son who is in the Middle school, and his old blind father are applicants for baptism.

While it is easy for the patients to confess an interest in Christian Truth while living in the hospital, it becomes a different thing upon their return to their native villages. Koi sim, a former patient who came again this year, told us that upon her return home last year, she informed her family that she had decided to become a Christian. Her son, the head of the family, made no objection until his neighbours jeered at him. They said, "We are over 4000 people in this village. Never till now has one of our clan left our ancient customs and gone over to the new teaching. But now, one has done so, and that one is your mother." This was more than the son could stand. Mortified and angry, he beat the old mother so severely that for ten days she was unable to walk. Since then he had not spoken to her. This is only a small part of what the poor women has had to bear. Upon hearing her story some one said to her —"Yes, Koi sim, you have had a hard time, why not give up worshipping God, and go back to the idols?" "No," she replied, "I want after death to go where God is and not again to be born into this world" [a Buddhist idea].

Among the applicants at one of the country stations this year was a blind man. Some years ago he had come to the hospital, hoping to have his sight restored. But this was impossible. He stayed, however, ten days or so, learning about the doctrine. He then returned to his home, and instituted family worship and the observance of the Sabbath. His wife, too, became a Christian. Upon his applying for baptism, he would have been received but for the fact that he still contributed towards idolatrous plays, being obliged to do so by his fellow villagers who would have expelled him from the village had he refused.

It sometimes happens that those who have heard something of the doctrine come to the hospital for no other purpose than to hear more. Such was the case this year with two women from a village remote from any chapel. They had heard some years ago from one of our Bible-women who had been sent to their village to visit old hospital patients. One had been so impressed at that time that she made chronic sore eyes an excuse with her mother-in-law to come to the hospital, so that she might receive further instruction. On her return home she endured patiently much persecution, and has remained steadfast ever since. This year, she and her friend came to seek admission to the church. They told how, for some time, some six or eight women had been meeting together on Sundays for worship,—the worship consisting of a hymn and a prayer, and then those who could read a few hymns tried to teach the others to read them also. These women were taken into the class for learning to read the romanised colloquial, and in six weeks one of them was able to read fairly well and intelligently—so well that it is hoped that now she has gone back to her home, she will be able to read such portions of the scriptures as have been printed in romanised colloquial, and also to teach the other women to do so when they meet on Sundays." It may not be out of place to remark, for the consideration of those who object to the use of romanised books in teaching Chinese converts, that it would have taken many months, if not years, for this woman to have learned to read a Gospel in Chinese characters.

SURGICAL OPERATIONS.

On the Eye:—

Operations for Entropion and Trichiasis	298
" " Pterygium	50
" " Anchyloblepharon	1
" " Hernia Iris	2
" " Anterior Staphyloma (abscission) ...	2
" " Hypopyon	2
Extraction of Cataract	19
" " " (Traumatic)	1
" " Foreign body in Cornea	1
Needling after Cataract Extraction	2
Iridectomy for Artificial Pupil	10
" " Glaucoma	1
Plastic Operation for Cicatricial Ectropion	1
Excision of Tumours, Cysts from Eyelids	11
" " Growths of Conjunctiva	4
" " Eyeball	3
" " Sarcoma of Orbit	1
Peritomy for Pannus	2
	411

On the Body generally:—

Operations for Harelip	33
" " Phymosis	10
" " Fistula in Ano	58
" " Repair of Split Lobule	54
" " Imperforate Anus	2
" " Short Frenum Linguae	1
" " Caries of Bone	6
" " Ganglion	7
" " Ranula	3
" " Paraphymosis	2
Lateral Lithotomy	3
Perineal Section	1
Laparotomy	1
Radical Cure of Hernia (Wood's)	1
Amputation of Fingers	5
" " Forearm	1
" " Arm	1
" " Leg (through Knee Joint)	1
" " Supernumerary Thumb	1
" " Penis (Epithelioma)	2
" " Elephantiasis Scroti	2
Excision of Callosities	17
" " Epithelioma of Lip	1
" " " of Skin	1
" " Wens	3
" " Epulis	3
" " Fatty Tumours	8
" " Cystic "	4
" " Fibrous "	4
" " Glandular "	1
" " Large Fibroma (Molluscum Fibrosum)	1
" " Sarcoma	4
" " Tumours of Breast	2
" " Part of Lower Jaw	1
" " Testicle	1
" " Fungus Testis	1
" " Sebaceous Cysts	16
" " Enlarged Tonsils	5
" " Polypus of Frenum Linguae	1
" " " Rectum	1
" " " Female Urethra	1
" " Papilloma of Prepuce	1
" " External Haemorrhoids	22
" " Supernumerary Auricle ?	2

Excision of Osteoma of Foot...	1
" " Os calcis and Astragalus (Caries) ...	1
" " 1st Metatarsal and Int. Cuneiform Bones (Caries)	1
" " Prolapse of Rectum (by thermo-cautery)	3
Extraction of Nasal Polypus	22
" " Urethral Calculus	1
" " Bamboo Splinters, Needles, etc. ...	6
" " Bullet from Patella	1
" " Sequestrum	22
Tapping Hydrocele	2
Tapping and injecting Hydrocele	22
" " " Lymphocele	1
" Cystic Tumours	2
Tying Internal Haemorrhoids	34
Plastic Operation for Congenital Malformation of Penis	1
Opening large Abscess	9
Incising Fissure of Rectum	1
" Sinuses	6
Incision into Hip Joint	1
Electrolysis of Keloid	2
" " Naevus	1
" " Warts	2
Aspirating Bladder	2
Needling for Sciatica	1
Cauterising for Disease of the Spine	1
Total	442
Extraction of Teeth	191

Besides opening abscesses, reducing dislocations, setting fractures, dilating urethral strictures, &c.

Cataract.—Nineteen cases of senile cataract were operated on with the following results:—Eighteen cases recovered without a bad symptom and with good vision; in the other case, *Iritis* supervened on the fourth day. This last operation was performed about the time of the setting in of the N.E. monsoon, and after a sudden fall in the temperature of the atmosphere, the patient had a smart attack of fever. After two days fever iritis set in. The other eye of this patient had been successfully operated on a few weeks before. In a case of injury of cornea, iris, and lens, it was attempted to save the eye by extracting the wounded lens, but unsuccessfully.

The operation performed was either the modified linear extraction, or the 3 m. m. flap, and accompanied with a moderately large iridectomy in all but one case. In seventeen cases the incision was made in the upper section of the cornea. Several times I employed the syringe to wash out cortical matter from the anterior chamber, but did not find this method superior to gentle manipulation in affecting this purpose. The application of thorough antisepses to cataract operations is a great improvement. The antiseptic used was a saturated solution of Boracic Acid.

The case in which no iridectomy was made was somewhat anomalous. The lens was expelled in its unbroken capsule. The eye was small, and possibly the incision was relatively larger than usual. Any how, as I was about to insert the iris forceps the patient moved his eye and the lens was expelled. The capsule was tough and the lens within was soft and almost liquefied. A satisfactory recovery and good vision resulted.

A needling operation was only performed twice. Some of the other eyes required this treatment, there being a few fine thread like bands stretching across the pupil; but the Chinese, I find, will rarely submit to this operation. They are satisfied with the amount of vision obtained, and do not wish any more meddling with the eye.

Plastic Operation for Cicatricial Ectropion:—The upper eyelid was drawn up and everted, exposing the eye which was inflamed. The cicatricial skin extended a considerable distance along the forehead and side of face; hence, a flap of healthy skin was not obtainable from that locality. The cicatricial tissue was dissected off the eyelid and side of face, a flap of skin was dissected up from the forearm, and applied to the raw surface of eyelid and face. Knowing the marvellous power of the Chinese to endure discomfort and pain, I left the flap attached to the arm which I bound firmly to the side of the face. The patient submitted to this uncomfortable arrangement for 36 hours or longer. The result was very satisfactory, a good serviceable eyelid being obtained.

Excision of Eyeball.—Every year many cases of painful shrunken eyeball and of anterior staphyloma apply for treatment. In the earlier years of my practice I used to urge such patients to submit to enucleation of the eyeball, but few would consent to this surgical procedure. The Chinese, however, do not seem specially liable to suffer from sympathetic ophthalmia, so I have ceased to press this treatment on them, and, in cases of anterior staphyloma, I generally only abscise the projecting portion of the eyeball.

Within the last few months two patients have come and asked me to enucleate a diseased eyeball and insert a glass one in its place. Not having artificial eyes on hand, I was not able to acceed to their request, but, on their urgent entreaty and at their expense, I have ordered some glass eyes from home, and next year they are to return for operation. One was a girl near the marriageable age, and doubtless the prospect of getting more dollars for her induced the father to bring her to the hospital. Perhaps before long we will have patients desirous of being relieved of diseased limbs if artificial ones are supplied in their place!

Major Amputations.—Three such operations have been successfully performed during the year;—one, through the forearm, one, of the arm above the elbow, and the third, of the leg through the knee joint. This last case, a weak debilitated man who was suffering from a large sarcomatous tumour of the ankle, is still under treatment. Part of the long anterior flap sloughed and this has delayed his recovery.

Lateral Lithotomy.—Five cases were admitted with vesical calculus, but of these only three submitted to operative treatment. Lateral Lithotomy was performed in all of the cases with successful results. The first case was that of a boy, aged 3 years, from whose bladder a calculus weighing 120 grains was extracted; the second was a boy of 7 years, the calculus being 80 grains in weight. The third case, a man aged 41, was the most interesting one. On examination there seemed to be a large calculus filling the upper part of the bladder. The lithotrite was passed and an endeavour made to crush it, but the mass was so friable that the blades of the lithotrite passed through it on the slightest pressure. Lateral lithotomy was then performed, and it was found that a large portion of the posterior wall of the bladder was thickly coated with a calcareous deposit. This was scraped off by means of the scoop and the finger. About two ounces of debris was removed. The wound was kept open for a fortnight and the bladder washed out daily with an antiseptic lotion. Patient made an excellent recovery, and, four months afterwards, he returned to report himself in good health and free from any bladder trouble.

Urethral Calculus.—A calculus about the size of a marble was removed from the urethra in the glans penis. It had been lodged in the urethra for ten years.

Large Fibroma.—This patient, a woman aged 46,

was admitted with a large pedunculated tumour, growing from the posterior aspect of the right shoulder just below the spine of the scapula, the huge mass reaching nearly to the hip and measuring about 2½ feet in circumference at its widest part. Its weight was so great that frequently on sitting down patient would lose her balance and fall backwards to the ground. It commenced to grow six years ago. The isthmus and right lobe of the thyroid gland were also enlarged, causing slight pressure symptoms, but there were no fibrous nodules or tumours in any other part of the body. The patient's general health was good, but mentally she was somewhat childish. After removal the tumour weighed 23 lbs. The patient proved very refractory. A few days after the operation she could not be kept in bed. Nevertheless, the wound, to a great extent, healed by first intention, and patient was well enough to run away from the hospital in about a fortnight, out running her husband on the way. These tumours are not infrequently met with in this part of China. The back is a favourite site. Other varieties of molluscum fibrosum are also met with.

Laparotomy.—This operation was undertaken for the relief of chronic intussusception of the large bowel. The patient, a boy of seven years, had been ill for four months. Two months before operation he was under our care. Then, we distended the bowel with air and the intussusception seemed to disappear. He improved very much, was taken home, and continued in fairly good health for a month when the symptoms returned. On admission the second time the child was evidently fatally ill. On opening the abdomen, we found a large mass of intussuscepted bowel lying on the left side which we failed to reduce, it being firmly bound by adhesions. An artificial anus was made, but patient died 13 hours after operation.

Excision of part of Lower Jaw.—A young man, 18 years old, was admitted for a myeloid tumour of the lower jaw, situated to the left side of and implicating the symphysis. It was endosteal, and had expanded both the outer and inner plates of the bone. The whole mass was as large as a medium sized orange. An incision along the edge of the jaw was made, the soft parts dissected up, the bone on either side of the tumour divided, and the mass removed. Patient made a good recovery.

Perineal Section.—The patient on whom this operation was performed came to be treated for a traumatic stricture of the urethra. Some years before the urethra had been injured by a fall on the perineum. No 1 bougie was passed on two occasions. The second passage of the instrument was followed by a severe attack of urethral fever with complete retention of urine. The bladder was aspirated several times, but as the fever continued and the patient was becoming seriously ill, I performed perineal section. No instrument could be passed. After a long illness patient recovered, the urethra easily admitting a large bougie. Any attempt to dilate traumatic strictures by means of instruments is apt to be followed by urethral fever, more or less grave, much more so than in cases of stricture following gonorrhoea. I find much difficulty in getting Chinese patients to undergo operative treatment for this affection.

Tumour of Male Breast.—The breast was excised in two cases for tumour. In one case, a young lad of 17 years, the tumour was sarcomatous and was very large, measuring fully 18 inches in circumference. In the other case the gland was hypertrophied.

Elephantiasis Scroti,—There were only two cases operated on this year, the tumours weighing after removal 25 lbs 10 oz. and 9½ lbs respectively. The wound healed by first intention in both cases.

Supernumerary Auricle (?).—Two cases of a small congenital growth situated anteriorly to the tragus of the ear, and resembling it in structure, applied for treatment. Supernumerary thumbs and fingers are common, but these are the first cases of this kind of congenital deformity, I have come across.

Imperforate Anus.—In one case the operation was unsuccessful. The bowel could not be found. The child defecated per urethram.

Excision of Tarsal and Metatarsal Bones.—Of three such operations, two were followed with a good result, but in one case, that of the os calcis and astragalus, the disease (caries) returned in some of the other bones. The patient in still under treatment.

A Series of Accidents.—Severe injuries are comparatively uncommon, but in October last we had a regular run of cases, a list of which we give below, as such experiences are rare in hospital work in China.

From the 13th to the 27th october we admitted the following cases:—

Contusion of Eyeball from blow.—eye destroyed.

Two Cases of Fracture of Humerus.

Fracture of Spine.—Patient was struck by the falling mast while sitting in a crouching attitude on the deck of a boat. When taken away from the hospital a month later, the lower limbs were still paralysed.

Fracture of Skull.—Died in a few hours.

Crushed Foot.—The soft structures on the dorsum and side of the foot were lacerated or torn off and several of the bones smashed. Amputation was refused. About two thirds of the foot eventually sloughed away.

Wound of Abdominal wall with prolapse of bowel. A boy of 6 years was gored by a buffalo, the wound being on the left side near the ribs. The bowel had ruptured, and all the faeces were discharged though the artificial anus thus formed.

Dislocation of the Shoulder.

Wound and severe injury of the knee joint caused by falling from the top of a house.

Dislocations.—A backward displacement of the femur at the hip is the most common dislocation we are called upon to reduce. In one case an unfortunate occurrence happened in attempting to do this. The patient, a boy aged 8, was thrown from a pig's back and his hip dislocated backward. Two months afterwards he was brought to the hospital, and the dislocation was comparatively easily reduced by manipulation. In three months more the child was brought back suffering from the same displacement which was caused in the same way as before. No difficulty was anticipated as the injury was only of a few days standing. The first attempt by manipulation brought the head of the femur down, but it caught on the rim of the acetabulum. On attempting to complete the reduction (and not much force was used) the femur snapped in two.

Dislocation of the Wrist Backward.—A well marked case of this injury was seen. The humerus was also fractured.

Foot Binding.—A girl, aged nine, was admitted suffering from the effects of somewhat vigorous treatment during the process of foot binding. Her mother being desirous of very small feet for her daughter, had "hammered" the toes and feet to "make the bones soft," and then bound them tightly, with the result that the anterior half of one of the feet sloughed off, leaving an unhealthy granulating surface. The foot will likely require to be amputated.

We have often been struck by the infrequency of congenital deformities of the feet among the Chinese [e.g. in Chao-chow prefecture]. The common varieties of Talipes are even seldom seen. It may be that the people do not think it worth while to bring their children for treatment for such affections, but in going among the people in Swatow and in the country, I have rarely seen any one with congenital talipes or other pedal deformity.

The Chinese have bound the feet of their women and girls, it is said, for at least 1000 years; hence, one would naturally expect, in consequence of this long continued mutilation, that queer freaks of nature would be often seen with regard to the shape and size of the feet. The Chinese, however, seem to have as large feet in proportion to their size as other people among whom this savage custom is unknown. The rite of circumcision, it is said, has not caused any congenital shortening of the prepuce in the Jewish race, and it appears to me that foot binding has not effected any permanent shortening of the foot among the Chinese generally.

LIST OF DISEASES.

General Diseases.

Intermittent Fever :—		Struma	46
Quotidian	9	Rickets (?)	1
Tertian	15	Rheumatism	240
Quartan	99	Anaemia	55
Irregular	12	Do. with enlarged Spleen	20
Febricula & simple continued Fever	88	General & Malarial Debility	109
Typhoid Fever	1	Beriberi	25
Cholera	140	Alcoholism	2
Erysipelas	1	Goitre	3
Syphilis	221	Starvation	1
Do. Congenital	9	Opium Smokers for cure ...	81
Leprosy	251	Do. poisoning (suicidal)...	3
		Masturbation	5

Diseases of the Respiratory System.

Coryza	2	Bronchitis	114
Laryngitis	5	Phthisis Pulmonalis	101
Asthma	17	Acute Pneumonia	2
Emphysema	5	Haemoptysis (only)	5

Diseases of the Genito-Urinary System.

Chronic Nephritis	5	Urinary Fistula	3
Haematuria	2	Traumatic Rupture of Urethra	1
Suppression of Urine	1	Gonorrhoea, Gleet	35
Incontinence of Urine	3	Spermatorrhoea	18
Retention of Urine	1	Balanitis	1
Vesical Calculus	5	Orchitis	3
Calculus in Urethra	1	Hydrocele	37
Enlarged Prostate	1	Varicocele	3
Phymosis	13	Syph. Enlargement of Testicle	3
Paraphymosis	4	Tumour of Testicle	1
Epithelioma of Penis	9	Fungus Testis	5
Chancres and Syph. Ulceration of Penis and Scrotum	84	Wart, Papilloma of Prepuce	2
Stricture of Urethra	9	Congenital Malformation of Genital Organs	1

Leucorrhoea	8	Chancres of Vulvum	2
Amenorrhoea	5	Condyloma of Do.	1
Dysmenorrhoea	2	Pruritus of Do.	2
Metrorrhagia	3	Gonorrhoea	2
Irregular Menstruation ...	2	Vesico-recto—Vagnial Fistula	1
Uterine Polypus	1	Polypus of Urethra	1
Ovarian Tumour	1	Carcinoma of Vagina	1

Diseases of the Lymphatic System.

Elephantiasis of Scrotum	15	Enlarged Glands in Groin (Elephantoid)	4
Do. of Leg	32	Lymphadenoma	2
Do. of Leg and Scrotum	3	Bubo	3
Lymph Scrotum	4		

Diseases of the Digestive System.

Epithelioma of Lip	1	Constipation	3
Gumboil	4	Haematemesis	1
Dental Sinus	3	Vermes	21
Ulcerated Gums	5	Hernia—Inguinal	38
Stomatitis	1	Epigastric	1
Enlarged Papillae of Tongue	2	Umbelical	2
Short Frenum Linguae	1	Faecal Fistula	1
Cleft Palate	5	Ulceration of Rectum and Anus (Sodomy)	37
Harelip	34	Epithelioma of Anus	2
Congestion of Fauces	9	Fistula in Ano	72
Granular Pharyngitis	9	Haemorrhoids—Internal	50
Ulceration of Fauces	11	Do. External	16
Chronic Tonsillitis	10	Stricture of Rectum	6
Stricture of Œsophagus	4	Prolapse of Do.	6
Dyspepsia	379	Polypus of Do.	1
Dilated Stomach	1	Fissure of Do.	3
Colic	6	Liver—Unclassed	9
Dysentery	34	Ascites	5
Diarrhoea	22		

Diseases of the Skin.

Callosities	17	Pemphigus	2
Epithelioma	5	Keloid	3
Ulcers	186	Herpes Zoster	2
Condyloma	7	Scabies	24
Ecthyma	5	Seborrhoea	1
Eczema	76	Intertrigo	1
Tinea—Circinata	148	Melanoderma	1
Favosa	4	Prickly Heat	1
Imbricata	7	Molluscum	1
Pityriasis	15	Onychia	5
Psoriasis	19	Pruritus	6
Lichen	21	Syphilides	45
Leucoderma	5	Rodent Ulcer	1
Acne	3	Alopecia	2
Lupus	7		

Diseases of the Nervous System.

Paralysis of one side of face	4	Insanity	9
Do. of one arm	3	Imbeciles	2
Hemiplegia	11	Deaf Mutes	3
Paraplegia	1	Pseudo-hypertrophic Paralysis	1
Neuralgia	19	Locomotor Ataxy	1
Epilepsy	8	Spinal unclassed	2
Neuritis	3	Local Anaesthesia	20
Hysteria (?)	1		

Diseases of the Circulatory System.

Cardiac—Valvular	15
Unclassed	4
Anaeurism	2
Naevus	1
Varix	5

Tumours.

Sabaceous Cyst	11
Dermoid Cost	2
Fibrous	10
Cystic	8
Ranula	4
Glandular	4
Chondroma	1
Osteoma	4
Fatty	10
Epulis	2
Wen	2
Ganglion	10
Papilloma	7
Lymphangiectasis Cavernous	1
Molluscum Fibrosum	4
Hypertrophy of breast	1
Unclassed Innocent	5
Congenital	1
Sarcoma	19
Carcinoma	11
Do. of female breast	5
Malignant unclassed	25

Diseases of the Eye.

Conjunctivitis—Catarrhal	62
Purulent	25
Phlyctenular	7
Granular	476
Pterygium	53
Conjunctival Growths	3
Ulcer of Cornea	24
Slough of Cornea	6
Abscess of Cornea	2
Leucoma	39
Do. Adherens	47
Foreign body in Cornea	1
Anterior Staphyloma	24
Hernia Iris	16
Keratitis	13
Panus	7
Iritis	8
Irido—Choroiditis	1
Corneo—Iritis	8
Occlusion of Pupil	15
Hypopyon	6
Cataract	33
Do. Traumatic	2
Lenticular Opacity	3
Glaucoma Chronic	15
Destruction of one or both Eyes	49
Panophthalmitis	4
Wounds, Injuries of Eyeball	8
Atrophy of Optic Nerve	3
Amaurosis	15
Haemorrhage into Retina	1
Night Blindness	4
Paresis of Ext. Rectus Muscle	1
Myopia	2
Symblepharon	2
Anchyloblepharon	1
Entropion and Trichiasis	215
Ectropion	4
Ophthalmia Tarsi	14
Ptosis	2
Cysts, Tumours of Eyelids and Eyebrows	9
Epithelioma of lower lid	2
Malignant of Orbit	6
Abscess of Eyelid	1
Burn of Eyelid	1
Wounds of Eyelid	4
Œdema of Eyelid	1
Hordeolum	1
Chalazion	2
Hypertrophy of Tarsal Cartilage	1
Stricture of Nasal Duct	6

Diseases of the Ear.

Slit Lobule	42
Aural Sinuses	3
Otorrhoea	12
Non Suppurative Catarrh of Middle Ear	4
Deafness	4
Inflammation of Ext. Meatus	1
Wax in Ext. Meatus	1
Abscess of Auricle	1
Cysts of Auricle	2
Supernumerary Auricle	2
Congenital Deformity of Auricle	1

Diseases of the Connective System.

Whitlow	11	Sinus	20
Inflammation	21	Boils, Carbuncles	22
Abscess	64	Gumma	6

Diseases of the Nose.

Ozaenia	7	Ulceration of Mucous Membrane	9
Epistaxis	2		
Polypus	19	Hypertrophy Mucous Membrane	1
Do. Fibrous	1		
Closure of Anterior Nares	1	Deviation of Nasal Septum	1
Ulceration of Nose	16		

Diseases of the Locomotory System.

Periostitis	5	Bursitis	1
Ostitis	11	Strumous disease of hip joint	12
Caries	28	Do. do. of other joints	6
Necrosis	41	Anchylosis	5
Spinal Curvature	8	Gangrene of toes and fingers	7
Synovitis	27	Do. of leg	1

Local Injuries.

Wounds	74	Scalds and Burns	9
Do. Gunshot	2	Splinters, Needles, &c. lodged	6
Wound of Abdomen with Protrusion of Bowel	1	Bullets lodged	2
		Bites	19
Injuries, Bruises	61	Dislocations	12
Sprains	36	Fractures	10

Unclassed.

Midwifery	3	Muscular Twitching	4
Supernumerary Thumb	1	Do. Contraction	2

The above list is only approximately correct. It indicates rather the diseases for the relief of which patients came to hospital than the actual number of each disease treated. Many diseases have been treated in greater numbers than we have indicated. Thus, such skin diseases as Tinea Circinata, Scabies, might be numbered by hundreds. Again, at least 70 per cent of the cases of granular conjunctivitis were complicated with other diseases of the eye as keratitis, ulcer of Cornea, pannus, Hernia Iris, Trichiasis &c.

Typhoid Fever.—A typical case of this disease was under treatment. Typhoid fever is rarely seen in Swatow. My senior native assistants recognised the disease as one occasionally but rarely seen in this Region. The system of open drainage in vogue in Chinese villages, however objectionable it may be to the olefactory nerves of foreigners, appears at any rate to prevent the development of such fever as typhoid.

FINANCIAL.

As we have already mentioned in the Report, we undertook the medical care of the Foreign Community for nearly three months. The fees received amounted to $973.46, and the expenses (wages of five boatmen and jinricksha coolie) to $102.37, leaving a balance on hand of $871.09. Of this sum I handed to Dr. Cousland $370.07, and the remainder ($500.12) I have placed to the credit of the Hospital (see list of contributions). We beg to thank most heartily all the friends who have contributed towards the support of the Hospital.

SUBSCRIPTIONS for 1888.

Messrs. Bradley & Co.	$50,00
„ Butterfield & Swire.	50.00
„ Jardine, Matheson & Co.	50.00
„ Lauts & Haesloop.	25.00
China Sugar Refinery Co,. Ltd. per J. M. & Co.	50.00
Rev. Wm. Ashmore D. D.	50.00
R. H. Hill (special donation)	50.00
A. Silent Donor	50.00
Miss. Byworth	35.00
Jas. R. Brazier	30.00
Baron von Seckendorff	30.00
Rev. George Smith, M.A., ...	30.00
Otto Asverus	25.00
P. B. Cousland, M.B., C.M.	25.00

Rev. W. Duffus	25.00
Rev. J. C. Gibson, M.A., ...	25.00
A. Lyall, M.B., C.M.	25.00
H. Matchitt	25.00
Mrs. Wm. Pollock	24.00
D. C. Byworth	20.00
M. H.	20.00
L. Grunhuer	20.00
Schaar & Co.'s Estate, balance of, per Messrs. Lauts & Haesloop	19.01
Rev. H. L. Mackenzie, M.A., ...	15.00
W. E. Allum	10.00
A. Frater	10.00
Miss. Fielde	10.00
S. Leslie	10.00
Chas. B. Quelch	10.00
C. H. Palmer	10.00
Rev. S. B. Partridge	10.00
R. L. Richardson	10.00
J. De la Touche	10.00
Drummond Anderson	5.00
W. Bond	5.00
F. W. Dyere (fee)...	5.00
J. Featherstonehaugh	5.00
F. W. Focken	5.00
Rev. J. M. Foster...	5.00
W. F. Inglis	5.00
T. Kerr	5.00
J. J. McGrath	5.00
F. McQuire	5.00
J. O'Neil (fee)	5.00
W. Pollock	5.00
E. A. Roberts	5.00
W. H. Wilkinson	5.00
E. Benson (fee)	3.00
C. A. Maasberg	3.00
A. Bryson	2.00
M. G Nahmen	2.00
A. L. Piersdorf	2.00
A. Brosowsky	1.00
"Fine" per W. H. W.	1.00
Share of Fees for Medical attendance on Foreign Community	500.12
	$1447.13

CHINESE.

Liao Foo Sang	$25.00
Lim Yam Seng	25.00
Presbyterian Church (Native) Swatow	25.00
Tsan Tai Wan	20.00
Yuen Seng Huat	10.00
Siao Ah Kim	10.00
Kho Buey Tso	10.00
Wong Sew Heuk	10.00
Ee Kee	10.00
Low Cheang Yee	10.00
Ding Shao Lin	5.00
Ko Leang Sz	5.00
A Chhim	5.00
Kho-Po Seng tng	4.00
Lam Tat Hing	3.00
C. Aruyew...	2.00
Ho Pin Wen	2.00
See Buan	2.00
Sim Kye Pang	2.00
Ang Seng	2.00
Tshuat Thai	2.00
Kwai Fung	2.00
Lau Su Keng	2.00
Patients	24.40
	$217.40

RICE AND CASH TICKETS.

Tang, Ngnan Seng 5000 tickets	$147.700
Hiap-li	2.70

STATEMENT OF INCOME AND EXPENDITURE.

To Wages	$327.00	By Balance	$590.93
„ General Expenses	156.53	„ Contributions and fees from Foreigners	1,447.10
„ New Buildings & Repairs	639.33	„ „ „ „ Chinese	217.43
„ Medicines bought in Swatow and Hongkong	272.12	„ Receipts from Opium Smoker	68.00
„ Medicine bought in London	191.15	„ Rent of Small Ward	12.85
„ „ „ „ paid by Missionary Committee in Edinburgh	864.23	„ Sale of Medicines, Trusses, Milk, less cost and Expenses	358.29
„ Aid to poor Patients	32.94	„ Grant from Missionary Committee in Edinburgh	864.23
„ Burial Expenses	14.09		
„ Oils	84.20		
„ Lards	23.60		
„ Cotton Wool	57.63		
„ Water	42.22		
„ Cloth	32.81		
„ Paper	46.23		
„ Washing Wards	10.03		
„ Balance on hand	764.18		
	$3558.29		$3,558.29

CH'AO-CHOW-FOO

MEDICAL MISSION

UNDER THE CARE OF

P. B. COUSLAND, M.B., C.M.

CH'AO-CHOW-FOO.

Temporary premises having been at length obtained in this city, and the necessary repairs and fittings seen to, a Dispensary was opened on the 18th of November, 1888. From that time until the end of the year, 1660 patients were seen, including a few who were visited at their homes.

The dispensary was open every day, and in a short time we had as many patients as we could attend to. It was noticeable that those who came first had, in some way or other, known about the Swatow Hospital. A few had been there themselves, others had had friends who had been there, and most of them had heard of it. In this way we made a good start, and it was not long before others, hearing of us from those who came, began to show their confidence by attending.

A good feature is the large proportion of women who came,—500 being registered on the books, i.e. nearly one third of the total number of patients. This surely shows some little confidence in us and our methods.

A daily morning service was conducted with the assembled patients by a native preacher, and after it, he availed himself of the opportunity to enter into conversation with those in the waiting room.

STATISTICS.

Individual Patients	1660
Including in-patients	20
„ Females	500
Subsequent visits of out-patients	721
Number of operations	55

In addition, more than 300 patients were seen during a visit paid to the city in spring.

OPERATIONS.

Operations for Entropion and Trichiasis	...	27
Needling Congenital Cataract	... ...	2
Operation for Pterygium	... ...	1
,, ,, Stricture of Nasal duct	...	1
,, ,, Nasal polypus	... ...	4
,, ,, Harelip	... ...	3
,, ,, Slit ear lobule	... ...	9
,, ,, Phimosis	... ...	3
,, ,, Wen	... ...	1
,, ,, Callosities of Sole	... ...	1
Extracting coin from Œsophagus	... ...	1
Opening chronic abscess of Leg	... ...	1
Removal of fatty tumour of back (Weight ℔s12;12 ozs.)	... ...	1

PHILIP B. COUSLAND.

REPORT

OF THE

MISSION HOSPITAL

AT

SWATOW

IN CONNECTION WITH THE

PRESBYTERIAN CHURCH OF ENGLAND,

UNDER THE CARE OF

ALEXANDER LYALL, M.B., C.M.

For 1890.

PRINTED BY KWAI-FUNG, SWATOW.

REPORT.

FROM various causes I have been hindered from submitting earlier a report of the work that has been done in the Swatow Mission Hospital during the past year. It is not necessary to enter into details. The Statistics given below will show that a good deal of work has been accomplished, and on the whole it has been a successful year.

STATISTICS.

Number of Individual Patients:—		
In-patients	2958	
Out-patients	2926	
Total	5884	
Females included in above		1017
Visits to Chinese patients in their own homes ...		227
Daily average number of In-patients...		180
Average attendance of Out-patients on dispensary days		55
Total number of visits of Out-patients to the Dispensary (Incomplete)		8913
Number of Surgical Operations		1026

Dr. Henry Layng has regularly throughout the year helped greatly in the Surgical work; and assistance was rendered by Dr. Cousland at various times when not engaged in his own mission work in the city of Ch'ao-chow-fu.

A Chinese merchant in Swatow, who has taken a

deep interest in the hospital for many years and whose wife was under my treatment some time ago, has asked me to build a number of wards for women, entirely separated from the General Hospital for men, and towards the cost of which he offered to give $1000. His offer was accepted by the Mission. Since then he has collected more than $2000, which, I understand, has been placed in the Bank and will be handed over to me as soon as I see my way to begin building. The only condition he makes is that a number of small wards be provided for renting to women belonging to the wealthier classes, so that they need not mix with all and sundry. So far, I have not been able to build owing to the difficulty of getting additional ground near the present Hospital, and, also, as I wish to obtain a considerably larger sum in order to make various alterations in the administrative department which will enable me to manage the work more easily.

The liberal contributions of the Foreign Community have enabled me to end the year with a favourable balance in hand. To them and to the Chinese subscribers my thanks are due for their kindly help.

I purpose, with the consent of my colleagues, withdrawing a sum of $500 from the general fund and placing it to the "Women's Hospital" fund. This sum was originally received for medical services rendered to the Foreign Community, and was placed by me to the credit of the Hospital.

I take this opportunity of thanking Tang-nguan-seng for his annual contribution of rice and cash tickets for distribution among the poorer patients. These to the value of more than $100 were received during the year, and many poor patients were thus enabled to remain in the hospital until their cures were completed.

EVANGELISTIC.

Since the year closed the Hospital has lost a good and true friend by the death of the Rev. George Smith. Whenever in Swatow Mr. Smith allowed nothing to interfere with his missionary work among the patients, and he was unwearied in his efforts to teach those who were interested in the Gospel.

Besides the usual services by Missionaries and native assistants, classes for the women and boys have been regularly carried on during the year, principally by the Misses Black and Harkness. These efforts have been attended with a considerable amount of success. Notes of some of the more interesting cases of conversion have been already published in the China Medical Missionary Journal.

SURGICAL OPERATIONS.

On the Eye:—

Operations for Entropion and Trichiasis	357
" " Trichiasis (by Electrolysis)	42
" " Ectropion	4
" " Hernia of Iris	3
" " Hypopyon	1
" " Symblepharon	1
" " Cicatricial Contraction of upper Eyelid	1
" " Pterygium	58
Peritomy for Pannus	4
Cataract.—Extraction of	17
" Needling after Extraction	2
" Iridotomy " "	2
Iridectomy	14
Excision of Subconjunctival Growths	5
" " Sebaceous, Dermoid Cysts etc. from Eyelid	9
Enucleation of Eye	1
Abscission of Anterior Staphyloma	3
Incision of Meibomian Cysts...	3
Canaliculus—Slitting up	2
	529

On the Body generally:—

Lateral Lithotomy	2
Extraction of Vesical Calculus in Girl	1
Perineal Section	4
Operations for Harelip	31
,, ,, Fistula in Ano	77
,, ,, Phymosis (Circumcision)	18
,, ,, Caries	4
,, ,, Repair of Split Ear	27
,, ,, Ganglion	8
,, ,, Sinuses...	7
,, ,, Stricture of Anus	1
,, ,, Hypospadios	1
,, ,, Buboes...	3
,, ,, Fissure of Rectum	1
,, ,, Cicatricial Occlusion of Nostrils ...	1
,, ,, ,, ,, ,, Vagina ...	2
,, ,, Ununited Fracture of Humerus ...	1
,, ,, Cyst of Antrum	1
,, ,, Cystic Goitre	1
Plastic Operation on Ear	2
,, ,, ,, Nostril...	1
Amputation of leg	1
,, ,, Foot (Choparts')	1
,, ,, Foot (Syme's)	1
,, ,, Penis	8
,, ,, Forearm	1
,, ,, Fingers	3
,, ,, Supernumerary Thumb	1
,, ,, Toes	3
,, ,, Elephantiasis of Scrotum	4
Extraction of Nasal Polypus...	14
,, ,, Sequestra	30
,, ,, Bamboo Splinters &c...	3
,, ,, Fish Bone from Oesophagus	1
Arthrectomy of Knee	1

Tapping Hydrops Articuli	1
„ Ovarian Cyst	1
„ and Injecting Hydrocele	37
Tying Internal Haemorrhoids	46
Exploratory Incision	1
Opening large Abscesses	6
Excision of Callosities	11
„ „ External Haemorrhoids...	19
„ „ Scars of Face	2
„ „ Epithelioma of Skin	1
„ „ „ „ Prepuce...	1
„ „ „ „ Lip	1
„ „ Cuneiform & 2nd & 3rd Metatarsal Bones	1
„ „ Condylomata	4
„ „ Epulis	2
„ „ Soft Fibroma	1
„ „ Fibrous Tumour...	1
„ „ Glandular „	4
„ „ Fatty „	8
„ „ Sarcomatous „	3
„ „ Sebaceous Cysts &c.	19
„ „ Dermoid Cyst	1
„ „ Granuloma	4
„ „ Papilloma of Rectum	1
„ „ „ „ Tonsil	1
„ „ Polypus of Rectum	3
„ „ Cystic Tumours	3
„ „ „ „ of Tongne (Congenital)	1
„ „ Hydrocele of Neck	2
„ „ Scirrhus of Female Breast	3
„ „ Sarcoma „ „ „	3
„ „ Recurrent Tumour of Female Breast ...	1
„ „ Parotid Tumour...	1
„ „ Soft Fibroma of Vulvum	2
„ „ Tumour (Unclassed)	4
Electrolysis of Keloid...	3
„ „ Naevus	2
Sundry Minor Operations	30
	497
Extraction of Teeth	138

The above list represents substantially the surgical work accomplished on operation days—Wednesdays and Saturdays. A considerable amount of minor surgery, such as opening abscesses, stitching wounds, skin grafting, dilating urethral and rectal strictures, setting fractures, reducing dislocations, etc. was done on other days, but of this work no record was kept. There were two deaths after operation during the year. (1) A case of complete obliteration of vagina after difficult parturition nineteen years ago. The operation performed was a pretty severe one, and was followed by a low form of pelvic peritonitis. The patient was removed from the hospital in a moribund condition about a fortnight after the operation and died shortly afterwards. (2) Died from Tetanus after amputation of the forearm for injury of the hand. The hand had been literally blown to pieces by the bursting of a small dynamite bomb. Amputation through the forearm was performed, and the wound was healed except a small sinus where the drainage tube had been inserted, when tetanus set in on the eleventh day. These "toy" dynamite bombs are sometimes used by the Chinese for killing fish in the village ponds, and last year no fewer than four cases of severe injury of the hand, caused by the bursting of these bombs from incautious handling, were under treatment.

Internal Haemorrhoids.—Since 1880 we have treated 415 cases of Internal Haemorrhoids by operation, mostly by trying. I have tried various other methods of treatment but have always reverted to the old one of tying, which, in my experience is as successful as any other. So far as I can recollect no complication beyond a temporary retention of urine has occurred in any case.

Vesical Calculus.—Three cases. (1) A boy of six years, calculus 85 grs. in weight removed by lateral lithotomy. (2) A young man, aged 26 years, who had suffered from urinary symptoms since his third year. I crushed the calculus by means of the lithotrite, but during the operation the gum-elastic aspirator gave way Three or four days afterwards lateral lithotomy was performed, and the bladder was cleared out with some difficulty. The patient made a good recovery, but a perineal fistula remained for three months which eventually healed all right. The calculus weighed 2 ozs. 4½ drms. (3) A girl aged eight years, the urethra was slightly incised, then dilated, and a calculus 280 grains in weight was extracted. No incontinence of urine resulted.

Large Tumours.—The following large tumours were sucessfully removed:—

Elephantiasis of Scrotum	......12 lbs	in weight.
,, ,,	...... 7 lbs 2 ozs	,,
,, ,,	...... 4 lbs 13½ozs	,,
,, ,,	...... 2½lbs	,,
Cysto-Sarcoma of Female Breast	12⅓lbs	,,
Parotid Tumour	.... 2 lbs 5 ozs	,,
Soft Fibroma of Groin	........., 2½lbs	,,
,, ,, ,, Labium	...... 5 lbs 13½ozs	,,

Cataract.—Seventeen cases. In one case some vitreous escaped during the operation and Iritis set in on the third day Iridotomy was twice performed on the eye with a fairly good result. In another case the operation was a failure. In fifteen cases the result was satisfactory.

SUBSCRIPTIONS FOR 1890.

Rev. Prof. Blaikie, D.D., L.L.D. (£10)	$61.73
Messrs. Lauts & Haesloop	75.00
„ Bradley & Co.	50.00
„ Butterfield & Swire	50.00
„ Jardine, Matheson & Co.	50.00
China Sugar Refining Company, Limited	50.00
R. H. Hill	50.00
Thank Offering	50.00
E. Eagger	30.00
Mrs. W. E. Allum	30.00
Rev. P. J. Maclagan, M.A.	30.00
Rev. George Smith, M.A.	30.00
A Silent Donor	25.00
M. H.	25.00
Ivo Streich	25.00
H. Matchitt	25.00
Wm. Paton	25.00
Rev. J. C. Gibson, M.A.	25.00
Dr. Henry Layng	25.00
Dr. A. Lyall	25.00
W. E. Allum	20.00
Mrs. Wm. Pollock	18.00
Otto Asverus	15.00
E. B.	15.00
A. Frater	15 00
J. W. Innocent	15.00
Rev. H. L. Mackenzie, M.A.	15.00
David Landale	10.00
C. H. Palmer	10.00
L. Grunauer	10.00
Dr. John Stewart, Pictou, Nova Scotia	6.14
Flower Show Fund—balance of—per R. L. R.	6.78
Drummond Anderson	5.00
F. Barre	5.00

J. J. Ruben	5.00
A. G. H. Curruthers	5.00
G. B. A. Castro	5.00
A. Johnsen	5.00
E. P.	5.00
King Yung	5.00
F. Cartman	3.00
Geo. A. Forsaith	3.00
Unknown Contributor	2.00
Swatow Presbyterian Church	25.00
Tsan Tai Von per B. & Co.	25.00
Lim Yam Seng...	25.00
A Patient (fee)	20.00
Siao A Nap per Messrs. L. & H.	15.00
Liao Too Sang	15 00
Yong Seng Fat per Messrs. B. & S. ...	10.00
Kho Buey Tso „ „ „	10 00
Wong Seu Yeuk „ „ „ ...	10.00
Chip Seng	10.00
Ben	5.00
Fong To Pui	5.00
Ho Pin Wen	5.00
Tai Tsze Keng	5.00
Lam Tat Hing	5.00
Ding Shao Lin	5.00
Ko Leang Sz	5 00
Ho Kam Un	3.00
Lan Tek	2.00
Lau Su Keng	2.00
Kwai Fung	2.00
Wong Tai	2.00
Tshai Nguan	2.00
Patients	2.00
Hospital Box	4.00
	$1180.25

STATEMENT OF INCOME AND EXPENDITURE.

By Balance from last year	$1014.74
„ Donations European	960 65
„ Do. Chinese	219.60
„ Grant from Mission Committee in Edinburgh (Drugs)	406.00
„ Receipts from Opium Smokers	62.94
„ Rent of Wards	33.87
„ Sales of Drugs, Trusses, &c.	948.28
	$3646.08

To Wages	$326.11
„ General Expenses	148.10
„ Repairs on Buildings	24.51
„ Aid to poor patients and burial expenses	112.94
„ Cloth, Wools, Oils, Lard, &c.	234.84
„ Water	131 94
„ Drugs, Rectified Spirit bought in China	477.65
„ Drugs, Surgical Dressing, Instruments, etc. from London	1230.15
„ Balance in hand	909.84
	$3646.08

Audited and found correct.

D. MACIVER.

REPORT

OF THE

MISSION HOSPITAL

AT

SWATOW

IN CONNECTION WITH THE

PRESBYTERIAN CHURCH OF ENGLAND,

UNDER THE CARE OF

ALEXANDER LYALL, M.B., C.M.

For 1891.

Printed by KWAI FUNG,
SWATOW.

REPORT

THE year 1891 has been the most unhealthy of all the years I have lived in Swatow. The statistics, however, show a slight decrease in the total number of patients applying for treatment in the Mission Hospital. This was due to the prevalence of Cholera during the summer, which practically stops patients coming from the more distant parts of the Region. Thus, in the months of September and October when usually the work is very heavy; it was this year comparatively light. As in former Epidemics of Cholera, the hospital remained comparatively free of the disease, though it was prevalent in Swatow for two or three months. Some cases were brought to the hospital, a few patients were seized with the disease, but it did not spread in the wards.

I have to acknowledge with grateful thanks the generous subscriptions from the Foreign Community and from a number of Chinese friends towards the support of the work; and, also, the kindly assistance of Dr. Henry Layng who has come regularly twice a week to help in the Surgical work. Dr. John Lang took charge of the Hospital during the month of July. Our thanks are also due to all who have helped in the Christian work which has been regularly carried on among the patients, and for the gift of rice and cash from the Tang Nguan Seng hong for the benefit of poor patients.

In last year's report I mentioned that it was my intention to build a separate Hospital for the women. I am sorry to report that no progress has been made towards the fulfilment of my desire, owing to the difficulty of obtaining a suitable site. The Tao-tai has refused us the site adjoining the hospital which I wished to obtain, so we will require to look elsewhere for what we wish.

Below, I give the Statistics for the year and shall leave them to speak for themselves.

Number of Individual Patients:—

In-patients	2670
Out-patients	2991
Total	5661

Females included in above	847
Visits to Chinese patients in their own homes	300
Daily average number of In-patients	172
Average attendance of Out-patients on dispensary days	55
Total number of visits of Out-patients to the dispensary (Incomplete)	10106
Number of Surgical operations	845

SURGICAL OPERATIONS.

On the Eye:—

Operations for Entropion and Trichiasis	221
" " Trichiasis (by Electrolysis)	54
" " Pterygium	30
" " Symblepharon	1
" " Hernia Iris	3
" " Anterior Staphyloma	7
" " Hypertrophied Tarsal Cartilage	5
Peritomy for Pannus	1

Iridectomy for Artificial Pupil	33
„ Glaucoma &c., ...	6
Cataract.—Extraction of	7
Excision of Subconjunctival Growths	2
„ Cyst of Eyelid	1
Incision of Meibomian Cyst	4
Canthoplasty	4
Plastic Operation on upper and lower Eyelids ...	1
Slitting up Canaliculus	1
Excision of Fungating Tumour of upper Eyelid ...	1
„ „ Malignant Tumour of Eye	1
Extraction of Foreign body from Cornea	2
	385

On the Body generally:—

Lithotomy—Suprapubic	1
„ Lateral	1
Urethral Calculus lodged—Extraction of	2
Perineal Section	2
Operations for Harelip	24
„ „ Repair of Split Ear	24
„ „ Fistula in Ano	99
„ „ Phymosis (Circumcision)	16
„ „ Recto—Vaginal Fistula	1
„ „ Cicatricial Occlusion of Vagina ...	2
„ „ „ „ „ Nostrils ...	1
„ „ „ Contraction of Knee ...	1
„ „ „ „ „ Hip ...	1
„ „ Imperforate Anus	1
„ „ Salivary Fistula	1
„ „ Cyst of Antrum	1
„ „ Ununited Fracture of Humerus ...	1
„ „ Sinuses	17
„ „ Ganglion	6
„ „ Ranula	1

Operations for Compound Fracture of Leg	1
,, ,, ,, Dislocation of Finger	1
,, ,, Wound of Tongue	1
,, ,, Fissure of Rectum	1
Excision of Callosities	12
,, ,, External Haemorrhoids	24
,, ,, Testicle	2
,, ,, Congenital Hypertrophy of Gum	1
,, ,, Polypus of Rectum	1
,, ,, Tumours.—Lipoma	7
,, ,, ,, Sebaceous Cysts	7
,, ,, ,, Granuloma	3
,, ,, ,, Epulis	4
,, ,, ,, Fibroma	1
,, ,, ,, Parotid	4
,, ,, ,, Cystic	5
,, ,, ,, of Palate	1
,, ,, ,, Malignant of Female Breast	3
,, ,, ,, ,, ,, Male ,,	1
,, ,, ,, Sarcoma	2
,, ,, ,, Unclassed	6
,, ,, Compound Palmar Ganglion	1
,, ,, Ganglion	1
,, ,, Fungus Testis	1
,, ,, Submaxillary Glands	2
Amputation of Fingers	3
,, ,, Toe	2
,, ,, Thigh	1
,, ,, Lower $\frac{1}{3}$ of Leg	1
,, ,, Penis (Epithelioma)	3
,, ,, Elephantiasis of Scrotum	4
,, ,, Leg	1
Extraction of Nasal Polypus	7
,, ,, Sequestra	30
,, ,, Fish Bone from Oesophagus	1

Tapping Ovarian Cyst	1
„ Hydrops Articuli	1
„ and Injecting Hydrocele	22
Aspirating Knee Joint	3
Tying Internal Haemorrhoids	47
Opening large Acute Abscesses	7
Hip Joint Disease—Enlaging Sinuses and Draining	1
Electrolysis of Naevus	2
Sundry minor operations	27
	400
Extraction of Teeth (incomplete)	101

SUBSCRIPTIONS FOR 1891.

Messrs. Bradley & Co.	$50.00
" Butterfield & Swire	50.00
" Jardine, Matheson & Co.	50.00
" Lauts & Haesloop	50.00
China Sugar Refining Co., Ltd. per J. M. & Co.	50.00
Rev. P. J. Maclagan, M.A.	30.00
Miss Black	25.00
Miss Harkness	25.00
Rev. Wm. Duffus	25.00
Henry Layng, M.R.C.S.	25.00
A. Lyall, M.B.C.M.	25.00
Wm. Paton	25.00
Ivo Streich	25.00
H. G. Dowler	20.00
O. Asverus	15.00
A. Frater	15.00
Rev. H. L. Mackenzie, M.A.	15.00
C. Lenox Simpson	15.00
W. A. Cruickshank	10.00
J. H. C. Günther	10.00
J. W. Innocent	10.00
David Landale	10.00
J. D. Munro	10.00
Rev. J. Spencer Norvell	10.00
Captain Sellar	10.00
H. E. Shadgett	10.00
F. Barre	5.00
P. F. Grovedon	5.00
J. Ruben	5.00
Henry Sage	5.00
G. A. Forsaith	3.00
V. Ferreira	2.00
J. Martin	2.00

G. B. A. Castro	1.00
E. Milbe	1.00
Cash per H. Sage	1.50
"Fine" per E. Milbe	4.00
Fees per Dr. Lyall	18.00
Flower Show Committee per D. Landale ...	3.23
	$670.73

CHINESE.

Tsang Tai Wen	$25.00
Ee-Kee Tang Sing Huat	25.00
Swatow Presbyterian Church	25.00
Siao Ah Kim	20.00
Siao Ah Nap	15.00
Steam Launch Company, per Sim Kye Pank ...	10.00
Liao Too Sang	10.00
Chip Sing	10.00
Chan Yeak Ying	5.00
Ko Leang Sy	5.00
Ben	5.00
Fong To Pui	5.00
Tai Tze King	5.00
Tan Pi	5.00
Ho Kam un	3.00
T. Lam	2.00
Seng	2.00
Kwai Fung	2.00
Eng Tshai Nguan	2.00
Tan Kin Cheng	2.00
Leung Yee San	1.00
Ki Peng	1.00
Patients	0.30
	$194.30

Tang Nguan Seng Hong Rice and Rice Tickets to the value of more than $100.00.

STATEMENT OF INCOME & EXPENDITURE.

To Wages	$377.00	By Balance from 1890	$909.84
,, General Expenses	137.20	,, Contributions and Fees as per List ...	865.03
,, Repairs on Buildings	169.33	,, Donation from Messrs Lauts & Haesloop for patient	9.25
,, Drugs bought in China	384.82	,, Sales of Drugs	999.98
,, Drugs, Surgical Dressing and instruments from London	919 11	,, Sales of Trusses, Bottles and Sundries	124.45
,, Do. paid by Mission Committee in Edinburgh	493.75	,, Payments from Opium patients	84.00
,, Aid to poor patients	32.84	,, Rent of Private Wards	16.90
,, Burial Expenses	57.29	,, Grant from Mission Committee in Edinburgh	493.75
,, Cotton, Wool, and Bandage Cloth ...	139.79		
,, Water for Hospital	129.90		
,, Lard, Wax and Oils	129.10		
,, Paper	15.61		
,, Transferred to New Building a/c	500.00		
,, Balance in hand	17.46		
	$3,503.20		$3,503.20

Audited and found correct.

D. MacIver.

NEW BUILDINGS A/C.

By Donation from Miss Scott, London ...	$ 19.20
,, Transferred from General Hospital Funds	$500.00
	$519.20

Audited and found correct.

D. MacIver.

REPORT

OF THE

MISSION HOSPITAL

AT

SWATOW

IN CONNECTION WITH THE

PRESBYTERIAN CHURCH OF ENGLAND,

UNDER THE CARE OF

ALEXANDER LYALL, M.B., C.M

For 1892 and 1893.

Printed by Kwai Fung,

Swatow.

REPORT.

No Report was published for 1892. Therefore in this Report will be found the Statistics, names of Subscribers, and a statement of Income and Expenditure for 1892 and 1893. In both years the work has been very heavy, and at certain seasons the number of applicants for admission quite outnumbered the available accommodation,—though Mission Hospitals in the South of China are somewhat elastic and Chinese patients not difficult to please in the matter of space. This explains why, with a considerably greater total number of patients, the number of in-patients has not materially increased. I am glad to say that sufficient funds are now in hand for a separate Women's Hospital: but a suitable site is still to be found. The foreshore to the west of the present buildings would satisfy most requirements; but the native authorities refuse to rent us this ground. In the collecting of the money at home for the proposed new Hospital I am entireiy indebted to Miss Black; and I now tender her my grateful thanks and trust we shall make a good use of the funds obtained through her kind advocacy.

STATISTICS.

Number of Individual Patients :—

	1892	*1893*
In-patients	2544	2766
Out-patients	4115	4586
Total	6659	7352

	1892	1893
Females included in above	1209	1317
Visits to Chinese patients in their own homes	325	371
Daily average number of in-patients ...	157	176
Average attendance of out-patients on dispensary day	67	73
Total number of visits of out-patients to the dispensary (incomplete)	11872	13237
Number of Surgical Operations	984	1118

Lately we have added to the staff a native colporteur and a biblewoman. Some ten years ago we employed a colporteur for some time to follow up old patients. His work was not a success. Being employed exclusively in travelling about the country he was not recognised by old patients as belonging to the Hospital, and so lost any advantage which connection with the Hospital might have given him. This time we are going to try another plan. It is proposed that he give a good part of his time to work in the Hospital, selling books, teaching patients—individually and in classes—to read some Gospel tracts and the Hymn book. Occasionally, also, he will take trips into the country to look up old patients, especially those who have shown some interest in the Truth, and whom he has helped to teach. We hope that thereby he will be recognised as belonging to the Hospital staff and treated as an old friend by those whom he visits. The B. and F. Bible Society have undertaken to pay half of his salary.

The work of the biblewoman is thus sketched by one of the ladies of the Mission. "To work among the women a Biblewoman has been engaged whose duties are in the main two-fold. One is to teach the brighter ones to read simple tracts, and the Hymn book, or as much of it as may be learned during their limited stay in the Hospital. To this work the Biblewoman is expected to devote the afternoons, while her morning hours are given to work in the wards among those who cannot leave their beds; the old, the stupid, the blind, and the partially deaf being her special care. It is hoped that through the faithful discharge of her duties few women will leave the Hospital without some knowledge of the Gospel. The Biblewoman is herself one of the fruits of the Hospital. Less than six years ago she entered it as a heathen, and was for months intellectually convinced of the Truth of the Gospel before her heart was touched. Since then she has made such advancement in intellectual and spiritual knowledge that she commended herself as suitable for the work indicated. In connection with the evangelistic work, classes have been maintained during the years by the agents of the W. M. A.; and other ladies have more or less constantly visited the females' wards, and have done good work.

As in previous years Dr. Henry Layng has helped in the Surgical work, and for two months in 1893 he kindly took a general oversight of the Hospital during my absence in Japan. Dr. Cousland has also helped at times when not engaged in Ch'no-chow-foo.

To the subscribers towards the funds of the Hospital we tender our grateful thanks. The Tang Nguan Seng hong have continued their gift of rice and cash tickets for impecunious patients. Annually this amounts to about $100; but when one supply of tickets is exhausted another is at once forthcoming, so the limit of their generosity has never been reached. It is unnecessary to point out that this benefaction is greatly valued by those patients who participate in it, and also by myself.

In the beginning of March I leave on furlough, and during my absence Dr. P. B. Cousland will be in charge.

SUBSCRIPTIONS FOR 1892.

Messrs. Bradley & Co.	$50.00
„ Butterfield & Swire	50.00
„ Jardine, Matheson & Co.	50.00
„ Lauts & Haesloop	50.00
China Sugar Refining Co., Ltd. per J. M. & Co.	50.00
Rev. P. J. Maclagan, M.A.	30.00
Proportion of Fine per Messrs. J. M. & Co. ...	25.00
Miss Harkness	25.00
Henry Layng, M.R.C.S.	25.00
A. Lyall, M.B.C.M.	25.00
Wm. Paton	25.00
Ivo Streich	25.00
murdo Rev. ~~H.~~ L. Mackenzie, M.A.	20.00
Billiard Handicap prize per D. R. Law	15.30
A. Frater	15.00
C. Lenox Simpson	15.00
J. H. C. Günther	10.00
J. W. Innocent	10.00
J. D. Munro	10.00
A. Bryson...	10.00
Do.	5.00
W. Ford (Fee)	10.00
D. R. Law...	10.00
F. Barre	5.00
G. A. Bowman	5.00
Rev. J. Carlin, D. D.	5.00
V. Larsen	5.00
P. E. Milhe	5.00
Graham Rome	5.00
H. E. Shadgett	5.00
J. Williams	5.00
S. Wakefield	4.00
F. A. Cartman	3.00
V. Ferreira	3.00
J. Martin	2.00

CHINESE.

Tsan Tai Von	$25.00
Swatow Presbyterian Church (native)	25.00
L. Yam Seng	25.00
Siao Ah Kiam	20.00
Siau Tai Loan	15.00
Tai Tze Kim	10.00
Chip Seng	10.00
Ko Tai Chu	10.00
Liao Tsze Sang	10.00
Tshua Si Lau	9.00
Anonymous	8.00
Chau Yeuk Ying	5.00
Ko Leang Sy	5.00
Ben	5.00
Fang To Pui	5.00
Ding Shao Lin	5.00
Wong Tai Ping	5.00
Tan Siau Huan	4.00
S. Kye Pang	3.00
Ho Kam im	3.00
Lam Tat Hing	3.00
Kwai Fung	2.00
Eng Tshai Nguan...	2.00
Ngau M	2.00
Ki Iau	2.00
Chie Tsu Tek	2.00
Tang Seng Sim	2.00
Ma Seng	1.00
A. Sui	1.00
Patients	**11.00**
Hospital Box	**3.82**

(6)

STATEMENT OF INCOME & EXPENDITURE for 1892.

To Wages	$397.69	By Balance from 1891	$17.46
„ General Expenses	79.42	„ Contributions and Fees as per List	876.12
„ Repairs on Buildings	261.12	„ Sales of Drugs	963.24
„ Drugs bought in China	214.25	„ Sales of Trusses, Bottles and Sundries	113.46
„ Drugs, Surgical Dressings and instruments from London	719.94	„ Payments from Opium patients	85.00
„ Do. paid by Mission Committee	648.00	„ Rent of Private Wards	16.95
„ Water	140.14	„ Grant from Mission Committee	648.00
„ Cotton, Wool, and Bandage Cloth	150.69	„ Balance ~~in hand~~	136.82
„ Lard, Wax and Oils	118.08	due Treasurer	
„ Paper and Sundries	40.80		
„ Aid to poor patients	48.22		
„ Burial Expenses	38.70		
	$2,857.05		$2,857.05

New Building Account.

By Cash in hand $519.20

Audited and found correct.

J. Steele.

SUBSCRIPTIONS FOR 1893.

Dr. Henry Layng	$75.00
Messrs. Bradley & Co.	50.00
„ Butterfield & Swire	50.00
„ Jardine, Matheson & Co. per D. M. ...	50.00
China Sugar Refining Co., Ltd. Do. ...	50.00
A. Lyall, M.B.	50.00
Rev. T. E. Sandeman, M.A.	50.00
Messrs. Lauts & Haesloop	40.00
Rev. J. L. Milne B.D.	30.00
Wm. Paton	27.00
Miss Harkness	25.00
D. R. Law	10.00
B. C. George Scott	25.00
Rev. J. Steele, B.A.	25.00
Ivo Streich	25.00
W. B. Porter	20.00
C. Lenox Simpson	20.00
Donation per Mrs. Foster	15.00
Rev. H. L. Mackenzie, M.A.	15.00
H. Asverus	10.00
L. Grunauer	10.00
J. H. C. Günther	10.00
A. E. Hodgins	10.00
J. W. Innocent	10.00
Graham Rome	10.00
F. Barre	5.00
Rev. W. H. Brodt	5.00
G. C. Bowman	5.00
A. Bryson	5.00
Alex. W. Cross	5.00
S. Wakefield	5.00
V. Ferreira	3.00
Fee per D. L.	10.00
	770.00

1892—1893年汕头福音医院报告

CHINESE.

Tan Hou Teng (for medical attendance) ...	$100.00
Siau Tai Loan per L. & H.	40.00
Tsan Tai Von per B. & Co.	25.00
L. Yam Seng	25.00
Swatow Presbyterian Church	25.00
Compradore, J. M. & Co. per D. M.	20.00
Ng Boon Po per L. G.	20.00
Ko Tai Chu ,, ...	10.00
Ko Leang Sy ,, ...	10.00
Tai Koo ,, ...	10.00
Lim Hee	10.00
Tai Tze Keng	10.00
Chip Seng	10.00
Chia Siah In	10.00
Sim Chi Hun (patient)	8.00
L. C. J. T.	8.00
Lim Pai Lam per L. & H.	8.00
Chin Tai Li	8.00
Ding Shao Lin per L. G.	5.00
Chau Yeuk Ying ,, ...	5.00
Wong Tai Peng ,, ...	5.00
Ben	5.00
Phua Sin-se	5.00
Fang To Pui	5.00
Ho Kam-iin	3.00
S. Kye Pang	3.00
Lim Tat Hing	3.00
Eng Tshai Nguan...	3.00
~~Kwei Fang~~	~~2.00~~
Ma Seng	2.00
Sim Tsong	2.00
Chhiu Tshing-tsha	2.00
Pho Ti	2.00
Tan Nie-meng	2.00
Khou-Kim-zu	2.00
Ki Iau	1.00
Patients	31.05
	445.05

STATEMENT OF INCOME & EXPENDITURE for 1893.

To	Balance from 1892 a/c	$136.82	By Contributions and Fees as per List	$1213.05
,,	Wages	421.98	,, Sales of Drugs	935.82
,,	General Expenses	124.99	,, Sales of Trusses, Bottles and Sundries	162.77
,,	Repairs on Buildings	49.59	,, Payments from Opium patients	51.00
,,	Drugs bought in China	191.32	,, Rent of Private Wards	19.95
,,	Drugs, Surgical Dressings and instruments from London	392.54	,, Grant from Mission Committee	744.00
,,	Do. paid by Mission Committee	744.00		
,,	Paper and Sundries	55.36		
,,	Aid to poor patients	30.47		
,,	Burial Expenses	48.17		
,,	Water	131.97		
,,	Lard, Wax and Oils	174.54		
,,	Cotton, Wool, and Bandage Cloth	202.07		
,,	Rectified Spirit for Finctures &c.	248.26		
,,	Balance in hand	174.51		
		$3,126.59		$3,126.59

New Building Account.

By Cash in hand $519.20

Audited and found correct.

JOHN STEELE.

SURGICAL OPERATIONS in 1892.

On the Eye:—

Operations for Entropion and Trichiasis	272
,, ,, Trichiasis (by Electrolysis)	43
,, ,, Pterygium	44
,, ,, Hernia Iris	3
Cataract.—Extraction of	26
Iridectomy for Artificial Pupil	27
,, ,, Glaucoma	2
Peritomy for Pannus	1
Excision of Sub-Conjunctival Growths	3
,, ,, Cysts &c. of Eyelids	7
Abscision of Anterior Staphyloma	1
Plastic Operations on Eyelids	3
Extraction of Foreign Body from Cornea	4
Incision of Meibomian Cysts	5
	441

On the Body generally:—

Lithotomy—Median	1
,, Lateral	2
Urethral Calculus lodged—Extraction of	2
Ovariotomy	1
External Urethrotomy	5
Internal ,, ...	1
Sequestrotomy ~~Urethrotomy~~	42
Operations for Harelip	20
,, ,, Fistula in Ano	84
,, ,, Split Ear Lobule	33
,, ,, Cicatricial Contraction of Urethral Orifice	1
,, ,, ,, ,, Nostrils ...	1
,, ,, ,, ,, Anus ...	2
,, ,, Epithelioma of Upper Lip	1
,, ,, ,, ,, Skin	1
,, ,, ,, ,, Fingers	1
,, ,, ,, ,, Wrist	1
,, ,, ,, ,, Knee	1
,, ,, Imperforate Anus	1
,, ,, Polypus of Ear	2
,, ,, Aural Fistula	1
,, ,, Paraphymosis	2

Operations for Phymosis (Circumcision)	18
,, ,, ,, (slitting up)	1
,, ,, Ranula	3
,, ,, Sinuses	14
,, ,, Haematocele	3
,, ,, Procidentia Recti	2
Amputation of Fingers	7
,, ,, Hand (partial)	1
,, ,, Forearm	2
,, ,, Supernumerary Thumb	1
,, ,, Penis (Epithelioma)	3
,, ,, Leg	2
,, ,, Toe	1
,, ,, Elephantiasis Scroti	7
Excision of Callosities	19
,, ,, External Haemorrhoids	15
,, ,, Testicle	1
,, ,, Tumours—Sebaceous Cysts	26
,, ,, ,, Mucous Cysts	3
,, ,, ,, Hydrocele of Neck ...	1
,, ,, ,, Dermoid Cyst	1
,, ,, ,, Bursa	3
,, ,, ,, Cyst of Female Breast ...	1
,, ,, ,, Angeioma	2
,, ,, ,, Haematoma	2
,, ,, ,, Enlarged Tonsils	3
,, ,, ,, Epulis	3
,, ,, ,, Polypus of Rectum ...	2
,, ,, ,, Lipoma	3
,, ,, ,, Papilloma	1
,, ,, ,, Sarcoma	4
,, ,, ,, Granuloma	2
,, ,, ,, Parotid	4
,, ,, ,, Fibroma	4
,, ,, ,, Glandula of Neck	1
,, ,, Head of Femur	1
Extraction of Nasal Polypus	23
,, ,, Large Naso-pharyngeal Polypus ...	1
,, ,, Bullets lodged	4
,, ,, Splinters, Needles	9
,, ,, Fishbone from Oesophagus	2
Tying Internal Haemorrhoids	50
Tapping and injecting Hydrocele	15
,, ,, ,, Cystic Goitre	1

Plastic Operation on Forehead	1
" " on Nose	1
" " on Lip	1
" " on Ear	1
Stretching Ulnar Nerve for Leprosy	1
Sundry Minor Operations	60
	543

Extraction of Teeth 224

SURGICAL OPERATIONS in 1888.

On the Eye:—

Operations for Entropion and Trichiasis	229
" " Ectropion	1
" " Pterygium	47
" " Symblepharon	5
Cataract—Extraction of	[illegible]
" Secondary Operations	[illegible]
Iridectomy	28
Excision of Cyst of Orbit	1
" " Eyelids	7
" of Congenital Growth of Cornea ...	1
" of Malignant " Orbit ...	1
Enucleation of Eye (Staphyloma)	1
Abscision of Anterior Staphyloma	3
Peritomy for Pannus	1
Canthoplasty	2
Plastic Operation on upper Eyelid	1
Minor Operations unclassed	6
	490

On the Body generally:—

Tying Internal Haemorrhoids	**48**
Tapping and Injecting Hydrocele	**38**
" " " Goitre	**1**
" Ascites	**1**
" Acute Synovitis of Knee Joint	**1**
Sequestrotomy	**40**
External Urethrotomy	**6**

Lithotomy—Lateral	3
Ovariotomy	1
Laparotomy	2
Electrolysis of Keloid	3
Plastic Operation on Ear	1
Arthrectomy of Knee Joint	1
Plastic Operation on Palate	1
Amputation of Arm	1
" " Fingers and Toes	3
" " lower 1/3 of Leg	2
" " Foot (partial for Congenital Hypertrophy) ...	1
" " Supernumerary Thumb	1
" " " Toe (6th) ...	1
Excision of Elephantiasis Scroti	7
" " Lymph Scrotum	1
" " Epulis	3
" " 1st and 2nd Metatarsal Scaphoid and Astragalus Bones ...	1
" " Hypertrophied Male Breast	1
" " Angeioma	1
" " Neuroma	1
" " Carbuncle	1
" " Callosities	23
" " External Haemorrhoids	25
" " Sebaceous Cysts	33
" " Haematoma	2
" " Lipoma	3
" " Epithelioma of Prepuce	2
" " Strumous Glands	3
" " Pericondrial Cysts	2
" " Parotid Tumours	2
" " Fibroma	4
" " Sarcoma	5
" " Granuloma	3
" " Sublingual Cysts	2
" " Testicles (Sarcoma)	2
" " Glandular Tumours	3
" " Tumours unclassed	8
" " Elbow Joint	1
Operations for Fistula in Ano	103
" " Phymosis (Circumcision)	18
" " " (Slitting up)	1
" " Harelip	30

Operations for	Slit Ear Lobule ...	... ...	38
„ „	Caries of Bones...	... ...	8
„ „	Sinuses	... ...	9
„ „	Cicatricial Contraction of Anus	...	2
„ „ „	Occlusion of Auditory Canal		1
„ „ „ „	of Nostrils	...	2
„ „ „	Contraction of Knee and Ankle		1
„ „	Congenital small Anus	... ...	1
„ „	Hip Joint Disease (Draining)	...	5
Extraction of	Polypus of Nose	... ...	18
„ „	Needles and Splinters	... ...	5
„ „	Fish Bone from Oesophagus	...	1
Sundry Minor	Operations	... ...	92
			628

Extraction of Teeth 240

Ovariotomy.—Two cases have been operated on, one successfully, the other ending fatally on the 27th day after operation. The successful case was certainly the more difficult operation, there being many adhesions. The cause of death in the second case was doubtful but it pointed to an inflammatory complication of the large bowel. There were few adhesions, but the tumour was sessile and adherent to the uterus, and the lower portion of the large bowel was greatly distended. It seemed almost to fill the pelvic cavity after removal of the ovarian mass. Fever set in shortly after the operation, followed later by diarrhœa, with pain and slight induration in the line of the descending colon. A fortnight later a small swelling appeared near the upper end of the abdominal wound which had healed by first intention. This eventually proved to be a foecal fistula. Evidently the greatly distended lower bowel had got injured in some way. Patient died from exhaustion on the 27th day. Apart from this bowel complication neither Dr. Layng nor I could find any explanation of the symptoms.

REPORT

OF THE

MISSION HOSPITAL

AT

SWATOW

IN CONNECTION WITH THE

PRESBYTERIAN CHURCH OF ENGLAND

UNDER THE CARE OF

P. B. COUSLAND, M.B., C.M.

For 1894.

Printed by Kwai Fung,

Swatow.

REPORT.

1894 has been a trying year for the people of Tiê-chiu. The failure of the summer rice harvest, from drought followed by floods, coming after the bad harvests of 1893, with the stoppage for a time of the importation of rice from the North, increased the price of all food stuffs and caused much distress. The climax was reached in October, and it looked at one time as if a rice riot were imminent. Fortunately the timely arrival of steamers relieved the acuteness of the situation. People were seen in the streets of Swatow actually jumping for joy at the sight of the steamers coming into the harbour.

This scarcity and dearness of eatables prevented some patients coming to the Hospital and shortened the stay of others. Wild rumours as to the dreadful practices of foreign doctors in Hongkong on plague patients, and perhaps the vague idea that China was fighting some other country have also had some effect on the attendance.

The demands of the in-patients on my time were so great that out-patients were restricted as much as possible to the regular dispensary days, i.e. Tuesdays and Fridays. This has helped to cause the reduction in their numbers.

The state of Dr. Lyall's health necessitated his leaving on furlough at the beginning of March and I was removed from Ch'ao-chow-fu to undertake the superintendence. The large amount of surgical work and the oversight of so many in-patients, besides the Dispensary department, Medical care of Schools, College and Foreign Missionaries, and a share in general mission work are too much for the strength of one man, and it is a subject of much gratification that the Foreign Missions Committee have promised to send a second medical man to Swatow.

As in previous years Dr. H. Layng rendered much

valuable help, and to him and those members of the Foreign and Chinese Community who have by their contributions enabled us to bring health and comfort to so many we accord our most hearty thanks. The head of Tan Nguan Seng hong gave us tickets to the value of $364.00 representing 15,000 substantial meals for destitute patients. He also signalised the Chinese new year's day by the gift of a day's rice to each patient, an offer that was taken advantage of by 94 of the 97 patients remaining in the Hospital.

The only change of importance in the buildings during the year under review was the rebuilding of the latrine on a new and improved system at a cost of $89.

Three of the junior assistants and four students were under instruction during the year, the subjects studied being Anatomy, Chemistry and Physiology, with some drill in reading and writing Prescriptions in Latin.

STATISTICS.

Number of Individual Patients :—

In-patients	2317
Out-patients	2746
Total	5063
Females included in above	994
Visits to Chinese patients in their own homes	173
Daily average number of in-patients. ...	151
Average attendance of out-patients on dispensary days	62
Total number of visits of out-patients to the Dispensary	10583
Surgical Operations	920

These figures represent the work done during the regular hours. In addition about 2000 cases of minor ailments have been seen by the Senior Assistants out of hours.

EVANGELISTIC.

Some idea of the pains taken to teach the patients

that there is something even better than bodily healing may be gathered from the following table :—

8. 30 A.M.—Morning Service in Hospital Chapel.—*Missionary or Senior Assistant.*

9. 15 A.M.—Short service with the female patients.—*Miss Black and Biblewoman.*

2—3 P.M.—Women's Reading Class.—*Miss Harkness and Biblewoman.*

3—4 P.M.—Women's Reading Class.—*Biblewoman.*

2—3 P.M.—Boys' Reading Class.—*Miss Black and a Christian Lad.*

7 P.M.—Evening service in Chapel.—*Sen. Assistant.*

In the wards, conversation and teaching men to read, the Hospital Colporteur and Miss Black's assistant.

In the wards, conversation and teaching women to read, the Biblewoman, the Ladies of the Mission and some native Christian women.

Selling of Gospels and Tracts, the Colporteur.

Sunday, 3 P.M.—Meeting for examining and instructing applicants for baptism, conducted by a missionary.

Those who are young and bright and are making a prolonged stay in the Hospital are taught the Romanised Colloquial, as putting within their reach a large part of the New Testament, many tracts, and the Church monthly newspaper. Others are taught the Hymn book and Ten commandments in Character Colloquial, and those who cannot learn to read memorise more or less.

As compared with my former term of superintendence ten years ago there is much more teaching carried on now, and both those who become Christians and those who do not should leave with a clearer knowledge of Christianity, and with helpful books and tracts, the contents of which they are to some extent acquainted with. I do not know that I notice much difference in the number of those who definitely decide to break with idolatry and join the Church. The classes and ward work are subsidiary to the preaching at the morning and evening services, and we have much reason to thank God for two so earnest and capable evangelists as the senior assistants. The Christian influence these two men have exerted on their fellow countrymen in this region during the past twenty years must be deep and widespread.

The Colporteur and Scripture Reader entered on his duties in March. He was sent on several expeditions to visit ex-patients in 2 or 3 Districts, but most of his time was spent in the Hospital wards and men's class room, and in selling Tracts and Gospels to the out-patients. He met with a better measure of success in his sales in the Hospital than when out visiting.

During the year about one hundred men and women applied for baptism. Some of these we suspect may be insincere, others we fear will yield to the force of village opinion when they go home, but some we have good reason to hope are both sincere and by faith will stand out against all persecution.

A number of old patients were baptised at the country chapels, and two or three in the Hospital. It is encouraging to know that some of these had not applied for baptism here, and yet on going home had destroyed their idols and attended service at the nearest chapel. An extract from a letter written by one of the ladies of the Mission after visiting a country station will illustrate how the influence of the Hospital is multiplied. "The woman who was baptised had heard the doctrine in the Hospital when she was there with her son who had his foot amputated. On their return home, the husband was quite willing to listen, and he and a young son also became applicants. This younger son my husband did not baptise, but he had the pleasure of receiving the husband and wife, eldest son, and little baby, all of one family, as well as another young man. We hope this family may be the means of bringing many others to worship as their home is in a village where as yet there are no Christians."

Among the converts there are occasionally some who, although relatives of Church members, have not become Christians at home, but are awakened and brought to decision by the more concentrated and continuous Christian influence and preaching in the Hospital.

Nine *Deaths* occurred in the wards. (1) Young man under treatment for Necrosis of Tibia. Pernicious Malarial Fever. Cardiac failure. (2) Phthisis Pulmonalis. Sudden Fatal Haemoptysis. (3) Man returned from Singapore. Alcoholic subject. Debility and Cardiac failure. (4) Young man under treatment for Trachoma. Fever and Constipation, then severe colicy pains for a day or two. Pain improved. No vomiting, tympanites, or abdominal tenderness, but pulse steadily failed. (5) Young man. Beri-beri? Neuritis? Cardiac failure. (6) Elderly man, opium smoker. Ruptured urethra and extravasation of urine in Scrotum from fall. No healing power, scrotum sloughed, bedsores and sloughs formed wherever the least pressure. Nourishment, opium and alcohol of no avail. Septic fever and death. (7) Elderly man. Chronic dysentery. Fell down in ward at night and found dead in the morning. Cardiac failure? (8) Elderly woman. Severe Dysentery. (9) Opium smoker, crushed by fall under a bag of sugar. Haemorrhage from nose and left ear. Third day better, ran away. Brought back in two days. Temp. 105°, delirium, death. There were no deaths after operation.

Bubonic Plague.—Swatow and neighbourhood were fortunately spared a visitation of the Plague in spite of the immigration by land and water from Hongkong and Canton. To the heavy rains which succeeded a long period of drought, and to the inspection of all steamers from the infected ports our immunity was in all probability largely due. The steamers were inspected by Dr. H. Layng, and all suspicious cases sent to a mat-shed Hospital erected by the mercantile community, and placed under the care of a native physician appointed by the Chinese authorities. This plan was found to work well, the native doctor proving a pleasant man to work with, and his presence preventing the rise of evil rumours. Of the *Eleven* cases landed two recovered. One of them when being conveyed ashore jumped overboard to escape a dreadful fate at the hands of the foreigners. He recovered.

In spite of all precaution a few cases occurred in Swatow, and as late as the end of August I was called to see one of the clerks in the Telegraph Office suffering from a fatal attack of this disease.

Influenza was prevalent in the early months of the year, and again during the last two months. The latter occurrence was not very severe, and differed somewhat from earlier epidemic outbreaks by the frequency of tonsillitis as an early symptom, and the comparative rarity of backache and other pains. The patchy pulmonary congestions and cough with tough scanty sputum were as characteristic as usual. Attacks did not leave the same prostration as formerly.

A widespread **Epidemic of Acute Catarrhal Conjunctivitis** passed over the Prefecture in the autumn, children especially being affected. None of the cases coming under observation were followed by serious sequelae.

A well marked case of **Haemophilia** was met with in a boy six years of age who was brought for treatment of a bleeding cut on his head. Before the slight wound finally healed haemorrhage occurred several times, and it was noticeable that when it was arrested ecchymosed spots appeared on his limbs. He had the history of a regular bleeder including haematemisis. His deceased brother was the same. No hereditary history could be elicited.

One patient involved his whole family most disastrously by his sin. He attended for a few days with gonorrheal ophthalmia but suffering much from the pain of panophthalmitis in one eye he went home. Two months afterwards he returned bringing with him his father and brother. The former had lost both his eyes and the latter one eye. We were able to save the other. He reported his mother as being quite blind. All had received the infection from his eyes.

Two **Spinal cases** made surprisingly good recoveries. The first was a man aged 52 who fell and injured his back. No lesion could be felt, but there was complete paraplegia and loss of control over the sphincters. On the fifth day there were evidences of returning power in his legs. He left on the eight day able to walk and with control over his sphincters. He was treated with ergot and K. I. on the supposition that it was a case of haemorrhage.

The history of the second case, a man aged forty, was that four months before admission he had an attack of 'fever' which was followed by paraplegia, which advanced for a fortnight and then gradually improved. On admission he could not stand, but had some control over his sphincters. Anesthesia had passed off. No history of syphilis. Various remedies were tried. K. I. always brought on clonic spasms of affected muscles, but a prolonged course of Hydr. Perchlor., Ergot and Belladonna was followed by marked improvement. He himself could always tell from the effects produced when he was getting this prescription. In six months he could walk out without a stick. Here we have a case evidently of congestion and tendency to sclerosis.

Among the more uncommon diseases met with during the year were the following:—

Leukaemia, in a boy, prop. of white cells to red, as 1 to 5.

Raynaud's Disease, young man, tips of the toes of both feet, duration five months.

Diabetes Insipidis, boy of 16, sp. gr. 1000, 320 ozs. in the 24 hours, duration six years. No treatment availed.

Acute Diabetes, one middle aged man.

Chronic Diabetes, elderly stout man, here last year, complained this time of Diabetic neuritis, relieved by Sod. Salicyl.

Hysteria, one case, a young woman.

Multiple Adenomata of Rectum and Anus. The Rectum as far up as could be felt was a mass of these little tumours.

Ectopiae Vesicae and Hypospadias in a boy of 8.

Coloboma of Iris (downwards)	1	Conical Cornea	1
Leprosy	162	Bubonic Plague ...	1
Asthma	25	Syphilis from Sodomy ...	75
Locomotor Ataxia	1	Vesical Calculus ...	5
Paralysis Agitans	1	Penile Calculus ...	2
Epilepsy	12	Elephantiasis of Leg ...	36
Beriberi	1	Do. of Scrotum	18
Goitre	7	Do. of both ...	2
Lymphadenoma	1	Molluscum Fibrosum ...	1

In one case of Elephantiasis of the leg the affection was entirely confined to the adductor side of the thigh, and in a scrotal case the transition from lymph scrotum to Elephantiasis was well demonstrated.

For the last two years the hypodermic administration of Morphine has been extensively used by natives in this Prefecture, ostensibly for the cure of the opium smoking habit. For a time it was very popular as it appeared to offer the prospect of a cure without either the suffering or the loss of time experienced in the plan of abruptly breaking off the habit. When it was found that the dose of Morphine could not be diminished beyond a certain amount without bringing on the pains of the "craving," the method fell into discredit and the administrators in some cases had rather a hot time of it. I have not been able to hear of a single cure effected, but many of the victims have come to the Hospital to undergo our method. They had all very bad arms, some pustulated, some keloidal. Evidently no care had been taken to keep the solutions or syringes clean. A number still employ this method finding that a return to the pipe did not satisfy them as well as the injections.

SURGICAL OPERATIONS in 1894.

On the Eye:—

Operations for Entropion and Trichiasis, upper ...	206
" " " lower ...	96
" for Ectropion	1
" " Pterygium	50
" " Ptosis	1
Cataract—Extraction of	17
" Secondary Operations	2
Iridectomy	40
Iridotomy	2
Cauterising Rodent Ulcer of Cornea	2
Excising and curetting Hypertrophied Conjunctiva	3
Excision of Orbital Tumour	1
Enucleation of Eye for Malignant Tumour ...	1
Operation for Chalazion	3
Electrolysis of Angeioma of Inner Canthus ...	1
Miscellaneous Operations	2
	428

On the Body generally:—

Abscising External Haemorrhoids	27
Tying Internal "	55
Tapping and Injecting Hydrocele	33
" " " Lymphocele	1
" Goitre	3
" Ascites	1
Sequestrotomy	29
External Urethrotomy	3
Lithotomy—Lateral	2
Tonsillotomy	1
Scraping Caries, Lupus, Ulcers, Glands, etc. ...	38
Incising Anal Fissure	3
Tying Umbilical Polypus in a child	1
Plastic Operation for Partial Restoration of Ear ...	1
" " " Restoring Nasal Column ...	2

Amputation of Arm for Caries (circular) (A) ...	1
" " Fingers	2
" " Leg for Caries (large post. flap) ...	1
" " Foot (Syme's) for Caries	1
" " Toes and Congenital Tumour ...	1
" " Supernumerary Thumb	4
" " Great Toe (B)	4
" " Elephantiasis Scroti (C)	7
" " Lymph Scrotum	1
Excision of Epulis and portion of Lower Jaw ...	2
" " Angeioma of Scalp	1
" " Rectal Adenomata	3
" " Callosities	10
" " Sebaccous Cysts	18
" " other Cysts	3
" " Lipoma (D)	3
Excision of Epithelioma	1
" " Tuberculous Glands	1
" " Keloid	2
" " Exostosis (E)	2
" " Fibroma (F)	3
" " Sarcoma (G)	6
" " Ganglion	2
" " small Tumours	10
" " Malignant Tumours, unclassed ...	4
" " Submaxillary Glands (Leper) ...	1
" " Tibia	1
" " Head of Humerus	1
Operation for Fistula in Ano	51
" " Phimosis (circ.)	14
" " " (slitting up)	3
" " Harelip	25
" " large Chronic Abscesses	2
" " Slit Ear Lobule	30
" " Tarsal Caries	1
" " Sinuses	3
" " Congenital Atresia Ani	1

Opening and Stuffing Haematocele	2
Straightening Ankylosed Knees	3
Reducing Dislocations, Hip, Shoulder, Jaw ...	3
Extraction of Nasal Polypi	8
Snaring Aural Polypi	1
Extraction of Needles and Splinters	3
Sundry Minor Operations	46
	492
Midwifery, ...	3
(one case of Internal Version for Placenta Praevia lateralis, child dead, mother recovered).	
Extraction of Teeth	201

A considerable amount of Minor surgery performed in the wards or out of the regular hours is not included in the above list.

Notes on the Surgical Work.

Iridectomy.—This operation was performed for the most part for artificial pupil. The other cases were for Glaucoma, Rodent Ulcer of Cornea, and Iritis due to anterior senechia. It is often a matter of great difficulty to know whether to operate in cases of anterior senechia or not. Some do very well if left alone. In one of these cases operated on the result was extremely satisfactory, the irritability entirely disappearing.

External Urethrotomy was required in three cases of traumatic rupture of the urethra with extravasation of urine. The seat of rupture was cut down upon, a catheter passed into the bladder and tied in. This accident is fairly common. Several other cases came under treatment where a catheter could be passed without operation. One of these ended fatally as mentioned among the deaths.

Lithotomy.—Lateral. The calculi weighed 14 drachms and 3½ ozs. respectively.

The first case illustrates the efficacy of rectal irrigations in Dysentery. After the operation all went well for a week, when his temp. rose to 104 F., and by the 11th day Dysentery of a not very characteristic type was fully developed. There was no blood in the stools, and they some times seemed half diarrhoeic, half dysenteric. The usual remedies per os failed to check or modify the course of the disease. On the 15th day his condition was very grave, temp. A.M. 101.8, P.M. 104, pulse almost imperceptible, delirious. Free stimulation with ammonia and alcohol, hypodermic injections of Digitalis to the amount of 70 M. in the course of the day of no avail. In the evening irrigated large intestine with 3 pints of $\frac{1}{2}$ % Creolin solution. 16th, Temp. A.M. 98.6, sweating, pulse stronger. Took plenty of milk but little stimulant during the day, reirrigated; P.M. Temp. 100.2, four stools. 18th, Temp. A.M. and P.M. 98; three motions.

We had to stop the irrigation owing to the patient's objections, and each time the temp. began to rise and the stools become more frequent. Irrigation again produced marked improvement. 33rd day, first formed motion. Perineal sinus had to be cauterised three times before it closed. Patient a centurion, aged 41, of remarkably strong constitution.

(*A*) Through middle of upper arm, very spry old man. Down stairs on the third day bringing on secondary haemorrhage. Wound healed rapidly. (*B*) All young women. Footbinding had caused low vitality of the part and the great toe was badly ulcerated. Amp. is the best treatment. The wound unites rapidly. (*C*) Smallest 1$\frac{3}{8}$lb, largest 4$\frac{1}{2}$lb. Small flaps left to cover testicles in each case. (*D*) Of scapula 8 lb, of shoulder 2$\frac{5}{8}$ lb. (*E*) One, pedunculated, cauliflower like, of lower end of shaft of femur. The other of second metatarsal bone. Both 2 ozs. by weight. (*F*) Fibroma of breast, 19 ozs., old woman. Of shoulder 1$\frac{1}{2}$ lb in a man. (*G*) Cystic, of thigh in young woman 5 lb. Spindlecelled of breast, elderly man, been removed twice before. Sarcoma of breast in woman.

One case of suicidal cut throat came under observation. The wound in the larynx was sutured, but the patient, who was insane, left in a few days.

A boy was brought with necrosis of the whole shaft of the tibia from Acute Suppurative Periostitis, a disease seldom seen here. The bone was removed up to the Epiphyses with great improvement to the patient's general health, but new bone was very slowly formed, and five months afterwards the new shaft was still too weak to be of use.

Chloroform was administered only eighty times as the Hoklos, or people speaking the Ch'ao-chow vernacular, have remarkably little sense of pain.

SUBSCRIPTIONS FOR 1894.

Dr. A. Lyall, ...	$60.00
Messrs. Bradley & Co.	50.00
„ Butterfield & Swire	50.00
„ Jardine, Matheson & Co.	50.00
China Sugar Refining Company, Limited ...	50.00
Rev. P. J. Maclagan, M.A. (2 years) ...	60.00
Rev. J. C. Gibson, M.A. (2 years)	50.00
Rev. J. Steele, B.A.	30.00
Rev. J. L. Milne, B.D.	25.00
B. C. George Scott	25.00
D. R. Law	25.00
Dr. Henry Layng	25.00
Wm. Paton	25.00
Miss Harkness	25.00
P. B. Cousland, M.B., C.M.	25.00
B. & F. Bible Society, half wages of Colporteur	22.25
Miss Black	20.00
C. Lenox Simpson	15.00
J. H. C. Günther	10.00
Mrs. Asverus	10.00
O. Tiberii	10.00
W. Ford	10.00
Rev. H. L. Mackenzie, M.A.	10.00
Thank offering for recovery of child (for poor patients)	10.00
A Friend	10.00
Messrs. Bradley & Co., account patient ex S. S. *Siam*	10.00
H. E. Shadgett...	5.00
Graham Rome	5.00
Alex. W. Cross	5.00
G. Lange	5.00
L. Grunauer	5.00
J. W. Andrews	5.00
P. E. Millie	5.00
Anonymous Donation	2.00
Sale of Photographs per Dr. C.	43.97
	799.22

Hou-teng-iâ (medical attendance)	$100.00
Tsan Tai Von	25.00
Siaŋ Ah Kim	25.00
Lim Yam Seng	25.00
Koe Choon Long	25.00
Swatow Presbyterian Church	25.00
Lim Ching King	15.00
Jin Seng Hang	10.00
Chip Sing	10.00
Liao Tsze San	10.00
Tai Tsze King	10.00
L. C. I. T.	10.00
H. B. M. Consulate and Post Office gigmen per H.B.M. Consul	10.00
Ben	5.00
Fong	5.00
Ding Shao Lin	5.00
Chan Yen Kying	5.00
Wang Tai Ping	5.00
Phua Pin Kheng	4.00
Goû Tüa-te	4.00
Kwai Fung for 1893	2.00
Smaller sum from friends and patients	23.24
	$358.24

STATEMENT OF INCOME & EXPENDITURE for 1894.

Expenditure		Income	
To Wages	$477.24	By Balance from 1893	$174.51
,, General Expenses	94.10	,, Subscriptions and Donations	1157.46
,, Drugs etc. from London	902.86	,, Fees from Opium patients	59.00
,, Do. ,, Mission Committee	876.00	,, Rent of Private Wards	7.00
,, Do. ,, China and Hongkong	207.84	,, Grant of Drugs etc. from Mission Committee	876.00
,, Spirit for Tinctures &c.	186.99	,, Sales of Drugs, etc.	1051.33
,, Lard, Wax and Oils	135.96	,, Balance due Treasurer	171.03
,, Cotton, Wool, and Cloth	190.77		
,, Aid to poor patients	63.35		
,, Repairs on Buildings	114.47		
,, New Latrine	89.00		
,, Water	112.62		
,, Paper and Kerosine	34.99		
,, Burial Expenses	5.14		
	$3,496.33		$3,496.33

New Building Account.

By Cash in hand $519.20

REPORT

OF THE

SWATOW MISSION HOSPITALS

IN CONNECTION WITH THE

PRESBYTERIAN CHURCH OF ENGLAND,

For 1913.

PRINTED BY
KWAI FUNG,
PRINTER, BOOKBINDER & STATIONER,
SWATOW,
1914.

STAFF

GENERAL HOSPITAL

Dr. A. Lyall M.B.C.M.

Dr. G. Duncan Whyte M.D. (absent)

Dr. A. Wight M.B.C.M. (acting)

Ie Huai-Kun

Tan Sui-Tsho

Tshu Hui-Chiang

Kuan Hien-Theng

WOMEN'S HOSPITAL

Dr. Nina H. Beath M.B.C.M. (absent)

Dr. Marguerette Ross M.B.C.M.

Tan Peng-Kui

Tan Mui-Chhin

Phe Un-Thong

汕頭福音醫院之佈告

本院之設原不獨爲醫人疾病亦以播傳福音眞理勸人悔改歸順上帝信賴耶穌以期民德歸厚爲宗旨故凡就醫有年少并病勢須在院日久者亦敎之讀書冀其聽道更易也溯本院開創自英國醫學博士吳君威凜至今已閱五十周年病人來院就醫者起初尚少而越久越多是故院屋宜逐漸推廣計自初創至今改建或推廣已凡四次且於十年前增設女院并蒙西女醫士來駐以專醫婦孺由此就醫益便而就醫人數更見日衆查現年就醫人數計總院住院者男女三千四百零八名不住院者男女八千三百九十三名請往其家診視者七百九十七名合共一萬二千五百九十八名女院住院者一千三百八十八名不住院者二千二百零九名請往其家診視者三百四十四名合共三千九百四十一名不住院者若以其至院診視次數計之則男院二萬六千八百三十一人女院七千六百一十五人以上就醫之人其須用刀針剖割者男女計共一千九百二十九人此外請往接生者一百九十人拔齒牙者七百五十九人注射防鼠疫及吐瀉者共三千零三十九人至人來院就醫住總房者日惟取食費銀一毛住稅房者每月取房租銀四元醫費俱分毛不取不住院者若逢拜二拜五對期就醫亦不

取分文惟不對期者則每人取銀二毛亦不過藉以整秩序省時間耳非所謂醫費也茲將全年進支數目列左計

收銀七千九百九十九元零三弌

出銀八千零九十六元零三弌

欠銀九十七元

火食數目

收銀四千零三十八元零九分

出銀四千零八十六元二弌

欠銀四十八元一弌一分

以上數目惟總院女院不包在內

竊維就醫日衆費用日繁苟非中外　仁慈君子官紳士庶同發婆心隨緣慨助源源不絕奚能長此不息以垂永遠哉故凡捐助本院者或給貧病之人以食費者本院同人莫不感謝靡暨如就醫者以報爲施捐題不拘多少亦甚歡喜感謝茲將一千九百十三年捐助芳名列左以表謝忱

中華民國二年　　福音醫院總理來愛力謹告

REPORT.

1913 is the Jubilee Year of the Swatow Mission Hospital.

Medical Missionary work was commenced at Swatow by Dr. Wm. Gauld in the month of November 1863. A Chinese house was rented and fitted up as a dispensary and hospital, and three days a week set apart for receiving patients.

In his first report for the years 1864 and 1865, Dr. Gauld gives the total number of patients treated in this improvised hospital, and, on visits to mission stations, as 1967 in 1864,-of whom 200 were in-patients and 312 were women and girls; and as 1779 in 1865, of women 250 were in-patients and 343 were women and girls. These patients came from 500 different towns and villages. The report ends with an appeal for contributions towards the building of a new hospital, a site for which had been obtained.

Appeals for a "New Hospital" have been frequent throughout these fifty years. In Dr. Gauld's hands, the hospital had three removes, and when he handed it over to his successor at the close of 1879, it was housed in a new building on a site adjoining the Mission compound, given by the, then, Taotai in recognition of professional services rendered to him.

In his last report, that for 1879, Dr. Gauld gives the total number of patients as 3108,-of whom 2028 were in-patients and 466 were women and girls. The average attendance of out-patients on dispensary days was 25. It is, also, mentioned that "ten of this year's patients had been baptized [in 1878 there were twelve baptisms] but there have been as many as ten applying for baptism at one time in the hospital". At one time during the year, there had been no fewer than 250 patients living in the larger and the smaller [the leper] hospitals, and in referring to this, Dr. Gauld remarks, "We can well remember the gratification we felt in commencing work in Swatow, 16 years ago, at having half-a-dozen patients in the hospital, which was at that time an ordinary Chinese dwelling. The work has grown since then with a steady growth, year by year, through the blessing of Him for those cause it is carried on".

The in-patient department had increased out of all proportion to the out-patient department. The out-patients were still few. This was partly due to the fact that Swatow was then a small town and patients were drawn from all over the surrounding districts, and, for their accommodation and treatment, a combination of hospital and hostelry was required. Until now, the hospital has retained this feature, though to a much lessened extent; but in the future, the exigencies of the times, calling for better equipped hospitals and a higher standard of professonal work, the hostelry idea must entirely give way. A hostelry is now not so much required. There are now a considerable number of hospitals scattered throughout the Swatow region. The E. P. Church has hospitals at Wu-king fu, Chao-chow fu, Sua-bue, and Sam ho pa, and plans to open another at Shong-hong in a year or two. The American Baptist Missionary Unior has hospitals at Kakchieh, Kioh-yang and plans to oper others at Chao-yang, Ho-po and Ng-kng. The Base mission has one in Kia-eng city. From all of these places, patients used to come to the Swatow Hospital and, indeed, still come, but now the majority of such patients are of a kind requiring not merely house accommodation but the best hospital care and treatment that we can give them.

Ten years ago, the hospital was rebuilt on a much larger scale than the earlier ones; and, alongside it, a woman's hospital was erected and placed under the charge of a Lady medical missionary. In these two hospitals, fairly good accommodation for 300 patients is provided.

Below, I give the statistics for the year ending Oct 31st 1913. of both the General Hospital and the Women's Hospital.

It has been a busy year, and during three of the summer months there was, in these two hospitals, a daily average of 400, or more, under treatment.

STATISTICS.

		General Hospital		Women's Hospital
In-patients,	male	2879		
„	female	529	*Women & Children*	1388
Out-patients,	male	5716		
„	female	2677	do.	2209
Patients seen in their homes	male	402		
	female	395	do.	344
Total individual patients		12598		3941

Total visits of out-patients to the Dispensary	...26831		7615
Total visits to patients in their homes	1822	*(incomplete)*	536
Midwifery cases	 11		146
Operations on the Eye,	... 456		382
,, general	 907		184
,, obstetrical and gynecological	11		179
,, Dental	 657		102

Inoculation for plague, and Vaccinations, 2990, Inoculation for cholera &c. 49.

Of the above operations 531, mostly major operations, were performed under Chloroform.

THE GENERAL HOSPITAL.

In-patients—are charged ten cents a day for their food, but no charge is made for medicine or other treatment.

A number of small wards are available for such patients as do not care to go into the general wards. A charge of four dollars per month is made for these wards. All of them have been continuously occupied during the year, and several hundreds of dollars have thus been added to the income of the hospital.

Out-patients—on two days of each week, Tuesday and Friday, out-patients are seen, and such medicine and treatment as is necessary, given to them free of charge. Accident cases and emergency cases are seen and attended to without charge, at all hours.

Out-patients coming on days, other than fixed dispensary days, or outside of dispensary hours, are expected to pay twenty cents, unless manifestly poor. No poor patient is refused.

When Dr. Duncan Whyte, after a serious illness was invalided home in February, Dr. A Wight who was about to leave on furlough, was asked by the Swatow mission council to postpone his furlough for a year and take Dr. Duncan Whyte's place in Swatow. Dr. Wight readily consented and we are very grateful for all his kindness and help. Dr. R. Chalmers, also gave a helping hand for two or three weeks in the middle of summer.

The work in the hospital has been carried on month after month, throughout the year without interruption and we have had our hands full of work. We have not, indeed, been free from epidemic diseases which so often interfere with the coming of patients from outlying districts. In the spring and earlier summer months, Bubonic plague was rife in some parts of the district and there were cases in Swatow. There was a good deal of Cholera in august and september, and an epidemic of Dengue fever in the latter month when the three medical missionaries were for two or three days hors-de-combat at the same time with this somewhat painful fever. But the flow of patients was not interrupted by any of these prevailing diseases, neither did the "rebellion" in which our province of Kwang-tung took part, cause any disturbance in the Swatow region. This jubilee year is also a record year so far as number of patients is concerned.

It used to be difficult to get other than Hoklo or Hakka speaking Chinese to remain as in-patients in the hospitals. There always seemed to be a good deal of mutual distrust largely due no doubt to their inability to understand each others language. There is now a considerable change in this respect. We have now many Cantonese and men from other provinces among our patients. One ward has had to be set apart for soldiers who are mostly Cantonese or Mandarin speaking Chinese, and most of this class of patients have come for treatment of Venereal diseases. During the last two years there has been a great increase of syphilitic and other venereal diseases in Swatow. This is one of the deplorable results of these revolutionary times with its accompanying license and abandonment of moral restraints.

The number of out-patients continues to increase year by year. The accommodation available in a hospital limits to some extent the number of in-patients but the growth in the number of out-patients is not subject to any such natural limitations. The more rapid means of travelling to and from Swatow by steam launches and railway has brought a much wider area of country within the scope of the out-patients department, and on some dispensaries days the number of patients is difficult to cope with Much more efficient work-professional and missionary, is done among the in-patients, but as compared with 20 or 30 years ago the out-patient department provides much better opportunities now for evangelistic work. We have, for instance, in the course of a year, numerous cases of ulcers, granular lids, etc. coming regularly for a lengthened period of time, twice a week or oftener, for treatment of their special ailments.

There is one thing which never seems to chang and that is the daily continued, never ending, fight against dirt in all its forms.

EVANGELISTIC WORK.

In regard to the evangelistic work there is littl to be said different from what we have reporte on former occasions.

The various means employed in the past to give the patients an intelligent knowledge of the Gospel have been industriously pursued during the year. Missionary colleagues, our Chinese assistants and students have assisted the hospital preacher, Ng-Sin-Teng, to conduct daily morning and evening services, and various classes have been held for teaching the scriptures in Romanised and Chinese Character to such of the patients who were willing to learn.

The inquirers class is composed of those who have given in their names as applicants for baptism. This class has numbered 78 in the general hospital, not counting those who had applied before, and 96 in the Woman's hospital.

It is very difficult to follow up these applicants when they return to their homes. All of the plans which we have tried, to keep in touch with these people, sooner or later, break down, especially if left much to the Chinese helpers to carry out.

This year we have heard of 17 of the present year's applicants attending Church services near their own homes. Our inquiries have not covered the whole of the year's work nor all of the Chapels. My own opinion is that our Hospitals are as fruitful in spiritual results now as in former years.

Ng siu-teng, the preacher, has worked well. He is an ex-minister of the Chinese Church and he is himself a fruit of the hospital work. He was a patient in the summer of 1880

Another ex-patient, named Tan Hai-tien, who afterwards was ordained to the pastorate of the Chinese Church, was drowned by the capsizing of a steam launch during a typhoon in September.

FINANCIAL.

Once more we take the opportunity of tendering our grateful thanks to all who have helped us financially or otherwise during the passed year.

We would especially thank the following:—The Foreign community and many Chinese friends for their generous subscriptions, During all its fifty years, the hospital has always received generous support from members of the Swatow Foreign community, of many nationalities, and they have done much to relieve the financial strain on those who have carried on the work; Mrs. Lyall for a gift of $842 from her drawn-thread fund; Tshu sok hua and Tshu sok che for a donation of $250 to pay for bringing water into both hospitals.

When the electric light was installed in Swatow, the engineer in charge, suggested to some Chinese friends that they might take the opportunity of presenting the hospital with an X-Ray outfit. We have received, per Mr. Kwok lai chow, a sum of $297 (mex. $262) to be used for this or any other purpose we might decide. This sum, however, is not nearly sufficient to buy an X-Ray apparatus, and, in the meantime, it is carried on into next year's account. The Foreign mission committee of the E. P. Church has given £140 toward the supply of medicine and surgical dressing.

SURGICAL WORK.

The number of operations performed during the year is given in the column of statistics;—those of the Women's hospital are incomplete. A large amount of minor surgery, such as opening abscesses, stitching wounds etc. is performed in the dispensary, but no record of this has been kept.

The following is a list of the principal classes of operations which have been performed:—

	General Hospital	Women's Hospital
Operations for Entropion	259	333
" " Pterygium	64	15
Iridectomy (for artificial pupil)	41	6
Cataract Extraction	20	8
Excision of Tumours, cysts	112	26
" " Cervical glands (Tubercular)	10	15
" " Elephantiasis Scroti	5	
Operations for Cario-necrosis of bones	85	15
" " Vesical Calculus	9	
" " Cystic goitre	2	2
" " Phymosis	36	
" " Harelip	24	4
" " Hydrocele	29	
" " Haemorrhoids	95	27
External Urethrotomy	12	
Plastic operations	7	4
Amputations	36	6
Bullets Extracted	21	
Nasal Polypi "	18	4
Radical operation for Inguinal Hernia	5	
Ovariotomies		7
Operations for Vesico-Vaginal Fistula		15
" " Ruptured perineum		3

532 of the operations were performed under the influence of choroform which is the only general anaesthetic used. At the present time it may be of general interest to note that in the fifty years there has only been one death due to the anaesthetic, that of a young boy, about 20 years ago, who was being operated on for cario-necrosis of the tibia. My predecessor Dr, Gauld, was in the habit of calling in the doctor of the foreign community to give chloroform, but since 1880, it has been entirely given by chinese asistants, many of whom become quite skilful chloroformists. As a general rule, there is little or no trouble afterwards from vomiting, and I have never been able to detect anything like Post chloroform poisoning.

It is quite impossible to give anything like a correct idea as to the total number of chloroform cases during the past fifty years. No record at all was kept for 20 or more years. During the last ten years, there has been an average of about 500 annually in the two Hospitals. In the earlier years there was nothing like this number, but since 1880, the number of cases annually has been very considerable. Perhaps if we put the total number as 10.000 we will be within the mark.

Operations for entropion and trichiasis continue to be numerous. The condition must be very prevalent, for there are now other six hospitals and dispensaries in the Tie-hui-prefecture; and, besides, a large number of Chinese now perform such operations. It is almost entirely due to Trachoma.

Pterygium is also very common, and may be put down as largely due to the same cause.

Cataract,—is not very common. The number of operations continue much the same year by year: the largest in any one year was a little over forty.

Hernia,—our first attempt at a radial cure of Inguinal Hernia was made in 1888, when Woods' operations was performed in one case.

Our numbers still remain small, due chiefly to fact that most of the patients, who are, as a rule, in good health, are deterred by the prospect of a month's confinement to bed.

V. V. Fistula:—This class of case continues to increase every year and now, cases are successfully operated on which 20 years ago would have been rejected as hopeless. It is surprising what huge "holes" can be successfully repaired by one or two operations

Ovariotomy,—We very seldom get a patient suffering from ovarian tumour to consent to operation while the tumour is still small. Practically all our cases have tumours of large size, with their general health more or less weakened;—the results, however, are very gratifying. Of the seven cases this year, one had fairly large tumours of both ovaries, and a double ovariotomy was performed. And in another one, the operation could not be finished. It was a case of a very large unilocular cyst, The cyst wall seemed to be completely adherent all over; the patient's heart was in a bad condition, and it was quite evident her chances of recovery would be better if the operation was not completed; so no attempt was made to separate the cyst but drainage, as efficient as possible, was applied. The patient, after a long convalecsence, is now going about.

The first laparotomy performed in the hospital was in 1888 for chronic intussusception of the bowel: and in 1892, the first ovariotomy was performed. Later, this patient joined the church, and subsequently married again and bore two children. The elder of these children is now a promising student in the women's hospital.

False spina bifida,—Two of these Congenital Coccygeal growths were successfully operated on, one in an infant and the other in a child three or four years old. These tumours are rarely seen. Cases of true spina ifida are seen every year.

Club foot,—such cases are rarely seen in Swatow. A case of Talipes varus and another of Talipes equinus were operated on. These chlldren were taken from the hospital too soon to be assured of a satisfactory result.

Elephantiasis of the leg—In our time we have tried a considerable numbers of surgical procedures for this condition.

Two or Three years ago, Dr. Whyte and I tried Handleys "Thread" in a few cases, but even the immediate result did not seem to me more than what rest in bed would produce, and in one case we had septic mischief set up which did not improve matters. During the last 10 or 12 years we have in a number of cases performed an operations which I first saw done in Mr. Cantlies clinic, viz:-cutting out long, deep wedge shaped portion of skin and thickened tissue on both the outer and inner aspect of the leg. A deep scar was thus produced which was hoped would exert a resistance to the return of the oedema. While the immediate result of this operation was good, yet, I rear, the improvement was not permanent and the swelling would return, sooner or later, when the patient returned to his ordinary occupation.

This year we operated on one case atter Kondoleon's method and the immediate result was certainly excellent. A longitudinal incision was made in the outer and inner aspect of the leg, extending from the knee to near the ankle, the skin dissected up, and a long piece, three inches wide, of the thickered œdematons tissue removed right down to the muscles from both sides of the leg. The muscular aponeurosis was then excised to the same extent. This method deserves further trial.

Hydrocephalus—A case of Hydrocephalus in an infant, beginning after birth, with much distended head and severe, often recurring, convulsions, was treated by means of lumbar puncture. The operation was performed on three occasions and was followed by immediate cessation of the convulsions. After the first puncture the convulsions did not return in a severe form.

The child was recently seen again, when one year old, and five months after the third or last puncture He was a large will nourished child. There was no spastic paralysis, but the limbs were weak and flaccid and, although the child showed signs of Intelligence by noticing things, he had made no attempt to walk.

The disease seems to have been arrested by the treatment: anyhow, it was followed by a complete cessation of the convulsions.

STATEMENT OF INCOME AND EXPENDITURE.

By Balance from last year	$510.06
„ Donations fees	3.677.53
„ Sale of Drugs, Trusses etc.	923.97
„ Payments from patients	773.01
„ Rent of small wards	587.95
„ Grant from F. M. C. London for repainting wood work £15	154.37
„ From F. M. C. for support of Cots £12.7.10=	121.96
„ From F. C. M. for Drugs	1.250.00
„ Balance due Treasurer	97.18
	$8.096.03

To Wages	$1.652.48
„ Repairs on buildings white washing etc.	601.01
„ Electric Light and Water	927.43
„ Drugs bought locally	1.589.28
„ Drugs for London	1.465.27
„ Paper, Stationery etc.	330.34
„ Dressings, Lint, Oil, Lard, Cotton, Wool	1,253.04
„ General Expenses Ground Rent and Insurance)	132.00
„ Food to Poor Patients	145.18
	$8096.03

Audited by

A. Wight

A. W. Edmunds

GENERAL HOSPITAL

KITCHEN A/c.

Cr.

Receipts for Patients	$3.885.34
Donation per Mrs. Lyall	100.00
For Poor Patients	52.75
	$4.038.09
Debit balance	48.11
	$4.086.20

Dr.

Expenditure Food &c.	$4.086.20

DONATIONS, FEES, &c.

Mrs. Lyall from Drawn Thread Fund ...	$674.00
,, for Salary of Ng Siu-teng	169.00
Messas. Bradley & Co.	150.00
Drs Brangwin and Hobson	100.00
Messrs. Butterfield & Swire	50.00
,, Jardine, Matheson & Co., Ltd. ...	50.00
,, Lauts & Haesloop	50.00
,, The Standard Oil Co. of New York	50.00
,, E. V. S. Lim & Co. 源順公司 ...	50.00
,, Hock Cheang & Co. 福昌公司	50.00
The S'tow & C'chow Railway Co. 潮汕鐵路公司	50.00
The Sua Tie Kit S. Launch Co. 汕潮揭輪船公司	50.00
W. G. Lay	50 00
A. Razlag M.D.	50.00
do.	25.00
G. Duncan Whyte M.D.	50.00
Ang-Tshu Ji Thai	50 00
Yang Khi-phou 楊祺圃	50 00
Yong Hock Guan 榮福源	49.00
do. 榮福源	40 00
Tek Chhiang 德昌	45.00
Kim Nguan Long 錦源隆	40.00
Kuan Hong 方廣豐	40 00
Swatow Chinese Church 汕頭長老會 ...	40.00
Trade Mark Co. 商標公司	30.00
Tan Pou Seng 陳步新	30.00
Kwok Lai Chow 郭麗州	30.00
Jin Nguan Hong 仁源行	30.00
Thong Hong Siang (J. M. & Co.) 怡和行	30.00

Lim Pang Kiet 林邦杰	... ...	30.00
Rev. A. H. Page	... ...	30.00
Wm. Paton	....	30.00
Dr. A. Lyall	... ...	30.00
E. V. S Lim 林源順	... ...	25.00
The Kai Meng Electric Co. 開明電燈公司		25.00
Ko Seng Tsu 高繩芝	... ...	25.00
The Swatow Dispensary 汕頭藥房	...	25.00
The Swatow Water Works Co. 水公司	.....	25.00
Seng Nguan Ho 生源號	... ...	25.00
Messrs. Gebruder Roese	... ...	20.00
„ Ben & Co. 悅泰	... ...	20.00
„ Wendt & Co.	... ...	20.00
G. P. Pitzipios	... ...	20.00
H. von Borck	... ...	20.00
Eng Tshai Nguan 翁財源	... ...	20.00
Ho. Yeu 何耀	... ...	20.00
Nam Kee 南記	... ...	20.00
Lim Tek Khim 林德欽	... ...	20.00
Wun Huan Lu 溫猶立	... ...	20.00
Tshu Tsu I 徐主意	... ...	20.00
Lo Tek Mui 羅德美	....	20.00
Tng Siang Siu 湯祥壽	... ...	20.00
Li Jin Ki 李仁記	... ...	20.00
Li Thiang Hong 李天豐	... ...	20.00
Tan Iong Ki 陳榮記	... ...	20.00
Lou Cheng Koon 劉清崑	... ...	20.00
Jak Seng Dispensary 益生藥房	...	15.00
N. Kasai	... ...	15.00
Tam Fuk Yu 譚福曜	... ...	15.00
Be Thai Se per Tan Iak Theng 馬泰生	...	15.00

Seng Nguan	成源	15.00
Keng Seng So		15.00
Tan Eng (Tan sun hua)	陳順和	15.00
Treasurer. Teo-Chew flood Relief fund.		14.70
Khu Zui Hui		12.00
Greenlaw U. F. Sabbath School £1 =		10.02
J. Mc G. Forbes		10.00
J. H. R. Hance		10.00
Nguan Heng Seng Ki	元興成記	10.00
Ie Buan Kang	楊文江	10.00
M. O. Clark		10.00
Mrs. Asverus		10.00
W. Diehr		10.00
S. Perceboi		10.00
J. A. Greenfield		10.00
Li Kang Jiang	李康然	10.00
J. Skadiang		10.00
Von Ruffin		10.00
Tan Theng Khuang	陳照巖	10.00
Chin Tie Kong Si	振潮公司	10.00
Siau Chip Seng	蕭楫盛	10.00
Tan Sin Hu		10.00
Sim Kye Pang	沈開枋	10.00
Kai Sheng	祺昇	10.00
Khi Seng	祺昇	10.00
A. Holz		10.00
S. Nishigori		10.00
Chinese Telegraph Administration	電報局	10.00
China Merchants Co. per Sui Soak Chow	招商局	10.00
Tshua Tang Jiang	蔡坦然	10.00
Tie Bue Sui che Tshu	吳祥建	10.00

T K. Chiang 10.00
Mrs. Liang, Hongkong 黄良德嫂 ... 10.00
Ngan Seng Li 顏盛利 10.00
of Ng Khi village 10.00
Tio Lai Hah 張來學 10.00
Tan Che Chhe 陳芷青 10.00
Li Hang I 李翰院 10 00
Lo Tek Mui 羅德美 10.00
Lim Tsang Chee 林傳之 10.00
Te Soh Po 鄭雪波 10.00
An Huat 洪安發 10.00
of Huo Leng Village 10.40
Tsan Tso Chhiu 曾佐秋 10.00
Tie Kien Tsho 張建初 10.00
Khou Buan Kien 許萬經 10.00
Tsu A Un 10.00
Gek Po 10.00
Miss Alexander, Greenlaw £1= 9.56
Mrs. G. Alexander „ 10/- 4.79
Tshua Hang Nguan 蔡漢源 8.50
Chiu Ho Ang... ... ... 8.00
Sing Mi Sing 8.00
Hmang Kia M 6.00
Ng Thiam Hok 黄添福 6.00
C. Hodgson 5.00
A. E. Herdman 5.00
Sim Kye Lim 沈開林 5.00
Nguan Chhiang Kong Si 元昌公司 5.00
C. Wacker 5.00
S. H. Yong 辛向榮 5.00
G. Witte 5.00

Cheung Yam	5.00
J. S Than	5.00
E. G. Jamieson	5.00
H. Freer	5.00
Mark C. Lim 林馬可	5.00
Long Chhiang Sui Thai 隆昌瑞泰 ...	5.00
Po Púa 寶華	5.00
Chhiang Long 長隆	5.00
Jin An Dispensary 仁安藥房 ...	5.00
Po Tai Wo Dispensary 保太和 ...	5.00
Te Lu Seng 鄭魯生	5.00
Joh. Clausen	5.00
Pan Chiong Yong	5.00
Tou Tong Kee	5.00
Captain & Mrs. Milroy, Hongkong ...	5.00
Miss Barber do. ...	5.00
Kwai Fung 仁昌	5.00
T. Carr Ramsay	5.00
Fan Yong 范傑臣	5.00
Tung Ying Chih	5.00
Wai Gek Hun	5.00
C. L. Williams	5.00
Tan I	5.00
Nguan Sun Kong Si 源順公司 ...	5.00
Tou Sin Hun	5.00
Hok Leng	5.00
Kueh Su Khai	5.00
Sim Thiam Hang	5.00
Lim Kok Siang	5.00
Buan Thai 2 donations 萬泰	10.00
Gou Hong Huat	5.00
Sim Teo Soon	5.00
Gou	5.00

K. G. Kring	5.00
Nam Heng	5.00
Jong Hak zu	5.00
Tie Hue 張 花	5.00
Te Seng Khoi	5.00
Rev. W. Hughes	5.00
J. M. Du Cruz	5.00
Kueh Tia Bun 郭鼎文	4.00
Kuang Siu Chiang 鄺壽昌	4.00
Ang Cheng Suio 洪圻瑞	4.00
Jah Siu Dispensary 益壽藥房 ...	4.00
Sih Thong Thai	4.00
Ki Kang Kiang	4.00
Khou Tok Kheng	4.00
Tshua Mông Pang	4.00
Tsok Sim...	4.00
Tang Teng Bun	4.00
Gou Tek Jiet	4.00
Li Keng Sam	4.00
Eng Bi Soh	4.00
Chiu Ngiap	4.00
Gou Theng Hong	4.00
Nguan Chhiang	4.00
Mr. Bourne	4.00
Lim Lang Iu	4.00
In smaller Sums, or Names of donors not ascertained	250.60
	$3.962.07
Less grant to Women's Hospital and loss on	$—284.54
	$3.677.53

Special Donation per Kwok Lai Chow $297—
262.10 Mex. to be carried forward to next year

SUBSCRIPTIONS TO THE WOMEN'S HOSPITAL.

Khi Sin Tsu Kek	$30.00
Siao Chhe Liang	30.00
Peng So	15.00
Tan Chiap Hou	14.00
Khim Ton Chi	14.00
Kueh Nguan Thai	12.00
Kueh Cheng Tin	10.00
Tsap Sim	10.00
Tan Jang Theng	10.00
Goa Kia Meng	10.00
Tshu Ui Hau	10.00
Tan Hah Hua	10.00
Chiu Jim Hah	10.00
Tshu Khau I	8.00
Liang Kok Sim	8.00
Chhiang Mong Nguan	6.00
Tan Mong Li	6.00
Tai Ho Sim	5.00
Kh Tong Chiang	5.00
In smaller Sums, or, Subscribers' names not obtained	337.00
Total	$673.00

DONATIONS SPECIAL

Mrs. Lundie for Support of Student		$50.87
Milne fund	do.	39.81
Miss Greig	do.	50.00
Mrs Lyall, from Drawn thread funds	do.	18.00

WOMEN'S HOSPITAL

SUPPORTED BEDS

RECEIPTS;

The Succourer Bed (In memory of Mrs. Bristow)			$55.00
E. M. Mathews Bed (In memory of.)			50.00
Connie Nicol	„	do.	50.00
Agnes Fairbairn	„	do.	50.00
Highgate	„		50.00
Wollasey	„		51.70
Bed supported by friends of Dr. Ross			50.00
Balance November, 1912			51.60
		Total	$408.30

EXPENDITURE

Paid into Hospital funds	$369.52
Balance in hand	38.78
Total	$408.30

REPORT

OF THE

SWATOW MISSION HOSPITAL

IN CONNECTION WITH THE

PRESBYTERIAN CHURCH OF ENGLAND.

For 1914.

PRINTED BY
KWAI FUNG,
PRINTER BOOKBINDER & STATIONER,
SWATOW.
1915.
汕頭懷安街仁昌刷

STAFF.

A. Lyall M.B.,C.M. 來爱力

G. Duncan Whyte M.D. 懷敦幹

Ie Huai-Kun 楊懷璭

Tan Sui-Tsho 陳瑞初

Kuan Hien-theng 官獻廷

汕頭福音醫院佈告

汕頭福音醫院開創迄今歷有年所治病之效雖未得無病不袪無疾不愈之妙術然而所療各等病症成效頗見卓著故遠近赴院就醫者年益增多自民國二年十一月一號至民國三年十月三十一號所治各症計住院者男二千八百五十人女五百六十七人不住院者男六千零一十八人女二千七百三十九人其延請出院診治者男五百三十八人女九百零九人共計一萬三千二百一十七人較去年就醫者男多四百左右女多二百左右因就醫者年見增多故英國所派兩位醫士誠難獨肩重任幸有越安如醫士及楊官陳諸君暨住院學生協迺心齊迺力盡迺職共肩斯務故得如此之成效也且汕埠爲輻輳之區賓客萃會故至院就診者言語殊難周于應答院中諸君則熟習正音廣音客音藉以問答免失交通之誼裨益就醫誠不少也至於所治等症如眼科用割術者五百四十九人接生者七人其餘內外科用割術者九百五十四人嘗用迷藥者四百三十五人其他不須迷蒙者若外科之膿瘡刀傷流血者跌斷尿管者皆不在此列割症稍少用迷藥亦少故熏藥之法尚有缺點而今用迷藥日多本院已有熟習用

迷藥手術者七人皆稱妥善再查所治之病外科較多因患病者悞以西藥惟精外科耳故本院於內科更爲特別注意茲擇內科之最要者而討論之以解世之疑惑而造莫大利益其綱目如榀疫注射癨亂症肺癆症鈎蟲症

榀疫注射

榀疫爲世界最劇烈之傳染症害較他症爲更速是以文化早開之國醫學之研究日精一日印度醫士發明注射以防榀疫若種牛痘以防天花救活多人術傳其國近來潮州榀疫盛行死亡枕藉本院懷醫士有鑒於此故倡行注射之術初則就射者稀若晨星既而年多一年迨是歲之春注射之數已達三千三百四十一人亦可見藥之有效醫之若神矣其時或至院注射者或各處鄉村延至其家注射者又有慷慨善士林蘭友君痛人生患此症之慘酷因特捐項於醫院俾醫士至其屋而爲貧民注射其樂善之心爲何如乎惜就注射者亦有發疫者蓋緣其地發生此症如其人已受疫染伏毒在內未發而就注射注射之後必遲至數日藥力方能遍及週身而能可保無虞乃伏毒在內藥力未週而疫已發此注射之太遲非注射之無效也深盼各處明注射之理由先事預防不至窒礙注射之

前途以免人世久遭此苦其益詎淺尠哉夫若注射之事業關係匪輕故必有保薦始得注射之權六年前本醫院診症乏人不暇兼及來懷兩醫士同薦官君獻庭得印度醫士許其注射現年因就射者多因呈報印度醫士任注射者蕭惠榮林起陳益彰林性道廖獻成陳益庭杜景祺張健初楊懷瑾陳瑞初柳德生鄭曉初林章光林以澤曾憲章徐惠彰孔憲芳侯仰修謝之惠李業軒蕭曉初等

癨亂症

汕埠近年又癨亂流行死亡狼藉患者每越一日而亡因是症之急有非服藥可得而治者也本院乃施以注塩([illegible][illegible]充迴血管也)之術而效乃見活人不少矣現年春雨早至故是症發生較少僅注七十八人而已其中有注至三四次而愈者亦有服藥而愈者其有不可救者因求治太遲食物不慎耳然癨亂之症雖得注射之妙術而尚乏防染病院蓋防染病院之設必求寬闊以通空氣清潔以暢精神則於看護(専習看護病人者)無傳染之虞醫生亦得巡視之便而他人更免傳染之害防染病院誠不可無也迴憶前年癨亂最盛之時一日間求醫者十三人後得吳督辦暫假沙汕汛營為治疫室由是染者日少是後迄今更得存心善

堂在大峯廟備屋以予患是症者居住且極優待允宜欽佩者也

肺癆症

肺癆較他症尤爲危險以其傳染更易既染此症又難於醫治且患者文人獨多是以天下諸國益求良法抵敵此症以絕滅之毋俾人民遭此險譆我國病症亦莫不以肺癆爲甚故當竭力袪除以與各國共表同情庶幾肺癆之禍日就剗滅今既知其害而不早圖則蔓延之下其害愈不堪設想者矣查此症之傳染皆因唾痰在地面痰之微菌西名都比加(三字口旁)若由人之呼吸侵入於肺則肺癆之病旋生若由傷口侵入患病之骨則令其骨節病終身不治可不懼哉至於抵敵之法惟嚴禁癆者唾痰於地以絕傳染之原醫者以顯微鏡查病者之痰有無都比加(三字口旁)微菌有則以良法治之以良藥服之俾病者減其苦而除其菌現院中練習調染顏色以查此菌者已有五人自去年三月一號本院以顯微鏡查一百四十八人之痰中有癆菌者五十一人亦可謂患者多矣若不講求袪菌衛生肺癆之症不將徧染羣生乎

吮血鈎虫

本院創設多年奇難怪症雖無日無之而於鈎虫則罕見也乃至現年此症發現甚多且各處患此症者聞本院之醫術亦多來求醫尤以山尾華嶋及其左右鄉村爲衆數月間赴院就診者共五十六人而遠處尚未聞知也然調查患此病之處潮屬已占九縣之七矣夫鈎虫之害較痡虫尤甚虫長不及半寸體常勾而不直多至千餘條少亦數百餘條生於腸内以吮其血患此症者不第血虧面黃且被吮之處腸破血洩兩受其害居於熱帶之地患此症者其精神多不舒暢

敬告汕埠紳商注重福音醫院

（劉澤榮）

洪範六極二曰疾四曰貧夫貧雖非人人所同患而疾則統貧富尊卑所不能逃甚矣疾病之纏人也如影隨形依依若有不可離之勢也富戶閥閱千金之丹却病可也窮巷貧黎度生且竭而何有於治病也此貧困遘疾每多任其死生者也何幸仁人抱惻隱之懷求去極之方創施醫院俾貧疾者得以療治不至顛連轉乎溝壑意至仁舉至美其功德誠無量也

大英長老教會體好生之德本救世之仁傳教之餘創設醫院汕頭福音醫院之創亦經五十餘年擴張兩次矣所療疾病屈指難勝經費等需數亦甚鉅而醫士之拮据勤勞鞠躬盡瘁造福人世誠非淺鮮遐邇既沾仁澤咸知診治之良近悅遠來院常人滿查其就醫非盡貧困强半因醫之精而就療耳是以紳商善士僉知醫院之功樂意解囊以助廣施雖曰慈善之爲要亦人生所當盡之義務也且本埠商旅輻輳人煙稠密衛生之道絕少講求碍生之患時所常有核疫霍亂年年發現雖人事不齊亦天行之無可如何者也然而天演之理人治進則天行息泰西諸國汲汲於講求衛生蓋即此耳核疫霍亂爲症之最惡而極險者偶有所患即骨肉至親每亦懼而不敢前汕頭福音醫院醫士犧牲一己之生命以起死回生而止疫厲不惟汕埠人士得沾救濟即內地鄉市亦莫不同沐深仁而羣頌再造之德則我人對於醫士之感情應如何哉而對於醫院之感情又應如何哉

僅獻二端爲我紳商士庶告

一曰慷慨解囊以濟貧病也（甲）助醫藥福音醫院歷年醫藥雜費自英國善士認捐本埠紳商亦多贊助然因就醫日衆藥物雜費日見繁多自必廣呼將伯英

邦人士且慷慨樂捐博施遠人況我同胞同域其可慳吝而一毛不拔乎(乙)助衣食就醫者除醫藥不費外食用均自給也貧人患病度生無由稱貸微資曷足贍養每多病未愈而糧已竭因而回歸致疾不療實堪嘆也況病者衣食不足疾難早除委頓纏綿醫藥遲效前者陳雨亭翁閔念乎此廣施錢米貧病得沾厚澤而今繼武何人我紳商士庶足衣足食亦念乎顛連無告者乎

二曰協除傳染以救羣生也(甲)注射除毒滅生之毒莫甚於核疫霍亂福音醫院醫士已用注射術保存多命免遭疫毒蓋注射之液能使人身之血敵勝疫毒不爲所害然必先事預防更宜人人注射方無傳染之虞我潮多處已嘗注射獨惜信者仍少倘能同心協衆注射除毒疫當不除而自末矣自愛之士幸勿視爲等閒(乙)專院防染核疫霍亂既普傳染則人衆之區自不可忽泰西等處特設防染病所使免染病者均住其中既易於醫調復免乎傳染法至良也惜我邦人士徒懼傳染而不設法以絕染患亦甚矣爲今之計宜倡設防染病所布置得宜俾染病者安住受醫杜其傳染則疫毒不難袪除矣謹獻芻言爲我紳商與有地方之責者告

兹將全年進支數目列左計

收銀玖千零陸拾壹元叁毫陸分

出銀捌千玖百玖拾肆元捌毫柒分

存銀陸拾陸元肆毫玖分

火食數目

收銀肆千零壹拾元弍毫陸分

出銀肆千零弍拾伍元叁毫伍分

欠銀十肆元零玖分

REPORT.

The following table summarises the numbers of patients treated by the hospital during the twelve months ending 31st October 1914.

	Male.	Female.
In-patients (i.e. patients living in the Hospital.)	2850	567
Out-patients (i.e. those living in their own homes but coming to hospital for medicine or treatment.)	6018	2739
Patients who were visited in their own homes	538	505

Total numbers treated by the hospital 9406 male & 3811 female=13217.

Total attendances at the hospital 27137

Total number of visits paid to patients in their own homes=2246.

A comparison with the figures for last year shows that there is an increase of about 400 in the number of male patients treated, while the number of women has increased by about 200.

It is obvious that the large number of patients shown in the table could not be dealt with unless the European doctors were supported by an adequate Chinese staff. The senior assistant, Mr. Ie Huai-kun, has now been twelve years in the hospital and has shown that he fully merits the confidence reposed in him. By utilising his services, along with those of the other assistants (Messrs. Tan & Kuan) and the senior students, it is possible to secure that—no matter how many patients present themselves for treatment in the course of a morning—each patient can be examined with as much care and thoroughness as is required.

The fact that the assistants and senior students have learned Mandarin and Cantonese, as well as their own dialect of Chinese, has greatly facilitated the treating of many patients who were ignorant of the Swatow dialect.

During the twelvemonths under consideration Dr. Duncan Whyte has returned from sick-leave, and Dr. Andrew Wight (who was assisting Dr. Lyall in his absence) has gone home on furlough.

Mr. Tshu, who was fourth assistant last year, has now gone into practise at Ng-Kng.

The number of operations performed last year is given in the following tables, which show a substantial increase compared with last year,-fifty more "general" operations, ninety more eye operations, and an increase of sixty in the number of cases for which a general anaesthetic (chloroform) was required.

General	954
Eye operations	549
Midwifery cases	7
Operations under general anaesthesia ...	435
Inoculations for Plague	3341

In early years another European doctor was usually asked to give his assistance when it was necessary to administer an anaesthetic, but when chloroform is given to over 400 patients in the course of a year such an arrangement becomes impossible. At present 7 of the Chinese staff are competent to administer an anaesthetic.

The following is a list of the principal classes of operations which have been performed during the year.

Operations for Entropion..................	228
" " Pterygium	61

Iridectomy (for artificial pupil)		56
Glaucoma,-Elliot's trephining		5
Cataract Extraction		32
Peritomy		33
Ectropion, Plastic operation		4
Anterior Staphyloma, abscision of......		8
Operations for Vesical Calculus		9
,, ,,	Cario-necrosis of bone	92
,, ,,	Harelip	20
,, ,,	Phymosis	28
,, ,,	Hydrocele	30
,, ,,	Tubercular Disease of joints	12
,, ,,	Cystic goitre	2
,, ,,	Haemorrhoids	90
,, ,,	Fistula in Ano	68
,, ,,	Slit ear lobule	18
Extraction of Calculus lodged in urethra		9
,, ,,	Bullets lodged	9
,, ,,	Nasal Polypus	22
,, ,,	"Foreign bodies" from ear, nose, oesophagus & limbs	45
Amputations		24
External Urethrotomy		9
Radical operation for Inguinal Hernia		5
Excision of Tumours, Cysts &c.		120
,, ,,	Tubercular glands neck ...	19
,, ,,	Half of tongue (epithelioma)	2
,, ,,	Eleph. Scroti......	7

Beyond the number of operations shown above, there is an uncounted number of minor surgical procedures, opening abscesses, tying bleeding arteries stitching wounds, setting fractures, withdrawing collections of fluid (e.g. ascitis) etc., etc.

Last year's report was especially devoted to the surgical side of the work but, in view of the belief that was formerly so widespread, even amongst educated Chinese, that the method of treatment practised by

European doctors was only of benefit in Surgical cases, it may be of interest if this report directs attention especially to the *medical* side of work.

PLAGUE—During the Spring of 1914, 3341 individuals received prophylactic inoculation against plague. In some cases, the people came to hospital to receive these injections, but in most cases either Christian communities, or enlightened village elders, sent a request that some one might be sent to their own village to carry out the treatment. For this purpose, journeys were made North, South, East and West of Swatow, in some cases, a two days' journey being necessary to reach a group of villages that had combined to make the request.

As this is the fourth year in succession in which several thousands of cases have been reported under this heading, it is obvious that the method has passed beyond the experimental stage, and that prophylactic injections are demanded, *not* because they are recommended by a foreign doctor, but because thousands of villagers have proved from their own experience that Haffkine's vaccine does afford some degree of protection from plague. Unfortunately, in many cases, people do not ask to be inoculated till the disease has actually appeared in their town or village, so that probably some of those who come to be inoculated are already infected and may fall victim to the plague bacillus some days after the inoculation has been received, but before it has had time to afford any protection. When such a calamity occurs, a man dying from plague a few days after receiving inoculation, the neighbours are apt to have their faith in Haffkine's method weakened, but the more enlightened are now realising that the way to prevent these accidents is to have inoculation performed *before* plague makes its appearance in the neighbourhood.

One would like to put on record the action of

Mr. Lim of Tat thau pou who made a donation to the hospital for every day that a competent assistant remained with him, while he advertised over a wide area that poor people desiring to receive inoculation could come to his house and receive it free of charge.

Some wealthy merchants from Tsng-lim also arranged for such a scheme to be put into operation at the time that plague was raging near their home.

Some years ago, by arrangement with the European doctors of the Port and the Indian Medical Department (which manufactures and sells the prophylactic). Mr. Kuan Hien-theng was licensed to carry out inoculation against plague; but early in this year it became obvious that it was impossible for the European doctors and Mr. Kuan to do all the inoculating that was demanded. Therefore, advantage was taken of a plan which the doctors in South Fokien had made (with the acquiescence of the Indian Medical Department) to increase the number of authorised inoculators. Under this scheme, twenty-four ex-students and assistants of the Swatow and Chao-chow-fu hospitals have been authorised to administer prophylactic inoculations against plague.

CHOLERA—It is fortunate that this year the conditions as to rainfall, etc., have not been such as to lead to a widespread epidemic of cholera. In about 78 cases it was necessary to introduce saline solution into a vein (the method described by Leonard Rogers of Calcutta), and, although in some of the cases, this operation had to be repeated 3 or 4 times, yet, in the vast majority of the cases, the result was entirely satisfactory. When small children are attacked with choleraic diarrhoea there may be difficulty in exposing a vein that is large enough to permit of an intravenous injection being given. In such cases, as well as in some adults, the fluid was introduced directly into the abdominal cavity, with results that were all that could be expected. The fatalities were mostly due either to the doctor being called in too late, or the patient disregarding the directions that had been given as to diet, etc.

In addition to the 78 patients above referred to, there were scores of other cases in which milder measures sufficed to bring about complete recovery.

In this connection it cannot be too strongly insisted that what is most urgently required for the health of Swatow is a *Hospital for the treatment of infectious disease*—an isolation hospital.

One cannot refrain from expressing one's appreciation of the kindness and helpfulness of those administering the charities of the Tai-hong temple (on the opposite side of the road to the mission Hospital.) By their courtesy most of the cholera patients were treated in the small rooms which they benevolently provide as "Homes for the Dying." An infectious diseases hospital, however, should provide much more accommodation and a staff of trained attendants under the supervision of a European doctor.

Two of the minor benefits of such an institution would be, that the patients at such a hospital would be cared for by properly trained attendants better than by their ignorant, if affectionate, relatives. Secondly, the doctor would be able to visit all his patients more easily, and, therefore, more frequently, if they were gathered together in one place.

The community at large would be greatly benefited by an infectious diseases' hospital. At present, people are constantly exposed to the risk of infection from the illness and death of their neighbours of such diseases as plague and cholera. The risk would be greatly minimised if those, suffering from these diseases, were gathered together in one place, and separated from their fellowmen. No better proof of this could be afforded than the record of the cholera epidemic in this port two year ago. The number of fresh cases showed an increase every week till General Wu granted the use of the old fort (which has since been renovated) as a cholera hospital. At once all the sick were brought together in one place, and so ceased to be a danger to their families and neighbours. From that date the epidemic began to show a decline which was rapid and continuous.

TUBERCULOSIS of the lung ("consumption") is probably the commonest cause of death amongst the student class in China, and tuberculosis of the bones and joints is a very common cause of ill-health amongst the working classes, leading to months or years of invalidism and often to permanent deformity or impairment of function.

If any country ever needed a crusade against tuberculosis and against the habit of spitting which so often conveys the infection from the sick to the healthy, that country is China. Later generations will blame us if, realising as we do how much suffering and death are to be attributed to tuberculosis, we do not endeavour to check the spread of the disease. / To check the ravages of this disease, it is essential that indiscriminate spitting should be stopped, and that patients who are infected should be diagnosed early, while the disease is still in a curable stage. The indisputable evidence that a patient is suffering *not* from a cold or bronchitis but from tuberculosis, is the presence in his sputum of the tubercle bacillus. Five of the student-assistants are now competent to discover the presence of the bacillus in the spit, to stain it properly, and recognise it under the microscope. Out of 148 specimens of sputum examined last year the tubercle bacillus was present in 61.

ANKYLOSTOMIASIS. Another disease that has brought some hundred patients to the hospital during the past year is ankylostomiasis-"hook-worm disease"-a condition of which a good deal has been heard recently, in consequence of the endeavour of the United States to prevent the entrance into North America of immigrants who harbour this parasite.

This is not the place to enter upon a detailed description of how these intestinal parasites, like the fabled vampires, suck the blood of their victims and so enervate the inhabitants of vast areas of the tropics. The worm is barely half an inch long and does not require much blood for its sustenance, but as a patient may harbour from 300 to 1000 of them, and the blood may ooze for a long time from the puncture that each has made, it is obvious that the worms may cause a very considerable loss of blood.

It is curious that though a good many years have elapsed since the first patient was treated for ankylostomiasis in the Swatow Mission Hospital, yet it is only within recent months that the inhabitants of some of the villages nearest to Swatow have discovered that treatment in the mission hospital will cure their anaemia (native drugs are valueless) and give them back that joy in living and capacity for working which have alike been lost in the lethargic weakness to which the worm gives rise.

One hundred and twenty patients have been treated for ankylostomiasis during the past year; 56 of these came from Swabue, Hau-u, or one of the neighbouring villages,—the remainder were distributed over seven of the nine districts into which the Chao-chow prefecture is divided.

G. D. W.

FINANCIAL.

The receipts from all sources for the year amount to $9061.36 and the expenditure to $8994.87, leaving a balance of $66.49 in the hand of the treasurer.

We beg to offer our hearty thanks to all who have helped by contributions and otherwise to the upkeep of the hospital. We also thank those,—English and Chinese,—who have helped in the Evangelistic work daily carried on among the patients.

STATEMENT OF INCOME AND EXPENDITURE.

By Donations, Fees &c.	$5047.79
„ Sale of Drugs; Trusses;	1044.88
„ Payments from patients	977.19
„ Rent of small wards	622.50
„ From F. C. M. for drugs £130	1358.00
	$9061.36

To Debit balance from last year	$ 97.18
„ Wages	1656.74
„ Repairs on buildings	369.37
„ Drugs, Rectified spirit &c. bought locally	1747.01
„ Drugs from London	2543.11
„ Dressings Oil, Cotton Wool, Lint &c.	1001.49
„ Stationery, Paper & Sundries	335.93
„ General Expenses (Ground Rent, Insurance &c.)	139.46
„ Lighting and Water	757.99
„ Help and Food to poor patients	346.59
„ Balance in hand of Treasurer	66.49
	$9061.36

Audited by
G. DUNCAN WHYTE.

A. LYALL *Treasurer.*

KITCHEN A/C.

Cr.

By Receipts from Patients	$3844.67
„ From Hospital Funds for Poor patients ...	346.69
Balance due Treasurer	14.09
	$4025.35

Dr.

To Expenditure on food, wages, Coal &c.......	$4025.35

DONATION, FEES, &c.

Drawn Thread fund per Mrs. Lyall ...	$727.00
Gou Meng Seng 吳明成	150.00
Gou Meng Seng 吳明成	150.00
Messrs. Bradley & Co. 德記洋行	150.00
Anon 無名氏	120.00
Mrs. Lim Nguan Sun	100.00
Per Miss. Greig	100.00
Ko Laû Phûa	100.00
Drs. Braugwin & Hobson	100,00
Low Cheang Yee 榮福源	100.00
Anon. 鄭順益	62.80
American Baptist Mission	60.00
An Tshù	50.00
Anon 學心氏	50.00
Tsng-lîm per Tē Sun Seng 鄭順成 ...	50.00
Kueh tè sì hí mêng	50.00
Dr. & Mrs. Duncan Whyte	50.00
Dr. & Mrs. Lyall	50.00
Lim Tuang Chee 林傳之	50.00
Messrs. Jardine, Matheson & Co., Ltd. 怡和洋行	50.00

Messrs. Butterfield & Swire 太古洋行...	50.00
,, Hock Cheang & Co. 福昌公司 ...	50.00
,, Lauts & Haesloop 元興洋行...	50.00
W. G. Lay	50.00
Yang Khi Phou 楊祺圃	50.00
The Swatow & C'chow Railway Co. 潮汕鐵路公司	50.00
The Standard Oil Co., of New York 三達洋行	50.00
The Bank of Taiwan Ltd. 臺灣銀行 ...	50.00
The Suà Tie Kit S. Launch Co. 汕潮揭輪船公司	50.00
E. V. S. Lim & Co. 源順公司代理華商輪船公司	50.00
The Asiatic Petroleum Co. per T. K. Brownrigg	50.00
Tek Seng	40.00
Swatow Chinese Congregation	40.00
Anon 隱名氏	40.00
Lim Tuang Chee 林傳之	40.00
Iê Ki Hiang 姚繼賢	30.00
Dr. Omata	30.00
Nguân Nguan Hong 源源茶行	30.00
I Hûa Hang 怡和行...	30.00
Lim Pang Kiet 林邦杰	30.00
Kwok Lai Chow 郭麗洲	30.00
The Swatow Kaiming Electric Co. 開明電燈公司	30.00
The Swatow Waterwork Co. 自來水公司	25.00
J. A. Shore	25.00
The Swatow Dispensary 惠安藥房 ...	25.00
Ko Un Khim 高蘊琴	25.00
Tē Hong Chiu 鄭豐周	24.00
Ng Hu Tsu 黃輔之	24.00
Per Captain Wolff S. S. "Rajaburi" ...	20.45
Ang Hiap Sang 洪協生...	20.00
Siau Iu Khim 蕭友琴	20.00
Ko Iu Huat 高有發	20.00
Li Tsak Lim 李作霖...	20.00
Tshu Tiā	20.00

Kong Iah Seng 公 益 成	... ...	20.00
Heng Siau Zu 王 少 瑜	... ...	20.00
Teng Zu 應 如	.. ..	20.00
Iô Tsu Huang	... ...	20.00
Chiu Seng	... ...	20 00
Miss. Harkness	... ...	20.00
Kuan Tek Heng	... ...	20.00
Mrs. Tan Chiang Yong 陳 章 榮	... ...	20.00
Mr. Kirrman & Dr. Benoit	... ...	20.00
Tan Hah Li 陳 合 利	... ...	20.00
Siau Iu Khin 蕭 友 琴	... ...	20.00
Chiu A Chieh (Hapsua)	... ...	20.00
Chiu A Chieh	. ...	20.00
Ie Iah Ki 楊 益 記	... ...	20.00
Ie Iah Ki 楊 益 記	... ...	20.00
Gwan Chiang	... ...	20.00
Nam Kee 南 記	... ...	20.00
Messrs. Gebr. Roese 新 昌 洋 行	... ...	20.00
G. D. Pitzipios	... ...	20.00
Messrs. Ben & Co. 悦 泰	... ...	20.00
Tshu Tsu I 徐 子 祥	... ...	20.00
Eng Chai Nguan 翁 財 源	... ...	20.00
Heng Khi Kuan	... ...	20.00
I Hing 怡 興	... ...	15.00
Tsng-lîm Luang Hng 樹 園	... ...	15.00
Hûa Huat 和 發	... ...	15.00
Tsu Sok U 朱 雪 吾	... ...	15.00
T. K. Chang 張 廷 鑒	... ...	15.00
Seng Nguan 成 源 正 記	... ...	15.00
Iak Seⁿ Ièh Pang 益 生 藥 房	... ...	15.00
Tan Sun Hua 陳 順 和	... ...	1500
Tam Fuk Yu 譚 福 曜	... ...	15.00
Bé Thai Seⁿ 馬 泰 生	... ...	15.00
Chie Tsàn Phoù 章 俊 浦	... ...	10.00

Mien Seng (Tekseng)	10.00
Rev. H. W. Oldham	10.00
Cheng Sêng	10.00
Tie^{n} Liang Kî	10.00
Bôu Iâ	10.00
A. W. Edmunds	10.00
Iê Li Phīan 姚利賓	10.00
Miss. Craig	10.00
Iê Kiam Seng	10.00
Kong Huat 公發	10.00
An Huat 洪發	10.00
Captain Hodgins 海陽船主	10.00
Buān Thai 萬泰	10.00
U Kang Iang	10.00
Iâm Tsaù	10.30
Li Nguan Tek	10.00
Tan Iông Ki	10.00
Sim Lou Tuang	10.00
Ko Su Che 顧樹齋	10.00
Lou Se^{n} Hang 盧世翰	10.00
Ng Tsu Chheng 黄之清	10.00
Hong Chhiang	10.00
Tê$_{n}$ Sun Seng 鄭順成	10.00
Ng Hu Tsu 黄輔之	10.00
Lîm Tsang Sin 創垂堂	10.00
Cheung Yum	10.00
Kek Heng 吉興	10.00
Pao Chen Dispensary	10.00
Gou Tok Ngi 吳卓儀	10.00
Gou Siang Hue 吳祥輝	10.00
Thng Meng Tsu 湯銘之	10.00
Sam Seng 三盛	10.00
Seng Keng Siu 辛經受	10.00
Gek Hong Zu	10.00

Uang Hiang Poú	王向甫	10.00
Sim Heng Thuan	沈興端	10.00
Sim Heng Thuan		10.00
Sim Heng Thuan		10.00
Iû Khiam Ti	游劍池	10.00
C. S. Holdsworth		10.00
Tek Kee Bue Tsang	德記煤棧	1[illegible]
Jameson McG. Forbes		10.00
W. F. Alway		10.00
Chinese Telegraph Administration		10.00
F. K. Brownrigg		10.00
Ie Bun Keng	楊文江	1.000
Nguan Heng Seng Ki	元興成記	10.00
Messrs. Wendt & Co.	興盛洋行	10.00
Li Khang Jien	李康然	10.00
W. Wagner		10.00
H. Féer	法國領事	10.00
N. Kasai	日本領事	10.00
Tshûa Than Jien	蔡坦然	10.00
Mark C. Lim	林俊良	10.00
W. T. Ching	曾會同	10.00
Compradore Geb. Roese	新昌辦房	10.00
Chin Tie Kong Si	振潮公司	10.00
Chua Hang Nguan	蔡漢源	10.00
Siau Chiao Seng	蕭捷盛	10.00
D. Percebois		10.00
W. H. Page		10.00
China Merchants Co. per Siau Soak Chew	蕭叔椒	10.00
Chiap Li	捷利	10.00
J. Skadiaug		10.00
Siau Chhiu Lam	蕭秋南	10.00
Pue Nguan Tshng	培源莊	10.00
Lim Tek Hak	林德合	8.00
Tan Teng Eng		5.00

Tie^{n} Khiang Meng	5.00
Li A Buc, Nam Ie	5.00
Li A Buc ,, ...	5.00
Li Kang Jien 李康然	5.00
Buān Thai 萬泰	5.00
Mrs. Worley	5.00
Tsu Kia Chiu	5.00
Phua Kí Thien 潘其珍	5.00
Ko Toa Ko	5.00
Li Kang Tsho	5.00
Chiàu Ngam	5.00
Tê Sun Seng 鄭順成	5.00
Lîm Lang Kai 林蘭階	5.00
Kueh Phêng 郭平	5.00
Khou Tsün 許俊	5.00
Chiu Liang Sang	5.00
Captain Suà Buc Launch	5.00
Anon 無名氏	5.00
Khou Tsun 許俊	5.00
Lau Tsun Tsho 劉俊初	5.00
Mr. J. P. Anderson	5.00
S. Barker	5.00
J. M. de Cruz	5.00
S. Kye Lim	5.00
C. Hodgson	5.00
A. E. Herdman	5.00
J. Thun	5,00
T. Carr Ramsay	5.00
H. W. Hosking	5.00
H. G. Fletcher	5.00
R. H. Strangman	5.00
V. Ruffin	5.00
Mrs. Asverus	5.00
Long Chhiang Sui Thai 隆昌瑞泰 ...	5.00

Fan Yung 范榮	5.00
Ang Chung Suey 洪增瑞	5.00
Sing Mi Sing	5.00
Tan Theng Kheng	5.00
Po Tai Wo Dispensary 保太和	5.00
S. Wyatt Smith	5.00
Woo Gek Hua	5.00
M. S. Myers	5.00
Chhiang Long 長隆	5.00
Nang Seng Li 顏盛利	5.00
Kwai Fung 仁昌印務處	5.00
Kuang Siu Chhiang 廣壽昌	5.00
Iak Siu Dispensary 益壽藥房	5.00
Ang Cheng Ngou 洪增熬	5.00
Buan Thai 萬泰	5.00
Kheng Seng Heng 慶新興	5.00
Tek Heng Khuang 得興館	5.00
K. B. Fontaine	5.00
O. Witte	5.00
Messrs. Lee Brothers & Co. 維記公司	5.00
Tan Gek Tshan 陳玉鏘	5.00
S. Nishigori 西郡宗三郎	5.00
J. S. Than	5.00
Tan Tek Kun 陳德君	5.00
Tan Pù Jiang	4.00
Patient Pang Khoi	4.00
Tai Chhiang 泰昌	4.00
Lim Sok Leng	4.00
Sì Huat Sim 四發嬸	4.00
Tsok Só 袁足嫂	4.00
Khou Tok Keng	4.00
Hu Hong	4.00
Patient Phû Iê Chhi	4.00

Ko Iong Se^{n}		4.00
Teo-Chew Flood Relief Fund per F. C. Butcher & Sim Kye Pang		4.00
Zuah Thai	悅泰	4.00
Zu Tshai	裕才	4.00
Heng Siau Zu	王少瑜	4.00
Tsu Song	子松	4.00
Li Heng I		4.00
Thòng Thai		4.00
Tshua Hong Nguan	蔡丰源	4.00
Jin Seng (Sin hie^{n})	仁成	4.00
Tie Tsu Iah	張之益	4.00
Gui Soi^{n} Meng	魏先明	4.00
Lîm Ou Khi	林胡祺	4.00
Tsok Hong	足丰	4.00
Hong Huat		4.00
In smaller sum, or names of donors not ascertained		$336.41
	Total...	$5516.46
Less grant to Women's Hospital and loss on dollars...		$468 67
		$5047.79

The following donations, collected by Tie Kien Tsho and handed to me towards the end of the financial year, will appear in next year's accounts.

以下張健初先生經手繳到太遲該欵
入在一千九百一十五年數內

Kia Huat	嘉發莊	15.00
Long On	隆安莊	10.00
Iah Long	益隆	5.00
Iong Huat	榮發	5.00
Lou Bun Ki	盧文記	10.00
Siam Heng Li	暹興利	10.00
Hu Hong	阜豐莊	20.00
Lou Hau Tshuan	盧浩川	5.00
Tan Tek Seng	陳德成	10.00
Tshu Che Lam	徐星南	10.00
Phou Thong Dispensary	普同	5.00
Tek Hua	德華	2.00
Tsun Chhiang	峻昌	1.00
Li I Sin Se^{n} Nie	李員先生娘	10.00
Iah Leng	益齡藥房	4.00

REPORT

OF THE

SWATOW MISSION HOSPITAL

AND OF THE

SWATOW WOMEN'S HOSPITAL

IN CONNECTION WITH THE

PRESBYTERIAN CHURCH OF ENGLAND

For 1915.

PRINTED BY
KWAI FUNG
PRINTER, BOOKBINDER & STATIONER,
SWATOW.
1915.

STAFF.

GENERAL HOSPITAL

A. Lyall M. B. C. M.

G. Duncan Whyte M. D.

Ie Huai Kun

Tan Sui Tsho

Kuan Hien Theng

Li Ngiap Hun

Siau Hiau Tsho

WOMEN'S HOSPITAL

Nina H. Beath M. B. CH. B.

Tan Peng Kui

Phe Un Thong

汕頭福音醫院一千九百十五年之佈告

本院之設原不獨爲醫人疾病亦以播傳福音眞理勸人悔改歸順上帝信賴耶穌以期民德歸厚爲宗旨故早晚有禮拜講道而凡就醫病勢須在院日久者亦敎之讀書識字冀其聽道更易明也溯本院開設至今已閱五十三年接續無間而就醫者年多一年故院屋宜逐漸推廣自初創至今改建或推廣已凡五次査現年就醫人數計住院者男二千九百二十八名女六百四十一名不住院者男六千七百八十五名女三千一百六十一名請往其家診視者九百八十名合共一萬四千四百九十五名比上年多一千二百七十八名不住院者若以其至院診視取藥之次數計之則爲四萬二千三百八十一次請往其家診視者若以次數計之則爲一千四百一十四次以上就醫之人其須用刀針剖割者眼症六百一十八人其餘各症九百一十三人此外又有請往接生者三人至院拔牙齒者六百三十五人注射防疫者九百四十四人又女院住院者一千五百三十二人不住院者二千二百二十一人請往其家診視者五百三十九人合共四千二百九十二人不住院者若以其至院診視取藥之次數計之則爲九千一百六十四次請往其家診視者若以次數計之則爲六百六十七次其中用刀針剖割者各

症共二百二十六人眼症三百五十六人婦人病四十四人請接生一百七十五人至院拔牙齒者一百六十四人就醫者如此之多其住總房者每日惟取食費銀一毛一分住舊稅房者每月取房租銀四元住新稅房者每禮拜取房租銀二元醫費俱分毫不取不住院者若逢拜二拜五對期就醫亦分文不取惟不對期者則每人取銀三毛貧乏者亦不之討取銀三毛者不過藉以整秩序省時間耳非所謂醫費也如是就醫者衆則藥物與他項費用自多且現年各物騰貴常用之藥多有不但價貴而且得之最難者故費用益巨如此巨費何處籌充此爲敝同人之所罣慮者也乃蒙中西諸位仁德君子慷慨捐助迨至年終結數竟不但足敷所用而且存有餘款此敝同人不勝感激稱謝捐助諸君不已也不第此也本院稅房原間數無多一遇多人求租每有不能應付之嘆乃榮福隆頭家劉長意君慨捐巨款大銀二千一百元以建新稅房又蒙諸善士樂捐湊至七兌銀五千七百四十二元即龍銀五千四百四十三元八毫五建成三層樓屋一座上下計共房廿三間并安置電燈水管每房眠床兩具就醫者租爲養病之所不但適宜且合衛生敝同人又感謝捐建諸君不置也自汕頭創立電燈公司之始其機師曾向數富商提及易士透光電鏡之益勸之集款購買以贈本院爲驗病之用

於是三年前由郭麗洲君送來銀二百九十七元即龍銀二百六十二元特爲買此物之用但未足可買故其銀至今尚存凡有心帮助本院者敝同人莫不感謝之也兹將全年進支数目列左

進　欵

收捐銀六千七百二十三元八毫七

收賣藥及牛乳腎風帶共銀一千六百元零八毫零五

收就醫者所還銀七百四十八元九毫四

收房租銀五百九十九元一毫五

共銀九千六百七十五元六毫

英會出買藥銀一千三百元不在其内

支　欵

束金與工資共銀一千八百七十六元五毫二

地租保險共銀一百三十一元八毫六

修整院屋共銀四百三十一元零六分

倫敦買藥共銀三百二十八元七毫三

本地買藥共銀四千一百六十二元二毫四
布棉花油共銀一千一百零八元四毫三
紙與各等雜費銀三百三十七元三毫七
電燈及水費共銀七百八十六元
帮助貧病者共銀一百八十七元七毫四
共銀九千三百四十九元九毫九

總　結

原銀六十六元四毫九
收銀九千六百七十五元六毫
出銀九千三百四十九元九毫五分
存銀三百九十六元五毫五分

懷敦幹
來愛力
楊懷瑾
謹白

REPORT.

This report covers the work done from November 1st. 1914 to October 31st. 1915. The hospital books are always closed at the end of October in order, to coincide with the financial year of the E. P. Mission.

The year under review has been one of steady uninterrupted work. There was no cholera epidemic and less Bubonic plague than usual in the district of which Swatow is the centre. In the city of Swatow itself, for some years, few cases of Bubonic plague have been seen; but in the early spring of this year there was a small outbreak of Pneumonic Plague, confined to one street, mostly occupied by Cantonese. Fortunately it did not spread,—the means used to combat the disease, being aided by the opportune occurrence of a spell of warm weather.

Ways and Means.—The question of "ways and means" has given us much concern. The cost of almost everything has greatly increased. Many drugs in daily use have not only enormously increased in price but. also, have been difficult to obtain.
The increasingly large number of patients means, of course, the consumption of much medicine and much expenditure of other kinds. How to obtain the requisite supplies has given us much trouble and concern. We are thankful to end the year with a balance in hand, and we are truly grateful to the large number of friends, both Foreign and Chinese, who have generously contributed to the funds of the hospital. Some have even increased their usual subscriptions. We venture to hope that the contributions for the coming year may not be less liberal.

The Foreign Mission Committee of the Presbyterian church of England has continued their grant of £120 for drugs and £10 towards the upkeep of the hospital buildings and, in connection with these grants, we desire specially to thank Dr. Bruce Low and the congregation of St George's Presbyterian church, Sunderland.

We have also to acknowledge with hearty thanks the receipt of a box of useful articles from Liverpool per Miss Heyworth.

The Swatow Waterworks Co. has continued to supply water at half price, a most practical way of helping the hospital in its beneficent work among the suffering Chinese around us.

For some months we had the help of Dr. M. S. Ross until he went to Chao-chow-foo to take charge of the medical missionary work there. Drs. Chalmers and W. C. Dale, also, gave some assistance in September.

New Block of private wards.

There is a great demand for private wards by people who are a little better off or more educated than the generality of our patients, and are willing to pay for the privilege of having a small room to themselves. We had 14 small wards available for this purpose, but the accommodation was much too limited to meet the demand.

Last summer, an old friend, Low Cheang Yee of the Yong Hock Guan Hong, offered us a sum of $2100.00 towards the expense of building additional private wards. We accepted the gift which was made as a thank offering for medical services rendered to him for many years. Other donations from Chinese friends brought the total amount up to $5742, Swatow Currency, (Mex $5443.85). A three-storeyed block has been erected, all the rooms furnished, the electric light installed, and water brought in at a cost of Mex $5469.27.

On the first and second storeys there are, in all,

12 wards each with two beds, two rooms for Chinese nurses, and two Kitchens for the patients. A rent of $2 per week is charged for each room. On the top storey there are one room for microscopic work and six rooms for medical students. We tender our grateful thanks to the Chinese friends who supplied the funds, and it must be gratifying to them to know that since the building was completed and opened, all the wards have practically been constantly occupied.

X. Ray apparatus Wanted

When the eletric light was installed in Swatow, the Engineer in charge, suggested to a few of the more prominent Chinese merchants that they might take the opportunity of presenting the hospital with an X Ray outfit. A beginning was made to collect funds for this purpose, and three years ago a sum of $297.00 (Mex $262.00) was handed to us by Mr. Kwok Lai-Chow. Since then nothing more has been done, and the need for an X Ray outfit is year by year being more urgently felt, not only for the Hospital work, but also for the Port, There is no X Ray apparatus in Swatow. The present, we know, is not an opportune time to appeal for funds, but we would strongly recommend this scheme to any Chinese who may wish to do a service to the Hospital and to medical work generally in Swatow. We have made no estimate, as yet, of the amount required but in addition to the $262.00 in hand, at least $1000.00 more would be needed, for in order to take advantage of the electric light current, transformers and accumulators will be necessary. For half of the year the electric current is not on during the day so accumulators will be necessary to have the X Ray apparatus available at any moment.

STATISTICS

The following are the statistics for the year:—

In-patients, male	... ...	2928
do. female	... ...	641

Out-patients, male	6785
do. female	3161
Patients seen in their own homes... ...	980
Total number of individual patients ...	14495
Total attendance of outpatients	42381
Total visits to patients in their homes	1414
Inoculation against Bubonic Plague ...	944
Surgical operations, on the eye	618
do. do. general	913
do. do. obstetrical	3
do. do. Dental	635

Of the above operations 452, mostly major operations, were performed under chlorofrom.

The total number of individual patients treated was 14495, an increase of 1278 over last year's number.

There has been a marked diminution in the number of cases of inoculation against plague. The number is less then one third of last year's. This is partially accounted for by the fact that plague was not prevalent in some districts in which a lot of inoculations was done in previou years.

On another page, a summary of the principal surgical operations performed during the year, will be found; but, beyond this, no attempt will be made in this report to portray the large amount of medical and surgical work which has been overtaken. It has been no light task to the two medical missionaries in charge, even with a comparatively large Chinese staff to help them.

The Chinese staff, exclusive of nurses and servants, consisted of five assistants, eleven students, a preacher and a Bible Reader. On them necessarily devolves much of the routine work of the hospital and this they have done in a satisfactory manner.

In-patients,—The daily average of inpatients each month has varied from 119 in february to 296 in october.

In-patients are charged eleven cents a day for their food, but no charge is made for medicine or other treatment.

As has been already indicated, there are now two sets of pay wards for such patients as do not care to go into the general wards. A charge of four dollars per month is made for one set of fourteen wards, and two dollars per week for the other set of twelve wards.

Out-patients—The average attendance of out-patients on out-patient days has varied from 136 in February to 370 in October.

On two days of each week, Tuesday and Friday. outpatients are seen, and such medicine and treatment as is necessary, given to them free of charge, but those coming on days, other than fixed dispensary days, or outside of dispensary hours, are expected to pay thirty cents, unless manifestly poor. No poor patient is refused.

Accident cases and emergency cases are seen and attended to without charge at all hours.

Evengelistic Work—The missionary side of the hospital work, we endeavour to keep in its proper place of prominence. As the Chinese church develops, changes in missionary methods are, no doubt, called for, to take advantage of new opportunities arising from ever changing conditions brought about by many influences in the course of the passing years. But for purely evangelistic efforts, the hospital provides opportunities as yet surpassed by few of the many forms of Christian work employed on the mission field. We regret that these opportunities are, for many reasons, not always fully taken advantage of.

For the greater part of the year, we had no hospital preacher, The one appointed to this office, broke down in health and was obliged to retire.

The Colporteur's duties are, primarily, to work in the outpatient clinic in the forenoons, and to visit the wards in the afternoons to converse with and read to the patients,—especially those who are entirely confined to bed. He has done his work in a fairly satifactory manner.

The daily morning and evening services in chapel have been conducted by the Pastors of the Swatow Congregations, the Assistants in the Schools and College, the Theological students and the hospital staff.

Two biblewomen, under the superintendence of Miss Harkness, have conducted classes in the afternoons for the benefit of the patients. These classes have been well attended,—The attendance varying from 30 to 50 throughout the year.

As the people attending these classes were, of course, continually changing, a very considerable number of men and women, must pass through them in the course of a year. A good many from these classes have applied for admission to the church.

The applicants for Baptism and any others who may care to come and listen, are called together on sunday afternoon for examination and instruction. This class has, for the most part, been conducted by Ng Siu-teng.

Five former patients were admitted to the Swatow Church during the year, but there has been no opportunity of examining the records of the 40 or 50 other churches scattered throughout the Swatow region. The biblewomen say that they rarely visit a station in the country without coming across women who have been taught in the hospital

SURGICAL OPERATONS,—A SUMMARY OF—

On the Eye,

Operations for Entropion & Trichiasis ...	284
„ „ Trichiasis (by Electrolysis)	124
„ „ Pterygium	42
Iridectomy	52
Cataract	25
Peritomy	10
Abscission of Anterior Staphyloma	5
Enucleation of Eyeball	4
Glaucoma, Elliot's trephining	3
Symblepharon	4
Canthoplasty	3
Plastic operations on Eyelids...	6
Excision of cysts, growths	26
„ of nasal duct	1

On the Body of Generally,

Operations for Vesical Calculus *mostly suprapubic*	12
„ „ Cario-necrosis of bones ...	110
„ „ Internal Haemorrhoids ...	88
„ „ External Haemorrhoids ...	15
„ „ Fistula in ano	78
„ „ Harelip	15
„ „ Hydrocele	24
„ „ Rectal prolapse	1
„ „ Slit ear lobule	22
„ „ Sinuses	45
„ „ Imperforate anus	3
„ „ Narrow anus	2
„ „ Empyema	1
„ „ Hypertrophied oscalcis ...	2
„ „ Epithelioma of lip	2
„ „ Elephantiasis of leg	1
Plastic Operations	5
Amputations	19
Radical operation for Inguinal Hernia ...	3
„ „ Congenital „ ...	1

Radical operation Femoral Hernia	1
Abdominal Section for gunshot wounds ...	2
„ „ Intussusception of bowel	1
Enucleation of Thyroid cyst	1
Extraction of bullets lodged	12
„ Calculus lodged in Urethra ...	6
„ Polypus of nostrils	21
„ Rectal Polypus	3
Foreign bodies from nose, ear œsophagus &c.	11
Excision of Tonsils	18
„ Callosities	11
„ Female breast	1
„ Male breast	1
„ Cyst of breast	1
„ Epulis	5
„ Branchial cyst	2
„ Meningocele of neck	1
„ Cysts, sebaceous &c.	42
„ Tumours	36
„ Cervical glands and tumours ...	33
„ Elephantiasis scroti	5
Tapping Ascites	19
„ Pleural Effusions	6
External Urethrotomy	2

STATEMENT OF INCOME AND EXPENDITURE

Income		Expenditure	
Balance from last years	66.49	Wages, assistants & Servants	1,876.52
Donations, Fees, less grant to Women's Hospital and loss on dollars	6,723.87	General Expenses (Ground Rent & Insurance &c.	131.86
Sale of Drugs, milk, Trusses	1,608.05	Repairs on Buildings, Furnishing	431.06
Payments from Patients	748.94	Drugs from London paid by Hospital...	328.73
Rent of Small wards	599.15	Drugs Rectified spirit, milk bought locally	4162.24
	9746.50	Dressings, Cotton Wool, Oils, Lint	1108.43
		Paper, Stationery, and Sundries	337.37
		Lighting and Water	786.00
		Help to poor patients	187.00
		Balance in hand of Treasurer	396.55
			$9.746.50

Audited and founde orrect
G. Duncan Whyte
J. C. Smith

GENERAL HOSPITAL
KITCHEN A/C.

Total Receipts	$4114.77
Total Expenditure	3.960.28
Balance in hand of Treasurer	154.49
	$4.114.77

NEW BLOCK OF PRIVATE WARDS:

STATEMENT OF ACCOUNT:

Slow Currency.

劉 長 意

By Low Cheang Yee donation		... ...	$2.100.00
Tan Tau Nam	,,	陳道南 ...	500.00
Tan Thong Hou	,,	陳桐侯 ...	400.00
Low Koon Yee	,,	劉坤意 ...	300.00
Kueh Tsu Pheng	,,	郭子平 ...	200.00
Tan Siu Sua	,,	陳秀山 ...	200.00
Tan Ngang Chhiu	,,	陳雁秋 ...	200.00
Tan Hue Zu	,,	陳晦如 ...	200.00
Li Tsu	,,	李芝 ...	200.00
Tan Jiak Phang	,,	陳若帆 ...	200.00
Tie Hau Tek	,,	張孝德 ...	200.00
Tan Tsai Hng	,,	陳栽園 ...	200.00
Lou	,,	劉干 ...	162.00
Kueh Pek Hiang	,,	郭柏香 ...	100.00
Kueh Zui It	,,	郭惟乙 ...	100.00
Tan Sui Ki	,,	陳垂記 ...	100.00
Tan Tek Seng	,,	陳德成 ...	100.00
Kueh Tshun Phou	,,	郭春圃 ...	100.00
Tan Iong Kheng Tng	,,	陳永慶堂 ...	100.00
Lim Kok Liang	,,	林國樑 ...	50.00
Siau I Ek Tng	,,	蕭燕翼堂 ...	20.00
Puo Nguan Teng	,,	培源莊 ...	10.00
			$ 5.742.00

=Mex $ 5.443.85

Debit Balance Charged to Hospital a/c. 25.42

Mex $ 5.469.27

To Cost of Building in cluding Painting Mex$4333.66

Rebuilding boundary wall, and

renewing part of courtyard 167.58

Green Island cement	82.60
Furnishing the wards	565.92
Electric Light Installation	224.31
Laying down Water pipes	33.20
Memorial Stones	62.00
	Mex $ 5.469.27

Subscriptions and Fees—

For Medical Service per G. D. W. ...		$ 500.00
Drawn Thread fund per Mr. Lyall ...		308.70
Lim Huang Soi	林放先 ...	200.00
Mess. Bradley & Co.		150.00
Lou Cheang Yee	榮福源 ...	150.00
Tia Hong	鼎豐 ...	150.00
Tang Long Chhiang	東隆昌 ...	100.00
Peh Mong	柘茂 Unclaimed balances	
Kueh Hang Seng	郭漢陞 ...	
Swatow Keng Tshat Kek	汕頭警察局	100.00
Kwok Lai Chow	郭麗州	100.00
Low Koon Yee	劉坤意	100.00
Tie Siam Kai	張蟾階	100.00
Drs. Brangwin & Hobson		100.00
Yang Khi Phou	楊祺圃	60.00
Mess. Lauts & Haesloop		50.00
Miss. Harkness		55.50
Te Sun Seng	鄭順成	50.00

Hak Sim Si.	學心氏	50.00
Gek Hiang	... ...	50.00
Chia Chiah	謝 石	50.00
Pai Tai Wo	... ...	50.00
Dr. Ross. part of Fee	... ...	50.00
Mess. Jardine Matheson & Co.,	... ...	50.00
,, Butterfield & Swire	... ...	50.00
,, The Standard Oil Co. of New york	,	50 00
,, The Asiatic Petroleum Co.	... ...	50.00
,, E. V. S. Lim & Co.	源順公司 ...	50.00
,, Hock Cheang & Co.	福昌洋行	50.00
,, The Bank of Taiwan	台灣銀行	50.00
Sua Tie Kit S.S. Co.	汕潮揭輪船公司	50.00
C. Chow & S'tow Railway Co.	潮汕鐵路公司	50.00
W. G. Lay	... ...	50.00
Dr. A. Lyall	... ...	50.00
Dr. Whyte	... ...	50.00
Rev. Floyd Bates	... ...	50.00
Fee, Khek Khoi	... ...	50.00
Sng Tshan Kek Png Seng Sai Tng	方承先堂	40.00
Swatow Chinese Congregation	汕頭禮拜堂	40.00
Tan Gek Kia Nai	陳玉經奶	40.00
Si Huat Sim	... ...	35.00
Cheng Heng (Heng Siam Zu)	王少瑜	60.00
Sam Iah Tsu	三益書莊 ...	150.00
Gwan Chhiang	元昌	30.00
E. Hua Hong	怡和行	30.00
Lim Thuan Tsu	林傳之	30.00
Kwok Lai Chow	郭麗州	30.00
The Swatow Dispensary	惠安藥房	30.00
Captain White s.s. Rosarii	... ...	25.00
Kaiming Electric Light Co., Ltd.	開明電燈公司	25.00
The Swatow Water Co.	自來水公司	25.00
British American Tobacco Co., per V. R. Vick		25.00
Rev. J. Steele	... ...	24.94
Leng Koh £2 =	... ...	23.20

Hah Li	合利	20.00
Chiu A Chiap, fees	... ...	40.00
Ie Iah Ki	楊益記	20.00
Chin Heng Kong Si	振興公司 ...	20.00
Chin Chhiang	振昌行	20.00
Cheng Heng	增興	20.00
Fung Chuh sim	... ...	20.00
Te Iong Khang	鄭永康	20.00
Tang Seng	東成	20.00
Chia Theng huang	謝騰芳 ...	20.00
Chia Zun Tsho	謝潤初	20.00
Png Su Jin	方樹人	20.00
Ki Hah Sun	紀合順	20.00
Tek Kee Bue Tsang	德記煤棧 ...	20.00
Li Hang Kue	李享衢	20.00
Nam Kee	南記	20.00
Mess. Ben & Co.,	悦泰	20.00
Chao Chow Chiu Sue Kek	潮州酒稅局	20.00
Tan Chhiang Yong	陳長榮 ...	20.00
Eng Tshai Nguan	翁財源 ...	20.00
Siau Iu Khim	蕭友琴	20.00
The Bank of China	中國銀行 ...	20.00
Iong Heng Hong	煒興行	20.00
Pue Nguan Tsng (Chiu Nam)	培源莊	20.00
G. D. Pitzipios	... ...	20.00
T. K. Chang	張廷鑒	20.00
Gebr. Roese	... ...	20.00
Compradore Gebr. Roese	... ...	20.00
Chip Hong	集豐	20.00
Tshun Hong	春豐	20.00
Ngan Seng Li	顏盛利	20.00
Lee Ngak Chhin	李岳臣	20.00
Tshu Sok Hua	徐椒和	20.00
Chia Chi Chieh	張泰祥謝靜石	20.00
Cheng Hong	增興	20.00

Gueh Po So		16.00
Mr. Ibsen		16.00
Kim To Tshan	金在田	15.00
Cheng Heng	增興	15.00
Sim Hiong Kiam	沈雄堅	15.00
P. S. Li		15.00
Mr. Paton		15.00
Khou Gek Tshuan	許玉川	15.00
Jih Seng	益盛	15.00
Jameson M. S. Forbes		15.00
Bo Thai Se	馬泰生	15.00
Tan Siau Ki	陳紹箕	15.00
Li Kang Jiang	李康然	15.00
N. Kasai		15.00
H. Von Borch		15.00
Yak Seng Dispensary	益生藥房	15.00
Chua Thang Jiang	蔡坦然	15.00
Seng Nguan	成源	15.00
Seng Mui	成美	15.00
Ie Kun Iang	楊君遠	14.00
Fee per G. D. W. Cheque $11.30		12.10
do. do. $11.53		12.36
Siong Hong	祥鋒號	12.00
Fee per G. D. W. Cheque $11.40		11.80
Tan Tshai Tsu	陳財書	10.00
Png Kui Piang	方季斌	10.00
Lok Su Li	洛士利	10.00
Lu Che Ia		10.00
Ng Tong Chhin	黃棟臣	10.00
"M"		10.00
Hong Hah	鴻合	10.00
Tan Tsu Tshan	陳書田	10.00
Li Su Tsu	李素芝	10.00
Tshua Tai Seng	蔡大升	10.00

Mr. Nielson	... ...	10.00
Chia Mng Tan Si	周門陳氏 ...	10.00
Mr. Lim (Phu Leng)	... ...	10.00
Kueh Keng Seng So	... ...	10.00
Iah Ang	益安行	10.00
Tek Kee Tsun Pang	德記船房 ...	10.00
C. S. Holdsworth	... ...	10.00
Sim Kye Pang	沈開榜	10.00
J. H. A. Hance	... ...	10.00
Li Seng Kong Si	勵成公司 ...	10.00
Chua Hang Nguan	蔡淡源	10.00
D. Perecbois	... ...	10.00
Mrs. J. Skadiang	... ...	10.00
J. Skadiang	... ...	10.00
I. H. L. Haesloop	... ...	10.00
Nguan Heng Seng Ki	元興成記 ...	10.00
Greenlaw F. W. Sabbath School £ 1	...	10.90
Chiu Kheng Tng	周肯堂 ...	10.00
Heng Zu Lang	王御蘭	10.00
Kim Hua ...	金和	10.00
Chia Tsu Hui	謝之惠	10.00
Patient, Liang Heng Li	... ...	10.00
Iong Heng Kong Si	永興公司	10.00
Fung Ying Chih	... ...	10.00
Ng Tong Sua	黃重山	10.00
Chen Au Chim	... ...	10.00
Tan Hah Li	陳合利	10.00
Tan Si Chiu	陳四周	10.00
An Huat	安發 (2 donations) ...	20.00
Tang Si Chiu	陳四周	10.00
Tan Nguan Tiam	陳元沾	10.00
Rev. Pere Vogel	... ...	10.00
Kai Shing (for 1914)	祺昇	10.00
Hah Li	... ...	10.00
Ji Muo	... ...	10.00

Khek Ti		10.00
Fung Ying Chih		10.00
Tsng Koh Tong	莊閣東	10.00
Anon		10.00
Gou Kui Seng	吳桂生	10.00
Phua Zu Tsu	潘如之	10.00
Tung Ying Chih		10.00
Ie Bun Kang	楊文江	10.00
Kai Shing	祺升 (2 donations)	10.00
S. Barker		10.00
G. F. Chin	陳玉璐	10.00
Mark C. Lim	林俊良	10.00
Chin Tie Kong Si	振潮公司	10.00
Khou Siu Leng	許修翎	10.00
Siau Chiap Seng	蕭捷盛	10.00
Jin Hong	仁豐	10.00
S. Wyatt Smith		10.00
H. Freer		10.00
Chinese Telegraph Administation		10.00
China Merchants N. S. Co.	招商局	10.00
C. H. Wood		10.00
Huang Hui Po	袁慧波	10.00
Lim Tsang Sui Tng	林創垂堂	10.00
Iah Ang	益安行	10.00
Ng Tsu Bue	黃作梅	10.00
Ng Zui Kang		10.00
Gou Teng Soh	吳穎椒	10.00
Pun Ki		10.00
Tsang Hiok Teng	曾旭亭 (2 donations)	20.00
Nguan Chhiang Li	源昌利	10.00
Tan Tau Lam	陳道南	10.00
Tie Gek Sang	張玉珊	10.00
Iap Khai Tiau	葉凱超	10.00
Chua Seng Choo	蔡成書	10.00
Te Theng Chhiu	鄭廷秋	10.00

Sim Bue Siang	沈梅仙	10.00
Tan Po Tsu	陳寶書	10.00
Mien Seng Hong	綿成行	10.00
Tang Nguan	... ...	8.00
R. B. McLachlan	... ...	8.00
Chiap Li	... ...	8.00
C. Hodgson	... ...	7.00
Kek Siang	吉祥行	6.00
Tang Tsu Keng	陳子乾	6.00
Iah Seng	益盛號	6.00
Ie Si	楊氏	6.00
Chhiang Long	長隆	6.00
Tan Tshai Tsu	陳財書	6.00
Siang Pong Ho	祥錄號	6.00
Chiu Choo Chai	... ...	5.00
Tan Chin Sam	陳震三	5.00
Lau Peng Hun	劉炳剛	5.00
Sih Khi Hun	薛啓煌	5.00
Lim Lang Kai	林閬階 (4 fees)	20.00
Tie Kim Thiam	張錦添	5.00
Li Peng Khuan	李炳光	5.00
Sim I Chheng	沈頤清	5.00
Heng Siam Zu	王少瑜	5.00
Tsong Khuan Gauh	什成樂	5.00
Pau Tai Hua Dispensary	... ...	5.00
Kwong Seng	... ...	5.00
Gow Chi Tong	吳紫東	5.00
Kang Ti Ki	江智記	5.00
Ang Cheng Iau	洪增耀	5.00
Ie Chiu U	楊照吾	5.00
Sim Tiau Sun	沈調順	5.00
Pai Tai Woo	... ...	5.00
Ng Seng Tek	黃盛德	5.00
Mrs. Worley	... ...	5.00
Tan Tia Hong (2 fees)	陳鼎豐 ...	10.00

Sim Kye Lim	沈開林	5.00
J. M. da Cruz		5.00
Hu Tsun		5.00
Tshuu Chhe Koh	蔡星閣	5.00
S. H. Yong	章向榮	5.00
G. Witte		5.00
F. K. Brownrigg		5.00
H. G. Fletcher		5.00
C. G. Asker		5.00
R. H. Strangman		5.00
Mr. Smith		5.00
Fan Yung		5.00
Ang Cheng Suee	洪增瑞	5.00
Ho Cheng Ung		5.00
Chen-Un Chin	陳元沾	5.00
Ang Ching Nou	洪增蔡	5.00
J. S. Than		5.00
T. Carr Ramsay		5.00
H. Unotoro		5.00
Lee Brothers	李維記	5.00
Kwai Fung	仁昌印務局	5.00
Eo Kee	怡記	6.00
Sing Wei Sing		5.00
Io Hun Thiu	楊雲濤	5.00
Yak Siu Dispensary	益壽藥房	5.00
Mrs. Asverus		5.00
W. T. Cheng	曾會同	5.00
Wei Gek Hua		5.00
G. C. Hanson		5.00
Buan Thai	萬泰源記	5.00
Kuong Siu Chhiang	鄺壽昌	5.00
Ngan Seng Li	顏盛利	5.00
J. Thun		5.00
Tan Chheng Nguan	陳清源	5.00
Tan Tek Khun	陳德君	5.00

Tan Chie Ngam	陳照岩	5.00
Iap Chie thong	葉照唐	5.00
Tsang Gauh	莊樂	5.00
A. H. Johnson	... ...	5.00
Lim Kok Liang	... ...	5.00
Tan Li Hah	陳利合	5.00
Phua Zu Tsu	潘如之	5.00
Ngi Chheng	... ...	4.00
Tsu Kau	之厚	4.00
Li Chhiang Chhe	李長青	4.00
Khou Tok Kheng	許琢卿	4.00
Goi Piah Tsu	倪璧芝	4.00
Sim Tsu Hng	沈滋園	4.00
Yue A Tong	... ...	4.00
Tie Lip Seng	張立新	4.00
Tshun Hua Ho	... ...	4.00
Gou Siah Khuang	吳錫光	4.00
Khou Tshun Mong	許春茂	4.00
Leng Kok Kheng	... ...	4.00
Tsu Tok Chin	... ...	4.00
Tshua Tshun Lim	蔡春森	1.00
Chia Tai Chiau	謝大朝	4.00
Lou Iong Pa	劉耀豹	4.00
Kuan Su Ia	... ...	4.00
Se Tie	... ...	4.00
Te Hua Seng	致和祥	4.00
Kueh Hua Hong	郭和豐	4.00
Sen Ie Jin	... ...	4.00
Gou Hiang Si	吳香時	4.00
Li Hun Siang	李雲祥	4.00
Nguan Chhiang	... ...	4.00
Ngan Seng Li	顏盛利	4.00
Tan Si Pou	陳四布	4.00
Thau Kak Zu	陶覺如	4.00
Siau Su Ia	... ...	4.00

Lim Ngi Ui	林毅偉	4.00
Li Tsua	利泉	4.00
Nie Su Ia	梁容光	4.00
Tshua Tek Chhin	蔡德臣	4.00
Lim Kong Kiau		4.00
Ie Tek Siang		3.00
Lim Lai Thiam		3.00
Tan Chiau Kim		3.00
Tan Zu Chin		3.00
Leung Ying Kuang		3.00
Wong Jung		3.00
Ek Sam		3.00
A Iau		3.00
Mrs. Hauser		2.90
In Smaller Sums, or Names of donors not obtained.		261.14
Per W. T. Ching	以下什會同先生經手	
Chong Yee Sang	張義生	50.00
Mrs. Lai Kee	禮記	10.00
Chue Ching Ho	徐清河	5.00
Chong Ng Kong	什梧岡	10.00
Tong Siu Chow		3.00
Yong Kwai Ngok	楊季岳	2.00
Ng Koon Put	吳君弼	1.00
Yap Tit Ng	葉鐵吾	1.00
Lai Chee Ho	黎子和	2.00
Cheah Mong Chee	謝夢池	200.00
Cheah Yee Kiao (2 donations)	謝逸橋	20.00
Ko Peng Cheng	高鵬程	5.00
Kim On, Contractor	建安	5.00
Siu Hua Seng	新和盛	5.00
Sun Hing	三興	4.00
Miss Looker	裕記	2.00
Mrs. T. W. Ching	什會同先生娘	10.00

Per Tie Kien tsho:--以下張健初先生經手

Kia Huat	嘉發	15.00
Long An	隆安	10.00
Iah long	益隆	5.00
Iong Huat		5.00
Lou Bun Ki		10.00
Siam Heng Li	暹興利	10.00
Hu Hong	阜豐	20.00
Lou Hau Tshuan		5.00
Tang Tek Seng		10.00
Tshu Che Lau		10.00
Phou Thong Dispensary		5.00
Tek Hua		2.00
Tsun Chhiang		1.00
Tsok Hong	祝豐	5.00
Zu Huat	裕發	5.00
Iah Leng		4.00
Li I Sin Se Nie		10.00

Per Messrs. Ben & Co.—以下悅泰經手

Lee Jim Lee	李任勵	20.00
Lou Cheng Koon		5.00
Heng Tok Leng		1.00
Lou Long Teng	倚南深處	50.00
Lou Yam Huat	劉炎發	15.00
Lou Long Yam	劉隆炎	15.00
Sih Wang Lou	薛蔚樓	20.00
Poh Tong Chun		5.00

Per Tow Keng Kee:—以下杜景祺先生經手

Tou Keng Kee	杜景祺	5.00
Lim Siau Ngo	林小忠	5.00
〃 Ngam Chieh	林雁石	5.00
〃 Ngi Seng	林毅誠	2.00
〃 Hong Tshai	林宏材	2.00
〃 Thai Ma	林太媽	2.00

Lim Li Si	林李氏	...	...	...	3.00
„ Sim Si	林沈氏	...	...	...	2.00
„ Gou Si	林吳氏	...	...	...	2.00
„ Khou Si	林許氏		...	...	2.00
„ Sim Si	林沈氏		...	...	2.00
Sua Sin Su	沙慎思		...	...	10.00
Lim Ngi Eng	林毅英		...	...	5.00
Lim Siau Bue	林少枚		...	...	5.00
Lim Phuan Tsho	林盤初		...	...	5.00
Lim Ngiong Chiu	林仰周			...	2.00
Lim Kia Chhiu	林鋭秋		...	...	20.00
Tsu Chhe Lam	徐星南		...	...	5.00
Lim Ang Ki	林安記		...	...	5.00
Kou Su Ki	許仕記	...	...	...	10.00
Tsai Hong	再豐號	...	...	...	5.00
Kou Jiat Pang	許若鵬		...	...	5.00

WOMEN'S HOSPITAL

STATISTICS

Inpatients	1532
Outpatients	2221
Patients visited in their own Homes ...	539
Total Individual Patients	4292
Total Visits of Patients to Dipensary ...	9164
Total Visits paid to patients in their own Homes	667

OPERATIONS

General	226
Eye	356
Gynecological	44
Obstetrical	175
Dental	128
Chloroform administrations	164

Fees, Donations to Oct. 31st 1915.

Tie Pu Iong	$4.00
Tshua Mia Chieh	20.00
Lim Kuang Ki	6.00
Tan Kim Chiu	4.00
A. Hong Nng	6.00
Lim Ngak Zu	10.00
In Sim	6.00
Li Hai Tong	15.00
Kien Tong Sim	4.00
Tie Sin Khi	5.00
Sim Tshun Hua	10.00
Nguan Tau Pheng	15.00
Ng Ngi Huang	5.00
Teh Hu	4.00
Phou Thong Tsang	10.00
Su Mien thou Chhien	10.00
Pu Hong Ho	5.00
Tit Ti Sim	10.00
Tan Mong Li	20.00
Kheng Hong Ho	20.00
A Sou Nng	4.00
Meng Teh	4.00
Lim Kuang Ki	6.00
Cheng Heng Hang	20.00
Tie Hah Thih	4.00
Tsun Iong	10.00
Ngiam Sin Se	5.00
Lau Si Huat Sim	35.00
Gou Iong Seng	4.00
Hak Ti	4.00
Ie Seng	8.00
Sit Iah Sim	6.00

Tan U Sim	3.00
Ngou Chhiang	8.00
Sok Hiang Nng	4.00
Kui-Iong	5.00
Ni Ang Sim	5.00
Gou Thai Nguan	4.00
Zu Iong Nng	6.00
A Tek	10.00
Bun Sim	3.00
Sai Sim	4.00
Li Eng Zu	4.00
Khou Thiam Su	10.00
Teh Li Sim	10.00
Tie Hue Sim	4.00
Siau Lim Bak	4.00
Siau Hok Sim	20.00
Tan Tan Nam	50.00
Siang Li	5.00
Sa Kou	5.00
Soi Mue	4.00
Hieh Siang Tsang	20.00
Smaller Sums	81.00
Tan Seng Li	3.00
Midwifery fees, &c.	326.00
Special collected funds	50.00
Mrs. E. V. S. Lim	50.00
Per Mrs. Lyall	57.00
Rev: J. Steele	25.00
Share of General Subscriptions	405.00

REPORT

OF THE

SWATOW MISSION HOSPITAL

AND OF THE

SWATOW WOMEN'S HOSPITAL

IN CONNECTION WITH THE

PRESBYTERIAN CHURCH OF ENGLAND

For 1916.

PRINTED BY
TSUAN CHING & Co.
PRINTERS, BOOKBINDERS & STATIONERS.
SWATOW
1917.

STAFF.

GENERAL HOSPITAL

A. Lyall M.B.C.M.

G. Duncan Whyte, M.D.

Ie Huai-Kun

Tan Sui-Tshio

Kuan Hien-Theng

Tan Tiau-Thong

Tshua It. Siang

WOMEN'S HOSPITAL

Nina H. Beath M.B.Ch.B.

F. W. Heyworth L.R.C.P. & S.

Li Mok-Seng

Ie Zui-Gek

REPORT

FINANCE. In presenting the report of the Swatow Mission Hospital for the year ending 31st. October 1916 one cannot but put in the first place an expression of thankfulness that in spite of all the difficulties that have arisen, difficulties especially of obtaining drugs and other hospital supplies, it has still been possible to carry on the work of the hospital: and the number of patients treated has been larger than ever. In spite of the increased cost of living at home and the many urgent calls that have been made for subscriptions there the generosity of our friends has enabled the Foreign Missons Committee to continue its annual grant of £130 to the purposes of the Hospital.

The special feature of last year s report was its reference to the new block of rented wards which had been built on the initiative of Mr Lau Cheng Yee at a cost of over four thousand dollars. Probably the special feature of *next* year's report will be the installation of the new X-ray apparatus, that is being given to the Hospital. For this year it will suffice to put on record the unstinted generosity of our Chinese supporters in raising money for this object.

No sooner had the cost of the new block of wards been fully subscribed than Mr. Kee Buan Sun came forward—to be assisted later on by Mr. T.M. King—to act upon the suggestion contained in last year's report viz. "The need for an X-ray outfit is year by year being more urgently felt." These two gentlemen have raised over two thousand dollars and this, together with sums previously in hand and other sums that have been subscribed for this object, should be enough to cover the cost of a good piece of apparatus and provide adequate accommodation for it in the hospital.

It is only fair to say that last year as well as this these extra sums of money have been collected without in any way interfering with the regular increase in the value of the Chinese fees and subscriptions to the running expenses of the Hospital, which have never been so large as they are for the year at present under review. Some of these donations may represent a return "for services rendered" but many of them are signs of that spontaneous generosity which is content to do a good deed and hopes for nothing in return.

The names of all the subscribers to the X-ray outfit will be published when the apparatus is ready for use. The list of the subscribers to the ordinary hospital expenses will be found, along with an audited statement of the accounts for the past year, in the last pages of the Report. A comparison of this balance sheet with that for last year shows that, as a result of the erection of the new block of rented wards, the income derived from this source is practically double. All the wards are almost continually in use.

PATIENTS Turning to statistics regarding patients we find that over 15,000 patients, men, women and children, have been treated in the hospital during the past twelve months. Of this large number 90 % have not been asked to pay anything for drugs, or surgical dressings, or professional advice. It is only by the continued generosity of the subscribers to the hospital that so many people are able to receive free healing. Five hundred of the inpatients required an operation of such seriousness as to demand a general anaesthetic.

About 3000 visits have been paid to other patients in their own homes. Of these only a few can pay an adequate fee, but the majority are able to make a small contribution to the cost of their medicine, while some are too poor to do even this.

It is unnecessary to draw special attention to any other items in the detailed statistical statement which is given in the adjoining table.

STATISTICS

1st Nov. 1915 to 31st. Oct. 1916.

In-patients male..	3112
do. female..	640
Out-patients male..	7170
do. female..	3147
Seen at their own homes male	581
do. female..	530

Total individuals male	10,863
do. female	4317
Total attendances of outpatients, first and return	42990
Total visits to patients in their own homes ..	2975
*Operations :—	
General	967
Obstetric	8
Eye	532
Dental	738
Vaccinations etc	799
Opium smokers treated	30
Hospital beds	252.

SURGICAL. From the professional point of view there are always developments in the work. The increasing confidence of the Chinese enables us to carry out operations to which they would not have consented a few years ago. e. g. this year has seen an enormous cystic tumour of the kidney removed by Dr. Lyall from a small child and the first operation for chronic peritonitis with ascites, another for a large aneurism, as well as the more usual operations for calculus, hernia (two of the herniae were strangulated) goitre etc. In spite of the proverbial good nature of the Chinese we have every year many cases of assault and this year there have been two rather exceptional injuries. One man received a deep

*545 of the operations were performed under a general anaesthetic.

stab in the abdomen with perforation of the viscera which also prolapsed through the wound; he was brought at once to the Hospital where the wounds were closed and he made a complete recovery. Another man was a warder in the local prison on whom the prisoners (possibly as a result of the preaching they have every Sunday!) repeated the experiment that Jael performed on Sisera. When Dr. Lyall arrived at the patient's bedside he found that the nail had been driven into the skull for an inch and a half. This patient too made a complete recovery.

MEDICAL. One is glad to notice an increasing belief in the value of "Western Medicine" in non-surgical cases. There is an increase in the number of cases of valvular and other diseases of the heart that come to hospital, while an increasing number of pleural effusions are found that require to be tapped and of empyoemas that must be drained.

Leprosy. During the year a few cases of leprosy have submitted to the treatment recommended by Dr. Heisser of Manila. This is somewhat painful and has to be carried out week by week for several months, but in spite of these drawbacks patients who have persevered with the treatment have been very well satisfied with the results obtained. The treatment depends, partly, on the use of the oil of gynocardium (chaulmoogra) which is obtained from a seed that has long been used by Chinese doctors in the treatment of leprosy. Recently Leonard Rogers has been experimenting with a new preparation derived from the same source, viz. Sodium gynocardate, which can be injected into a vein without causing much pain. The use of this drug in India has been followed in some cases by apparent cure, so a supply of the drug has been ordered from Calcutta.

Diphtheria. Till a few years ago diphtheria was unknown in the Swatow region, but it must now be regarded as a regular cold weather visitant. This is doubly unfortunate because firstly the Chinese doctors, having had no experience of the disease, are not in a position to diagnose the condition and, secondly, they have not yet at their disposal a remedy to compare in effectiveness with the diphtheria antitoxin, which has reduced the mortality due to this disease in Europe from about 33 % to less than 10 %.

In Chinghai and Chaoyang as in Swatow itself cases are constantly occurring, and those which receive early and sufficient treatment with this antitoxin may be expected to make a good recovery.

Hookworm Disease. During the twelve months 800 cases of hook-worm disease (ankylostomiasis) have presented themselves at hospital and most of these have required two or three treatments to eradicate all the worms. Increasingly from year to year we find how densely the whole of this prefecture is contaminated with this disease. It is not as though only a few men in each village were infected with the parasite. Amongst the farmers from 70 % to 80 % suffer from ankylostomiasis, each individual harbouring perhaps some hundreds of these minute worms, which, by their attack on the lining membrane of the gut, not only drain away the patient's blood but also seriously interfere with his absorption of nourishment. It is no exaggeration to say that tens of thousands of men in this region are less energetic, less able to do a proper day's work than they should be, and are unable to earn a full day's wage, because they are infected with this parasite.

Cancrum Oris. A new line of treatment that has been tried in the past year is the use of "606" in cases of Cancrum oris. This is a gangrenous ulceration which begins in the cheek and spreads on to the face; it only attacks children in enfeebled health and usually ends fatally. Two out of three cases treated with this drug have made a complete recovery.

EVANGELISTIC. The directly evangelistic work of the hospital is carried on in five different ways.

(1) Every morning there is a service in the Hospital Chapel which is attended by the

outpatients and by such of the inpatients as are able to leave their beds. On Tuesday and Friday (when the service is conducted by the teachers in the Theological College, and the out-patients are treated for nothing) the attendance frequently exceeds 300. On other days this service is conducted by the minister of the Chinese church, by the Chinese treasurer of the mission and by some of the foreign missionaries.

(2) After the forenoon service the colporteurs may spend two or three hours in informal talks with groups of patients in the Chapel or in the wards with patients who are confined to bed. These informal conversations are also held in the wards in the afternoon.

(3) After the patients have had their mid-day meal those who care to do so gather in the Chapel again where some are taught to read the Gospels in "Romanised", the simplest way in which a Chinaman can be taught to read, while others learn by heart the simpler hymns. For the supervision of this part of the work we are indebted to Miss Harkness.

(4) In the evening worship is conducted in the Chapel of by one of the colporteurs or some other member of the Hospital Staff.

(5) On Sunday afternoons a meeting is held for the examination and instruction of those who have expressed a desire to enter the Church. This meeting is attended by many who are not yet professed "applicants" but are interested. "Haply they may feel after Him and find Him, though [in very truth] He is not far from any one of us."

SURGICAL OPERATIONS,-A SUMMARY OF-

On the Eye,

Operations for Entropion & Trichiasis ..	261
Do .. Do (by Electrolysis) ..	30
,, .. Pterygium	46
,, ,, Glaucoma, Iridectomy ..	1
Do Elliot's ..	2
Iridectomy (Artificial pupil)	53
Cataract Extraction	20
Do Soft..	5
Do Secondary operation..	1
Peritomy	28
Symblepharon	2
Abscission of Anterior Staphyloma ..	3
Enucleation of Eyeball	7
Operations for Prolapse Iris	5
,, ,, Hypopyon	5
,, ,, Ectropion (plastic) ..	2
Excision Lachrymal Sac	2
,, Cysts, Growths	37
Extraction of foreign bodies	5
Unclassed	17

On the Body Generally,

Operations for Vesical Calculus	9
,, ,, Harelip	37
,, ,, Slit Ear lobule	12
,, ,, Cario-necrosis of bones ..	116
,, ,, Fistula in ano	82
,, ,, Internal Haemorrhoids ..	60
,, ,, External Do	30

,,	,,	Rectal prolapse	3
,,	,,	Imperforate anus	4
,,	,,	Narrow anus	2
,,	,,	Phymosis	32
,,	,,	Paraphymosis	5
,,	,,	Hydrocele	46
,,	,,	Hypospadias	2
,,	,,	Sinuses	23
,,	,,	Empyema	3
,,	,,	Liver abscess	2
,,	,,	Do (Exploratory) ..	1
,,	,,	Salivary fistula	1
,,	,,	Suppurating Knee Joint ..	2
,,	,,	Intussusception of Bowel ..	1
,,	,,	Gunshot Wound of Bowel ..	1
,,	,,	Bayonet Do Do ..	1
,,	,,	Do Do Abdominal wall	1
,,	,,	Elephantiasis of leg (Kondolien's)	1
,,	,,	Ununited fracture of Patella	1
,,	,,	Suture of ulnar nerve ..	1
,,	,,	Aural Suppuration (Stacke's)	1
,,	,,	Cut Tendo Achilles	1
,,	,,	Gunshot Wounds, mostly of bones	10
,,	,,	Anchylosis of Joints ..	7
,,	,,	Large diffuse Aneurism of thigh	1
,,	,,	Aneurism of forearm ..	1
,,	,,	Tying Femoral artery (for Haemorrhage)	3
Excision of Tonsils			16
,,	,,	Callosities	17
,,	,,	Elephantiasis Scroti ..	4

,, ,, Tubercular Glands	.. ..	27
,, ,, Epithelioma of lip	.. ..	3
,, ,, Do Tongue	.. ..	1
,, ,, Do Penis	.. ..	7
,, ,, Large Cystic growth of Kidney		1
Plastic Operations	.. ..	6
Amputations	.. ..	21
Inguinal Hernia, Strangulated,	.. ..	2
Do Radical Cure	.. .. ..	10
External Urethrotomy	.. .. ..	8
Aspirating for Pleural Effusion	.. ..	14
,, Knee Joint	.. .. ..	2
Tapping Ascites	... .	13
Extraction of lodged Urethral calculus	..	4
,, ,, Nasal Polypus	.. ..	20
,, ,, Adenoids	.. .. ..	2
,, ,, Bullets lodged	.. ..	11
,, ,, Needles, splinters and foreign bodies from Oesophagus, Ear, Nose &c.		32
,, ,, Rectal Polypus	.. ..	4

Tumours:—Excision of

Lipoma	.. ..	8
Epulis	.. ..	5
Fibroma	.. .. ..	4
Granuloma	.. .. ..	7
Osteoma	.. .. ..	1
Enchondroma of toe	.. ..	1
Cysts,-sebaceous &c.	.. ..	26
Ranula	.. ..	2
Haematoma	.. .. ..	2
Branchial Cysts	.. ..	3

Hydrocele of Neck	3
Adenoma of female breast ...	2
Recurrent of female breast ...	2
Malignant „ „ ..	1
Angeioma	6
Parotid Growth	1
Large Congenital, of-Shoulder	1
Malignant	8
Unclassed	8
Enucleation of Thyroid cyst..	1
Excision of Elbow Joint	1
Electrolysis of Keloid &c.	14
Unclassed	137

STATEMENT OF INCOME AND EXPENDITURE

RECEIPTS

Balance from last year	396.55
Donations: Fees	
A. Foreign	3318.72
B. Chinese	5233.74
Sale of Drugs, milk, Trusses	1498.84
Payments from Patients	1156.98
Rent of Small wards	1264.00
Balance due Treasurer	975.07
	13843.90

Audited and found correct

G. Duncan Whyte

Thomas Bowen Partington

Note.—In addition to the above the hospital received a grant of £130 from the Foreign Missions Committee of the E. P Church for drugs.

EXPENDITURE

Wages:— Assistants & Servants	2214.41
General Expenses (Ground Rent & Insurance) &c.	117.79
Repairs on Buildings. Furnishing &c.	1034.05
Drugs from London paid by Hospital.	405.08
Drugs, Rectified spirit. milk	6885.65
Surgical Dressings. Cotton Wool, Oils	1107.53
Paper, Sundries,	442.80
Lighting & Water	989.75
Help to Poor patients	212.56
Share of Public Subscriptions to W. Hospital	434.28
	13843.90

A. Lyall

Treasurer

GENERAL HOSPITAL
HOSPITAL KITCHEN A/C.

balance from last year	154.49
total Receipts	4141.16
	4295,65

total Expenditure	$4290.60
balance in Treasurer,s hand	5.05
	$4295.65

A. L.

Treasurer.

Donations and Fees.

The following list contains the donations and fees received from November 1st 1915 to October 31st, 1916. The letter "f" after a name indicates fees.

We are very grateful to all who have helped us financially or in other ways. We beg to acknowledge specially the very generous donations from The Deli Planters' Vereeniging received through the kindness of Mr. van Izeren.

	Mex.	T.P.
The Deli Planters Vereeniging per M. van Izeren ..	1000.00	
Dr Brangwin and Hobson ..	775.00	
Drawn Thread Fund per Mrs. Lyall	432.00	
Mission Catholique (f.)	300.00	
The Deli Planters Vereeniging per M. van Izeren ..	250.00	
Roger S. Greene	217.70	
R. B. Stewart, Glasgow	196.87	
Messrs. Bradley & Co. 德 記 行	150.00	
Gou Mui Ki (f.) 吳 美 枝		150.00
Dr. Brangwin & Hobson	100.00	
Ko Uan Kum		100.00
W. G. Lay	75.00	
Yang Khi Phou 楊 祺 圃 ..	60.00	
Messrs. Butterfield & Swire 太古行	50.00	
,, Jardine Matheson & Co. 怡和行	50.00	
,, The Sandard Oil Co. of New York 三 達 公 司	50.00	
The Asiatic Petroleum Co. 亞 細 亞 公 司	50.00	

		Mex.	T.P.
.. British America Tobacco Co.	英美煙公司	50.00	
.. Hock Cheang & Co.	福昌	50.00	
.. E. V. S. Lim & Co.	源順公司	50.00	
.. The Bank of Taiwan	台灣銀行	50.00	
.. Yong Hock Guan	榮福源		50.00
M. Van Izeren		50.00	
G. Duncan Whyte, M.P.		50.00	
A. Lyall M.B.		50.00	
A. "Fine" per W. G. Lay ..			50.00
Te Sun Seng (f.)	鄭順成	50.00	
Sua-Tie-Kit S. S. Co.	汕潮揭輪船公司		50.00
C. C. & S'tow Railway Co.	潮汕鐵路公司		50.00
Swatow Tng-Hue	汕頭禮拜堂	50.00	
Chia Nguan Jiang	謝元讓		50.00
Pang Keng Siang	馮敬常		50.00
Png Ni Hun	方泥雲 ..	50.00	
Hak Sim Si	學心氏		50.00
Chua Seng Chow	蔡成之		50.00
Ie-Po-Bun	楊波文		50.00
Anon			50.00
Ton Zui Ngou (f.)	杜維五		50.00
Miss Harkness		41.60	
Lim Thuan Tsu	林傳之 ..		40.00
Chua Seng Chow	蔡成周		40.00
Tou Zue-Ngou (f.)	杜維五 ..		35.00
Chiu a Chieh	周石 ..		30.00
Tsu Ka-Kau	朱膠交	30.00	
Iu Piah Kheng	尤璧卿		30.00
Heng Mien Soi (f.)	王綿先		30.00

		Mex.	T.P.
Cheng Heng (f.)	增興	60.00	
Guan Chiang	元昌		30.00
E. Hua Hong	怡和行		30.00
Messrs. Ben & Co.	悅泰	30.00	
The Swatow Dispensary	惠安樂房	30.00	
Kwok Lai Chow	郭麗州		30.00
Lim Ngien Chiu	林仰周 (f.)		30.00
Tshu Sok Hua	徐淑和	30.00	
Tshua Tek	蔡德	30.00	
R. Tiefermann		25.00	
Kai Ming Electric Light Co.	開明公司	25.00	
Swatow Water Works Co., Ltd.	水龍公司		25.00
Uang Iang Chhiu	袁遠周		25.00
Per Miss Greig, London		23.00	
Lim Kia Chhiu	林鏡秋	18.00	
Rev. H. W. Oldham		20.00	
Rev. T. W. Douglas James		20.00	
Dr. R. Chalmers		20.00	
Leng Kok Liang			20.00
Chie Sun Seng	章順成		20.00
Kueh Siah Kui	郭錫奎		20.00
Tshu Sok Che	淑靜姊	20.00	
Kou Iong Seng (f.)	許永誠		20.00
Tan Song Teng (f.)	陳松亭	20.00	
Li Ngi Siu	李宜修	20.00	
Siau Iu Khim	蕭友琴		20.00
Ie Khai Chi			20.00
Tan Tek Li	陳德利		20.00
Tshai Nguan Ki (f.)	蔡元記		20.00

		Mex.	T.P.
Tshua Mong Lam	蔡明南		20.00
Kuang Seng (f.)	廣成		20.00
Cheng Hong	增興莊		20.00
Gou Thai Khiang	吳太堅		20.00
Tek Ki Bue Tsang	德記煤棧		20.00
Lee Hang Kue	李亨衢		20.00
Nam Kee	南記	20.00	
Bank of China	中國銀行	20.00	
Pue Nguan Tsng	培源莊		20.00
Lim Pue Ngou	林飛五	20.00	
Eng Tshai Nguan	翁財源	20.00	
Mitsu Bussan Kaisha Ltd.			20,00
Tan Chhiang Yong	陳章榮	20.00	
Tshu Tsu Siang	徐子祥	20.00	
Tan Hok Lam (f.)	陳旭南		20.00
Gou Tie Khim (f.)	吳潮欽		20.00
Lim Kia Chhiu	林鏡秋		12.00
Gou Teng	吳亭		12.00
Ki Meng Siu	紀明修	14.00	
Gow Hong Heng (f.)	吳豐興		15.00
Tan Tsu Liet	陳子烈		15.00
W. Paton		15.00	
Captain Jansen		15.00	
F. C. Butcher		15.00	
C. S. Holdsworth		15.00	
Jameson Mc G. Forbes		15.00	
J. H. R. Hance		15.00	
M. O. Clark		15.00	
T. J. Chua		15.00	
Jak Seng Dispensary	益生藥房	15.00	

		Mex.	T.P.
F. K. Cheng	張廷鑑		15.00
Li Khien Jiang	李康然	15.00	
Seng Nguan	成源		15.00
W. E. Ford		15.00	
Li Tshun Hui (f.)	李春耀	15.00	
Khou Ngo Khoi (f.)	許愚溪		15.00
Heng Goi Phon	王藝圃		10.00
Seng Mui (f.)	成美		10.00
Lim Pue Ngou	林培五		10.00
Kue Huah	瓜發	10.00	
Tan Peng Chhiang	陳炳章		10.00
Uang Hui Po	袁惠波		10.00
Lim Hou Sua	林雨山		10.00
Lim Hok Liang	林福連		10.00
Ie Chin per K Hien Theng	楊振	10.00	
An Huat	安發		10.00
Tah Ngiak Chhin	陳業岸		10.00
Tan Bun Leng	陳文龍	10.00	
Ou Ki Chhin	吳岐岸		10.00
Chin Kiu	振球		10.00
Tan Peng Chhiang	陳炳章		10.00
Tan Po Tsu (f.)	陳寶壽	10.00	
Tshu Cheng Ho (f.)	徐清何		10.00
Ng Gek Kui	黃玉桂 (f.)		10.00
Ang Tsu Bun	洪子文		10.00
Nguan Chheng Li (f.)	源昌利	10.00 &	10.00
Ie Kek An	楊吉安	10.00	
Lau Tshai Seng (f.)	劉財成	10.00	
Hiang Siang Zu (f.)	王少瑜		20.00
Cheng I Sui (f.)	鍾意修	10.00	

		Mex.	T.P.
Tan Gek Siam	陳玉嬌	10.00	
La Seng Kong Si	勵成公司	10.00	
Bradley & Co's Shipping Department	德記船務	10.00	
S. Barker		10.00	
C. Hodgson		10.00	
Sim Kye Pang	沈開榜		10.00
J. Skadiang		10.00	
Nguan Heng Seng Li	元興成記	10.00	
Ie Bun Kang	錫文江	10.00	
K. H. Strangman		10.00	
Ngan Seng Li	顏[illegible]利	10.00	
Sieo Sock Chow	蕭淑椒	10.00	
Siu Leng Dispensary		10.00	
S. Wyatt Smith		10.00	
H. F. King		10.00	
Chua Hang Nguan		10.00	
Buan Thai	萬泰行		10.00
Khi Seng			10.00
Chin Tie	振潮公司		10.00
Pau Tai Wo	保太和		10.00
R. Soulange Teissier		10.00	
H. Von Booch		10.00	
Gai Si Mue	倪四妹		10.00
Mark C. Lim	林俊良	10.00	
Siau Chiap Seng	蕭捷成		10.00
Jin Hong	仁豐		10.00
Sun Seng Ie Hang	潤成		10.00
G. T. Chen			10.00
Mui Li Ie Hang	美利洋行		10.00

		Mex.	T.P.
Per Dr. Ross (f.)		10.00	
Tshua Seng Tsu (f.)	蔡成書		10.00
Chia Chin Seng	謝振成		10.00
Ek. Soon & Co. (f.)			10.00
Ngang Khuan	源宏		10.00
Zu Li	裕利		10.00
Greenlaw U. F. Sabbath School		9.50	
Khou Buang Khiang		8.00	
Gek Siang Sam Nai	吉祥三奶	8.00	
Khu A. Keng	邱阿敬	8.00	
Te Hai Liang (f.)	鄭海良		8.00
Kuang Siu Chhiang	廣壽昌		8.00
Chip Li	集利	8.00	
Mrs. Lotz, Australia		8.00	
Kuang Iah	光益		6.00
Kueh Tsu Seng	郭子升		6.00
Ie Tsu Meng	楊子明	6.00	
Tsok Sim	足嬸	6.00	
Te Siau Iau (f.)	鄭紹耀	6.00	
Un Kim Che	温金	6.00	
Chhiang Long	長隆		6.00
Kuang Tek	廣德	6.00	
Tshua Chhe Koh	蔡星閣		5.00
Kuang Iah Zu (f.)	光益裕		5.00
Heng Siau Bun (f.)	王少文		85.00
Tshua Chheng Seng	蔡臣盛		5.00
Cheng Heng (f.)			35.00
Li Ngia Thi (f.)	李雅特		5.00
J. M. De. Cruz		5.00	
Sim Kye Lim	沈開林		5.00

	Mex.	T.P.
Hu Tsun 許俊		5.00
Y. A. Kou 游劍池		5.00
F. M. Young	5.00	
S. H. Yong 辛向榮	5.00	
F. K. Brownrigg	5.00	
T. M. Heng	5.00	
Kwai Fung 仁昌	5.00	
Mrs. Pang	5.00	
J. S. Than	5.00	
Tan Theng Khuan 陳廷光	5.00	
T. Carr Ramsay	5.00	
Tsu Ke Kau 朱家奎	5.00	
Tan Po Chi 陳寶書	5.00	
Goo Kang Kok 吳江谷	5.00	
Gou Huang Siau (f.) 吳芳紹		5.00
Li Soi Chow 李樹照	5.00	
Kwok Wai Nam 郭煒南	5.00	
E. A. Cavaliere	5.00	
Kwan Tek Hui 官德惠	5.00	
Wang Tse Kia 王治家	5.00	
Fun Yung 范榮	5.00	
Lu Heng Pu 盧興富		5.00
Tung Yung Chih		5.00
Lin Shao Chien		5.00
Wong Juong 王驤		5.00
Kwok In Kai 郭今階		5.00
Chinese Telegraph Administration 電報局	5.00	
Chin Huat (f.) 振發	10.00	
Khiu Keng Chiu		5.00

		Mex.	T.P.
Ie Chie U.	楊照香 (f.)		15.00
Gou Chhit Nai	吳七奶		5.00
Tie Sie Kia	張新加	5.00	
Khou Sia Ku	許聲舉		5.00
Tang Tek Seng (f.)	陳德成		5.00
Li Eng Phou	李應炮	5.00	
Tan Hong	東方		5.00
Hu Hong (f.)	阜豐		10.00
Pou Siang Teng	傅善亭		5.00
Tan Ngiap Cheng	陳業臣		5.00
Ie Hui Phou (f.)	楊惠普		10.00
Tie Pheng	張平		5.00
Tan Tek Li (f.)	陳德利		10.00
Mrs. Worley		5.00	
Tsang Ki (f.)	贊記		40.00
An Iong Heng	洪榮興		5.00
Tsu Piang Ia	書邊爺 (f.)	5.00	
Tshua Tsu Pien (f.)	蔡子邊		5.00
Yung Ying Chih		5.00	
Tan Gek Chiam (f.)	陳玉簪		5.00
Ie Hiang Tsu (f.)	姚獻之		5.00
Tan Kou Theng (f.)	陳觀澄	5.00	
Ie Tsu	楊書	5.00	
Tou Keng Kee	杜景祺		5.00
Kueh Siu Sun (f.)	郭壽純		15.00
Sek Sek Lu (f.)	適適廬		5.00
Liang Ku Cheng	連顧鐘		5.00
Teng Liang Tshun (f.)	鄧連存	5.00	
Keh Siang Hong (f.)			10.00
Khou Loi Ngi (f.)	邱禮儀		5.00

	Mex.	T.P.
Tau Tai Hua		5.00
Mrs. Asverus	5.00	
G. C. Hansen	5.00	
Wee Gek Hua		5.00
F. D. Bisseke	5.00	
Iak Siu Dispensary 益壽		5.00
S. Tanaka	5.00	
Ang Cheng Ngou 洪增鰲	5.00	
Ie Hun Thiu 楊雲濤		5.00
Messrs Lee Brothers & Co. 維記		5.00
Gou Teng (f.) 吳丁		5.00
Tan Tek Seng		5.00
Tan Iak Cheng (f.) 陳約臣	5.00	
Ki Thai Ma 紀太媽		5.00
Chheng Chhiu 鐘樹		5.00
Lim Liang Hui 林良霏		5.00
Chia Peng Seng (f.) 謝秉生	5.00	
Tong Siau 中霄		5.00
Ti Meng Kong Si (f.) 智明公司		5.00
Kok Hiang (f.) 國賢		5.00
Khuan Nguan Chhiang 廣源昌		5.00
Phou Theng Dispensary		5.00
Gek Siang (f.) 玉祥		10.00
Chia Su 謝序	4.00	
Sng Iu Meng 孫友仙	4.00	
Gou Chhe Su 吳青史	4.00	
Gou Iau Tsho 吳耀初		4.00
Tan Tshai Tsu 陳材之	4.00	
Buan Seng 萬盛	4.00	
Tie Sok Ge 張淑牙	4.00	

	Mex.	T.P.
Tshua Tshai Kuang 蔡財廣 ..	4.00	
Iau Kui (f.) 瑤貴	16.00	
Lim Tshai 林財	4.00	
Sun Su Heng Chhim (f.)	36.00	
順裕興昌		
Sim Hiong Khiang 沈榮堅 ..	4.00	
Ie Pek Khiang 楊伯慶		4.00
Heng Tua Ti 王大弟	8.00	
Sng Song Sam 孫宋三 ..	4.00	
Gou Siam Tshai 吳叁財 ..	4.00	
Li Jiau Ki (f.) 李然記 ..	4.00	
Gui Soi Meng 魏細明 ..	4.00	
Koh Liang Teng 閣連亭		4.00
Li Si Long (f.) 李時隆		4.00
Lim Iu Sua 林友山	4.00	
Chia Chi Tek Hng 謝濟德堂 .	4.00	
Tek Li (f.)		4.00
Li Theng Kuang 李廷光 ..	5.00	
Pue Kim Hiang 飛錦賢 ..	4.00	
Ie Pek Ngam		4.00
A. Lak 阿陸		4.00
Hang Ngi 翰院	4.00	
Tshu Thien Ho 徐天河 ..	4.00	
Quak Hua Hong 郭和豐		4.00
Kueh Tu	4.00	
Zu-Li		4.00
Iu Mui Kai Ai		4.00
Lim Huai Tek 林懷德		4.00
Tan Khiang 陳強		4.00
Tie Tong Siang	3.00	

		Mex.	T.P.
Li A. Bue		3.00	
Khou Si		3.00	
Chen Ah Chim		3.00	
Iau Peh			3.00
Kim Chhe Kong Si			3.00
In Smaller Sums or Name of Donors Not obtarned			253.16
Per Tie Kien Tsho:—			
Hu Heng	阜豐		20.00
Po Seng	寶成		15.00
Tek Seng	德成		10.00
Tia-Heng	潮豐		10.00
Kia-Huat	嘉發莊		15.00
Ie Heng Tsok	楊恆足		5.00
Kuan Iah Zu	光益裕		5.00
Lou Hai Tshuan	盧海全		5.00
Pau Chin	保真		10.00
Iah Long	益隆		5.00
Long An	隆安		10.00
Iah Leng	益[illegible]		4.00
Siam Heng Li	暹興利		10.00
Kia Huat (For 1915)	嘉發		15.00
Hu Heng (Do)	阜豐		20.00
Iah Leng (Do)	益隆		5.00
Long An (Do)	隆安		10.00
Siam Heng Li (Do)	暹興利		10.00
Pau Chin (Do)			10.00
Per C. F. Chuang:—			
Chong Wo & Co.	中和公司		10.00
C. F. Chuang	莊子[illegible]		10.00

		Mex.	T.P.
Lee Tong Bank	利通莊	..	..10.00
Sin Tai Hong	新太行..	..	..10.00
Y. S. Chuang	莊荣升..	10.00	
Liang Ngan Chor	梁雁初	..	..5.00

WOMENS' HOSPITAL

STATISTICS

Inpatients	1362
Outpatients	2518
Total Individual Patients	3880
Total Attendances	9258
Patients Visited in Their Homes	435
Visits paid to patients in their Homes	750

OPERATIONS

General	195
Eye	327
Obstetrical	167
Gynecological	43
Dental	141
Chloroform administrations tered	170
Minor Operations (Incomplete)	113

N. H. Beath

Donations and Fees to Women's Hospital.

Tie Nguan Nng	$2.00
Tshai Tshuan	4.00
Li Hap Sun	4.00
Bun Sui	2.00
Sih Kok Khiu	10.00
Kheng Hong Hang	2.00
Ng Sin Se	2.00
Su Ho Chheng	20.00
Li Nng	12.00
Tsu Ka Kau	30.00
Sun Hah Ie	20.00
Tan Sin Se	4.00
Chiu Nng Chhiang	4.00
Chiap Hah	2.00
Sia Huat Ki	10.00
Tou Chhie Sang	4.00
Ng No Jit	2.00
Su Hiang	5.00
Tie Tsun Mong	2.00
A. to	2.00
Phou Thong Tsang	10.00
Sim Siang Kuang	60.00
Tsu Ai Sim	1.00
Tie Zui Sim	10.00
Tan Kang Heng	2.00
Tiet Pheng	200.00
Tshua Tsang Mong	4.00
Tan Chhiu Iam	4.00
Ie Tsu Khim	12.00
Ng Tsang Eng	10.00

Chin Hua Heng	20.00
Li Hua Hong	4.00
Tan Sam Ie	20.00
Tsu Bun Nng	6.00
Tshua Tia Huang	6.00
Tie Meng Sin	1.00
Sia Ki Sua	30.00
Ki Hap Sun	10.00
Eng Tsua Kim Heng	2.00
Tan Mng Si	2.00
Khou In Song	2.00

汕頭福音醫院週年報告

（一千九百十五年十一月）
（至十六年十月三十一日）

本醫院開創歷有年所就醫者日益衆而費用日益繁洎自歐戰發生藥物昂貴雖由大英長老會捐助金磅一百三十爲藥劑費幸得樂善諸君解囊相助是以醫務得以支持非賴諸君博施濟衆之力詎得若此更荷劉長意君倡捐建築新宿舍故現年所收之房租較去年加倍藥劑之費益有所賴今養病舍雖已增多而定租者每有不敷之嘆將來勢必擴張以應就醫者之用旋又荷紀萬順王德茂諸君捐銀二千餘元以購易士鏡一具並建適宜之房舍以安置之諸君樂善不倦非僅如是而已卽常年捐亦逐年增多誠感佩之靡既矣至一年中就醫之男婦老幼統計一萬五千人十之九乃受濟者不收其分文其寄宿在院者男三千零十二人女六百四十八人照醫期來就醫者男七千一百七十人女三千一百四十七人到院領藥共四萬二千九百九十次用割術者一千五百十二人其中大症用迷蒙藥者五百四十五人拔牙者共七百三十八人種痘者共七百九十

九人眼科需割者五百三十二人戒煙斷癮者三十人接生八人延至其家診症者男五百八十一人女五百三十八人週年間醫生至病家診症共三千次

玆將一年間治痊之症就其最著者論之如左

外科用割術者

就醫者衆而信者亦多嘗有患內腎瘤者㾓臟者血囊者均用割術而癒其餘常見者有若砂淋腸疝脾核瘤等亦皆割治而癒另有特異者一人之腹部被刺頗深腸露且破血流如注卽至本院療治而癒又審判廳監犯一名頭部被釘釘入寸許猶得醫治而痊

內科等症

就醫者日增故心病肺病腦病肺胞膜積㾓肺膿等症較平時尤多餘如痲瘋疥症虧血勾虫口頰疖等症今一一述之

痲瘋

現年本院之治此症常以大風雜油射於患者之皮下治法較之服藥尤覺辛苦且當每星期射藥一次然尚有願就射藥者故獲效不少

痳症（俗名白喉）

昔年汕中不見此症近數年來於冬令常見之從前歐洲患此症而死者百之三十三其後發明一種特效之藥名敵痳盟注射於患者之皮下而死者少矣在潮州此症發生未久故中醫驟見此症或不認識雖能認識苦無良藥束手無策今潮陽澄海汕頭等處此症已屬常見苟有患者立至醫院就診得射此藥之足分劑其效如神試驗不爽

虧血勾虫（俗名黃沙）

此症在潮循各處可謂多矣匪直一鄉有之甚或一家數人同患者病甚者精神痿靡筋骨懈怠不能操作因虫住腸內嘬血令人血虧故也潮循之患此症者爲數不少矣其害豈淺尠哉現年此症就醫者數滿八百間有服殺虫藥一次不能癒當服數次方癒者

口頰疳

前患此症者每苦無藥療治現有新藥名六百零六射之有效然用之者仍少也

就醫須知

更有一事不得不貢獻於諸君者即患病者多有誤以上午就醫者衆恐醫生應接不暇而察驗不周迨至上午則驗病必詳故常有於下午到院求醫者孰知不然蓋本院之診症斷不因就醫者衆而生厭煩致有苟且診視之弊惟時迨下午醫生各有定務或門出巡病更無閒暇也此後就醫者雖喜出診金亦盼望均在上午勿於下午反有不便特此佈聞

汕頭福音醫院

懷敦幹
來愛力
楊懷瑾 謹白

Subscriptions toward X-Ray Apparatus.

以下係捐買易士鏡諸君芳名

紀萬順君經手勸題開列

豐遠輪題	五十元
怡和洋行題	五十元
豐盛輪題	三十元
老寶琴題	一百元
福昌洋行題	三百元
林光齡題	五十元
榮成利題	十元
王協利題	十五元
黃玉和題	二十元
蕭紀臣題	二十元
仁昌題	二十元
林子達題	三十元
順成洋行題	三十元
豐茂輪題	五十元
豐美輪題	五十元
紀萬順題	一百元
豐發題	二十元
吳信記題	二十元
光榮成題	十元
怡德和記洋行題	十元
悅泰公司題	二十元
藍裕錦題	十元

姚德順題	十元
張葵賓題	五元
厚豐	五元
德豐題	五元
萬合題	五元
紀祿記題	五元
勝豐題	五元
新南興題	五元
孔明齋題	五元
陳包氏題	四元
李湘圃題	十五

高鵬程題	十元
蕭兩初題	五元
南盧題	五元
捷美題	五元
合福盛題	五元
玉裕題	十元
隆成題	五元
協和題	十元
南發題	五元
陳成美題	十元

共題銀一千一百五十四

王德茂君經手捐款

郭麗州題	一百元
陳桐候題	一百元
隱名氏題	二百元
公發號題	一百元
廣成興題	五十元
三達公司題	二十元
辛向榮題	十元
宏安公司題	二十元
裕發號題	十元
文發行捐	五元
許兆豐捐	五元
陳鵬秋題	二百元
張蟾階題	一百元
公興號題	一百元
廣合公司捐	五十元
王德茂題	五十元
陳業臣題	十元
嘉發莊題	三十五元
英發行題	十元
大發行捐	十元
祥發行捐	五元
公發行捐	十元

共捐銀一千二百元

郭麗州捐龍　二百六十二元一式半

陳玉晉捐　二百元

宋景州捐　五十元

范斯蘭捐　五十五元

合共　龍銀三百一十七元一式半

直銀二千六百雰四元

REPORT

OF THE

SWATOW MISSION HOSPITAL

AND OF THE

SWATOW WOMEN'S HOSPITAL

IN CONNECTION WITH THE

PRESBYTERIAN CHURCH OF ENGLAND.

For 1918.

PRINTED BY
KWAI FUNG,
PRINTER BOOKBINDER & STATIONER,
SWATOW.
1919.
汕頭永安街仁昌刷

HOSPITAL STAFF.

as in July 1919.

福音女醫院

WOMEN'S HOSPITAL

N. H. Beath M.B.
S. Winifred Heyworth L.R.C.P. & S.E.
李穆誠 Li Mok Seng
曾德徽 Tsang Tek Hui
張步周 Tie Pou Chiu

汕頭福音醫院醫生

SWATOW MISSION HOSPITAL

來愛力 A. Lyall M.B.,C.M. *(on Furlough)*
懷敦幹 G. Duncan Whyte M.D.
羅瑪鑑 Malcolm S. Ross M.B.
楊懷瑤 H. C. Yang
蕭曉初 Siau Hiau Tsho
陳兆桐 Tan Tiau Thong
蔡逸翔 Tshua It Siang

REPORT.

The following table summarises, in the briefest possible fashion, the work done in the Swatow Mission Hospital during the twelve months ending 31st. October 1918.

After a brief consideration of this table a few notes will be given on the medical and surgical conditions dealt with, and, finally, the financial situation will be reported upon.

STATISTICS. 病彙表

In-patients	Male	2407	男	留醫
do.	Female	539	女	
Out-patients	Male	6307	男	門診
do.	Female	2270	女	
Patients seen in their own homes	Male	602	男	外診
do. do.	Female	394	女	
Total Individual Patients ...	Male	9316	男	總數
do. ...	Female	3203	女	
Total Attendances, first and return		44179	門診	重診
Total Visits to patients in their own homes		2302	外診	

Operations:- General	580	普通科	解剖
„ Eye	612	眼科	
„ Dental	314	牙科	
„ Under Chloroform	445	施蒙藥	

There are 232 beds in the Hospital.

A comparison with the figures for the previous year shows that there is a slight decrease under most of the headings, which is not unnatural considering the number of troubles that have disturbed Swatow and the Hospital since 1st. Nov. 1917.

First of all in December, there was the fighting between the Northern and Southern armies, culminating in the triumphal entry of the Southern soldiers into Swatow with the looting of shops and the murder of policemen. For some months both before and after this climax the political atmosphere of Swatow was so troubled that many sick people were unwilling to leave the peace of their own homes even to receive the benefits of Hospital treatment. Both when the Northern Army fled in December and when the Swatow troops of the Southern army fled (temporarily) in June the Hospital was glad and able to take adequate measures for safeguarding the wounded soldiers who were left behind by the retreating armies.

It is many years now since mat-sheds and a wood-yard were erected on part of the China Merchants' Company's land adjoining the Hospital, and Dr. Lyall has frequently pointed out to those responsible the risk to which the Hospital was exposed by the proximity of these highly inflammable structures. In January 1918 his fears were realised and a big blaze, happily of short duration, seriously threatened the existence of the Hospital. Through the vigorous action of the Fire Brigades and many other friends the Hospital buildings were preserved from serious damage and only some hundred and twenty dollars had to be expended on repairs. We have received assurances that these structures which were burnt down will not be rebuilt.

In February the earthquake came, and although that brought us hundreds of patients on the 13th. of February and the following days, yet the instability of some of the upstairs wards and the "fear of living upstairs" which so many people had at that time, prevented the number of patients from being so large as it would otherwise have been.

For all these reasons–fighting, fire earthquake–and, also on account of the absence of Dr. Lyall for the last half of the year, it will not seem strange that the number of patients is less than last year, and yet 42418 * visits to the hospital are recorded. One would especially emphasize the fact that in

* It is obvious that this enormous number could not be dealt with if the efforts of the foreign doctors were not supplemented by those of competent and experienced Chinese.

all but 7% of this enormous number (i.e. in the case of 39,354 visits) advice was given, treatment was administered. the necessary medicines, dressings and bandages were supplied, **without any cost to the patients.** The only demands we make of the out-patients are that they shall arrive in time (i.e. before 9 a.m. on a Tuesday or a Friday) and that they provide for themselves suitable receptacles to hold their medicine. Accidents and other urgent cases are, of course, treated whenever they arrive, and one of the senior members of the Chinese staff is in constant attendance, day and night, to supervise the treatment of such cases. The only expenditure which the in-patients (who are admitted at any time) are asked to make is thirteen cents a day to cover the cost of their food, if they can arrange to have appropriate cooked food brought to the hospital thrice daily **no charge is made whatever.**

Of course there are out-patients who do not wish to arrive in time, and they pay the small sum of .30 cents for advice and medicine. Similarly there are inpatients who wish to have a ward to themselves, and this they are able to secure for a rent varying from four dollars a month to three dollars a week. With these insignificant exceptions (and treatment with neo-salvarsan or one of its substitutes) all treatments in the Hospital, including operations, are carried out for nothing.

During the latter part of the year under review arrangements were made whereby all children, whether brought by the father or the mother, are seen by the doctors before the treatment of the adult patients is begun. This enables the little ones to be taken back to their own homes without undue delay.

MEDICAL NOTES.

Consumption. It has been felt for long that adequate accommodation should be provided for those suffering from Pulmonary tuberculosis. It is not right that patients suffering from this disease should be treated in the same wards either with medical or with surgical patients, and one has not the heart to refuse to give as much relief as one can even to the most hopeless consumptive. A small ward with a Southern aspect, (ventilated by four windows which cannot be closed) has now been prepared for the accommodation of five patients, and already some of those who have been treated there have showed the benefit of the open air treatment and of the better food which they have received. No disease is more curable than consumption if the treatment is begun when the disease is in its earliest stages. Unfortunately in many of the patients who come to us the disease is too far advanced for a cure to be possible.

Hookworm. Of the various diseases we are called upon to treat there are few that present a greater variety of symptoms than ankylostomiasis. Some patients complain of abdominal discomfort, some of general weakness. others of anaemia or breathlessness on exertion, while the more advanced cases may have swelling of the legs. However diverse their symptoms may be all agree in the response they make to treatment, they improve wonderfully as soon as they have been freed from these blood-sucking parasites. During the year some 600 patients have been treated for ankylostomiasis. the majority of them requiring two or three treatments completely to clear out the worms.

Cerebro-spinal meningitis caused us much anxiety in the spring of 1918 when there were many cases of the "fulminant" variety i.e. one who was in good health in the morning might be dead by sunset. As the disease was unknown to most of the Chinese physicians. and as many patients we treated were considerably relieved by the withdrawal of the fluid that was pressing on the brain and spinal cord ("lumbar puncture"), we were called to a large proportion of these cases, many of whom recovered.

As the epidemic of cerebro-spinal meningitis was passing off, cases of **typhoid fever** began to make their appearance, and throughout the summer months we were never without cases of this disease in the Hospital, both soldiers and civilians. Unfortunately Dr. Ross (who had been left single-handed for three weeks) received so severe an infection that it was two months before he was well enough to leave the Port.

Apart from these special conditions we have treated large numbers of medical cases both in the hospital and in their own homes e.g. valvular and other diseases of the heart, (as well as conditions of the arteries varying from a temporary hyperpiesis to an advanced degree of arterio-sclerosis,) diseases of the lungs, bronchi and pleurae (we seem to be seeing more cases of empyoema, pleurisy and pleural effusion every year): along with the various diseases that affect the alimentary canal, and the different forms of Bright's disease. There would be no lack of variety in one's daily routine even if one confined one's attention to the purely medical side of the work.

One of the most interesting patients, professionally, exhibited in most characteristic fashion the symptoms of a tumour in one half of the cerebellum. He got so tired of being asked to demonstrate "diadococinesia" that he went home!

SURGICAL.

The operations performed during the year are shown in the following table which has been prepared by Dr. Ross.

LIST OF OPERATIONS.

Operations on Bones and Joints. 骨與骨節之施割術者

Cario-necrosis of Humerus ... 8 死骨之屬於肱骨者
,, Radius ...... 1 䯁骨
,, Carpus ...... 1 捥骨
,, Ilium .... 1 骼骨
,, Sacrum ...... 1 骶骨
,, Femur ...... 16 䯊骨
,, Tibia .... 37 骭骨
,, Tarsus ...... 13 跗骨
,, Maxillae ... 18 牙牀骨

Fractures and Dislocations 骨折及節脫

Humerus, compound .... 2 肱骨折及皮破
Separation of epiphysis .... 2 骺分離
Clavicle .... 1 䯝折
Radius............................ 1 䯁折
Femur............................. 4 䯊折
Tibia .... 1 骭折
Tibia, compound.................. 2 骭折及皮破
Fractured patella, sutured ...... 2 縫合髕折
Dislocation of hip .... 2 髀節脫
do. shoulder .... 1 肩節脫

Amputations 施截斷術者

Through upper arm .... 1 全上臂
Through forearm .... 2 全肘者
Finger............................ 4 指
Above knee........................ 9 膝上
Below knee .... 8 膝下
Toes.............................. 3 趾

Operations on the Skin 皮膚之施割術者

Plastic operations .... 18 施修補術者
Scraping ulcers .... 20 刮瘍
Scraping sinuses.... .... 10 刮骨孔
Keloid .... 2 瘢瘤
Corns .... 2 釘胼

Sebaceous cysts .... 24 脂袋瘤

Operations on Glands 腺之施割術者

Neck .... 12 頸

Groin .... 3 脥股處

Operations on Mouth, Fauces etc. 喉及喉門等之施割術者

Tonsils and Adenoids .... 3 喉門棚及鼻後棚

Pharyngeal abscess............... 1 喉生膿

Tracheotomy .... 1 總氣管剖術

Draining Antrum .... 1 頄穴引流

Nasal Polypi .... 7 鼻瘜

Cicatricial contraction of nose 2 鼻孔塞

Operations on Thorax 胸部之施割術者

Aspiration of fluid .... 4* 抽出流質者

Pneumothorax .... 1 胸積氣

Stab wound...................... 1 刺傷

Amputation of breast............ 1 截斷肬

Empyema .... 5 胸統膜積膿

Operations on Abdomen 腹部之施割術者

Ascites, tapping.................. 4* 水膨症放液刺術

Subdiaphragmatic abscess ...... 1 膈下生膿

Liver abscess .... 1 肝瘻

Faecal fistula .... 1 糞瘺

Colostomy .... 1 胴剖成口術

Gall stones .... 1 膽石

Appendicectomy................. 1 割取闌尾

Inguinal Hernia................. 1 脥疝

Operations on Ear 耳部之施割術者

Haematoma .... 1 血瘀

Granulations .... 4 成粒

Operations on Bloodvessels 絡部之施割術者

Ligature of Brachial artery ... 2 縛肱衇

Ligature of Transversalis colli 1 縛頸橫衇

Brachial aneurism .... 1 肱衇囊

* These number are obviously incomplete

Femoral aneurism .... 1 股道脈囊

Operations on Tendons 脲中腱之施割術者

Tenectomy .... 1 肌腱

Tumours 割瘤

Epithelioma .... 2 膚疽

Sarcoma .... 3 疕.

Rodent ulcer .... 1 蝕瘍

Cartilagineous.................... 1 肕瘤

Vascular .... 1 絡屬瘤

Lipoma .... 4 脂瘤

Dermoid .... 2 雜膶袋瘤

Fibroma .... 2 筋瘤

Cysts .... 11 袋瘤

Granuloma .... 1 粢瘤

Epulis .... 1 牙座筋瘤

Operations on Genito-urinary system 生殖尿具部之施割術者

Phymosis .... 18 包皮狹窄

Paraphymosis .... 3 包皮勒莖

Amputation of penis .... 8 截斷陽莖

Elephantiasis of penis .... 3 陽莖象皮症

do. scrotum ...... 1 陽囊象皮症

Fungus testis .... 4 精腺脫露

Excision of testicle.............. 2 割取睾丸

Hydrocele .... 8 精腺膜疢

Lithotomy, perineal .... 1 胱石會陰割取

,, suprapubic .... 8 胱石骱上割取

Urethrotomy .... 4 尿脜剖術

Urethral stricture .... 1 探尿脜狹窄

Scraping phagoedenic ulcer ... 1 陽莖生死肉

Operations on Rectum & Anus 肛及肛門之施割術者

Haemorrhoids...................... 52 內外痔

Fistula in ano.................... 41 肛門瘺

Scraping Condylomata .... 3 脂痔
Peri-anal abscess .... 1 肛圍瘺
Artificial anus .... 1 假肛門
Stricture of rectum .... 7 肛狹窄
Rectal polypi .... 1 肛瘜瘤
Removal of bullets, needles, splinters etc. 22
割取子彈針木屑等

Operations on the eye. 眼部之施割術者

Meibomian cysts.................. 15 瞼瞤袋瘤
Repair of eyelid .... 1 修補瞼
Cyst of eyelid..................... 2 瞼袋瘤
Excision of lachrymal sac ...... 1 割淚囊
Entropion, upper ....118 上瞼內捲
Entropion, lower .... 28 下瞼內捲
Electrolysis for trichiasis ...... 50 睫毛擦眼電化
Degeneration of tarsus.......... 1 瞼扁變壞
Peritomy............................ 9 膵圍割除術
Hypertrophy of conjunctiva ... 2 膵膶過長
Pterygium .... 19 膵翳
Staphyloma........................ 1 眼壁凸
Rupture of Sclera .... 1 肝膜疝
Hypopyon .... 3 瞭炎
Iridectomy .... 16 睛簾剜割術
Glaucoma .... 2 青光眼
Cataract .... 7 瞕
Enucleation of globe .... 2 剜割眼球
Evisceration of globe .... 4 肝內剜眼球

The patients treated during the year have been classified under the headings shown in the following table. "Children" means "up to the age of 15 years."

TABLE

Where treated	Total No	Medical	Surgical	Eye	Children
At the Hospital	12519	32 %	32 %	10%	26 %
In their own Homes	996	51 %	7 %	1 %	41 %

每年診病之人數

來醫院就診者合共人數

一萬二千五百一十九人

計內科每百人中有三十二人

計外科每百人中有三十二人

計眼科每百人中有十人

計兒科每百人中有二十六人

外診者九百九十六人

計內科每百人中有五十一人

計外科每百人中有七人

計眼科每百人中有一人

計兒科每百人中有四十一人

NAMOA. This section of the report should not close without reference to the relief work carried out at Namoa after the Earthquake. On the invitation of the Civil Magistrate a party of workers from the Hospital and from the "Red Cross" members of the Boys' Brigade, as well as Drs. Kwan & Tan, went to Namoa City, equipped with drugs, splints, bandages and all sorts of hospital requisites; we stayed there for the best part of a week, setting fractures, reducing dislocations, amputating gangrenous limbs as well as attending to other sorts of injuries.

An appeal to the Foreign Community in Hongkong and Swatow brought in over $ 6000 which was mainly expended in providing rain-proof roofs for 1900 homeless families. Less than $1000 was required for the upkeep of an "emergency hospital" from which Drs. Chia & Tan ("graduates" of the Swatow Hospital) administered medical relief in and around the City for two and a half months.

There was a small unexpended balance of this Relief Fund: one half of this appears in the list of donations to the Hospital, the other half was given to the Boys' Brigade.

FINANCIAL.

EARTHQUAKE. On another page will be found the statement of the expenditure of the money that was collected by Messrs. Tshua Ngan-su, Ie Hai-lau and Chia Tok-khuan to cover the cost of the damage done to the two Hospitals by the earthquake. " It was stated, in the appeal which these gentlemen took round, that any unexpended balance was to be spent in preparing a suitable place for the Mission Hospital's X-ray apparatus: " the amount of $1000. was accordingly transferred to the X-ray fund. THE X-RAY ACCOUNTS are printed on another page, but we must take this oportunity to express our gratitude to Messrs. Kee Buan Soon, T. M. King and Siau Siau Lam who collected the money that has enabled us to procure a really excellent X-ray apparatus, which is now working very well.

One cannot but be impressed with the extraordinary generosity exhibited by the many friends of the Hospital as it is revealed in the preceding paragraphs. Two suitably inscribed stones are being inserted in the wall of the Hospital to commemorate the help given by the above named gentlemen in collecting these monies.

On the GENERAL FINANCIAL SITUATION it must be confessed that in spite of the very generous response made to the Hospital's appeal last summer it proved to be impossible to keep "expenditure" within "income". Although Dr. Lyall had been able to open the year's account with a credit balance of more than four hundred dollars, when the books were closed there was a deficit of almost $ 300, showing an excess of ordinary expenditure over ordinary income of about $ 700. It is only fair to say that Mr. Wang Shing Hsien (王廷獻) came to our rescue then and collected in Hongkong over $ 2000* (of which $ 500 was passed on to the Women's Hospital) but even with that help the Hospital's position remains most precarious. A very heavy burden is thrown on the funds by the high prices of drugs and of materials for Surgical Dressings, as well as the large increase in the item "salaries and wages" necessitated by the increasing cost of living.

One is glad to be able to record many kindnesses shown to us throughout the year. In accordance with an understanding made when Electric Light was introduced into the Hospitals, the Kai Ming Company will never charge the Hospital more than 20 cents per unit; while the Water Company, without any bargaining on our part, has allowed us for many years a rebate of 50% on our monthly account: when extra water is required Mr. Tan Chiang Yong also generously supplies it to us at half price.

For many years past the patients have been made glad every Christmas time by the receipt of oranges. Two hampers of these are sent to the Hospital at that time by Mr. Tung Hong Seang (唐宏祥) of Jardine, Matheson & Co. and Mr. Tan Chhip Ngiau (陳緝堯) of Messrs. Butterfield & Swire. the former gentleman accompanying this gift with a box of tea.

---

* This gift will find its place in the accounts published at the end of the current year.

Throughout the year the doctors frequently receive presents of eggs for which they are grateful. Friends of the Hospital may be glad to know that few gifts could be more acceptable. Eggs are invaluable for providing that extra nourishment which is needed by so many patients, especially by the consumptives and those suffering from beri-beri.

Formerly one of the Hospital's friends presented twenty cents to every patient who was in the Hospital wards at (China) New Year time but in recent years this practise has stopped, much to the regret of the patients. We will always be glad to act as agents for any who may wish at some festal time to give gladness to the sick poor in the Hospital.

EVANGELISTIC.

This is not the place to give a detailed account of the educational and evangelistic work carried on in the Hospital, but three classes of the patients may be distinguished.

First, a large number, probably most, of the patients go home with their old superstitious fears weakened, if not shattered. Second, many of the more chronic cases (who may have been absolutely illiterate when they came to the Hospital) learn enough before they go home to be able to read the New Testament and "The Pilgrim's Progress" etc for themselves.

Finally, year by year, an appreciable number take the momentous step of definitely turning "from idols to serve the Living and True God" for which we must indeed give thanks.

SWATOW WOMEN'S HOSPITAL, ACCOUNTS.

RECEIPTS.		EXPENDITURE.	
Chinese donations	$919.20	Deficit last year	$317.50
Earthquake donation (Chinese merchants)	150.00	Wages	782.21
Foreign Donations	627.25	Lighting	83.58
Sales	303.00	Water	42.94
Rented Wards	721.77	Medicines	1997.03
Bed grants to poor fund	110.00	Repairs	437.87
Donation from students fees	20.00	Hospital Necessaries	422.05
Interest on Deposit Receipt	6.97	Sundries	379.29
Grants from Home	1359.12	Loss on Exchange	95.66
Share of Public Subscription Money	495.73	Milk	108.55
Deficit	136.79	Fire Insurance	37.50
		Ground Rent, (2 years)	55.44
		Customs, freight, landing charges etc.	40.21
		Poor Fund to Kitchen	50.00
TOTAL	$4849.83	TOTAL	$4849.83

SWATOW WOMEN'S HOSPITAL STATISTICS.

1917-1918.

In patients	993
Out patients	2379
Patients seen in their own homes	538
Total individual patients	3910
Total attendances, first and return	9555
Total visits to patients in their own homes	989

OPERATIONS.

General	221
Eye	201
Gynaecological	29
Obstetrical cases	141
Dental (incomplete)	144
Under chloroform	145

N. H. Beath.

SWATOW MISSION

汕頭福音醫院

RECEIPTS. 進款

Balance from last year	上年存欵 ...	435.76
Grant of £ 140 from E. P. Mission	英會助銀	781.30
Share of Public Subscription List	捐銀	1806.85
Donations brought of Hospital		2553.58
Fees as per printed list	診金 ...	2349.74
Rent of small wards	房租	1859.80
Other payments from Patients	藥金 ...	624.75
Sale of Drugs, milk, etc	賣藥及牛乳腎風帶	1074.30
From Hongkong Fire Insurance Co. 火險公司所賠償之欵	...	120.25
Deficit	欠欵	281 67
	TOTAL	11887.70

Account books examined and found correct

A. Wight

A. Guthrie Gamble.

9th. Novemberf 1918.

HOSPITAL ACCONUTS
全年進支總數

EXPENDITURE	支款	Mex. 洋銀
Salaries & Wages	薪水與工資 ...	2196.82
Repairs	修整院屋	1040.81
Surgical Dressings	棉花布油	2243.52
Lighting & Water	電燈及水	1147.96
Drugs, Spirit, Milk etc.	本地買藥 ...	3914.61
Help to Poor Patients	帮助貧醫者	557.00
Stationery and other Sundries	紙與各等雜費	787.00
	TOTAL	11887.70

原四百三十五元七毫六分

收一萬一千一百七十元二毫七分

出一萬一千八百八十七元七毫

欠二百八十一元六毫七分

SWATOW MISSION HOSPITALS.

EARTHQUAKE FUND.

地震捐銀收整院屋之銀項

INCOME 進款

	T. P. 直銀
Donations Collected by :— 捐金表	
Tshua Ngan Su 蔡彥士先生經手 ...	2481.00
Kim Lun, Ie Hai Lau 錦綸楊寄滄經手	485.00
Chia Toh Khuan in Swatow 謝卓權先生於汕頭經手	1814.00
Chia Toh Khuan in Shanghai 謝卓權先生於上海經手	800.00
Donations brought to Hospital 親至本院題捐者	2904.00
Profit on converting Shanghai Contributions 出水銀	51.76
TOTAL	8535.76

EXPENDITURE 支款

	T. P. 直銀
Paid into Account of Women's Hospital 抹助女醫院之總數	150.00
Paid into Account of Mission Hospital 抹助福音醫院之總數 (For dressings & food for injured persons)	350.00
Earthquake repairs in Women's Hospital 女醫院地震收整院屋	2359.27
Earthquake repairs in Mission Hospital 福音醫院地震收整院屋	4592.43
Publishing names of Subscribers 登告報紙	37.20
Loss on Exchange & Bad Bank Notes 蝕水	46.50
Balance paid to X-ray fund 抹助易士鏡之數項	1000.36
TOTAL	8535.76

X-RAY FUND ACCOUNTS

易士鏡之數項

INCOME 進款		Mex.	T.P.
Donations collected by:—	捐金表	洋銀	直平
Kwok Lai Chow	郭麗州君經手	262.15	
Kee Buan Soon	紀萬順君經手		1154.00
T. M. King	王德茂君經手		1200.00
Siau Siau Lam	蕭少南君經手		343.30
Donation from G. T. Chen	陳玉潜捐銀		200.00
Huam Su Lan	范斯蘭捐銀	55.00	
Song Keng Chiu	宋景州捐銀		50.00
Balance from Earthquake fund	地震存欵抹出之數項		1000.36
Converted from T.P. Dollars ...	此洋銀係直平銀找換入	199.78	
TOTAL		516.93	3947.66

EXPENDITURE 支欵		Mex. 洋銀	T.P. 直平
Remitted to England	寄往英國買鏡	193.71	2138.06
Freight, Landing, Duty	船租 起貨 餉稅	139.34	
Fitting up the apparatus, and accessories	接電及購置家私	177.98	152.20
Electric current & other expenses, to end of April	電費	5.90	83.02
Converted into Mexican Dollars (at .76)	直平找換洋銀加入進欵洋銀數內		217.00
Balance in Hand	存款		1357.38
TOTAL		516.93	3947.66

Monies sent to England

In 1916		2000.00	realised	£236.2.6
In 1918	159.97	[illegible]	do.	£ 25.
In 1919	33.74	138.06	do.	£ 27.9.6
INTEREST	...	... ...	do.	£ 4.2.3
TOTAL	193.71	2138.06		£292.14.3

Donations and Fees to Women's Hospital.

福音女醫院捐銀與診金諸君芳名

Kang U Sim ...	$ 3.00
Meng Tsu	1.00
Ki Seng Sim ...	4.00
Ngui Sim	2.00
Chia Ti Tong ...	2.00
Tan Iang Ki ...	4.00
Hu Hong Tsang	20.00
Siu Khun ...	2.00
Sim Khang Leng	20.00
Sim Iong ...	2.00
Chiap Seng ...	4.00
Chiu Iam ...	6.00
Sin Un	1.00
Sia Ki Sua ...	5.00
Tan Tai Tsho ...	20.00
Tie Sin Se Nie ...	8.00
U Li Thang ...	5.00
Nap Nng Su ...	8.00
Lim An Huat ...	10.00
Jin Sim	6.00
Li Sim	4.00
Sim Gueh Po ...	10.00
Gek Hiang ...	5.00
Ki Hah Sun ...	10.00
Nie Siu Cheng ...	2.00
Li A. Kin ...	40.00
Tan Sim ...	2.00
Heng Huai ...	2.00
Tan I. Lam ...	30.00
Tan A Su ...	2.00
Tan Keng Ngi ...	20.00
Un Seng Tien ...	5.00
Mong Nng Su ...	3.00
Siau Hok Iong	20.00
Liang Kia ...	4.00
Mong Siu Se ...	20.00
Ng Sim Hah ...	$ 2.00
Li Si Long ...	4.00
Ji Kou Nie ...	5.00
Tan Ue Ki ...	50.00
Tan Sim	4.00
Li Jin Li ...	30.00
Lim Kiu Lim ...	2.00
It Tong ...	2.00
Sim Nng ...	4.00
Bi Sim	5.00
Ie Nng	2.00
Chia Kam Tsua	20.00
Tan U Si ...	12.00
Be Hiap Thai ...	15.00
Lau Sin Se Nie	2.00
Tan Liang Meng	6.00
Chia Sim Hah ...	2.00
Ti Hia	4.00
Ho Kai Zu ...	6.00
Lim Ngon ...	2.00
Un Mia Li ...	20.00
Pang Nng ...	1.00
Sia Ki Sua ...	30.00
Tsai Zu Tsang ...	10.00
Ang Seng Khiang	2.00
Tie Thuan Hua	20.00
Ie Li Kien ...	2.00
Huat Sim ...	4.00
Ie A Meng ...	2.00
Zu Chek ...	4.00
Tshua Jit Tsu ...	2.00
Heng Siau Ek ...	30.00
Tie Mui Chhiu ...	4.00
Tsu Kia Kau ...	30.00
Tan Hu Se ...	4.00
Jiet Phang ...	200.00

(21)

PUBLIC SUBSCRIPTION LIST 1918

本院向各善士捐題者

		Mex. 洋銀	T. P. 直銀
The Deli Planters Vereeniging	十二公司	250.00	
Messrs. Butterfield & Swire (including fines & penalties)	太古洋行		213.92
Messrs. Bradley & Co.	德記行	200.00	
Drs Brangwin & Hobson	連亨咧藥房	100.00	
A. Macgowan Esq.	德記主人	50.00	
I. M. Moorhead Esq.	稅務司	50.00	
W. G. Humphreys Co.	紹昌洋行	50.00	
British American Tobacco Co.	英美煙公司	50.00	
The Asiatic Petroleum Co., Ltd.	亞細亞公司	50.00	
Alex Ross & Co.	囉士洋行	50.00	
Messrs. Standard Oil Co. of New York	三達公司		51.92
Messrs. Jardine, Matheson & Co., Ltd.	怡和洋行		51.92
The Bank of China	中國銀行		50.00
The Bank of Taiwan, Ltd.	臺灣銀行		50.00
Messrs. Hock Cheang Co.	福昌洋行		50.00
Messrs. E. V. S. Lim Co.	源順公司		50.00
Swatow Chaochowfu Railway Co.	潮汕鐵路公司		50.00
The S. K. T. Launch Co.	汕潮揭輪船公司		48.39
Lim Thuan Tsu	林傳之		40.00
Gwan Chiang	元昌		30.00
E. Hua Hang (Tung Hong Seng)	怡和洋行		30.00
Capt. G. St. M. Stocker		25.00	
G. D. Pitzipios Esq.	英領事官	25.00	
Swatow Presbyterian Church	汕頭堂會	25.00	
James M. Forbes Esq.	怡和主人		25.75
Kaiming Electric Light Co.	開明電燈公司		25.00
Swatow Water Works Co.	自來水公司		25.00
M. S. Myers Esq.	美領事官	20.00	

		Mex. 洋銀	T. P. 直銀
Tshu Tsu Siang ...	徐子祥	20.00	
Tie Soon Seng ...	張順成洋行	...	20.00
Lee Hang Kue	李亨衢	...	20.00
Tan Chiang Yong ...	陳長榮	...	20.00
T. K. Chang	張廷鑑	...	20.00
Tek Kee Bue Tsan ...	德記煤棧	...	20.00
Tek Kee Shipping Dept	... ...	...	20.00
Nam Kee	南記	...	20.00
Mitsui Bussan Kaisha Ltd	三井洋行	...	20.00
Pue Nguan Tsng ...	培源莊	...	20.00
S. Barker Esq.	... ...	15.00	
C. S. Holdsworth Esq. ...	... ...	15.00	
J. Robinson Esq. ...	... ...	15.00	
C. Humphreys Esq. ...	... ...	15.00	
R. K. Sharp Esq. ...	... ...	15.00	
H. Griffin Esq.	... ...	15.00	
T. M. King Esq. ...	... ...	15.00	
Poal Barantzen	... ...	15.00	
Chiap Lee	洽利	15.00	
The Swatow Dispensary	惠安藥房	15.00	
G. Thornton Esq. ...	... ...	15.00	
J. H. A. Hance Esq. ...	... ...	...	15.60
J. K. Oliver Esq. ...	... ...	10.00	
V. A. Maunder Esq. ...	... ...	10.00	
S. Tanaka Esq.	... ...	10.00	
K. J. Holm Esq. ...	... ...	10.00	
Lim Chiang Heng ...	... ...	10.00	
Eng Tshai Nguan ...	翁財源	...	10.50
Iah Siu	益壽	...	10.00
Mark C. Lim	林俊良	...	10.00
S. Kye Pang	沈開榜	...	10.00

		Mex. 洋銀	T.P. 直平
Tie Sok Siam	張淑蟾	...	10.00
W. T. Ching Esq.	曾會同	...	10.00
Siau Chiap Seng	蕭捷盛	...	10.00
Jin Hong	仁豐	...	10.00
Ngan Sang Li	顏盛利	...	10.00
Nia Tang Dispensary	嶺東藥房	...	10.00
Kai Shing, Tailor	祺昇	...	9.73
T. Carr Ramsey Esq.	... ...	5.00	
J. M. da Cruz	... ...	5.00	
S. Klubien Esq.	... ...	5.00	
E. Miyamura Esq.	... ...	5.00	
Sa Yik Wun	佘燡筠	5.00	
Chua Than Jien	蔡坦然	5.00	
Kwai Fung	仁昌	5.00	
E. A. Ozoric	... ...	5.00	
H. A. Ozorio	... ...	5.00	
S. Kye Lim	沈開林	...	5.00
Kwok Wai Nam	郭煒南	...	5.00
Tshua Chhe Koh	蔡星閣	...	5.00
Ie Hun Thiu	楊雲濤	...	5.00
Ang Cheng Ngau	洪增鰲	...	5.00
Lim Hu Tsu	林輔之	...	5.00
Man Shing	萬盛	...	5.00
Kuang Chek Dispensary	光澤藥房	...	5.00
Hu Tsun	... ...	...	5.00
Sun Jui Chi	孫瑞芝	2.00	
Kuan Te Hui	官得惠	2.00	
Iah Seng Dispensary	益生藥房	2.00	
Wei Hsien Ming	魏先明	1.00	
Ng Sun	黃順	1.00	
Hung Chiau Shun	孔昭恂	1.00	

				Mex. 洋銀	T.P. 直平
Loo Yik Fan	羅逸凡	...	...	1.00	
Kwan Un Shui	開元瑞	...	...	1.00	
Chia Siu Min	謝壽民	...	...	1.00	
Te Theng Ko	鄭庭槐	...	...	1.00	
Tan Leng Hui	陳龍惠	...	...	1.00	
Tshu Siau Bun	徐紹文	...	...	1.00	
		TOTAL		1240.00	1140.73

Mex. 洋龍	T.P. 直平	
$263.78	$243.65	Paid to Women's Hospital 抹助女醫院
$976.22	$897.08	Paid Mission Hospital 抹助福音醫院
$1240.00	$1140.73	

T.P. $ 897.08 = Mex. $ 830.63 (@756)

Mex. $ 976.22

Total to Mission Hospital $ 1806.85

(as on page 17)

Donations Collected in **Hongkong** by **Mr Wang Shing Hsien** (Heng Siau Bun) towards the current expenses of 1918-1919.

捐助本院諸君芳名王少文廷獻先生於香港經手

承興行王少文	貳百元
添和成行	壹百元
乾泰隆行	壹百元
裕德盛行	五拾元
王少瑜	五拾元
泰順昌行	五拾元
容星橋	叁拾元
太源洋行	弍拾元
許同泰號	弍拾元
廣昌盛行	弍拾元
成發莊	壹拾元
許鳴泰號	壹拾元
吳彩堂	壹拾元
元成發行	壹百五拾元
華暹公司	壹百元
廣安泰行	壹百元
廣美盛行	五拾元
振裕號	五拾元
裕錦行	叁拾元
王少平	叁拾元
誠信號	弍拾元
周宗興號	弍拾元
亞利馬打律師	壹拾元
南記莊	壹拾元
楊恒益號	壹拾元
敬昌號	壹拾元
元發行	壹百元
成順行	壹百元
廣源盛行	陸拾元
方養秋	五拾元
鳴裕泰行	五拾元
裕隆號	叁拾元
福泰祥行	叁拾元
廖源和	弍拾元
王少咸	弍拾元
南福莊	壹拾元
富珍齋	壹拾元
東和號	壹拾元
陳廣興號	壹拾元

福和興號　壹拾元
萬發莊　壹拾元
聚興號　壹拾元
陳順成棧　壹拾元
順成公司　壹拾元
成順泰號　五元
林熾南　五元
謙盛號　五元
金興隆號　五元
周贊成號　五元
和美棧　五元
源昌莊　五元
廣順利號　五元
裕和號　五元
泰和豐號　五元

美利號　壹拾元
許振興棧　壹拾元
公棧莊　壹拾元
元興甡號　壹拾元
加記號　五元
盈茂號　五元
崔典初　五元
桂興號　五元
勳記號　五元
曾雲記　五元
廣萬和號　五元
榮茂莊　五元
四海通莊　五元
梁蘭甫　五元
同安公司　五元

志泰號　壹拾元
炳記莊　壹拾元
德盛號　壹拾元
嘉發莊　壹拾元
榮記莊　五元
同豐號　五元
南棧號　五元
明德泰號　五元
捷成豐號　五元
陳足記號　五元
義興莊　五元
仁利號　五元
成昌莊　五元
崔肇基　五元

東興隆號　壹拾元
公和棧　壹拾元
蔡興利號　壹拾元
順福成莊　壹拾元
南盛莊　五元
劉芳臨　五元
再興號　五元
陳煥夫　五元
楊開興號　五元
萬裕號　五元
成豐莊　五元
蔡臣盛號　五元
安源號　五元
陳厚卿　五元

OTHER DONATIONS

各善士親至本院捐題者

From 1st Nov. 1917 to 31st Oct. 1918.

陽曆一千九百一十七年十一月一號即陰曆九月十七日
至一千九百一十八年十月三十一號即陰曆九月廿七日

		Mex. 洋銀	T.P. 直銀
Chino Siam Shipping Co.	華暹輪船公司	...	521.31
Transferred from earthquake account		...	350.00
	暹壺嶠俱樂部	...	265.00
Tang Heng Long ...	東興隆	...	117.16
Chua Seng Chow ...	蔡成珠	...	100.00
Li Buan Tek	李萬德	...	100.00
Fine per Commissioner of Customs ...	稅務司抹罰欵	...	100.00
Part balance Namoa Relief Fund $68 71 (@727)			=71.36
Fine per S.S. Kin Hua (C.N.C.)	金華輪船罰欵		70.00
Mrs. E. V. S. Lim	林源順先生娘	...	60.00
Png Ngian Hun ...	方儼雲	50.00	
Dr. Lyall		50.00	
Fine per Butterfield & Swire	太古洋行抹罰款	4.00	45.00
R. Soulange Teissier Esq.		40.00	
Capt. Jensen		40.00	
Miss Harkness		40.00	
Miss Travers		30.00	
Captain G. St. M. Stocker		25.00	
Rev. R. T. Capen		25.00	
Siau Iu Khim	蕭友琴	20.00	
Tshu Sok Che	徐淑靜	20.00	
Rev. A. H. Page		20.00	
Siau Tek Meng ...	蕭德民	20.00	
Ng Siang Leng ...	黃翔龍	...	20.00
Heng Siau Zu	王少瑜	...	20.00
Long Iam Ia	隆炎爺	...	20.00
Png Siau Ui	方少緯	...	19.46

		Mex. 洋銀	T.P. 直平
A. W. Edmunds Esq.	...	15.00	
W. M. Paton Esq.	...	15.00	
Anglo Chinese College	華英學校	10.00	
Chia Ku Tek	謝居得	10.00	
Ngiam Ia Pu	嚴亦富	10.00	
Tan Kam Theng	陳鑒澄	10.00	
Hang Hun	...	9.10	
Chia Un Zu	謝蘊如	...	10.00
Seng Phuan Chieh	辛盤石	...	10.00
Tan Hah Heng	陳合興	...	10.00
Ie Huan Sin	楊煥新	...	10.00
Tie Li Tong	趙禮中	9.10	
Phua Zu Tsu	潘如之	8.00	
Sia Sui Tshun	佘瑞春	8.00	
Tan Ek Meng	蔡逸民	...	8.00
Tie Hiang Su	張香士	6.00	
Gou Gek Sian	吳玉仙	6.00	
Heng Keng Sia	王景城	...	6.00
Li Kang Jien	李簡然	5.00	
P. C. Tan Esq.	陳賓書	5.00	
Sng Tong Liang	孫仲良	5.00	
Kho Hi Thiam	柯喜添	5.00	
Kueh Tek Hui	郭德惠	...	5.00
Li Siau Peh	李少白	5.00	
Lou Siau Phang	盧少帆	...	5.00
Tshua Jin Hah	蔡仁合	...	5.00
Ng Liang Hah	黃兩合	...	5.00
Huai Tek Tng	懷德堂	...	5.00
Chia Sui Eng	謝瑞英	...	5.00
Te Soon Seng	鄭順成	...	5.00
Lim Mui Tien	林美珍	...	5.00

				Mex. 洋銀	T. P. 直銀
Png Ki Jin	...	...	方繼仁	...	5.00
Kueh Hui Mong		...	郭惠茂	...	5.00
Tie Po Tien	...	...	張寶珍	...	5.00
Mong Jiang	...	...	茂　讓	...	5.00
Ng Siah Leng	...	...	黃錫齡	...	5.00
Chia Loi Kek	...	...	謝禮吉	...	5.00
Lim Hiang Chhin		...	林顯臣	...	5.00
Tie Song Hun	...	...	張松軒	...	5.00
Tan Ke Pang	...	...	陳家榜	...	5.00
Png Ki Jin	...	...	方繼仁	...	5.00
Tan Un Tso	...	...	陳恩助	2.00	2.00
Phou Thong	...	...	普　通	4.00	
Ng Theng Tsho	...	...	黃勝記	4.00	
Tan Ui Mong	...	...	陳偉懋	...	4.00
Anonymous	...	...	隱名氏	4.00	
Anonymous	...	...	無名氏	4.00	
Anonymous	...	...	無名氏	...	4.00
Si A Tie ...	...	...	施亞潮	...	4.00
Te Hiok Tsoo	...	...	鄭旭初	...	4.00
Ng Chiau Tong		...	黃昭仲	...	4.00
Hong Seng Chhiang		...	鴻盛昌	3.70	
Li Toh Zu	...	...	李卓如	3.00	
Ng Iong Hai	...	...	黃榮海	3.00	
Ie Iau ...	...	...	楊　瑤	...	3.00
Ng Hau Sip	...	...	...　...	2.00	
Tie Ie Song	...	...	張楊松	2.00	
Hui Ai ...	...	...	惠　愛	2.00	
Tie Ka ...	...	...	張　敎	2.00	
Ng Ngi Tshan	...	...	黃義創	2.00	
Tshu Mui Hua	...	...	徐美和	2.00	
Nguan Heng	...	...	元　興	2.00	

		Mex. 洋銀	T.P. 直平
Cheng Tsu Tshan ...	鐘子田	2.00	
Khu Siu	邱修	2.00	
Tie Iam Ki	鄭炎記	2.00	
Li Theng Hah	李廷合	2.00	
Hui Sim	惠嬸	1.00	1.00
Iang Sin Si	養心氏	2.00	
Thau Huang Hng ...	陶芳園	...	2.00
Ang Chhiau Ki Sim ...	洪朝枝嬸	...	2.00
Cheng Tsu Tshan ...	鐘子田	2.00	
Khou Kia Ki	許嘉記	...	2.00
Ah Fuat	... ...	...	2.00
Tan Tshun Kang ...	陳春江	...	2.00
Gou Iau Tsho	吳耀初	...	2.00
Khiok Kiong	克恭	...	2.00
Anonymous	無名氏	...	1.00
Ng Tek Chhiang ...	黃德昌	1.82	
Ie Chheng Sim ...	楊親心	1.00	
		582.72	2064.29

T.P. $ 2064.29 @ 733 $ 1970.86

TOTAL Mex. $ 2553.86

(as on page 17)

LIST OF FEES RECEIVED

診金一覽表

From 1st Nov. 1917 to 31st Oct. 1918.

陽厤一千九百一十七年十一月一號卽陰厤六年九月十七日
至一千九百一十八年十月三十一號卽陰厤七年九月廿七日

		Mex. 洋銀	T. P. 直銀
Drs. Brangwin & Hobson		600.00	
Tan Cheng Ui	陳振威	140.00	
S. H. Yong	辛向榮	...	130.00
Tan Kai Tong	陳介中	...	102.00
Be Thai Se	馬泰生	80.00	
Cheng Heng Tsng ...	増興莊	...	55.00
Mrs. E. V. S. Lim	林源順先生娘	...	51.00
U Suan Tsho	余選初	...	50.00
Tsu Kang	朱江	...	50.00
Tan Gek Ki	陳玉記	40.00	5.00
Ng Seng Jin	黃成仁	...	35.00
Lou Siau Phang ...	盧少帆	...	30.00
Kit Siang Hang ...	吉祥行	...	30.00
Hah Li Nguan	合利源	24.00	
Heng Siau Bun ...	王少文	...	20.00
Piah Zu	... ...	...	20.00
Siau Chhiu Phang ...	蕭秋帆	18.00	
Nam Kee	南記	17.00	
Li Siau Peh	李少白	10.00	7.00
Sim Sia Mien	沈聲綿	15.00	
I Huat Nguan Ki ...	怡發元記	...	15.00
Soon Seng Thai ...	順成泰	...	15.00
Lou Hut Ngan ...	盧佛眼	...	15.00

This fee is paid to the Mission Hospital by Dr. Brangwin in order that his patients may feel that they have every right to call for our help at any time when Dr Brangwin in not available himself.

			Mex. 洋銀	T.P. 直平
Tie Siam Kai	... ...	張蟾階	...	15.00
Heng Su Lim	... ...	王士林	...	14.00
E. Miyamura Esq.	...	... ...	12.00	
Te Keng Chheng	...	鄭景清	...	12.00
Kueh Chiap Sun	...	郭捷順	...	12.00
Tam Shui Wai	... ...	譚兆槐	10.00	
Jiau Hong Siang	...	饒鳳翔	10.00	
Anonymous	... ...	無名氏	10.00	
Kuang Iah Tsng	...	光益莊	10.00	
Gou Kuang Mui Tsng	...	吳廣美莊	10.00	
Li Tsu Iong	... ...	李子雍	5.00	5.00
Mien Huat	... ...	綿發	5.00	5.00
Siau Sia	... ...	蕭聲	...	10.00
Ang Eng Seng	... ...	... ...	...	10.00
Hua Kheng Tsng	...	和慶莊	...	10.00
Tan Gek Po	... ...	陳玉波	...	10.00
Tan Hun Thui	... ...	陳雲梯	...	10.00
Li Hai Sang	... ...	李海珊	...	10.00
Ou Sin Se	... ...	胡先生	9.09	
Nie Li Tsua	... ...	梁麗泉	9.09	
Lim Thuan Tsu	... ...	林傳之	2.09	7.00
Chiu Sia Thiu	... ...	周聲籌	8.00	
Phua Tua Mue	... ...	潘大妹	7.45	
Tshua Seng Tsu	...	蔡成書	...	6.00
Tan Sek Iu	... ...	陳式游	...	6.00
Hah Heng Mong	...	合興茂	5.00	
Kueh Hua Hong	...	郭和峰	5.00	
Zu Se Tng	... ...	裕生當	5.00	
Tan Cheng Hiang	...	陳振賢	5.00	
Tshua Siau Kheng	...	蔡少卿	5.00	
Li Thong Ngun Tsng	...	利通銀莊	5.00	

			Mex. 洋銀	T.P. 直平
Te I Kiong	... ...	鄭以恭	5.00	
Kueh Tek Hui	... ...	郭德慧	5.00	
Kueh Hua Chiang	...	郭華章	...	5.00
Li Sin An	... ...	李信安	...	5.00
Li Tsu Hien	... ...	李子香	...	5.00
Li Kang Phou	... ...	李簡甫	...	5.00
Li Sam Hah	... ...	李三合	...	5.00
Liang Siu Khiau	...	連修喬	...	5.00
Lim Tong Kheng	...	林仲卿	...	5.00
Lo Tiau Tshun	... ...	羅兆椿	...	5.00
Ng Kek Chhiu	... ...	黃吉秋	...	5.00
Sek Zu Sin Se	... ...	式如先生	...	5.00
Tie Hiang Su	... ...	張響士	...	5.00
Tan Tsong Hui	... ...	陳宗暉	...	5.00
Gou Tsong Tau	... ...	吳宗道	...	5.00
Hiap Heng	... ...	... ...	...	5.00
Heng Thai	... ...	亨　泰	...	5.00
Kou Tin Sai	... ...	古鎮西	...	5.00
Kueh Nguan An	...	... ...	...	5.00
Kuang Hong	... ...	廣　豐	...	5.00
Kuang U	... ...	廣　有	...	5.00
Ek Soon	... ...	宋廷琛	...	5.00
Other fees	... ...	... ...	75.27	366.51
		TOTAL	1166.99	1238.51

T.P. $ 1238.51 @ 733 $ 1182.75

TOTAL Mex. $ 2349.74

(as on page 17)

汕頭福音醫院章程

一本院逢拜一拜四診內宿拜二拜五診外宿拜三拜六爲割症日禮拜日停醫惟急症則不拘

一凡就醫者當於上午八句半鐘集齊聽講聖道然後領簽診病

一每日診病共分三期先診十歲以下之小孩繼診男人最後診女人

一凡依本院所定日期鐘點前來領簽者診病發藥不取分文

一凡逢醫期而無領簽或不遇醫期而欲就診者每人宜納診病費三角

一凡經有本院舊方而遺失或無帶來欲另開新方者每張宜納藥方費一角

一凡本院舊方非經本院醫生簽字而欲領藥者每劑納藥資四角

一凡非本院醫生所開藥方欲來取藥者每劑宜納藥資一元

一凡欲請本院醫生出診者每次宜繳診金五元外埠另議貧家與急症准予通融

一凡留宿本院病人每夜至八點鐘後則不許出入

一本院就醫者日多用費日鉅如有慈善君子樂意捐輸者本院格外歡迎

總房章程

一凡欲留宿本院者須先通報門房由其引宿何處不得擅自投宿

一凡留宿者早晚宜上講堂聽講聖道

一凡留宿者不得自行烹飪宜由本院廚房分給膳費依廚房所定之章程

一凡留宿者每逢拜一拜四均宜領簽候診惟重病則不拘

一凡欲入本院戒鴉片者每人宜先繳藥金二元

一　凡言語不通欲留宿本院者須有妥人挑保

一　凡眾界留宿本院者每禮拜每人醫藥膳費洋一元五角

租房章程

一　本院租房共分三等〔甲等〕一間每禮拜房租洋銀三元〔乙等〕每禮拜洋銀二元〔丙等〕每月洋銀四元租銀均宜先繳如租期未滿即欲移居者租銀不得領回

一　租房伙食准予自理惟當在廚房烹飪不得污穢他處

一　租房時所交之鎖匙須繳銀五毫作質至出院時銀匙兩交如鎖匙遺失則作質之銀不得取回

一　房內所有器物不得任意損壞

西歷一千九百十八年十一月

本院長重訂

汕頭福音醫院週年之報告

（自一千九百十七年十月起）
（至一千九百十八年十月卅日止）

連年以來地方多故兵燹之餘繼以地震本院際此困苦天年醫務之進行不無稍受影響爰將過去一年中之情形提綱絜要爲諸君子約畧陳之

一曰人數之減少

本院逐年就醫人數有加無已迨至今歲人數驟減揆厥原因盖有三故當十二月間南北之戰相持累月風聲鶴唳一夕數驚微論遠道聞風不敢抵汕即屬此間土著亦幾遷避一空此人數減少之一原因也泊乎北軍敗退劉使來鎮是邦地方秩序稍見安甯而土坪遭火本院幾被延燒雖經各界極力搶救得免於難然而外間傳說咸謂本院已成焦土傳聞失實病者裹足此人數減少之又一原因也詎料禍不單行不上一月而從來未有地震之鉅災忽而發現房屋倒塌傷斃人命災區之廣幾及全潮本院房屋雖未倒塌然而半傾未圮殊屬可虞病者既無處容身則就醫者自見其少且當此之時人心惶惶朝不慮夕除彼急不及待之症不得不求醫外苟可稍緩須臾誰肯輕離鄉井此人數減少之三大原因也

一曰財政之支絀

本院宗旨素抱博愛病家醫藥一概施贈其住院留醫者不過酌收膳費而已去年人數雖曰較少然而週年統計就診領藥者尚有四萬餘次之多藥費一項已自不貲況値此米珠薪桂之秋院內辦事人員又當酌添薪水至若電燈食水米鹽瑣屑之事無在而不需財雖經各慈善家解囊相助祇以費用浩繁入不敷出年終結賬尚虧七百餘元而地震屋壞修葺之費尚不在此數內此項虧空之彌縫尚有望於好善樂施之大君子焉

一曰醫務之進行

中土之視西醫也初不過以爲僅精外科補割之術而已內科非其所長近十餘年社會心理始一大變每年就醫之症內科猶不在外科之下畧舉其大端爲諸君告（一）肺癆症　世間百症莫烈於肺癆據有經驗者之調查全世界死亡之數癆症約居七分之一而中土爲尤甚按上海公共租界之調查華人住居公共租界內者四十七萬五千人死於癆症者年約千人以此推之全中國四萬萬人每年死於癆症者當有八十萬人平均計之每日死三千二百二十二人每一点鐘死九十三人也爲害之烈有甚於洪水猛獸故本院對於此症之治療異常注意特闢濱海樓房以爲肺病收留之所地方既通氣透光於病者大有裨益即此與人隔別

亦所以預防傳染茍在初程就醫多占勿藥惜乎就診者每在病入膏肓去死不遠時也(二)腦衣熱症此症爲潮梅罕有之症忽於春間發現患者發熱抽搐昏譫囈語終至脊腦變硬而死症極危急朝發夕死其嘗經本院醫生行脊腦針刺術得慶生全者頗不乏人且備噴汽滅毒之器使人吸之以防傳染乃不幾時該症遂息(三)曰黃疥症　此症患者面黃肌瘦困憊乏力胃口不佳日就枯萎致病之原係由一種小曲似鈎之虫寄生腸內以吮人血血薄則病發茍醫治不早恐有生命之憂本院之治斯症成績頗佳每年就醫得愈者恆在數百人以上云至若胃腎心腸以及肺部積膿積水等症每年就醫者亦以千百計近且購置葉克斯鏡一具藉電光之力照體內之骨其有助於內外各科之診斷醫治者不少總而言之舉凡有益於病人身體健康之物事本院無不竭力經營期臻完備俾脫疾病之痛苦而登斯民于壽域焉

南澳之救災

初地之震也災區雖遍全潮而最甚者厥惟南澳全城屋宇十九倒塌壓斃人命數以千計其幸而不死者亦皆焦頭爛額斷指裂膚滿目瘡痍慘不忍覩本院聞知登即派員赴救分遣醫員四出救護所全活者不少旋以院務冗繁未便久滯遂設臨時醫院以二人留守之餘人遂返惟是災黎徧野無處安身而春雨淋漓寒砭肌骨彼老弱殘廢之災民何以堪此本院乃向

港汕西人題捐共籌六千餘元除撥一千爲醫藥費用外其餘悉數充爲施篷盖屋之用非敢謂澤及災民不過聊盡救災恤鄰之天職已耳

本院之經費

本院常年經費除由院内房租及出馬診金少數收入外其餘欵項概由各界善士捐題而今年地震之損失葉克斯鏡之購置等特別經費則由蔡彦士楊寄滄謝卓權郭麗州紀萬順王德茂蕭少甫諸先生經手捐題而王少文君亦於香港捐二千餘元除抹五百入女醫院外其餘悉爲本院經費地方當喪乱之餘商場凋敝甚矣諸君子熱心公益奔走捐題而各大慈善家猶能仗義疏財樂善不倦不但病家受賜靡涯即敝院同人亦不勝欽佩之至茲將捐欵諸君芳名以及數項出入就醫人數臚列於左俾關心本院醫務諸君一省覽焉

餘音

本院每年電燈水龍之費若以全價計算幾占入欵十分之一爲數不可謂不多幸蒙該二公司均喜減收價錢有時水龍偶缺買水礐石該井主人陳長榮君亦算半價本院負擔藉以稍輕他如陳緝堯君唐宏祥君每於冬節送柑分給病人更有分給毫只鷄卵者事雖大小不同而好善樂施則一餘音之作所以誌謝忱也

REPORTS AND ACCOUNTS

OF THE

SWATOW MISSION HOSPITAL

AND OF THE

SWATOW WOMEN'S HOSPITAL

IN CONNECTION WITH THE

PRESBYTERIAN CHURCH OF ENGLAND.

WITH LISTS OF SUBSCRIBERS ETC.

For 1919.

PRINTED BY

KWAI FUNG,

PRINTER BOOKBINDER & STATIONER,

SWATOW.

1920.

汕頭儞安街仁昌承印

Telephone Nunber 64.

It is eighteen years since Mr. H. C. Yang entered the Mission Hospital, and for the last eight of these he has been the senior Chinese doctor there. The benefits from this appointment have been mutual: on the one hand the hospital is indebted to him for the active part he took in securing the gifts both of the "new" block (of rented wards) and the X-ray apparatus, as well as for other less obvious but very valuable services which he rendered to the hospital in planning new methods of helping the patients and in other ways.

On the other hand, during the many years in which he shared with the foreign doctors in the work of the consulting room and the operating theatre, as well as in the supervision of the hospital, he acquired a vast medical experience and a degree of surgical skill which should prove invaluable to him in his new venture. We wish every success to Dr. H. C. Yang, Tek Hua Dispensary, Chin Pang Street.

大英國長老會派駐

汕頭福音醫院徵信錄

中華民國七年

REPORT OF THE SWATOW MISSION HOSPITAL FOR THE YEAR FROM 1st NOVEMBER 1918 TO 31st OCTOBER 1919

The outstanding features of the year may be dealt with under the following headings

(1) The steady growth in the number of patients treated and the professional interest of many of the diseases seen.

(2) The epidemic of cholera.

(3) The continued generosity of the friends of the hospital.

(4) The very serious aspect of the financial situation.

(5) The installation of the X-ray apparatus.

(6) The evangelistic work in the hospital.

The statistics of the patients treated are set forth in the following table:—

STATISTICS OF PATIENTS: 病 彙 表

In-patients	Male	3256	男	留醫
do.	Female	545	女	
Out-patients	Male	7249	男	門診
do.	Female	2152	女	
Patients seen at their Homes ...	Male	611	男	外診
do. do. ...	Female	452	女	
Total Individual Patients ...	Male	11116	男	總數
do. ...	Female	3149	女	
Total Attendances, First and Return		42293	門診	重診
Total Visits to Patients in their Homes		1595	外診	
Surgical Operations: General ...		648	普 通 科	解剖
„ „ Eye ...		188	眼 科	
Operations with Anaesthetics ...		419	施 蒙 藥	
Opium Smokers Treated		41	改 鴉 片	

There are 232 beds in the Hospital, A comparison with the figures for last year shows that the male in-patients have increased by 800, and the out-patients by 900, over 11,000 men and boys have been treated during the year.

The Swatow Mission Hospital treats patients of every sort, and gladly receives women and girls as well as men and boys; but the accomodation set aside for women patients is very limited, and there is an excellent women's hospital next door under the care of an English lady doctor and a competent Chinese staff. In view of these special facilities provided for the women patients it seemed a little anomalous that in our hospital they should be treated **before** the men. so now the out-patients are dealt with in the following order **first**, children under twelve years of age, whether boys or girls: **second**, all the men and older boy patients and **third**, and women or older girls who prefer to be treated in our hospital. We generally have between thirty and fifty children, and have had as many as 115 women. This figure was reached when Dr. Ross was in charge early in September on a day when there were over 500 out-patients.

Although the majority of these patients suffer from the commoner illnesses, yet there are quite a number whose diseases are very rare and extremely interesting.

MEDICAL NOTES.

Encephelitis lethargica is a condition of which the most obvious symptom is sleepiness, which is usually accompanied by paralysis affecting the eyes and/or the face. The condition was brought prominently before the general public in 1918 when some hundreds of cases occurred throughout England. Three cases have now been recognised in Swatow, of which one proved fatal.

Cerebro-spinal meningitis and diphtheria are two other diseases which were unknown in Swatow a few years ago, but are now met with every cool season. In fulminant cases of the meningitic inflammation the diagnosis is obvious from the start and the foreign doctor is frequently sent for since it is known that the only measure that can be expected to give any relief is "lumbar puncture", i.e., the withdrawal of some of the products of inflammation through a hollow needle inserted into the spine. The combination of this method of treatment with the administration of anti-meningococcic serum (which we have received from Hongkong) has enabled us to save many patients whom one hardly dared to hope would get better.

Diphtheria is even more amenable to treatment than meningitis if only the diagnosis is made in time. Unfortunately in the patients we have seen the disease has often been so far advanced that tracheotomy (i.e., cutting a hole in the wind pipe below the larynx) has been necessary. We have now got an outfit for **intubation** whereby the difficulty of breathing (due to the blocking of the throat by diphtheritic membrane) can be relieved without any cutting. It is much easier to get the parents' permission for an intubation than for a tracheotomy!

In this connection reference may be made to a condition which often closely resembles diphtheria. It is known as **arachidic bronchitis** or "peanut" bronchitis, and is due to bits of peanuts ("monkey nuts") being accidentally aspirated into the lungs. One case has been recently met with, and the condition must surely be fairly common in this district where peanuts are plentiful and are given to quite small children. "Arachidic acid" is supposed to be the constituent of the peanut which is responsible for the diffuse tracheo-bronchitis which develops, and "the resemblance to the symptoms of those of diphtheria is sometimes most striking, and in a number of cases antitoxin has been administered".

The outstanding symptoms of **Thrombo angiitis obliterans** are the gangrene and falling off of fingers and or toes which may continue to take place for a number of years. It used to be supposed that this disease occurred almost exclusively amongst Russian Jews, but it has now been demonstrated throughout the length and breadth of China. Our wards are hardly ever without a patient suffering from this disease whose sufferings we try to relieve.

We have had a number of interesting **diseases of the nervous system** in many of which the patient has improved under treatment. A rapidly growing gumma (i.e. a syphilitic tumour) pressed on the part of the brain which initiates movements of the left arm and leg so that these became paralysed. Energetic anti-syphilitic treatment not only checked the spread of the paralysis, but actually restored power to the limbs which the patient had been unable to use.

In another patient successive attacks of paralysis were due to the blocking of some arteries of the brain by fragments of blood clot which, from time to time, were expelled from the heart, which was diseased.

In another patient the brain centres associated with the comprehension and utterance of speech stopped work for a few days. Thereafter the patient got better by well defined stages (1) He was able to understand what he heard: (2) then he could utter a few words, his power of speech improving rapidly from day to day: (3) later on he was able to read as well as to *copy* writing, but it was a long time before his recovery was complete and he was able (4) to write properly on his own initiative.

In spite of the largely vegetarian dietary of the people there are quite a number of men and not a few women whom we know to be going about in imminent peril of apoplectic strokes. The blood pressure is so high — over 200 m.m. of mercury — that, unless the heart fails, some one or other of the blood vessels in the brain is sure to give way sooner or later.

These patients form one of our most perplexing problems.

THE CHOLERA EPIDEMIC.

The Cholera Epidemic was the most striking feature of last year. Patients suffering from cholera cannot be admitted to the Hospital, and they cannot be treated properly in their own homes, but the temple opposite to the Hospital most obligingly puts its "rooms for the dying" at our disposal whenever cases of infectious disease occur. On this occasion however (as in 1912) the cases of cholera were so numerous that the temple accomodation was inadequate and the police officials — upon whom rests, theoretically, the responsibility for the health of Swatow — said they were unable to provide a place where these cases could be treated.

Dr. Beath isolated a block of the women's hospital for the treatment of cholera and kindly allowed us the use of part of this, but, even so, accommodation was inadequate.

Our friend Mr. Tshua Ngan Su then came to the rescue (as in 1912) and provided a large matshed for us on land quite near the hospital. There were three large wards with a wooden floor and some fifty beds, as well as a room for the nursing staff.

With the help of two hospital assistants (Messrs. Tshua and Chia) and five "nurses" we treated some 350 patients with a mortality of about 20%, a result which could not have been achieved without hard work on the part of every member of the staff.

By the time a patient with cholera came to the hospital he had already lost so much fluid by vomiting and copious evacuations that the eyes had sunk deep into the sockets and the whole body looked shrunken and the blood was so dried up that it could not easily pass along the blood vessels, and as a result the pulse could hardly be felt and the whole body was cold. The first requirement was, obviously, to supply fluid and this was easily done by the injection directly into a vein of 4, 5 or 6 pints of salt water, as a result of which the patient underwent a sharp reaction, the circulation was restored and the shrunken body filled out again to show the warmth and colour of life.

But the patient was not out of danger when this stage was reached, he might (and generally *did*) "collapse" again, whereupon more salt water would be injected into a vein: or on the other hand the *reaction* might proceed too far and the temperature rise so high that it would not come down again till the patient died! The surest way to prevent deaths from this cause is to be ever watchful for the beginning of the rise of temperature and to take means at once, by rubbing the patient with ice, to prevent its going too high.

We cannot express adequately our gratitude to Mr. Macgowan through whose generosity 100 lbs of ice was sent to the cholera hospital every day. It was because we were thus enabled to use the ice *without stint* that many patients were saved who would certainly otherwise have died from too high fever.

The generosity of the friends of the hospital.

This has been as remarkable as ever.

The subscription lists show the donations of money which we received — without this solid backing year by year from the whole Swatow community the work would, obviously, be impossible.

We must also express warm gratitude to the following gentlemen: To Mr. Tshua Ngan Su 蔡彥士 and his friends for the (temporary) Cholera Hospital.

To Messrs. Bradley & Co., 德記洋行 (per Arthur Macgowan, Esq) for 6000 lbs of ice for the same hospital.

To the Swatow Water Works, Ltd. and the Kaiming Electric Light Co., 自來水公司及開明電燈公司 who supplied water and light free of charge to the Cholera Hospital, and who allow a liberal discount to the Swatow Mission Hospital on the monthly accounts.

To Mr. Tan Chiang Yong 陳長榮 who also supplies water to the Hospital at half price.

To the Kwang Seng Hong 慶成興 for two cases of Asiatic Petroleum Company Candles.

To Messrs. Tung Hong Seang 唐宏祥 (of Messrs. Jardine, Matheson & Co.,) and Tan Chhip Ngiau 陳緝堯 (of Messrs. Butterfield & Swire) for their Christmas gifts of large baskets of oranges for the patients.

To the Swatow Telephone Co., 電話公司 for the free installation of a telephone in the Hospital, and for making no monthly charge either for that, or for the extension from there to the doctor's house.

To Messrs. Bradley & Co., and Messrs. Alex. Ross & Co. who provided cloth samples in such abundance that Mrs. Duncan Whyte was able to have a dozen "patch work" quilt-covers made.

To the Chinese ladies who actually made these quilt-covers for the hospital.

The seriousness of the financial situation:

While we are every grateful for all the generosity that is shown to the Hospital from year to year, yet we must draw attention to the fact that the subscriptions received are not enough, more money is needed. At the end of the year the books showed a debit balance of $800. of which $500. had been incurred during the year.

What is the explanation of this increasing deficit?

(1) The low value of the pound sterling (£1.0.0) means that we have received only a few hundred dollars from the Church in England, in place of the sum (well over a thousand dollars) which was the equivalent before the war of the grant from the Church.

(2) The increased cost of (Chinese) living in Swatow in reflected in the increasing bill for salaries and wages which is about $600. more than last year.

(3) The cost of drugs, cotton wool, lint *etc.*, has risen enormously in recent years

Over forty thousand treatments were given last year and it is obvious that these must cost a large sum of money. We are very reluctant to levy any charge for this on the poor patients — how could one refuse necessary treatment simply because the sufferer could not afford the fee ? but, unless the financial situation is relieved, some such step will be inevitable.

THE X-RAY APPARATUS:

During the course of the year the long awaited X-ray apparatus arrived from England. was fitted together and, eventually, put into working order. Thereafter it was exhibited first to Messrs. Kee Buan Soon, T. M. King, Siau Siau Lan. and the friends from whom these gentlemen had collected subscriptions for its purchase. Later on it was shown to the general body of Hospital Subscribers and on this occasion four hundred guests were present, including local officials, merchants, etc. The X-ray has proved invaluable both in medical and in surgical practice. Surgically, bullets or fragments of glass may be seen when they cannot be felt; fractures and dislocations may be accurately diagnosed even when there is *so* much swelling that the parts cannot be felt: the position of coins, metal buttons, etc., that have been swallowed can be clearly seen.

Medically, one is able to recognise alterations in the size and shape of the heart, as well as tuberculous disease (consumption) of the lung, pneumonia etc. By feeding the patient with opague drugs (such as bismuth and barium) one can see the size and shape of the stomach and intestines.

Some diseases of the skin are amenable to treatment by the X-ray, and perhaps the recurrence of cancer can be prevented by its means.

Unfortunately some people are reluctant to secure the benefits of the X-rays because they have been frightened by tales of the harm that the rays may do. To relieve this uncalled for anxiety it may be well to say :—

(1) The majority of such ill effects as have followed the use of X-rays — e.g. eczema, ulceration of the hands, sterility, etc., — have happened to the doctors and assistants who were working with the rays, *not* to the patients.

(2) In the case of our apparatus the tubes are so carefully screened by layers of lead or other impenetrable material that there is absolutely no reason for fear.

EVANGELISTIC WORK :

But all the hard work that is indicated by this report will have been relatively worthless and the hospital will have proved unworthy of its name, if it has not manifested love.

Why was medical mission work begun in Swatow ? Not only (1) to help alleviate the discomforts and cure the sicknesses of poor suffering Chinese, but also (2) to help rid the Chinese of the idea that they are at the mercy of stupid but malignant spirits who may often be tricked, but must certainly be propitiated. Further (3) to substitute for this, mistaken, idea the knowledge that the Supreme Ruler of the universe loves each one of us sinful men with a love that is more tender, more wise, and more ready to pardon that the love of any earthly parent : a love that was shown to men most clearly in Jesus Christ who went about doing good and healing all that were oppressed.

The object of the hospital is to show *love in action*, and no matter how much other work we may be busy with, we must not fail in *this* or our *raison d'etre* is gone. Shall past failure lead to our being contented with low aim ? No, we must still dare to keep our aim high and must resolve to be satisfied with nothing less than the manifestation of the love of God through the ministry of healing.

We have the greatest joy in recording that the hospital is being used to lead men and women into God's Kingdom.

(11)

福音女醫院

Women's Hospital Staff as in May 1920.

N. H. Beath M.B. (on furlough)

F. Winifred Heyworth L.R.C.P. & S.E.

李穆誠 Li Mok Seng

曾德徽 Tsang Tek Hui

SWATOW WOMEN'S HOSPITAL STATISTICS.

1918-1919.

In patients	1303
Out patients	3032
Patients seen in their own homes	672
Total individual patients	5007
Total attendances, incomplete	10,775
Total visits to patients in their own homes ...	1271

OPERATIONS.

General	215
Eye	333
Gynaecological	44
Obstetrical cases	176
Dental	175
Under chloroform	260
Minor incomplete	186

N. H. Beath.

F. W. Heyworth.

汕頭福音女醫院之出入數項

SWATOW WOMEN'S HOSPITAL ACCOUNTS 1918-1919.

RECEIPTS.

Chinese Donations Swatow	$1370.60
do. Shanghai	468.00
do. Hongkong	461.13
Foreign Donations	125.15
Singapore Coolie Steamer Dr's fee	150.00
Sales	300.12
Rented Wards	435.80
Student's fees	146.20
Grants from Home	654.69
Home poor fund money	154,50
Share of Public Subscription Money	649.72
TOTAL	$5215.91

EXPENDITURE.

Deficit from last year	$ 136.79
Fire Insurance	37.50
Lighting and Water	267.82
Medicines	1105.13
Surgical dressings	324.56
Repairs and Sundries	1103.70
Wages	753.20
Help to poor patients	226.83
Loss on Exchange	116.82
Student's Instruments etc.	179.60
Printing and Postage	33.25
Balance	931.31
TOTAL	$5215.91

List of Fees Received by Women's Hospital

福音女醫院診金諸君芳名

Cang Iau Hui	Ang pau ngun $	4.00
Te Kia Sun	do.	10 00
Ng Su Nai	do.	5.00
Tang Tsu Liat Sin Se ...	do.	5 00
Khien Thai Long	do.	2.00
do.	do.	2.00
do.	do.	2.00
do.	do.	5.00
Ng Su Nai	do.	5.00
Ng Sin Se	do.	5.00
Ng Su Nai	do.	5.00
Tang Su Nai	do.	2.00
Ng Su Nai	do	5.00
Lim Nie Ning	do.	10.00
Li Tet Mong Chhiang ...	do.	2.00
U Zai Tsun Sin Se	do.	3.50
Tsok Nng Su	do.	14 00
Tshu Chieh	do.	2.00
Te Sin Se	do.	5.00
Tsuan Ho Nng Su	do.	1.00
Kueh Nguan An Tsng ...	do.	12.00
Te Ti Sun	do.	10.00
Chhim Che	do.	2.00
Iong Hak Seng	do.	5.00
Hen Tan Ki	do.	10.00
Chia Pu Hong	do.	1.00
do.	do	1.00
do.	do.	1.00
Tai Kwang Kong Si ...	do.	2.00
Tang Meng Ki	do.	10.00
Sin Thai Liang	do.	20.00
Mong Sim	do.	5.00
Toh Si Leng	do.	7.00

List of Subscribers to the Women's Hospital.

福音女醫院捐銀諸君芳名

Li Chhiu Nam ...	$ 4.00	Hen Kui Phen	$ 10.00
Ke Song	2.00	Chie Sim ...	2.00
Bun Eng	4.00	Tsho Sia ...	4.00
Lu Bun Ki	4.00	Ie Siu Ni ...	8.00
Kueh Jin Kheng	200.00	Po Thai Sun	1.00
Nam Hua Heng Hang	100.00	Chia Su ...	8.00
Siau Zui Phong ...	4.00	Ang Sok Cheng	10.00
Tai Lien Tia Sim Chhiang	50.00	Jit Sin Chhiang	50.00
Thih Nia Jit Sin Chhiang	50.00	Tia Sin Chhiang	40.00
Tai Sam Ie Hang	10.00	Cheng Ki Kong Si	10.00
Hoh Ki	10.00	Tian Song Pheng	5.00
Iong Ki	10.00	Chia Toh Khuan	50.00
Lim Toh Li	30.00	Kien Seng Ho	50.00
Tai Se Ue	50.00	Hen Sui Hun	20.00
Cheng Seng Ho ...	20.00	Siau Siu Ngam	20.00
Chia Kia Nng ...	10.00	Sai Sim ...	4.00
Bun Ki	4.00	Sin Thai Hang	40.00
Sin Thai Hang ...	10.00	Ie Sin Hi ...	4.00
Go Iau Zu	8.00	Tang Seng An	4.00
Tang Hah Li ...	12.00	I Ki	4.00
Tshua Iak Tek Hang	5.00	Sun Chhiang Chi	5.00
Un Zui Tsun ...	10.00	Kou Piu Lan	8.00
Lim Mong Huat ...	2.00	Ie Sin Se ...	4.00
Liang Chhin ...	2.00	Khou Zu Thai	5.00
Ie Sin Se	6.00	Lau Hah Hong	4.00
Khuang Hng ...	2.00	Ka Hiang ...	5.00
Ku Seng Tsng ...	4.00	Tek Sun ...	4.00
Po Tek	4.00	Tie Ti Liang	8.00
Chek Ki	5.00	Cheng Ki ...	5.00
Han Seng Ki ...	4.00	Leng Heng ...	10.00

Kueh Hong	4.00	Un Mua ...	30.00
Chiu Si	12.00	Go Kuang Sun	6.00
Lip Ti	40.00	Khak Su Nai	8.00
Si Siñ Se Nie ...	20.00	Li Tok Tng	10.00
Tang Hng	10.00	Tit Sieh ...	10.00
Hng Sik Theng ...	5.00	Li Chi Tshuan	4.00
Chiau Soh	14.00	Chia Siu Se	100.00
Ngi Hai	6.00	Ng Li Che Khin	10.00
Hong Nguan ...	3.00	Teng Chen Ju	24.00
Li Hiang Kok ...	5.00	Tie Tsan Mong	2.00
Ng Jiak Hie ...	4.00	Kuang Sun Li	10.00
Tang Su Hai ...	4.00	Ie Bun Kang	4.00
Iong Chek	2.00		

(16)

SWATOW MISSION

汕頭福音醫院

RECEIPTS. 進款

		龍銀 Mex.	直銀 T.P.
Grant of £ 140 from E.P. Mission	英會助銀	244.85	420.11
Share of Public Subscription List	捐銀	634.30	1062.51
Donations brought to Hospital	捐銀	382.17	3751.62
Fees as per printed list	診金	1651.84	2154.47
Rent of small wards	租房 ...	2120.00	
Other payments from Patients	藥金	82.00	543.05
Sale of Drugs, etc.	賣藥及雜物等	535.83	258.07
Deficit	欵欠		779.55
	TOTAL	5650.99	8969.38
Balance on X-ray Account 1st. Nov. 1919			1032.46

Account books examined and found correct

A. Guthrie Gamble

13th. November 1919.

龍銀

原欠弍百捌拾壹元陸毫柒分

收伍千陸百伍拾元零玖毫玖分

出伍千叁百陸拾叁元零陸分

存陸元弍毫陸分

(17)

HOSPITAL ACCOUNTS

全年進支總數

EXPENDITURE 支款

		龍銀 Mex.	直銀 T.P.
Deficit 1st Nov. 1918	原欠 ...	281.67	
Salaries & Wages	薪水與工資	2774.31	
Repairs	修整院屋	371.78	227.78
Surgical Dressings	棉花布油 ...		2236.27
Lighting & Water	電燈及水 ...	870.51	535.39
Drugs, Spirit, etc.	本地買藥 ...	405.84	1546.44
Help to Poor Patients	幫助貧醫者	774.26	195.13
Stationery & other Sundries	紙與各等雜費	64.14	964.03
Cholera Epidemic	吐瀉費用	102.22	264.34
Balance	存欵	6.26	
	總共 TOTAL	5650.99	8969.38

直平銀

原無

收捌千壹百捌拾玖元捌毫叁分

出捌千玖百陸拾玖元叁毫捌分

欠柒百柒拾玖元伍毫伍分

PUBLIC SUBSCRIPTION LIST 1919

本院向各善士捐題者　於民國八年

		Mex. 洋銀	T.P. 直銀
The Deli Planters Vereeniging	十二公司	250.00	
Messrs. Bradley & Co. ...	德記行		207.71
Messrs. Jardine, Matheson & Co., Ltd	怡和洋行	50.00	
British American Tobacco Co.,	英美煙公司	50.00	
W. G. Humphreys & Co.	紹昌洋行	50.00	
Alex Ross & Co. ...	囉士洋行	50.00	
I. M. Moorhead Esq. ...	穆厚達	50.00	
Drs. Brangwin & Burrell	連亨喇	50.00	
Messrs. Butterfield & Swire	太古洋行		51.93
China Navigation Co. ...	太古船公司		51.93
Asiatic Petroleum Co., Ltd.	亞細亞公司		51.93
Standard Oil Co. of New York	三達公司		51.93
A. Macgowan Esq. ...	德記主人		51.93
Hock Cheang & Co. ...	福昌洋行		50.00
Iong Hok Nguan ...	榮福源		50.00
The Bank of China ...	中國銀行		50.00
The Bank of Taiwan, Ltd.	臺灣銀行		50.00
Swatow Chao-chow-fu Railway Co	潮汕鐵路公司		50.00
E Hua Hang (Tung Hong Seang)	唐宏祥		30.00
Guan Chiang	元昌		30.00
The Mitsui Bussen Kaisha	三井洋行		30.00
G. D. Pitzipios Esq. ...	英領事官	25.00	
James M. Forbes Esq. ...	怡和主人	25.00	
J. Robinson Esq.	德記大寫	25.00	
Swatow Water Works Co.	自來水公司		25.00
Kaiming Electric Light Co.	開明電燈公司		25.00
T. M. King Esq.	王德茂		25.00
Chas F. Richardson Esq ...	輝華洋行		25.00

		Mex. 洋銀	T.P. 直銀
Tshu Tsu Siang	徐子常	20.00	
M. S. Myers Esq ...	美領事官	20.00	
Nam Kee Hang	南記	...	20.00
Lee Hang Kue	李亨衢	...	20.00
Tek Kee Shipping Dept ...	德記船頭部	...	20.00
Tek Kee Bue Tsan ...	德記煤棧	...	20.00
Sun Seng Ie Hang ...	順成洋行	...	20.00
Light Railway Co.	汕樟輕便鐵路公司	...	20.00
Tan Chiang Yong Esq ...	陳長榮	...	20.00
J. A. Bloomfield Esq.	英美煙公司主人	15.00	
C. Humphreys Esq. ...	紹昌主人	15.00	
G. W. Thornton Esq. ...	囉士主人	15.00	
The late V. A. Maunder Esq.	怡和大寫	15.00	
Chiap Li	洽利	15.00	
The Swatow Dispensary ...	惠安藥房	15.00	
H Griffin Esq.	亞細亞主人	...	15.58
Laughland Esq.	太古大寫	...	15.58
J. H. R. Hance Esq. ...	太古主人	...	15.58
J. M. Goodeno Esq. ...	三達主人	...	15.58
C. F. Chuang	莊子峰	...	15.00
M. E. Summers Esq. ...	申陌士	10.00	
B. D. Tisdell Esq.	副稅務司狄詩樂	10.00	
S. Klubien Esq. ...	三等幫辦古祿彬	10.00	
E. Myamura Esq.	二等幫辦宮村榮仁	10.00	
E. Bernadsky Esq.	二等幫辦斐納璣	10.00	
Capt. J. S. Enright Esq.	頭等總巡恩萊	10.00	
G. A. Ozorio Esq. ...	何沙利	10.00	
Eng Chai Nguan ...	翁財源	10.00	
A. D. Keefe Esq. ...	三達大寫	...	10.38
Sim Kye Pang	沈開榜	...	10.00
Chiap Seng	捷盛	...	10.00

			Mex. 洋銀	T.P. 直銀
K. Sheki	... ...	石 機 松	...	10.00
W. T. Ching Esq.	...	答 侖 同	...	10.00
Tie Sok Siam	... ...	張 淑 蟾	...	10.00
Tshua Hang Nguan	...	蔡 漢 源	...	10.00
M. Taketoh	... ...	竹 籐	...	10.00
Hip Seng & Co.	...	協成公司	...	10.00
Jin Hong	... ...	仁 豐	...	10.00
Nia Tang Dispensary	...	嶺東藥房	...	10.00
Ngan Seng Li	... ...	顏 盛 利	...	10.00
Mark C. Lim	... ...	林 俊 良	...	10.00
Kai Shing	... ...	祺 昇	...	9.94
H. A. Ozorio Esq	...	... ...	5.00	
E. A. Ozorio Esq.	...	... ...	5.00	
J. Boyd Esq.		署理三等總巡博愛特	5.00	
Sa Zik Wun	... ...	佘 爗 筠	5.00	
P. C. Tan	... ...	陳 寶 書	5.00	
T. Carr Ramsey Esq	...	永慶主人	5.00	
G. H. Wee	... ...	黃 玉 和	5.00	
Ang Cheng Ngau	...	洪 增 鰲	5.00	
Tshua Than Jiang	...	蔡 坦 然	5.00	
Tek Hua Dispensary	...	德華藥房	...	5.00
Ie Hun Thiu	... ...	楊 雲 濤	...	5.00
S. Kye Lim	... ...	沈 開 林	...	5.00
Kwang Chek Dispensary		光 澤	...	5.00
Buan Seng	... ...	萬 盛	...	5.00
Kuan Tek Hai	... ...	官 得 惠	4.00	
Hu Tsun	... ...	許 俊	...	3.00
Iah Seng Dispensary	...	益生藥房	2.00	
Wei Hsien Ming	... ...	魏 先 明	2.00	
Li Sui Chuen	... ...	李 瑞 泉	...	2.00

		Mex. 洋銀	T.P. 直銀
Kwan Un Shui	關元瑞	1.00	
Long Hok Khun	隆福昆	1.00	
Hsu Shau Wen	徐紹文	1.00	
Loo Yih Fan	羅逸凡	1.00	
Chen Kun Wei	陳君蔚	1.00	
Fung Tsye Yuek	馮子煜	...	1.00
Hung Cihu Shun	孔昭詢	...	1.00

Donations collected by Sim Kye Lim and A. Macgowan Esq.

捐助本院諸君芳名德記主人與沈開林先生經手

Chip Seng Chhiang Ki ...	集成昌記	...	20.00
Chip Chhiang Khun Ki ...	集昌崑記	...	20.00
Tie Thai Siang	張泰祥	...	20.00
Hah Long Ho	合隆號	...	10.00
Li Tshuan San Ho ...	李全順號	...	10.00
Jim Hap Hua Ki ...	任合和記	...	10.00
Kia Hok Tng	嘉福堂	...	10.00
Chip Seng Huat	集成發	...	10.00
Kim Lun Ho	錦綸號	...	10.00
Long Chhiang	隆昌	...	5.00
Buan Thai Ho	萬泰號	...	5.00

Donations collected by Sim Kye Lim Esq.

捐助本院諸君芳名沈開林先生經手

Sei Yark Launch Co.	四益輪船公司	...	18.91
Li Si Hua	李時和	...	5.00
Sam Seng Iah Ki ...	三盛益記	...	5.00
Kheng Seng Huat ...	慶成發	...	5.00

Donations collected by Tan Iah Theng, (Physician)

捐助本院兩君芳名陳益廷先生經手

Ui Heng Hang	煒興行	...	30.00
Kan U Tsng	厚餘莊	...	5.00

	龍銀 Mex.	直銀 T.P.
Gross Receipts 本院向各善士捐題總數	893.00	1495.91
Sum paid to Women's Hospital ... 抹助女醫院	258.70	433.40
Net Receipts to Swatow Mission Hospital (as on page 16) 福音醫院所收入者(請看十六面)	634.30	1062.51

This sum will appear in the Women's Hospital Accounts for the current year 1919-1920

此上女醫院之數項即入現年之數至明年方有發白

OTHER DONATIONS

各善士親至本院向捐題者

From 1st November 1918 to 31st October 1919.

陽曆一千九百一十八年十一月一號即陰曆九月廿八日起
至一千九百一十九年十月三十一號即陰曆九月初八日止

		Mex. 洋銀	T.P. 直銀
Heng Siau Bun	王少文		2083.48
Te Iong Seng	鄭永成		100.00
Anonymous	隱名氏		100.00
Ko Theng Po	高澄波		100.00
British American Tobacco Co. being receipts from Sale of Hatamen Cigarettes (1st payment) 英美煙公司賣哈德門煙		60.26	
Heng Siau Bun	王少文		60.00
Png Ngian Hun	方爾雲	50.00	
Ie Kia Mien	楊家敏		50.00
Kuan Hien Theng	官獻廷		50.00
Anonymous	隱名氏		50.00
Tshua Khi Kien	蔡起見		50.00
Catholic Mission Swatow ...	汕頭天主堂		50.00
Anonymous	肆氏		50.00
Lak Hah	六合		50.00
Png Ki Jin	方繼仁		50.00
Tan Po Tsu	陳寶芝		50.00
Lak Hah	六合		50.00
Buan Zu	萬裕		50.00
Anonymous	無名氏		50.00
Tek Nguan	德元		50.00
Leng Song Che	甯頌靖		50.00
Anonymous	隱名氏		40.00
Heng Siau Pheng	王少平		30.00
Swatow Presbyterion Church	汕頭堂會	25.00	

		Mex. 洋銀	T.P. 直銀
Dr. Beath	米醫士	20.00	
Siau Iu Khim	蕭友琴	20.00	
Ng Hak Theng	黃學窗	20.00	
Anonymous	隱名氏		20.00
Tsng Cheng Zu	莊增裕		20.00
Lim Tong Kheng	林仲卿		20.00
Chua Seng Choo	蔡成書		20.00
Chiu Hiang Tsu	周顯芝		20.00
Lou Eng Chiang	盧用章		20.00
Rev. T. W. Douglas James ...	任杜力	15.00	
Gou Tai Lim	吳大林		15.00
Te Tsun Kheng	鄭俊卿		15.00
Kueh Sam Heng	郭三興	14.00	
Chia Kim Nguan	謝錦元		14.73
Mr. Suga	行成洋行	12.00	
J. M Forbes Esq.	怡和行		12.00
Eng Chi Chhiu	翁稚秋	10.00	
S. N. Liang Esq.	梁淑言	10.00	
Anglo Chinese College ...	華英學堂	10.00	
Tsok Ngou Si	祝五氏	10.00	
Dr. Everham	翁偉士	10.00	
Rev. E. S. Burkett	克明德		10.60
Tan Kiu Kau	陳九皋		10.00
Tan Tsu Liet	陳子烈		10.00
Kou Bun	古文		10.00
Li Hiang Kok	李香谷		10.00
Kuan Tek Zu	廣德裕		10.00
Ou Khi Mien	胡啓綿		10.00
Te Zu Nguan Huat	鄭裕源發		10.00
Gou Tsang Heng	吳贊助		10.00
Lim Tek Heng	林德興		10.00

		Mex. 洋銀	T.P. 直銀
Ang Sok Cheng	洪淑貞		10.00
Tsng Thien Iang	莊天燕		10.00
Ng Nguan Teng	黃元鎮		10.00
Gou Siang Hui	吳祥輝		10.00
Sim Iong Ki	沈榮記		10.00
Anonymous	無名氏		10.00
Anonymous	隱名氏		10.00
Tou Kai Tng	杜介堂		9.73
Lau Kheng Hun	劉慶雲	8.00	
Hai Nguan	海源	8.00	
Lim Kheng Chhiang	林慶昌		8.00
Sim Khai Lim	沈開林		7.80
Uan Jin Seng	袁胤新		7.00
Ie Khai	楊愷伯		6.00
Li Si Hieng	李世雄	5.00	
Gou Hun Theng	吳雲騰	5.00	
Ng Siah Leng	黃錫齡	5.00	
Tshua Ngan Su	蔡彥士	5.00	
Chiang Tan Si	章陳氏		5.00
Leung Yong Kwong	梁先生		5.00
Chia Loi Kek	謝禮吉		5.00
Lau Eng Kau	劉應高		5.00
Chek Ki	一記		5.00
Sim Pien Ki	沈彬記		5.00
Lau It San	劉一山		5.00
Huam Tek Tsu	范德滋		5.00
Tan Sang Iong	陳升榮		5.00
Li A Hien	李亞賢		5.00
Liu Cheng Iong	柳貞榮		4.86
An employe of A. Debeaux et Cie.	博泰洋行內	4.35	
Chiap Hong	捷豐	4.00	

		Mex. 洋銀	T.P. 直銀
Li A Ngou	李亞五	4.00	
Lim Si	林　氏	4.00	
Ie Lok	姚　祿	4.00	
Heng Keng Sia	王景城		4.00
Thng Liet Thau	湯冽韜		4.00
Ie Sun Seng	姚順成		4.00
Ie Tshun Tsu	姚存書		4.00
Gou Sai Hiang	吳賽香		4.00
Li Hang I	李翰院		4.00
Gou Huan Chiang	吳煥章		4.00
Li Phue Iong	李培榮		4.00
Khou Cheng Sun	許進順		3.78
Tan Hah	陳　合	3.00	
Chia Zu Kim	謝如金	3.00	
Tai Loi Hng	戴禮園		3.00
Te Hui Hun	鄭斐雲		3.00
Ng Kim Tsua	黃錦泉		2.84

The following gentlemen each contributed two dollars:—

以下各善士係每位捐題二元者

謝亞財	兩　海	林裕豐	林吉平
林嘉創	黃家敏	史　克	朱盛記
郭允發	如香嬸	許春茂	辛經足
美華公司	無名氏	吉　龍	陳爲周
吳滾明	蘇賽珍	洪紹强	陳渭周
許騰遠	賴月英女士	林　泉	楊　振
黃亞瞰	張　爭	洪俠生	鄭仰雲
鄭訓俗	蔡泰盛	蔡仁合	鄭廣園
海玉嬌	史　克	吳青史	廖來發
龎松齡			

(all the above) 25.00 49.00

		Mex.	T.P.
Other donations	其餘捐題者	8.56	3.80
	總共 TOTAL	382.17	3751.62

(as on page 16) 請看十六面

LIST OF FEES RECEIVED

診金一覽表

From 1st November 1918 to 31st October 1919.

陽厯一千九百一十八年十一月一號即陰厯九月廿八日起

至一千九百一十九年十月三十一號即陰厯九月初八日止

		Mex. 洋銀	T.P. 直銀
Drs. Brangwin & Burrell ...	連亨喇葯房	600.00	
Sim Kye Pang	沈開榜	290.00	5.00
Tam Shui Wai	譚兆槐	24.35	126.37
Ng Nguan Teng	黃元鎮	105.00	35.00
U Soi Min	余先民	...	125.00
Hongkong University, for services rendered as M. D. Examiner	香港大學酧謝主考	96.85	
Iong Khang Tsng	永康莊	...	100.00
Seng Seng Kong Si ...	誠信公司	...	80.00
Peng Heng Ji Lau ...	炳興二老	70.00	
Tan Hiau Zu	陳曉如	60.00	
Te Sun Seng Li	鄭順成利	...	60.00
Ie Hiang Tsu	姚献之	5.00	50.00
Iah Mui Hang	益美行	...	55.00
Iap Tsu Tshai	葉梓材	...	50.00
Tie Siam Kai	張蟾階	...	50.00
Tan Tsun Sam	陳俊三	15.00	25.00
Nguan Hong	源豐	...	40.00
Ko Ki Tsu	高繼祖	...	40.00
Tek Nguan	德元	...	40.00
S. Chilick Esq.	...	...	33.00
Khiam Hua Siang	謙和祥	32.00	

* This fee is paid to the Mission Hospital by Dr. Brangwin in order that his patients may feel that they have every right to call for our help at any time when Dr. Brangwin in not availahle himself.

		龍銀 Mex.	直銀 T.P.
Khou Pek Khim	許伯琴	...	30.00
He Sut Than	夏述唐	...	26.92
Heng Siau Bun	王少文	...	25.00
Lou Hut Ngan	盧佛眼	...	25.00
Thia Phong	程鵬	...	25.00
Li Peng Kui	李炳奎	...	23.70
M. Takata	竹籐峰治	22.00	
Mr. Suga	行成洋行	22.00	
H. Unotoro	鵜飼平三	2.00	20.00
Iong Hua Heng	永和興	20.00	
Ko Theng Po	高澄波	20.00	
Thai Kou Lam Ki	太古南記	5.00	15.00
Tie Thien Iah	趙天鎰	...	20.00
Lau Hang Chhin	劉漢臣	...	20.00
Hu Tsun	許俊	...	20.00
Kueh Siah Hia	郭錫邢	...	20.00
Siau Ki	紹記	...	20.00
Jin Chhiang	仁昌	...	19.00
Khian Seng	乾盛	...	17.00
Kousaka & Co.	幸阪洋行	15.00	
Nie Bun Eng	梁文英	15.00	
Tshua Tsu Pien	蔡芝賓	...	15.00
Tshua Seng Tsu	蔡成書	...	55.00
Hai Tsua Liang Ki ...	海泉連記	...	15.00
Cheng Tsu Tang	曾子東	..	15.00
Kueh Hua Chiang	郭華章	...	15.00
Sim Khai Lim	沈開林	...	15.00
Kuang Thai Lai	廣泰來	...	14.19
Tan Tia Chiang	陳鼎章	5.00	9.15
Cheng Keng Thang ...	鍾景棠	...	14.00
Students of Anglo Chinese College	華英學堂生	13.00	
Lim Tong Kheng	林仲卿	...	12.00
Hia Iong Chhiang	邢榮昌	...	12.00
Telephone Company	電話公司	4.35	6.89

		龍銀 Mex.	甯銀 T.P.
Lim Bun Chheng	林文清	...	10.52
Pue Nguan Tsng	培元莊	5.00	5.00
Tshu Sok Che	徐淑靜	9.35	
Kueh Li Chiu	郭麗洲		10.00
Iah Seng	葐成		10.00
Li Heng Khu	李亨衢		10.00
Chia Kim Nguan	謝錦元		10.00
Chip Mong Siang	集懋祥		10.00
Lim Iang	林楊		10.00
Chiang Seng Chiang ...	章成章		10.00
Nguan Heng Hang	元興行		10.00
Tu Kien Kek	潮州十屬房捐局		10.00
Png Ki Jin	方繼仁		10.00
Siau U'u Kheng	蕭韻鯨		10.00
Thong Zu	同裕		10.00
Tai Seng Kong Si	大成公司		10.00
Kueh Hong Zu	郭鴻裕		10.00
Light Railway Co.	汕樟輕便鐵路公司		9.92
Kai Shing	麒昇		9.45
Kuang Hok Hong	廣福豐		9.45
Khou Kuang Seng	許光成	1.35	1.75
Anglo Chinese College ...	... ...		8.92
Tan Li Hah	陳利合	6.00	2.00
Li Sek Hang	李植漢	6.00	2.00
Tie Kuang To.	張廣多	2.00	5.89
Tan Kai Jin	陳介人		8.00
Thong Thai	同泰	7.00	
Kueh Kien Bun	郭見聞	7.00	
Cheng Siu Tshan	鍾壽田		7.00
Li Khian Sam	李乾三	6.00	
Khou Ek Leng	許翼龍	6.00	
Tan Bun Pien	陳文彬	6.00	
Ku Ia Ge Khue	久野牙科		6.00
Ng Kim Tshuan	黃金全		5.69

	Mex. 洋銀	T.P. 直銀
Fees of $5.00 were received from each of the following 以下係每位出診金五元者		
此數係出五元之診金	90.00	290.00
Fees Received in Smaller sums 此數即診金不上五元者	31.70	98.07

黃勝記 龔師爺 仁元莊 同興 方蔚秋 林德興 楊百健 吳廣美 盧用章 松興 湯雲鵬 李子經 吳清益

仁元 增源莊 仁元建記 泰生 彭人菊 李春意 益昌莊 郭成才 增源莊 公發興記 陳大妹 黃世珍 集堅利

荷蘭領事官 林傳之 仁源生號 陳寶之 段永年 林双號 永合裕 孔昭詢 翁牧師 楊闢 侯作幹 土耳其人 廣成

龍廸里五號 洪榮興 五佐臣 陳鳳飛 同盛號 林鏡清 王如 紀明錦 翁隱 洪勉之 蔡等元 秦博洋行 邱梅巖

德興號 黎守忠 陳傳琛 石機松 胡義成 王廷献 桂昌 吳慶祥 馬賢信 徐德昌 鄭幹臣 郭和豐

誠信公司 馬時暉 陳錫周 石添記 胡義泉 華陀葯房 姚璧川 吳玉璋 馬育航 鍾壽仝 唐酢文 利發

	Mex 洋銀	T.P. 直銀
Total fees received for visits to patients in their own homes 此數係出門視病診金之共數	1627.84	2022.91
Fees for Certificates in Medico legal cases and fees from soldier in-patients 此數係本院向索留醫兵士之藥費并至本院證明驗傷單之數項	21.00	131.56
總共 TOTAL	1651.84	2154.47

as on page 16. 請看十六面

戊午年春地震倡捐八千餘圓修葺醫院諸君芳名

蔡彥士　楊寄滄　謝卓權

倡捐三千餘圓購置葉克斯鐳諸君芳名

郭麗州　王德茂

紀萬順　蕭少南

戊午年春地震倡損（捐）八千餘圓修葺醫院諸君芳名

蔡彥士　楊寄滄　謝卓權

倡捐三千餘圓購置道葉克斯鏡諸君芳名

郭麗州　王德茂

紀萬順　蕭少南

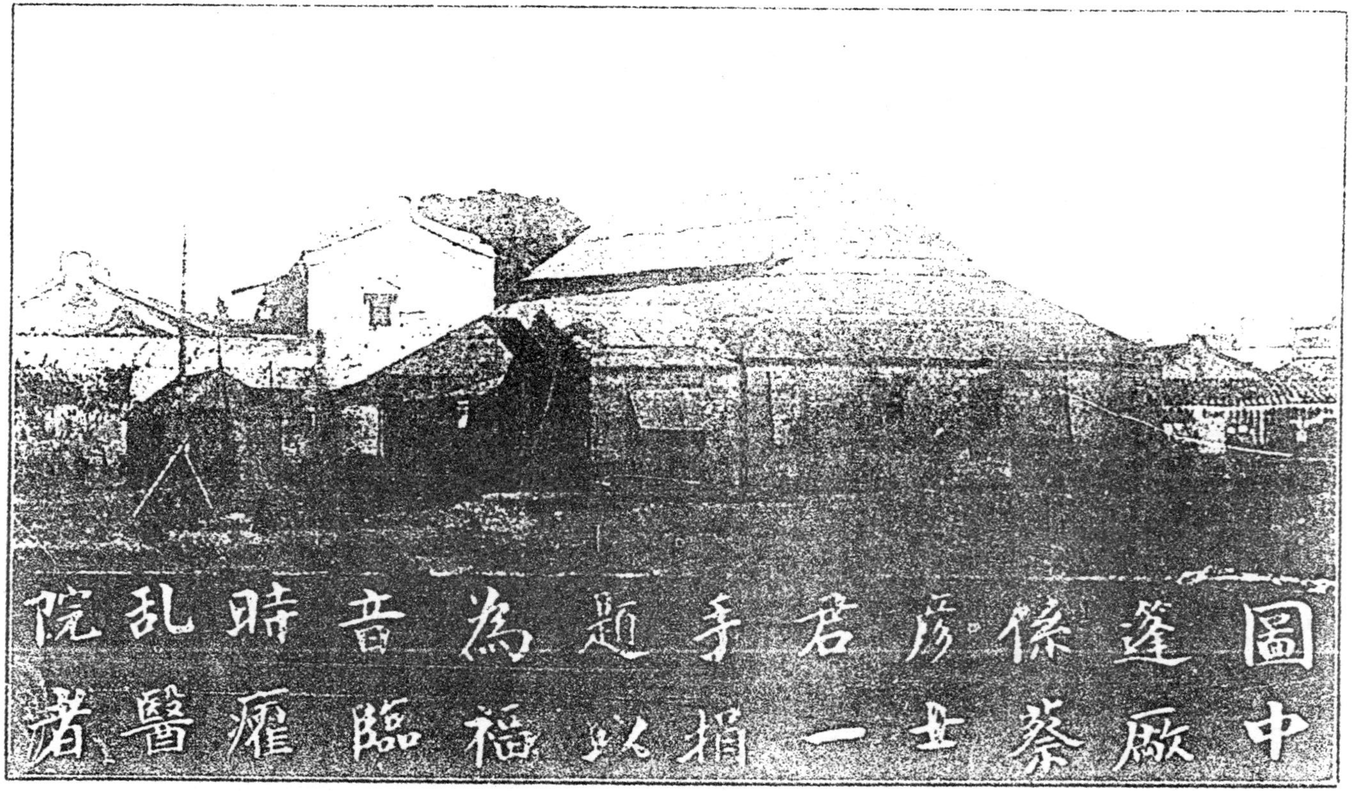

Temporary Cholera Hospital built on the initiative of Mr. Tshue Ngan-su, with funds collected by him. Recovery rate, 80 .

此圖係用影相機由葉克司鏡所攝出者骨骼臟腑無不畢現其兩旁横列似梯者為骱骨左畔黑影為心下畔黑影為肝及脾其色較白位於骱間者為肺

REPRODUCTION OF X-RAY PHOTOGRAPH OF THE CHEST OF A HEALTHY BOY.

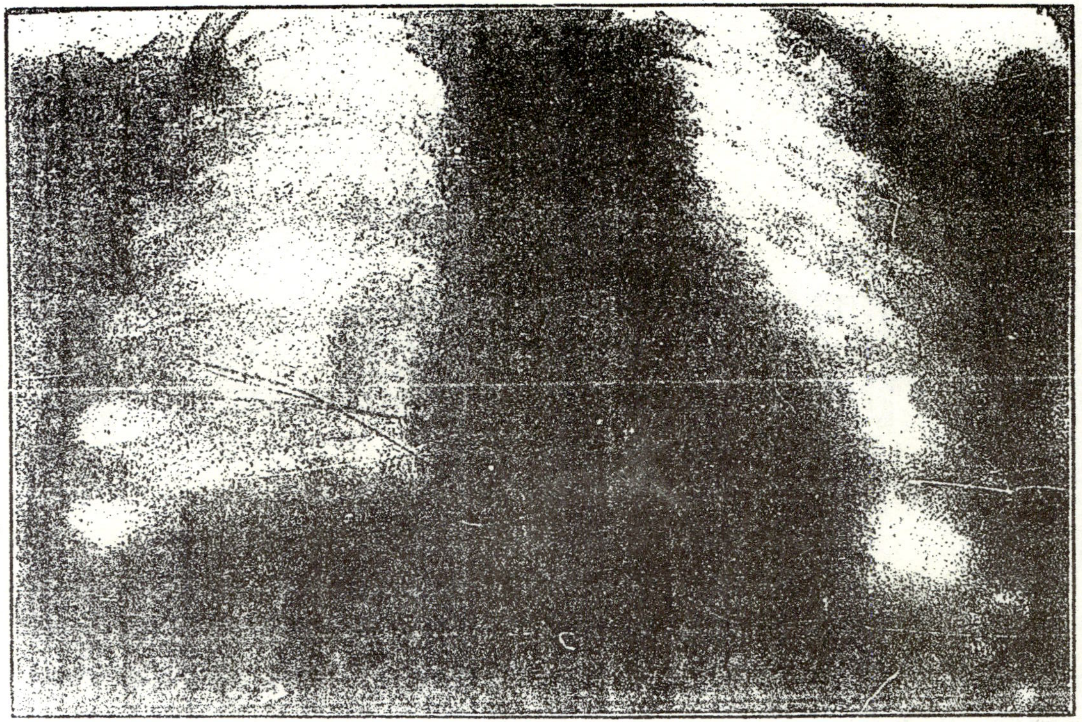

NOTE. The faint shadows of the ribs on both sides.
The dark shadows of the heart, in the middle and towards the left.
The dark shadows of the liver and the spleen at the lower part.
The lungs being healthy, throw no shadow, hence the clearness of the space between the ribs.

大英國長老會派駐

汕頭福音醫院徵信錄

中華民國八年

電話號數第六十四號

汕頭福音醫院醫生

Staff of Swatow Mission Hospital as in June 1920.

來愛力 A. Lyall M.B., C.M. *(on Furlough)*

懷敦幹 G. Duncan Whyte M.D.

蕭曉初 Siau Hiau Tsho

陳兆桐 Tan Tiau Thong

蔡逸翔 Tshua It Siang

葉世騰 Iap Si Theng

何志先 Ho Chi Soi

Dr. Andrew Wight 越愛如 of Chao-chow-fu and

Dr. Malcolm S. Ross 羅瑪鑑 of Swabue

both gave invaluable help during may months of the year under review.

For the first time in many years the name of Dr. H. C. Yang does not appear on this page: a farewell notice will be found over leaf.

前楊懷瑾先生任本院醫生多年現受德華葯房之聘已辭本院之職故現年其名不在此冊

汕頭福音醫院週年之報告

本醫院對於就醫人數進支欵項捐欵芳名及特別症之療治歷年皆有報告所以徵信用而昭愼重也茲將一千九百十九年一週年中經過情形挈其要綱以爲關心本院醫務諸君告

就醫人數

本醫院歷年就醫人數皆逐漸加增去歲因地方多故畧見減少前次報告經已提及茲不再贅惟至本年已復原狀統計週年就醫者約一萬一千餘人較之去歲合院內外宿計之共增一千七百餘人（詳情見後）女界就醫較前畧少故無特別之統計所[redacted]以然者因此鄰福音女醫院專爲女界而設有女西醫士主任醫務是以本院對於就醫婦女自無特加優待之必要故診病秩序先小孩次男人而後婦女在本院則以既有女醫院責有專任而女界則誤以有意爲難此所以女界漸少之原因也

葉克斯鏡

近世科學進步醫術日精於是葉克斯鏡乃應時而出葉克斯鏡者藉電光以照體內

之骨骼臟腑之鏡也古者扁鵲透視徵據乎謠傳今日此鏡澈照乃微之學理凡被燭照臟腑癥結莫能遁形骨骼損傷瞭如指掌在用以查驗肉內之子彈玻璃片以及療治皮膚膿瘡毒癰瘤等症猶其次焉從此醫士診病較有把握病者就醫易占勿藥其造益於民生實非淺鮮本院久謀購置特以款項無着遲遲不果幸蒙郭鹿洲紀萬順王德茂蕭少南諸先生力任捐題集三千餘金而斯鏡乃克如願購置大各界慷慨捐助樂善之心允堪欽佩而諸先生痌瘝在抱仗義疎財且不惜勞心費神籌斯鉅款共底於成其功德尤不可沒故敝院特為勒石紀念以垂久遠此鏡佈置完備乃於十二月十號開會延請捐款諸君暨官商各界參觀鏡搆之造及演照講解其功用是日赴會來賓四百餘人濟濟盈堂頗極一時之盛此置辦葉克斯鏡之大畧情形也抑更有進焉者本院為謀地方人士健康起見無論何人皆得照驗（簡章見後）俾各界瞭然於身軀內部之組織而益知更可察驗體內病症之所在惜乎未明此鏡之理者每懷疑懼或有誤聽損身之謠傳遂欲照而未敢豈知一切危險電機皆妥為封閉自無意外之虞縱有萬一之不測亦惟司理電機者受傷耳於就照者固無恙也疑懼胡為

霍亂臨時醫院之設施

頻年以來地方多故兵燹地震之餘而重以霍亂之症何我潮汕之不幸耶去春霍亂

流行勢甚劇烈死亡枕藉迥非昔比本院於症之初發即從事施救然療治有術而住宿無所蓋尚無傳染病院以居留患者雖存心善堂之養病室可以寄宿既而人衆而不能容本院乃商諸警廳迄無辦法不得已就女醫院特闢病室一所專治斯症然流行已盛被染者多又慮不足居住幸獲蔡君彥士等之贊助於本院對門曠地搭蓋蓬廠一座以爲療治癨亂臨時醫院一切醫務統由本醫院經理晝夜施治蔡謝二先生親到專任統計就醫病人共三百五十名平均愈者約十之八成績之佳頗見稱於社會焉

財政支絀

本醫院就醫者既日衆而費用亦浩繁雖蒙樂善諸君子慷慨捐助猶尚入不敷出揆厥原因蓋緣年來金融價跌英倫教會捐助之金匯作銀元年短數百元且值此荒歉之年米珠薪桂辦事人員應酌添薪水至若棉花絨布暨各種用品物物價昂統計週年就診領藥者共四萬餘次之多則藥費一項自屬不貲是以年終結賬共虧八百餘元除其中三百元係去年積欠舊數餘則本年所虧缺者不得不爲慈善諸君告至捐款諸君芳名以及一切進支詳細數目另列於後

捐助誌謝

本醫院開創五十餘年於茲矣所有經費多賴各界善士解囊相助是以醫務得以進行無滯夫豈惟患病者沾惠靡涯亦本醫院同人所深感佩者也至於本年癨亂臨時醫院實蒙蔡君彥士暨其諸友之贊助始克立成德記洋行則贈冰塊六千磅自來水公司開明公司亦各捐贈水票電燈即歷年本院亦蒙該二公司減收水電價錢或自來水偶缺碧石水井主人陳長榮君亦半其水價捐助電話公司則捐贈電話機一具置於醫院且免本院及院長住宅電話之月費慶成興行則贈臘燭二箱他如陳緝堯君唐宏祥君每於冬節備柑贈與病人羅士洋行及德記洋行贈送布樣以製被套更有婦女數人肩任縫衽事雖大小不同但樂善好施憐恤爲懷則一也本院感念之餘特代沾惠病人同聲稱謝

歉懷自勗

本院抱博愛之宗旨負施醫贈藥之責任對於就醫病人自應妥爲照料以免有出外朝朝難之嘆斯心境既泰然而藥石亦較有靈效但以就醫人多事冗務繁欵接容或不週良多懷歉以後自當特加注意冀貫徹所抱之宗旨而副各界之期望焉

特別症之療治

就醫者多則奇難危急之症亦常經診茲述其尤者如左

一　腦衣炎熱症　此症數年來始見於汕地前此固未之聞也今則每屆冬令有患之者矣症之急者數小時即可致命藥石無功醫士束手蓋傳染症之最劇烈者也今特用抽放炎液注射解毒盟於脊腦之法手術簡而收效宏苟患者能趁速療治則雖垂危亦多救活

一　腦炎　患者疲倦思睡第三對顱系攤瘓眼肌歪斜或不能展闔此症昔見於英國今則本院亦數經診治矣

一　痳症（俗名白喉）　病人若能及早就醫爲之注射敵痳盟則甚見功效惜乎就診者每在垂危呼吸道已閉塞故不得不施剖割術方能奏效惟本醫院近購置療痳特別器具可插喉間以通呼吸無須剖割因是病者就醫較爲妥便矣

一　落花生（俗名地豆仁）　肺氣管炎　症因落花生片誤入氣管中含一種酸素其毒能致氣管發炎甚至喉腫閉塞呼吸不通狀類痳症本院曾經診治之

一　脈炎絡塞　患者因或一部之脈管發炎凝血瀦塞該脈管以致血液難通而賴此血滋養之部因缺血育而變爲死肉久而爛脫疼痛特甚最常見者爲手指及足趾醫治之功奏效極緩昔則以爲惟僑居俄國之猶太人之特症今調查中國

一　各地亦多有患此症者

霍亂　當病者之就醫也其容顦悴其身瘦弱血枯脉微體溫低減究其原因則吐瀉過甚體內水分不足血稠凝滯所致也故主要之治法即入水以補其缺血內水分既足則患者霍然復甦矣惟多有反復不止一次間有熱度太高則以冰塊凉之就病施治以至健痊始已

一　至於腦部病症如疔毒瘤壓腦以致手足癱瘓或心病血凝凝塊塞腦內衇管以致不能語言及不能辨別語言以及失覺悟記憶才等症服藥後頗多見效而痊瘉

本院照鏡規則

一　凡有人欲照愛克司鏡可於拜二拜五下午五句半鐘至本院等開鏡每人每次收洋二元

一　如非拜二拜五欲請特別開鏡者每人每次收洋五元

一　如因骨折或傷而欲影其骨之形者每人每次收洋十元

一　如欲治病者每人每次收洋四元

汕頭福音醫院章程

外宿門診章程

一 凡外宿就醫者當於拜二拜五上午八句半鐘齊集講堂聽講福音然後領簽就診施醫發藥不取分文

一 凡急症至院就醫則不拘時刻

一 每日診病先診十歲以下之小孩繼診男人後診女人

一 凡逢醫期而無領簽或非醫期而就診者每人宜納診費藥費共三角以上午十二點前爲限如有人懼過繁雜可於下午四句鐘至本院候診每人收銀壹元

一 凡經有本院舊方或遺失或忘帶而欲另開新方者每張宜納葯方費一角

一 凡非本院醫士所開葯方而欲來取葯者每劑宜納葯費一元

一 禮拜日非急症一概停診

外宿出診章程

一 凡欲請本院醫士出診者每次宜繳診金五元外埠另議貧家與急症准予通融

內宿章程

一 凡欲留宿本院者不拘何日何時須先通報門房由其引宿何處不得擅自投宿

一 凡留宿者每拜一拜四上午八句半鐘齊集講堂聽講福音然後領簽就診施醫發葯不取分文

一 凡留宿非重病而能行動者早晚一聞欽聲應上講堂聽講福音

一 凡欲入本院戒鴉片者每人宜先繳葯金四元并不許擅自出入

一 凡留宿本院者每晚九點鐘後不許出入

一 凡言語不通而欲留宿本院者須有妥人担保

總房章程

一 凡留宿總房者不得自行煮飪宜由本院廚房三餐分給膳費則依廚房所定之章程

一 本醫院專爲平民而設凡軍界有重病者亦許留宿惟每禮拜每名繳膳費外須加補醫葯費銀六角

租房章程

一 本院租房共分三等每間（甲等）每禮拜洋銀四元（乙等）每禮拜銀二元（丙等）二禮拜銀三元租銀均宜先繳清楚如租期未滿而欲移居者房租不得領回

一 租房伙食准予自理惟當在廚房烹飪不得污穢他處

一 租房時欲交鎖匙須繳銀五毫作按出院時交還鎖匙即將五毫送回如鎖匙遺失則作按之銀毫不得領取

一 房內所有器物不得輕忽損壞

西歷一千九百二十年五月　　本院長訂

REPORTS AND ACCOUNTS

OF THE

SWATOW MISSION HOSPITAL

AND OF THE

SWATOW WOMEN'S HOSPITAL

IN CONNECTION WITH THE

PRESBYTERIAN CHURCH OF ENGLAND.

WITH LISTS OF SUBSCRIBERS ETC.

For 1925.

PRINTED BY
KWAI FUNG,
PRINTER, BOOKBINDER & STATIONER,
SWATOW
1926.
汕頭福安街仁昌承印

Telephone Number 64.

Women's Hospital Staff as in June 1925.

N. H. BEATH M. B. CH. B.
M. ROSS M. B. CH. B.
張步周 TIE POU CHOU
蔡韻秋 TSHUA UN CHHIU
劉集瑜 LAU CHIP ZU

Swatow Women's Hospital Statistics 病彙表 1924-1925.

In Patients	...1256	留病
Out patients	...2095	門診
Patients seen in their homes	... 339	外診
Total individual patients	...3968	總數
Total attendances ...	12397	門診 } 重診
Totsl visits to patients ...	...1377	外診 } 重診

OPERATIONS 解剖表

General	...455	普通科
Eye	...449	眼科
Gynecological	... 30	婦科
Under Chloroform ...	...187	施蒙藥
Obstetrical Cases ...	...278	產科

Staff of Swatow Mission Hospital rs in June 1925.

來愛力	A. Lyall	M. B., C. M.
越爱如	A. Wight	M.B. Ch, B. (on furlough)
羅瑪鑑	M. S. Ross	M. B. Ch, B.
裴義禮	Neil D. Fraser	M. B. Ch, B.
蕭曉初	Siau Hiau Tsho	
洪偉勳	Ang Ui Hun	

Report of the Swatow Mission Hospital for the year from 1st Oct. 1924 to 30th Sept. 1925.

STATISTICS OF PATIENTS 病彙表

In patients	Male	2571	男	留醫
do.	Female	638	女	
Out patients...	Male	8149	男	門診
do	Female	3785	女	
Patients seen at their homes	Male	423	男	外診
do.	Female	379	女	
Total individual patients ...	Male	11143	男	總數
do. ...	Female	4802	女	
Total attendences first and return		57426	門診	重診
Total visits to patients in their homes		2529	外診	
Surgical Operations: General ...		1115	普通科	解剖
do. Eye		766	眼科	
Operations with anesthetics ...		921	施蒙藥	
Opium smokers treated		12	改鴉片	

Report of the Swatow Mission Hospital for the year from 1st October 1924 to 30th September 1925.

The unsettled conditions obtaining in Swatow during the past few years, together with undiminished pressure of work on the hospital staff, more particularly on Dr. Lyall, have made it difficult to issue regular reports of the work of the hospitals and the financial statements.

We feel it due to our many friends and supporters in Swatow and elsewhere to issue now a brief report even though circumstances are not quite normal, and we shall endeavour to keep issuing reports from year to year in future, so that friends may be kept informed how the work progresses and how their gifts in money, or otherwise, are utilised.

On the financial side we include a statement showing how the various sums contributed to the Typhoon Relief Funds have been expended.

The ordinary accounts for the year 1924-1925 are also shown.

Brief as this report is it cannot go out without mention of the great loss the hospitals have sustained in the death of Dr. G. Duncan Whyte so long associated with Dr. Lyall in the General Hospital, and Dr. Nina Beath for nearly 20 years at the head of the Women s Hospital.

Dr. Duncan Whyte passed away in Nov. 1923 in Hongkong and was laid to rest in Kakchieh cemetery with every demonstration of honour and affection by Chinese and Foreigners alike. Dr. Nina Beath died in London in the Autumn of 1925, also deeply regretted. Many in Swatow and district have reason to remember with gratitude these two devoted workers.

Despite all the political changes and unrest of the past few years we are thankful that the hospitals have retained the confidence and good will of the people of Swatow and havebeen able to carry on their beneficent work without interruption.

We ask for a continuance of this good will and for such a measure of financial help as will enable us to serve still more effectively the sick and suffering, more especially the poor sick and suffering of Swatow.

We count it our highest privilege to minister to the need of body and soul in the spirit of Our Lord and Master Jesus Christ. Let those who would belittle the Christian religion reflect on this, that but for Jesus Christ and His teaching and example there would have been no Mission Hospitals in Swatow with their long record of service on behalf of needy suffering Chinese.

Our need of financial help is as great as ever and there are developments we should like to undertake so as to make the work of the hospitals still more efficient.

Mention may be made of the growth of our Leper work. From 12 to 20 who came a few years back, our members have steadily grown until now we have from 80 to 90 coming weekly for free treatment by the injection of the newer remedies that have proved successful in this dreaded disease. We ask your help to enable us to carry on and develop this very necessary and most hopeful side of our work.

The original X Ray installation given by Chinese friends was badly damaged in the typhoon and it had to be sent to England for repairs. Eventually, acting under expert advice the old machine was discarded and a simpler and more up to date set of apparatus purchased from Peking. This has been installed and is under the charge of Dr. Neil Fraser who took a special course in Radiology at the Peking Union Medical College. Dr. Fraser is gradually developing this side of the work and installing more apparatus as funds permit, and thereby increasing the usefulness of the X Ray Department to the hospital and the community.

We record our thanks to the Swatow Water Works Ltd., and to The Kaiming Electric Light Co. for a continuance of liberal discount on the monthly accounts.

(5)

Also to The Swatow Telephone Co. for the use of the Telephone without charge.

A. WIGHT.

DONATIONS 1925.

		Mex.	T. P.
Chiap Lee	洽利	15	
Anonymous	無名氏	8	
Ang Hien Tsu	洪獻書	20	
Shanghai Chamber of Commerce for Butterfield & Swire		98.90	
Sim Kye Lim	沈開林	5	
Ngan Gek Hua	顏玉華	8	
Rev. G. E. Lerrigo ...	... ...	25	
Tan Theng Po	陳燈波	6	
Rev J Speicher	... ...	10	
Captain Stocker	... ...	25	
Si Ti	世池	8	
Chua Seng Choo	蔡成書	20	
Tan Kiang Hun	陳健勳	10	
Tsu Soh U	朱雪吾	10	
Tan Song Thun	陳松儔	39	
Lau Soh Hu	劉淑漁	30	
Phua Min Sua	潘美山	10	
Tie Siau Bun	張紹文	20	
Ie Huai Kun	楊懷琨	10	
Tan Ngo Chek	陳虞澤	7.18	
Chiu Hua Heng	周和興	50	
A Lyall	來愛力	50	
Khai Tshan	開田	10	
Loo Ju Shun	盧如順	50	
Standard Oil Co., of N. Y.	... ...	...	50
Gou Hong Heng... ...	吳豐興	...	100
Thien Hi	天喜	...	40
Gou Iong Hieng...	吳永興	10	

		Mex.	T. P.
Rev. G. Waters	... ...	5	
Tshai Cheng Tsong Kek...	財政總局	...	141.43
Te Chia Si	鄭謝氏	10	
Messrs. Butterfield & Swire	太古洋行		578.17
It Tshun Uat Kun for Soldiers	粵　軍	99.46	
do. do.	... ...	9.33	
Chiap Lee	洽　利	8	
Railway Company for patient	潮汕鐵路公司...		45.00
Miss Greig	... ...	243.73	
Gou Sia Si	吳佘氏	20	
Tan Nguan	陳　元	50	
Chua Peck Beng... ...	蔡伯明	20	
Kueh Hau Khiam ...	郭浩謙	...	20
Tshu Tiau Khi	徐兆祺	20	
Kueh Theh	郭　宅	20	
Tai Zu Sim	大儒嬸	10	
Nam Kee	南　記	100	
Khou Tsong Si Leng for soldiers	許總司令	150	
do. do.	... ...	27	
Te Pek Bun	鄭伯文	10	
Sim Kia Liang	林佳祥	10	
Miss Harkness	候姑娘	10	
O. Hail	... ...	20	
Mrs. E. V. S. Lim ...	林　奶	100	
Kueh Tsu Pien	郭子彬	...	500
Chua Seng Chou... ...	蔡成書	...	20
Siau Hiok Kang	蕭旭江	...	5
Khua Ngo Khoi	柯悟溪	5	
Ngan Tsui	顏　水	...	[illegible]
Li Chek Jim	李澤壬	6	

		Mex.	T. P.
Ie Zu Nguan Hang ...	楊裕元行	5	
Mui Kiau...	美嬌	10	
A Patient...	病人	5	
Ko Jin Li	高仁利	6	
Chiu Ngon Chieh ...	周五石	...	... 5
Kho Ngo Khoi	柯恩溪	5	
Miss Harkness	候姑娘	50	
Tan Chin Thiam... ...	陳進添	10	
Iu Hun Pet Su	友雲別墅	20	
Gou Tsu Ki	吳子記	10	
Roman Catholic Mission	... ...	50	
Li Su Mien	李思敏	10	
Tshu Sok Che, Tshu Sok Hua	... ...	100	
Chia Loi Kit	謝禮吉	...	... 5
It Hah	逸合	...	50
Chiap Huat	洽發	4	
Gou Tian Lam	吳兆南	4	
U Sim Tshan	余心田	...	... 4
Patient	病人	4	
Lim Kang Ti	林江弟	4	
Lim Tsu	林珠	4	
Be Song Ki	馬松記	4	
Tshun Meng	春茂	...	... 4
Lim Tsu Bun	林書文	4	
Patient	病人	4	
Lim Tsun	林船	4	
Tshun Mong	春茂	4	
Lim Lai Hok	林來福	4	
Tang Ngmg Hong ...	莊腓荃	4	
Li Sam Ti	李三弟	4	

		Mex.	T. P.
Chiap Lee	洽利	4	
Patient	病人	...	...3.95
,,	病人	1	... .95
,,	病人	2	
Chiap Huat	捷發	1	
Tshua Hong Nguan	蔡豐源	2	
Tsan Mua Tsai	曾	2	
Heng Sim	興嬸	...	...2.99
Ie Kui Sua	楊桂山	2	
Patient	病人	1	
Tie Hiu Hua	張輝華	2	
Khou Iong Sang	許榮生	2	
Patient	病人	3	
,,	病人	2	
Te Zu I	鄭如意	2	
Patient	病人	1	
,,	病人	3	
Tan Peng Heng	陳炳興	2	
,,	陳炳興	...	...1
Tie Sin Se	張先生	2	...1 50
Tie Phek Iang	張碧陽	2	
Li Su Ui	李思偉	...	...1
Sng Tshau Sun	孫曹順	2	
Patient	病人	1	
Lim Si	林氏	2	
Khou Si	許氏	2	
Tan Tek	陳德	2	
,,	陳德	2	
Don.	... ...	2	...2.68
Lau Tek Tshai	劉得財	2	

			Mex.	T. P.
Hiap Seng Tsng ...	...	協成莊	2	
Donation ...	... ...	無名氏	2	
Tan Huat Kee	... ...	陳發記	2	
Tsu Hok Jong	... ...	朱學榮	2	
Donation ...	... ...	無名氏	2	
Kia Seng ...	... ...	佳成	2	
Donation ...	... ...	無名氏	2	
Lim Phek Chheng	...	林碧清	3	
Tie Li Si ...	... ...	張李氏	2	
Donation ...	... ...	... ...	2	
Hiap Seng Tsng ...	...	協成莊	2	

TOTAL............Mex. 1915.60
T P. 1589.03

$3504.63

SWATOW MISSION HOSPITAL ACCOUNTS

RECEIPTS 進欵	龍銀 Mex.
Grant of £50 from E. P. Mission 英會助銀	$438 77
Donations brought to Hospical 捐銀	3504.63
Fees 診金	4845.93
Rents of private wards 租房	2918.73
Other payments from patients 藥金	1050.68
Sales of drugs, milk etc., 賣藥及什物等	460.16
Deficit 欠欵	1794.31
總共 TOTAL	$15013.21

Account books examined and found correct

M. S. Ross

11th October 1925.

EXPENDITURE 支欵	龍銀 Mex.
Deficit 1st October 1924 原欠	$725.59
Salaties and Wages 薪水與工資	3595.68
Drugs, spirit, milk etc, 本地買藥	6171.65
Repairs & furnishings 修整院屋幷傢私	663.64
Lighting and Water 電燈及水	1413.66
Stationery and other sundries 紙及各等什物	904.32
Surgical dressings 棉花布油	1406.05
Help to poor patients 帮助貧醫者	132.62
總共 TOTAL	$15013.21

TYPHOON RELIEF ACCOUNTS
1922-1925.

RECEIVED

Aug.-Oct. 1922.	Mex.	T. P.
Swatow Municipal Relief Committee 100 hau		9.03
do. do. do. H.K. $50	50.00	
Tshua Khin Seng		50.00
Hongkong Chinese Chamber of Commerce		1000.00
Hongkong Tung Wah Hospital		1000.00
Swatow Relief Committee		5000.00
Li Si Hua 100 hau		9.03
Per Tan Un Mia (anonymous)		1021.42
Per Rev. Ng Siu Teng, Bangkok	371.00	
J. R. Wood Esq., Hongkong	20.00	
Swatow-Shanghai Relief Committee		10214.28
Sin Siu Tng		200.00
Per Rev. Ng Siu Teng, Bangkok	100.00	
Per Mrs. Hance from Tsingtao		349.65
Per Rev. Lau Chek Iong from Gou Song Suan, Bangkok.	100.00	
Goi Piah Tsu	20.00	
Per Rev. Ng Siu Teng Bangkok	25.50	
Total Receipts=	$686.50	$18853.41
Total expenditure to end of 1924.	$442.59	$14432.77
January 1925 Balance in hand	$243.91	$4420.64
March 15th 1926 Bank Interest		188.39
	$243.91	$4609.03

Total of both sums $4852.94.

TYPHOON RELIEF ACCOUNTS

1922-1925.

		Expenditure Mex.	T. P.
Aug.-Sept. 1922	Cleaning Hospital	30.31	
October 1922	Renewing electric light in Women's hospital	134.74	
October 1923	X. Ray apparatus to London for repair	62.21	2.26
December 1923	Repairs to Hospital assistant's house	105.67	
1922 and 1923	Re-roofing and other repairs to hospital		13122.50
	Repairs to assistants' house		20.80
1922	Repairs to Chaochowfoo hospital		276.00
July 1st 1924	Half cost renewing electric wires hospital		159.00
	Hospital Kitchen food for patients		792.80
	Sundry Expenses		59.41
Sept. 5th 1924	Duty on X Ray apparatus returned after repair	109.66	
Total Expenditure to end of 1924		$112.59	$14132.77

Accounts of Swatow Women's Hospital for year ending 31st October 1925.

RECEIPTS	Mex.	EXPENDITURE	
Balance	42.58	Salaries and wages	1557.81
Donations on the Field	778.00	Fuel and lighting	111.36
,, for special objects from England	277.24	Food and Milk	159.14
,, from Patients	908.16	Drugs	1005.56
Rents of private wards	908.20	Repairs and furnishings	304.22
Sales drugs etc.,	540.04	Hospital requisites	1003.10
Fees from Students	97.60	Sundries	77.00
Rickshaw earnings	132.05	Loss on exchange	3,05
Deposit Receipt and Interest	589.14	Water account	155.57
Treasurer (£110)	918.69	Freight, Customs etc.,	99.56
		Printing	8.10
		Credit Balance	707.23
TOTAL	$5191.70	TOTAL	$5191.70

I. E. BRANDER (Auditor)

8th February 1926.

TYPHOON RELIEF ACCOUNTS.

March 15th 1926	Balance in hand $1852.94	
	The use of part of the above balance in connection with the X Ray apparatus and the transfer of the remainder to the general account were specially authorised by Swatow Mission Council.	
	Special expenditure as above.	
April 20th 1925	Dr. Fraser's passage to Peking for X-Ray course	$95.00
	Do. other travelling expenses	35.00
	Paid to Dr. Fraser for X Ray a/c.	2000.00
	Bank commission on draft and exchange	77.19
Dec. 21st 1925.	Fitting X Ray room	18.55
February 3rd 1926	Dr. Fraser for X Ray outfit	219.46
		$2445.20

$4852.94
2445.20

Balance of $2407.74 transferred to Hospital general account.

In addition the General Hospital received in 1923 a generous gift of $3000 from Hongkong and Swatow Chamber of Commerce Typhoon Relief Committee for election of some building or purchase of any special apparatus required. No suitable opportunity has presented itself so far to justify the expenditure of this sum: but now a scheme for remodelling one of the hospital blocks to make an outpatient department is under consideration, and a large part of the money may be spent on such a scheme before the close of the year.

REPORTS AND ACCOUNTS

OF THE

SWATOW MISSION HOSPITAL.

AND OF THE

SWATOW WOMEN'S HOSPITAL.

IN CONNECTION WITH THE

PRESBYTERIAN CHURCH OF ENGLAND.

FOR

1926 & 1927.

汕頭福音醫院職員

Staff of Swatow Mission Hospital in June, 1926.

來愛力 A. Lyall, M.B., C.M. (on furlough).
越安如 A. Wight, M.B., Ch.B.
裴義禮 N. D. Fraser, M.B., Ch.B., D.T.M.
蕭曉初 Siau Hiau Tsho.
陳養頤 Tan Iang Hi.

汕頭福音女醫院職員

Staff of the Swatow Women's Hospital, 1926.

羅璇璣 H. Ross, M.B., Ch.B.
夏和平 F. Winifred Heyworth, L.R.C.P. & S.E.
張步周 Tie Pou Chiu.

汕頭福音醫院職員

Staff of Swatow Mission Hospital, June 1927.

如 A. Wight, M.B., Ch.B.
裴義禮 N. D. Fraser, M.B., Ch.B., D.T.M.
蕭曉初 Siau Hiau Tsho.
陳養頤 Tan Iang Hi.
李德夫 Li Tek Hu.
i/c laboratory. 化驗室管理
洪作樑 Ang Tsak Liang.
i/c dispensary. 藥房管理
李家隆 Li Kia Long.

汕頭福音女醫院職員

Staff of the Swatow Women's Hospital, 1927.

羅璇璣 H. Ross, M.B., Ch.B.
張步周 Tie Pou Chiu.
陳德馨 Tan Tek Heng.

汕頭福音醫院自一九二五年十月至一九二六年九月三十號佈告

Report of the Swatow Mission Hospital for the year from 1st October, 1925, to 30th December, 1926.

Statistics of patients. 病證表

In-patients	Male	2,255	留病
do.	Female	456	
Out-patients	Male	7,530	門診
do.	Female	3,406	
Patients seen at their homes	Male	254	外診
do.	Female	252	
Total individual patients	Male	10,039	總數
	Female	4,114	
Total attendances, first & return		50,749	門診 重
Total visits to patients in their homes		1,218	外診 診
Surgical operations	General	913	普通科
do.	Eye	500	眼科
Operations with anaesthetics		637	施蒙藥
Opium smokers treated		10	戒鴉片

汕頭福音女醫院報告

Swatow Women's Hospital Statistics.

1925-1926.

In-patients	1.433	院內病人
Out-patients	1,784	出外診病
Patients seen in their homes	356	巡視院外病人
Total individual patients	3,794	個人病人總數
Total visits to patients	753	外診總數

Operations. 解剖

Under Chloroform	156.	迷蒙藥
Minor	288	輕蒙藥
Eye	306	眼科
Gynaecological	39	婦科
Midwifery cases	221	產科
Teeth extracted	441	拔牙

汕頭福音醫院自一九二十六年十月在一九二十七年九月三十號報告

Report of the Swatow Mission Hospital for the year from October 1, 1926, to September 30, 1927.

Statistics of Patients. 病案表

In-patients	Male	1,622	男	留醫
	Female	78	女	
Out-patients	Male	6,581	男	門診
	Female	2,473	女	
Patients seen at their homes	Male	227	男	外診
	Female	73	女	
Total individual patients ...	Male	8,357	男	總數
	Female	2,624	女	
Total attendances, first and return ..		38,080	門診	重診
Total visits to patients in their homes		668	外診	
Cholera cases treated	about	200	霍亂症	
Opium smokers treated		7	戒鴉片	
Surgical operations	General	677	普通科	
	Eye	338	眼科	
Anaesthetics	General	461	施蒙藥	

汕 頭 福 音 女 醫 院 報 告

Swatow Women's Hospital Statistics.

1926-1927.

In-patients	1,341	院內病人
Out-patients	1,754	出外診病
Patients seen in their homes ..	491	巡視院外病人
Total individual patients	3,802	個人病人總數
Total visits to patients	1,294	外診總數
Operations.		解剖
Major, under chlorofirm	120	迷蒙藥
Minor ops.	225	輕蒙藥
Eye operations.		
Entropion—upper lid	652	剖眼上瞼
—lower lid	354	剖眼下瞼
Other conditions	24	剖眼其他情形
Midwifery cases	209	產科
Teeth extracted................	341	拔牙

REPORTS FOR THE YEARS 1926-1927.

A report covering two years of the work of the Swatow Mission Hospitals is herewith presented to our friends, bringing the record up to date.

In the first place we record with thankfulness that despite the frequently disturbed local conditions the hospitals have been able to carry on their work without interruption.

This work, we need hardly say, has continued to be what it has always been since the opening of the hospitals, an attempt to benefit both body and soul. Day by day the gospel of Jesus Christ has been presented to the patients, along with the ministry of bodily healing, and we know that to some the hospitals have proved to be a place of salvation in a double sense.

In March 1926 an event occurred which needs very special mention. This was the retirement from the field of Dr. Alex. Lyall whose name has been linked with the Swatow Mission Hospital for the long term of 47 years. Dr. Lyall came to Swatow from Scotland in 1879 to take over the Mission Hospital, which had been opened and had already begun to flourish under Dr. Wm. Gauld. These were the early years when many difficulties and prejudices had to be overcome. Dr. Lyall by his skill and kindliness gradually disarmed prejudice and secured the confidence of the people. As years went on his name and fame continued to draw patients in ever increasing numbers, and multitudes remember him to this day with gratitude. He left Swatow with many expressions of the affection and honour in which he was held by all classes. His name will ever be associated with the Swatow Mission Hospital.

Another valued worker retired during 1927, Dr. Malcolm Ross, whom many remember in Swatow. Dr. Ross was ordinarily in charge of the hospital in Swabue, where he had a deservedly high reputation, but from time to time he gave most valued help in the Swatow Hospital. We shall miss his experience and skill.

During the past summer Dr. J. H. Lamb of Yungchun, Fukien, gave us two months of much appreciated service in the hospital.

Elsewhere in this report Dr. Fraser deals in more detail with the Swatow General Hospital, and Dr. Hera Ross contributes a section on the Swatow Women's Hospital, so the present writer will conclude with an expression of sincere thanks to all friends, Chinese and foreign, who have helped in any way during these past two years. In addition to the names appearing in our donation lists we would record our thanks to the Swatow Waterworks Co. and to the Kaiming Electric Light Company for continuing to allow a liberal discount on the monthly accounts. Also to the Swatow Telephone Co. for the use of the telephone without charge.

Also to Dr. Henry Fowler, Medical Superintendent of the Mission to Lepers, Shanghai, for generous supplies of the drugs used in the injection treatment of leprosy.

Finally our friends may be reminded that in Chaochow-fu and Swabue, Mission Hospitals are being run on similar lines, in which good work is being done. For these hospitals we would solicit interest, sympathy and support.

A. WIGHT.

MEDICAL NOTES.

Leprosy.

Most encouraging results have been obtained by the use of the Ethel Esters of Chaulmoogra Oil, and Olive Oil. The injection is practically painless, and large numbers of patients have come up week after week with great regularity. One girl of 17 years old travels 3 miles by road then 30 miles by launch to continue the treatment she started having in Swatow. The average attendance is about 60 cases. Some few patients come up once or twice then cease their visits, but most, seeing the improvement in those who have been coming regularly over a period of time, are encouraged to do likewise.

Cholera.

As in former years a large share of the treatment of Cholera cases in Swatow has fallen to the hospitals, and thanks are due to the Tai-hong Temple for the use of the rooms which they benevolently provide as "Homes for the Dying." Without the use of these rooms it would be impossible for the hospital to undertake the treatment of Cholera cases. Some time after Cholera had appeared the Public Health Authorities opened a Cholera Hospital, and for a time we were relieved of this additional work. After the summer, however, the Cholera Hospital was closed, and for a further period of about two months part of our staff was occupied with this work. In all some 200 cases were treated by the hospital with hypertonic saline solution, with a good recovery rate.

Hookworm.

Appreciation of the treatment by Carbon Tetrachloride is shown by the fact that 1,300 patients were treated for Hookworm by the General Hospital last year.

There is no lack of opportunity for investigation into diseases of the heart and circulatory system, of the nervous system, and of the lungs, for they are seldom absent from the wards which we set aside for medical cases.

Surgical.

During the past two years we have had many gun-shot wounds to deal with, and bullets and other foreign bodies to extract. The periods during which some of our wards have not been occupied with soldiers have been but brief, for the tides of civil war have swept across this district in rapid succession, and at each ebb not a few wounded have been left stranded in the hospital. On one occasion when our wards were already full, dressers went from the hospital and treated over 200 wounded in a temporary dressing station.

An attempt made by certain military authorities to take over the hospital was fortunately averted, and the work went on without interruption.

The X-Ray machine has proved an invaluable aid in searching for bullets, needles and other foreign bodies, and also in the surgery of diseases of bone, of which we see many cases. Abscesses and cario-necrosis of bones, fractures and dislocations turn up day after day, and without the aid of an X-Ray picture operation would often be very much more difficult or even impossible. The hospitals have much cause to be grateful to those friends who made the installation of the X-Ray apparatus possible. One interesting case of a foreign body might be mentioned, although in this case X-Rays were not needed. A small boy came to hospital with a metal tube imbedded in his nose at the inner angle of one eye. A probe passed down the tube for two inches, and the tube would revolve on its own axis, but gentle traction would not move it. An anaesthetic was given, and by exerting a little more force a cartridge case was drawn out! The boy had been playing with gun-powder some six months before, and an explosion had driven the cartridge case into his face backwards !

X-Ray Department.

The use of the present X-Ray apparatus is limited to radiographic work—it is not suitable for fluoroscopic work nor for treatment. But the simplicity of the apparatus—as compared with that needed for treatment—combined with a large field of usefulness has, we think, justified this choice. As soon as the electric current supplied to the hospital improves—we hear that this will take place in the Chinese New Year—we hope to start using the X-Ray machine as an aid in the diagnosis of chest and abdominal conditions. The expenses in connection with the X-Ray department are heavy, and so a charge of $5.00 is made for small films, and of $10.00 for large films to those patients who can afford to pay. Much X-Ray work is done free of charge. As accurate interpretation of the films requires experience and constant practice, all films are retained by the hospital and are filed away for reference. In some cases patients wish to obtain a print, and for this a further charge of $5.00 is made.

Other arrangements can be made, if desired, by

Doctors in Private Practice who wish to have the benefit of the X-Rays for their patients.

N. D. Fraser.

Surgical Work.

List of Operations Performed in 1927. 一年割症目錄

Operations on bones. 骨割症	
Fractures, dislocations, abscesses and cario-necrosis 骨折 脫位 膿瘡 骨痨性	107
Amputations 截斷述	12
For bullets and other foreign bodies 檢傷異物	31
Tumours, simple 良性腫瘤	56
malignant 惡性腫瘤	32
Operations on rectum and anus 直腸並肛門之膿症	
Haemorrhoids. Fistula in ano. Stricture 內外痔 肛門痔 狹窄	68
Operations on Genito-urinary system 泌尿生殖的等症	
Phimosis. 包莖	
Amputation or penis 截斷陰莖	
Hydrocele 丸囊膜水腫	
Lithotomy. 截石述	
Stricture 狹窄	50
For Abscesses and Chronic Inflammatory conditions 膿瘡並炎性	68
Hare-lip 唇裂	14
Skin graft 植接皮	2
Operations on the eye 眼科諸症	338
Operations on the abdomen. 剖腹	
Gastro-enterostomy 腸胃吻合述	2
Hernia 疝	2
Liver abscess 肝生膿瘡	2

The Financial Position.

It has been the proud boast of the hospital for many years that the generous response on the part of the people of Swatow to the hospitals' appeals has made it possible to give advice and treatment without any cost to the majority of patients. Recently a slight change has been found necessary and those patients who can afford to pay, are asked to make a small contribution to the cost of their medicine and treatment.

Yet we would make clear that no case is refused advice or treatment on account of poverty or because they have not brought the money with them.

Patients are asked to pay 10 cents on registration, and the same for the first visit in each month during which it may be necessary to come to hospital for advice or treatment. Patients who have not brought enough money with them are not turned away, but are asked to remember to bring it next time. These charges cover consultation, medicines, and dressings, but actually pay for but a fraction of the cost. Accidents and urgent cases are, of course, treated when they arrive and one of the senior Chinese members of the staff is in constant attendance day and night to supervise the treatment of such cases.

Patients who register after 8.30 a.m. are asked to pay an additional fee of 40 cents: those who wish for an immediate consultation and those who come between the hours of 2.00 and 4.00 p.m. pay $1.00.

For the past year and more it has been found possible to hold an out-patient clinic daily, starting at 9.00 a.m. This practice has proved most satisfactory, and much congestion and consequent delay has been avoided, as the large numbers which in previous years were dealt with on Tuesdays and Fridays, are now spread over six days of the week.

Again we would appeal for a generous response from friends in Swatow, and especially from those who have received advice or treatment from the hospital. We start the year with a debit balance of over $700.00, and in addition have to meet very heavy bills for drugs and dressings. The increase in subscriptions has so far not kept pace with the rises in salaries and in the cost of medicines. The welfare of the hospital depends entirely on the support that it receives: a generous response would relieve us from a heavy financial burden and would enable us to devote our energies to increasing the efficiency of our services to the community.

Of the fund donated by the Hong Kong and Swatow Chamber of Commerce Typhoon Relief Committee for some special purpose in the hospital, part has now been used to refurnish three of the public surgical wards and to equip them with the necessary apparatus for efficient treatment. Each ward has cost roughly $150.00. One block of private wards has also been overhauled, and it is hoped that an opportunity will soon be found for fitting out the remainder in the same way.

Dr. Lyall.

Mention has been made of the retirement of Dr. Lyall after 47 years of service. Dr. Lyall's friends in England are hoping to raise a fund to commemorate the wonderful work that Dr. Lyall has done, and as a most suitable object the re-equipping of the opérating theatre has been suggested. If Dr. Lyall's friends in Swatow wish to express their appreciation in a similar way, no better purpose could be found than to provide a new operating theatre. Part of the Typhoon Relief Committee Fund was used to overhaul the present theatre—a small window being replaced by a larger one which gives much better light for surgical work, and a store room being converted into an instrument and sterilizing room; while the present operating theatre is all that can be desired for the treatment of casualties, of accidents and of septic cases, yet another theatre is urgently needed for aseptic surgery. To show how urgent the need is, it might be mentioned that our present theatre is in use almost every day of the week.

Dr. Duncan Whyte.

In the same spirit of commemoration, friends of Dr. Duncan Whyte have raised a fund in England for the re-equipment of the laboratory. An incubator has already been added to our apparatus and other articles will be bought from time to time. There are many diseases in the diagnosis and treatment of which an efficient laboratory service can be an invaluable aid. Under Mr. Ang Tsak Liang who has spent six months in the Institute of Hospital Technology at Anking, studying laboratory technique, we hope that as time goes on the laboratory will prove increasingly useful. Dr. Whyte's many friends in Swatow may wish to join in this expression of appreciation, and donations marked for this purpose will be used accordingly.

Need For New Buildings.

Perhaps this opportunity should be taken to mention the urgent need for new buildings, and for land on which to build. The widening and improvement of roads in Swatow is going on apace, and according to plan the hospital will need to sacrifice a block of fourteen private wards. Should the plan be altered to save the buildings, it would still be a most undesirable position, as the windows would open on to a wide and busy thoroughfare, and the noise and dust would be extremely bad for the patients.

We would urge the importance of securing for the hospital sufficient open spaces, that treatment may be carried out under the best possible conditions. A hospital closed in by surrounding buildings lacks the essential requirements of plenty of air and sunlight, and our present wards are in danger of being so closed in as to render them unfit for hospital purposes. Moreover the present buildings are not adequate for the numbers that come to us for treatment. The treatment of tuberculosis in all its forms demands above all fresh air and sunlight, yet in none of our wards can be meet these requirements. Near-by the hospital land is available; is Swatow prepared to secure this land where an up-to-date hospital might be built in ideal surroundings, as an extension of the present buildings? We look to Swatow to take action in this matter which concerns the welfare of the whole community.

Personnel.

Dr. Wight has for many years from time to time given up his work in Chaochow-fu to come to the aid of the Swatow Hospital when it was short-handed: and on the retirement of Dr. Lyall he agreed to take charge for a time. Dr. Wight feels however that he cannot longer delay resuming the charge of the hospital in Chaochow-fu, and accordingly when Dr. Fraser is joined by a newly appointed colleague, Dr. Wight will return to Chaochow-fu. We wish to express our appreciation of the valuable work that Dr. Wight has done during his residence in Swatow, and our regret at his departure.

We welcome the assistance of Dr. T. C. Pan, who has recently set up in practice in Swatow, and who has arranged to give two hours voluntary work to the hospitals each morning. The hospitals will greatly benefit from the skill and knowledge that Dr. Pan has acquire during his medical training in Glasgow, and his post-graduate work in London, Italy and Shanghai.

We would also extend a welcome to Dr. and Mrs. Worth who will have arrived in Swatow before this report is distributed. The addition of another doctor from home to the staff of the hospitals has made it possible to plan for further improvements and extensions of the work.

N.D.F.

RE-ORGANISATION OF WORK.

During 1927 the work of helpers in the hospital has been re-organised. Men have been taken on for four years, during which time they will receive practical instruction in all branches of the hospital work.

Under Mr. Ang they study the use of the microscope in the diagnosis of parasitic infections, and the essentials of bacteriology and of asepsis, in addition to the ordinary laboratory examinations.

Mr. Li Kia Long after a six months' course in Anking under the auspices of the Institute of Hospital Technology, has taken charge of the dispensary, where the helpers are given a systematic training in dispensary work.

Under the supervision of the assistants and the doctors the helpers perform the surgical dressings in the wards, and see that the instructions as regards treatment are understood and carried out by the patients.

In the operating theatre, which is in charge of Mr. Tan Sia Chhin, the helpers are trained to assist at all operations, in the preparation of instruments, sterilization of dressings—in each branch of theatre routine.

As these helpers become more efficient in the routine work of the hospital, we hope to find opportunity for giving further systematic instruction, and to arrange for a course on the First Aid Treatment of Emergency Cases.

So long as we have no trained nurses on our staff it is impossible for us to train these helpers to do all that is required for our in-patients, but their assistance renders it possible for us to cope with the large numbers that come to us for treatment.

And in the meantime patients bring a friend or relative to help look after them during their stay in hospital.

When our helpers have finished their four years' course, it is hoped that some of them will stay with us to take charge of one or other of the departments of the hospital work. Helpers will also be needed in our hospitals in Chaochow-fu and in Swabue, if it is found possible to keep these hospitals open.

N.D.F.

RE-BUILDING OF HOSPITAL ASSISTANTS' HOUSES.

A list of donations towards the re-building of the two houses which were pulled down to permit the widening of the road is appended. As the sum raised was not sufficient, a piece of land has been sold, the proceeds of which sale along with the donations, being used to build the houses on the remaining land. The work has already been begun, and it is hoped will be completed before long.

A balance sheet will appear in due course.

N.D.F.

SWATOW WOMEN'S HOSPITAL.

On the Women's side the statistics show a full two years of work.

As regards the diseases we treat, ankylostomiasis ("hookworm") is probably the commonest of the general disorders. Not only do we see patients in all stages of the disease itself, but the infection complicates other conditions in a great many cases, notably perhaps trachoma and leprosy. It lowers the resisting power of its victims very considerably. Pyorrhoea, and trachoma are exceedingly prevalent in this district, and we have to treat a large amount of entropion resulting from neglected trachoma. The operations for this condition are performed almost entirely by Miss Chang and Miss Chen.

Tuberculosis takes a heavy toll in these parts too, and one sees a sad number of young people with advanced phthisis. A great many children are admitted suffering from tuberculous bones and joints. During the summer months we had a good deal of typhoid and dysentery, and the cases this last year were of a severe type. In connection with the midwifery work it is interesting to notice that the majority of the cases are normal—a different story from earlier days, when people did not realise the wisdom of sending early for skilled help.

Some time ago certain alterations were made in tne surgical block of the hospital to provide bathrooms for the wards, and to make a new and wider staircase between them. Mrs. Ou Pek Thiu very kindly undertook to defray the cost of these alterations, and has collected a generous sum for this purpose. The details of this will be published in next year's financial report.

Soon after the completion of these alterations, the roof of one of the surgical wards collapsed. The disaster was caused by one of the large supporting beams giving way suddenly. The end of it which was buried in the wall had been eaten by white ants, and this had not been discovered in spite of periodical examinations of the roof. The patients mercifully escaped injury, and looking at the mass of beams and tiles and cement, and the twisted wrecks of the iron beds from which the patients were dragged, one felt that Divine protection had saved them. The cost of repairing this and other roofs which have since been discovered to be unsound has come to over $1,000.00. In connection with these repairs we have to thank Mr. Gumley, of Messrs. Butterfield and Swire, for the expert advice he very kindly gave us.

We join most earnestly in the appeal for more room and more buildings. We have to isolate our infectious cases in the private wards, and sometimes we have not one to spare. During a busy time also the accommodation is not sufficient for the ordinary cases, many of whom come from the country and have no friends in Swatow to go to.

During the spring and summer months of 1926 we were fortunate in having the help of Dr. Winifred Heyworth, who came out for a short term of service. We were very sorry to lose her, when she had to return home unexpectedly early for family reasons. We were very grateful also to Dr. Thacker of Chuanchow, who for a time was unable to be at her own station, and who gave us most welcome assistance.

A large part of the evangelistic work is carried on by voluntary help, and we thank the many Chinese and foreign friends who give ready and regular assistance in this way. On Sunday afternoons a Sunday School is held for the children in the hospital and the poorer children of the neighbourhood. During the past year and a half it has been conducted by Miss Paton.

We would like to record our grateful appreciation of Dr. Wight's help during the past months and our deep regret at losing him from Swatow.

We are also grateful to Dr. T. C. Pan, who has recently been giving valuable help in the clinical teaching of the senior students.

There are ten students assisting in the work of the hospital and two of these will graduate this summer. We are not admitting any new "medical" students, as we hope to start a course of nursing and midwifery.

H. Ross.

汕頭福音醫院全年進支總數

Swatow Mission Hospital Accounts.

1925-1926.

	Receipts.	進欵
Grant of £100 from E. P. Mission ..	$ 926.52	英會助欵
Balance of Typhoon Fund & interest..	2,407.85	八二風災存欵及利息
Donations to hospital	2,469.00	捐欵
Fees, Visits, and Consultations ...	2,810.16	診金
Injections, etc.	2,174.22	注射
Rents of Private Wards	3,218.82	房租
Sales of drugs, milk	654.61	賣藥及什物等
Sundry receipts ...	45.80	什費
	$14,706.98	總共

	Expenditure.	支欵
Deficit Oct. 1, 1925	$ 1,794.31	原欠
Salaries and wages	3,722.13	薪水與工資
Drugs, spirit, milk	4,750.39	本地買藥
Repairs and furnishings	707.93	修整院屋幷傢私
Lighting & water ..	1,527.28	電燈及水
Stationery & other sundries	777.57	紙及各等什物
Surgical dressings .	979.22	棉花 布 油
Help to poor patients	99.62	帮助貧醫者
Loss on exchange ..	87.28	失銀水
Balance on general account	261.25	存銀
	$14,7066.98	

Examined and found correct. 驗允

J. C. Smith. 28th October, 1926.

旅港潮州八邑商會汕頭賑災團捐款

Special Account.

Donation 1923 from Hong Kong & Swatow Chamber of Commerce Typhoon Relief Committee 原欵	$3,000.00
Bank interest to date 利息	182.24
	$3,182.24
Oct. 1, 1926.	
Balance in hands of treasurer 本利共	$3,182.24

爱克斯鏡房進支數目

X-Ray account, 1925-1926.

Receipts. 進欵	Mex.	Hong Kong
X-Ray fund per Dr. Lyall	$349.40	$2,000.00
Fees	184.50	
Gain on exchange		25.74
Donation. Mrs. Babcock		30.00
D. C. Fraser. £50		451.66
	533.90	2,507.40
	361.58	2,326.32
Credit Balance ...	Mex.$172.52	H.K.$ 181.08

X-Ray account, 1925-1926.

Expenditure. 支欵	Mex.	Hong Kong
Peking Union Medical College X-Ray installation		$1,200.00
Cook's, transport, customs		157.91
Eastman Kodak		370.86
Andersen & Meyer		597.55
Trav. expenses	$242.00	
Sundries	119.28	
	Mex.$361.58	H.K.$2,326.32

N. D. Fraser.

汕頭福音醫院捐款芳名

Donations, 1925-1926.

郭子彬	Kueh Tsu Pin	$ 500.00
	Military authorities	243.56
周古偉	Chiu Kou Thiu	200.00
楊	Ie	200.00
槙　記	Sek Ki	100.00
徐淑靜	Tshu Sok Che	100.00
羅懷榮	Lo Huai Iong	50.00
方劍衆	Png Kiau Tsua	50.00
朱遂生	Tsu Noi Seng	50.00
	Standard Oil Company	50.00
	Rev. R. W. R. Rentoul	50.00
蔡壽山	Tshua Siu Sua	50.00
	Mission Catholique	50.00
	Lon C. C.	40.00
	Miss Harkness	40.00
劉亦章	Lau Ia Chiang	36.35
	Mr. John	35.00
	Mr. W. A. Palmer	31.98
	Rev. G. E. Lerrigo	25.00
	Captain Wood	25.00
蕭友琴	Siau Iu Khim	20.00
羅懷榮	Lo Huai Iong	20.00
	Donation	20.00
陳鑽禹	Tan Tsang U	20.00
黃子朝	Ng Tsu Chiau	20.00
	M. O. Hall	20.00
竹　氏	Tsang Si	20.00
李質榮	Li Sit Iong	20.00
	A. L. Jones	15.00
鄭玉理	Te Gek Li	15.00
億合	It Hah	15.00
蔡德秋	Tshua Tek Chiu	12.00
許樹喬	Khou Su Khiau	12.00
英華	Eng Hua	10.00
顏輝記	Ngan Hui Ki	10.00
	Mrs. Francesca	10.00
吳奶	Gou Nai.　Ngun Ou	10.00
美嬌	Mui Khiau	10.00
先生娘	Au Sin Se Nie	10.00
	Miss Baker	10.00

李漢初	Li Hang Tsho	10.00
陳元利	Tan Nguan Li	10.00
辛來金	Sin Lai Khim	8.00
羅美玉	Lo Mui Gek	8.00
亞牛	A. Gu	8.00
張子材	Tie Tsu Tshai	8.00
黃淑卿	Ng Sok Kheng	6.00
林其遠	Lim Khi Iang	6.00
李俠先	Li Hah Sin	6.00
張河清	Tie Ho Cheng	6.00
楊掌卿	Chiang Keng	5.00
李	Li	5.00
莊　氏	Tsng Si	5.00
許俊明	Khou Tsun Meng	5.00
徐兆祺	Tshu Tiau Khi	5.00
美　璋	Mee Cheung	5.00
洪淑長	Ang Soh Cheng	5.00
陳亞國	Tan a I.	5.00
盧育桂	Lou Lok Kiu	5.00
張子松	Tie Tsu Song	4.00
蔡原英	Tshua Ngou Eng	4.00
林豐順	Lim Hong Sun	4.00
廖　氏	Liau Si	4.00
廖來興	Liau Lai Heng	4.00
徐育材	Tshu Iok Tshai	4.00
許張茂	Khou Tshun Mou	4.00
徐子安	Tshu Tsu Au	4.00
黃　平	Ng Pheng	4.00
戴先生	Tai Sin Se	4.00
珠能區	Tsou Leng Tsu	4.00
藍樹宏	Lan Su Hong	4.00
朱民鄒	Chu Ming Khu	4.00
林友能	Lim Iu Leng	4.00
	Sum of $2.00 and under	66.10
	Total	$2,469.00

汕頭福音醫院全年進支總數

Swatow Mission Hospital Accounts.

1926-1927.

Receipts. 進欵	Mex.$.
Credit Balance, October 1, 1926 存欵	261.25
Grant £100 form E. P. Mission 英會助銀 ..	979.61
Donations & Subscriptions 捐欵	3,219.19
Fees 診金	3,992.78
Rent of private wards 租房..	3,902.34
Sale of drugs, etc. 賣藥及什物	353.83
Sundry receipts 什費	276.27
Gain on exchange	84.66
Debit balance 存欵	766.40
	13,836.33

Expenditure 支欵	Mex.$
Salaries & Wages 薪金	4,846.60
Lighting & water 電燈及物	1,545.21
Repairs & furnishings 修整院屋并傢私 ..	592.77
Stationery 紙..........................	73.90
Surgical dressings 棉布油花	759.31
Medicines, etc. 藥物	5,048.04
Help to poor patients 帮助貧醫費	361.86
Sundries 什費	608.64
	13,836.33

Account books examined and found correct. 驗允

(Signed) J. C. Smith.

17th Oct., 1927.

葉克斯鏡房出入數目

Roentgenological Department Balance Sheet.

1926-1927.

Hong Kong Currency.

Cr.		Dr.	
Cr. Balance ...	$181.08	Eastman Kodak Co.	$306.91
Donation	27.20	Thos. Cook & Son	9.01
Sale of tube ...	174.94	Gen. Elec. Co. ..	35.00
Transfer from Swatow	350.00	To General a/c.	265.93
		Cr. Balance	116.37
	$733.22		733.22

Swatow Currency.

Cr.		Dr.	
Cr. Balance ...	$172.32	Local photo: goods	$ 18.77
Fees	613.00	Electric Light Co.	14.18
Dr. Balance ...	36.51	Customs duties	19.60
		Transfer to Hong Kong .	375.50
		To General a/c.	393.78
	$821.83		$821.83

旅港潮州八邑商會汕頭賑災團捐欵

Fund donated by Hong Kong & Swatow Chamber of Commerce Typhoon Relief Committee.

Receipts. 進欵

Oct., 1926.	Balance in hand 存欵	......	$3.182.24
Dec., 1926.	Bank Interest 利息	....	26.30
June, 1927.	Bank Interest 利息	....	8.96
			$3,217.50

Expenditure. 支欵

Reconstruction of wards with a view to converting them into a new Out-patient block 修整舊屋備作外診處取出欵	$1,610.65
Balance in hand 存欵	1,606.85
	$3,217.50

再建輔理醫生新屋住宅諸君捐欵芳名

Donations to fund for re-building Assistants' Houses.

		大洋 Mex. $
Li Hiang Kok	香谷	200.00
Nia Tang Ti Ngiap Co.	嶺東置業公司	50.00
Ngang Hui Ki	顏輝	30.00
Kwang Huat Co.	廣發司公	30.00
Lim Nguan Hong	林原豐	30.00
Cheng Nguan Co.	振源公司	30.00
Kuan Seng Co.	廣成公司	30.00
Thai Seng Co.	泰生公司	30.00
Chip Iah Bank	集益銀莊	25.00
Thong Hui Kong Si	同化公司	20.00
Chhin Seng Co.	臣盛公司	20.00
Lam Seng Co.	南生公司	10.00
Pheng Pheng Co.	平平公司	10.00
Kheng Hong Co.	慶豐金樓	10.00
Li Su Am	李素龕	5.00
		$530.00

小洋 Subsidiary Coinage.

The Mayor	汕頭市市政廳	$850.00
Swatow Chamber of Commerce	汕頭總商會	500.00
Kai Ming Elec. Light Co.	汕頭開明電燈公司	280.00
Swatow-Chaochowfu Railway Co.	潮汕鐵路公司	200.00
Swatow Waterworks Co.	汕頭自來水公司	150.00
Siang Hah	祥合號	100.00
Kia Hok Tng	嘉福堂	50.00
Bank of China	汕頭中國銀行公司	50.00
Hue Iang Kien	汕頭市花筵捐	20.00
Tai Ni Kong Si	糞溺捐大年公司	10.00
Jinricksha Co.	力車捐合華普益公司	10.00
Khua Heng Co.	菓商和益公所	10.00
Chhi Hu Hang	鮮魚行公所	5.00
Tsai Heng Kong Si	砂石捐再興公司	5.00
Iah Seng Hong Ki Co.	益盛豐記號	10.00
Swatow Light Railway Co.	汕樟輕便車鐵路公司	20.00
		$2,270.00

汕頭福音醫院捐欵芳名

Swatow Mission Hospital.

Donations. 1926-1927.

Kueh Tsu Pien 郭子彬	$ 500.00
Miss Greig per Dr. Lyall	440.43
Te Mui Seng 鄭美盛	200.00
E. C. Kueh	100.00
Lim Kui Chhiu 林桂秋	100.00
Shanghai Chamber of Commerce For Butterfield and Swire	98.25
N.D.F. ship's surgeon appointment	136.50
S. M. Cowles	75.00
Roman Catholic Mission	50.00
Gou Hong Heng 吳豐興	50.00
Lim Ki 林記	50.00
Standard Oil Company	50.00
Kaiming Electric Light Co. 開明公司	50.00
Jardine, Matheson & Co.	50.00
Indo-China S.N. Co.	50.00
Douglas S.S. Co.	50.00
Asiatic Petroleum Co.	50.00
J. A. Harrison	50.00
Sai Lou village 西爐鄉	40.00
Hua Ie Co. 華洋公司	40.00
Ie Chiang Kheng 楊長卿	40.00
Yew Kien Chee 游劍池	40.00
Mrs. Lee 利民學校	30.00
W. H. T. King	30.00
Tshu Sok Che 徐淑靜	30.00
Anon	25.00
Im Tien Seng 沈天生	25.00
Miss Macgregor per Dr. Lyall	21.42
Dr. Lyall 來醫生	21.42
Gebr. Roese	20.00
J. C. Frewin	20.00
Chua Seng Choo 蔡成書	20.00
Be Ki Bu 馬繼武	20.00
Khou Siau Pin 許少賓	20.00
Hong Seng 洪盛莊	20.00
Ngan Hui Ki 顏輝記	20.00
H. Palmer	20.00

"S. S. Archer"	13.00
J. C. Smith	10.00
Ti Ta So 知禾嫂	10.00
Lim Iu Leng 林友麟	16.00
Ang Tsun Huang 洪春芳	16.00
Hua Siang Li Tiam 華商旅店	10.40
Tan Nguan 陳元	10.00
Lau Tsun Tsu 劉船主	10.00
Boys Brigade per A. G.	10.00
Ng Tia T. Seng 黃傑生	10.00
C. B. Chamberlain	10.00
Tan Nguan Huat 陳源發	10.00
Te Seng Heng 鄭新興	10.00
Tię Kien Tsho 張健初	10.00
Ngan Iong Thong 颜永通	10.00
Khim Tsun 欽尊	10.00
Teng Kong Kuang 鄧公館	10.00
Kueh Iong Ki 郭永記	10.00
H. Duringer	10.00
H. M. Webb	10.00
R. Foster	10.00
T. Carr Ramsey	10.00
H. Donald	10.00
T. Poletti	10.00
G. E. Huygen	10.00
G. E. Huygen	10.00
Donations of less than $10	286.77
	$2,217.19

捐款自一九二七年十月一號

至一九二七至一九二八年再報告

Donation received since Oct. 1, 1927, will be entered in the 1927-1928 report.

汕頭福音女醫院進支總數

Accounts of Swatow Women's Hospital for year ending Sept. 30, 1926.

Receipts.		進欵
Balance	$ 707.23	總數
Donations on field	1,864.61	捐欵
Donations from England for special objects	161.16	英國長老會
Sales	345.85	售藥
Fees	200.00	學費
Interest and gain on exchange	141.00	滙水利息
Poor fund balance	400.00	濟貧總數
Kitchen	286.40	厨房
Ricksha earnings	38.00	車租
Rents	794.25	房租
	$4,938.50	總共數目

Expenditure.		支欵
Wages	$1,159.45	薪水
Fuel & Lighting	155.64	柴炭
Water	159.01	水費
Kitchen	432.46	厨房
Medicines	425.67	藥費
Repairs & furnishings ...	278.58	修整傢私
Hospital requisites	597.49	院內要需
Sundries	113.41	雜費
Credit Balance ...	1,616.79	總共數目
	$4,938.50	

Examined and found correct. 驗允

M. V. D. Paton

汕頭福音女醫院全年進支總數

Accounts of the Swatow Women's Hospital for the year ending Sept. 30, 1927.

Receipts.		進款
Balance	$1,616.79	總數
Donations on fiield	1,395.00	捐款
Donations from home for special objects	922.33	英國長老會捐款
Grant from E. P. Mission	1,476.65	英國長老會出款
Interest and gain on exchange	248.45	滙水利息
Students' Fees	40.00	學費
Sale of Medicines	365.55	售藥
Rents	949.90	房租
Kitchen	2,166.18	廚房
Ricksha earnings	2.60	車租
	$9,183.45	總共數目
Expenditure.		支款
Medicines	$ 656.04	藥品
Electric light re-wiring ..	235.00	修換電綫
Hospital requisites	797.67	院內要需
Carpenter	1,655.00	木工
Water	231.73	水費
Wages	1,656.15	薪金
Electric light	215.83	電費
Loss on exchange	21.19	滙水
Sundries	52.50	雜費
Kitchen	2,009.71	廚房
Credit Balance ...	1,652.63	總共數目
	$9,183.45	

Examined and found correct. 驗允

M. V. D. Paton.

Nov. 1927.

汕頭福音女醫院捐欵芳名

Swatow Women's Hospital Donations, 1925-1926.

Gou Kim Seng	吳錦成	$ 50.00
Gou Seng Heng	吳成興	50.00
Heng Sui Liu	王瑞鄰	20.00
Tou I Nam	杜以南	20.00
Hok Kou Me	福姑娘	15.00
Heng Zui Sam	王維三	14.00
Tie Thai Lai	張泰來	12.00
Bun Lo Gek	文羅玉	12.00
Un Lai Hua	溫來和	10.00
Tan Gek Un	陳玉恩	10.00
Tan Eng Ti	陳英智	10.00
Lim Un Tsu	林恩之	8.00
Tsang Si Mue	曾四妹	8.00
Tsang Lo Ki	曾四妹	8.00
Gou Peng Ti	吳炳智	6.00
Lo Thai Tsu	羅太珠	6.00
Gou Gek Ki	吳羅枝	6.00
Tan Si Gek	陳四玉	6.00
Ng Hiang Tsu	黃香芝	5.00
Lim A Ai	林亞愛	5.00
Te Ngi Iong	鄭儀容	5.00
Li Huang Tek	李芳德	5.00

汕頭福音女醫院捐欵芳名

Swatow Women's Hospital Donations.

1926-1927.

Tsu Tien Tsho	朱奠初	$ 50.00
Heng Kia Tsho	王加初	50.00
Tie Thai Thai	張太太	50.00
Heng Hua Chhe	王和星	50.00
Tie Kia Huat	張嘉發	50.00
Tie Kia Huat	張嘉發	50.00
Li Su Bo	李師母	30.00
Sng Ui Bun	孫渭文	30.00
Tan Gek Eng	陳玉英	30.00
Tan Si Huan	陳四芳	25.00
Tua Nai	大　奶	25.00
Ie Su Bo	楊師母	20.00
Hien Tek	賢　德	20.00
Nam Ki	南　記	20.00
Ke Iu	庚　寅	20.00
Lo Nng Su	羅女士	15.00
Gek Tshun	玉　春	14.00
Tan Heng Gek	陳恆玉	10.00
Kim Peng	錦　幷	10.00
Tshai Heng	彩　興	10.00
Bun Hua	文　和	10.00
Tie Su Nai	張師奶	10.00
Kia Heng	佳　興	10.00
Tan Po Tsu	陳寶書	10.00
Sim Kuan Siu	沈光瑞	10.00
Ng Tiau U	黃兆宇	5.00
Tan Tsu Khim	陳芝琴	4.00

弁言

本院常例年終即將進支各欵以及週年醫務造冊報告數年來因醫務浩繁本院職員應接不暇而以來醫生爲尤甚兼之時事糾紛多感困難是以報告之冊不能如常印發抱歉良深此後當逐年造冊報告俾捐助本院諸善士及關心本院諸好友得知本院年中經過情形所堪告慰者數年來雖政局屢變地方不靜然汕中人士對於本院之好意及信任心未嘗有異故本院之慈善事業得如常進行莫或間焉甚願此種好意年久常存同人等本吾主耶穌基督之精神竭其駑鈍以役事汕中病苦之人其貧乏而遇病苦者尤爲當務之急醫治其身體培養其心靈皆同人等所樂爲且視役事之工作爲無上之權利反敎之人盍試思之苟無耶穌基督之敎訓與其所遺之模範何有汕頭之福音醫院及其歷年所作役事病人之事業哉本院治病不拘種類以痲瘋而言就醫人數日見增加現在來院注射痲瘋者每禮拜計八十人以上因近年新發明注射之法其效甚大故也同人等甚願竭力以發展本院之事業然在在需財切望汕中及各處善士慷慨解

遂俾區區之念得以實現則幸甚本院前蒙中華諸友樂捐數千元購置葉克斯鏡一套藉電光以查察體內之骨骼臟腑惜該鏡爲八二風災所損壞近復由北京購來簡單之新式葉克斯鏡一套又有本院醫生裴義禮專司其事醫生曾在北京協和醫科大學專研究葉克斯光線之學其於該鏡之用漸謀推廣所需各種器具亦按財力之所及逐漸添設以期日臻完備不但本院可獨得其利且樂與闔境居民共沾其益本院數年來所經過有爲中西人士所同深哀悼者即懷醫生與米醫士之棄世是也懷醫生久與米醫生同勞竟於一九二三年卒於香港其靈柩則移葬於礐石米醫士長女醫院者將二十載去秋卒於倫敦兩位皆矢志一心鞠躬盡悴爲同人等所不能已於言者本院常年經費多蒙樂善諸君子捐資相助一九二四至一九二五年週年之進支數目列明於本冊八二風災由各方所得之賑欵亦順便列入並述明其用途本院所用電燈自來水每月還數蒙電燈公司及自來水公司准與折扣又本院所用電話蒙電話公司准與免錢一並提之以誌不忘

越晏如

汕頭福音醫院週年之報告

汕埠爲交通便利之區。士商萃會之地。本院創設於斯。歷有年所。療治各症。久著成效。故遠近負病就醫者接踵而來。現年病室。更時患不足。此固由於社會之心理。漸洞明西醫之精奥。能愈奇症。而起沈疴。尤足以徵社會之信仰本院者深矣。玆綜計一週年中就醫於本院者合內外宿數共一萬伍仟九百四十九。惟就醫人數。既日益增多。則一切醫藥等費。自必益鉅。本院得以維持醫務之進行。而免竭蹶滞碍者。實賴地方諸善士。慷慨捐助之所賜。此尤爲本院之所深感佩。而病家之所共同戴德者也。玆循向例。謹將捐欵諸君芳名。以及本院進支諸數目。與其他一切詳情。臚列於後。以貢諸樂善諸君鈞鑒。

本院照鏡規則

一　凡有人欲照愛克司鏡可於拜一拜五下午五句半鐘至本院等開鏡每人每次收洋二元

一 如非拜二拜五欲請特別開鏡者每人每次收洋五元
一 如因骨折或傷而欲影其骨之形者每人每次收洋十元
一 如欲治病者每人每次收洋四元

汕頭福音醫院章程

外宿門診章程

一 凡就醫者除星期日外當於上午八句半鐘齊集講堂聽講福音然後領簽就診施醫發藥不取分文遲到無赴領簽者每人收掛號銀四毫以上午十二点爲限
一 凡急症至院就醫則不拘時刻
一 每日診病先診十歲以下之小孩繼診男人後診女人
一 如有人懼過繁雜可於下午至本院候診每人收醫藥費壹元
一 凡經有本院舊方或遺失或忘帶而欲另開新方者每張宜另納掛號費一角

一 凡就醫者除星期日外當於上午八句半鐘到院領簽赴講堂聽講然後依次診病不收分文遲到無赴領簽者每人收掛號費銀四毫

一 倘有人懼過繁雜可於下午到本院就診每人收醫藥費銀壹元

一 凡因毆打姦淫等事到本院請驗給據者每人宜繳驗費銀五元

一 逢星期日非急症一概不診

一　凡非本院醫士所開葯方而欲来取葯者每劑宜納葯費一元

一　禮拜日非急症一概停診

外宿出診章程

一　凡欲請本院醫士出診者每次宜繳診金五元外埠另議貧家與急症准予通融

内宿章程

一　凡欲留宿本院者不拘何日何時須先通報門房由其引宿何處不得擅自投宿

一　凡留宿者每逢早晚禮拜時宜齊集講堂聽講福音然後領簽就診施醫發葯不取分文

一　凡欲入本院戒鴉片者每人宜先繳葯金四元并不許擅自出入

一　凡因毆打受傷等事至本院就醫如欲請驗給據者每名宜繳驗費銀伍元

一　凡留宿本院者每晚九點鐘後不許出入

一凡言語不通而欲留宿本院者須有妥人担保

總房章程

一凡留宿總房者不得自行烹飪宜由本院廚房三餐分給膳費則依廚房所定之章程

一本醫院專爲平民而設凡軍界有重病者亦許留宿惟每禮拜每名繳膳費外須加補醫約費銀六角

租房章程

一本院租房共分三等每間（甲等）每禮拜洋銀四元（乙等）每禮拜銀三元（丙等）每禮拜銀二元租銀均宜先繳清楚如租期未滿而欲移居者房租不得領回若有兩病人欲合租一房者租銀宜加一半

一租房伙食准予自理惟當在廚房烹飪不得污穢他處

一租房時欲交鎖匙須繳銀五毫作按出院時交還鎖匙即將五毫送回如鎖匙遺失

則作按之銀毫不得領取

一 房內所有器物不得輕忽損壞

西曆一千九百二十六年　月

本院長訂

SWATOW MISSION HOSPITAL.

REPORT 1930 -31

Men's Side.

The Years work can best be reviewed by a brief mention of the different departments.

General Medical & Surgical work.

A great part of the general medical & surgical work has been carried by the three hospital assistants; Mr Ang Ui Hun, Mr Tan Iang Hi & Mr Ang Tsak Liang. In all 838 operations have been performed ; of these 506 were under a general anaesthetic; and 230 were for eye conditions. Over 8000 patients have passed through the out-patient department and a total attendance of 39,500 is recorded.

The Leprosy Clinic.

The Leprosy clinic has been carried on by Mr Ang Tsak Liang. The attendance of the patients has been well maintained and further very encouraging results have been secured. In a number of cases all signs of the lesions have disappeared and the gradual progress of many other cases holds out good hope for their recovery. The total number of visits of Leper patients is 3704.

So far we have not found it possible to go forward with our plans for developing this branch of the work & establishing a small leper hospital, but we feel that the work we are doing is well worth while. Our thanks are due to the Mission to Lepers for the grant remitted to us for this work; and to the Chinese Mission to Lepers for their donation to cover the cost of Xmas gifts and tracts for every patient.

The Laboratory.

The laboratory under Mr Ang Tsak Liang and Lim Theng Hang has done very valuable work - over 2300 examinations have been made. The laboratory has also been used as a demonstration and lecture room for the nurses who have had instruction in Hygiene and Bacteriology, Anatomy and Physiology.

The X-Ray Work.

Unfortunately the X)Ray machine failed us in the middle of the year and it took us some months to replace the apparatus. The cost of this was met partly by special donations and partly by special funds in hand. Since tha new apparatus has been installed X-Ray work has been impossible for a time owing to the break down of the town generating plant. Before long however we hope to have things working smoothly again.

Evangelistic Work.

The Chapel services and ward visiting have been faithfully carried on by the hospital preacher & bible women. During the year the staff have formed a committee to arrange for devotional services and to increase the Evangelistic work amongst the patients. It is too early to report any results but the splendid start this committee has made promises well for the future.

Buildings.

During the year we have managed to go forward with the reconstruction in reinforced concrete of the verandahs, bridges and staircases for both sides of the hospital. As we anticipated it meant carrying on under difficulties while the work was going on, but we are now enjoying the advantages we looked forward to.

Financial Position.

The total local running expenses amount to $30470.00 Of this sum $8510 has been received as donations, and $12400. as fees for Private Wards and for Special Treatment.

Personnel

Mr Scott - our business manager - has spent a hard year on the language; we are looking forward to the time when he will be taking over a large share of our work. During his summer holiday he visited a number of Mission Hospitals and collected valuable data and experience that will be invaluable as we go forward with our plans.

Appeal For New Hospital.

We had hoped that by the end of this year our Appeal for funds for the New Hospital would be well under way, but the Flood Relief Work, followed by the troubles in Manchuria, drained the local merchants of funds and we have had to hold our hand. We still have strong hopes of making a start in the coming year.

Finally we would like to make clear that troubles in China mean more - not less - opportunity for missionary work. Doctors are still urgently needed and there is a hearty welcome and plenty of work awaiting them.

WOMEN'S BLOCK.

GENERAL MEDICAL AND SURGICAL WORK.

The general work of the hospital has carried on amazingly well in spite of the drawback and inconvenience occasioned by the demolition of a complete Ward-block comprising over 50 beds, and the demolition and replacement with re-inforced concrete of all old wooden verandahs and staircases. Accomodation for about 20 Hostel patients has been provided in the Chapel, but even so our "Bed Rating" has dropped from 11 to 7. More than 250 operations have been performed in the year of which, Dr. Chang was responsible for over 200. [illegible] major operations under General Anaesthesia were performed, and nearly [illegible] Maternity cases were conducted.

NURSING.

The level of treatment efficiency has been considerably raised already by the introduction of the Nursing System, and the patients are very quickly learning to adapt themselves to this innovation.

EVANGELISTIC WORK.

This is dealt with fully under the Matron's Report, but one would like to express the great joy one feels that we can now, with the introduction of nursing, do more to make use of the o[illegible]ortunities for such work.

MIDWIFERY AND GYNAECOLOGY.

With the possible exception of Children's work, Obstetrics and Gynaecology form the most important department in the Hospital, and our work in these subjects is probably more appreciated by our Chinese patients than anything else we do. Dr. Chang is responsible at present for the oversight of our Extern Midwifery work, and we have had two Midwifery Students working under her direction. Over 200 cases have been attended in the year, and a large number of these have been in the nature of Consultations, the cases being referred to us by outside Chinese doctors. In Gynaecology the operation for the removal of Ovarian Cysts still is called for more often than any other individual operation.

CHILDREN'S WORK.

The most important and certainly the most delightful piece of work we have to do. As our old Children's ward has been demolished, we have the children now in the general Medical and Surgical wards, where they bring a great deal of sunshine and laughter into the lives of the adults round them, and to the hospital staff as well.

Personnel.

One is continually amazed at the amount of sheer hard work which Dr. P.C. Chang gets through, and her skill and patience in dealing with a host of irritating details of hospital running lighten the work of the Foreign staff immensely.

Miss Macpherson was unfortunate in having to undergo a major operation during what should have been her Summer holiday. She is to be congratulated on the way in which in one short year, Nursing in Swatow has developed from a nebulous dream into a practical reality, which has obviously come to stay.

Miss Martin is doing well at the Language, and although not yet officially "in" the hospital, has made friends already with the Chinese Staff. We are looking forward to the day when she will be released from language study for the easier job of medical work.

We are looking forward to Mrs. Wallace's return from furlough, and hope that she will be able to help us again, especially in the Gynaecology work and Midwifery.

Last but not least, we must congratulate Dr. Fraser on his marriage to Miss Peggy Chesworth, formerly of Fatshan hospital. [illegible]

Nursing Report *Womens Block*

This year in Swatow has proved the opportunity to be as great as appeared when we began the nursing scheme. Things here are more advanced this being port and so close to Hong-kong, besides it is in the province of Kwangtung, from whose capital -- Canton -- most of the initiative in China proceeds. Educated girls are very ready to come in for nursing training, and we have had no need to camouflage by adding any other lines of training and study as pink sugar to the pill -- we were able to say 'like it or leave it' without fear of not getting enough staff to carry on the work of the hospital. That made all the difference to our morale -- and so we started with a flourish in April, by taking in three new Swatow-speaking probationers.

Of the five Chuanchow girls who came with me , two finished in the summer the other three have signed on to finish their training under the new syllabus that we have got out in Swatow. The two seniors had needed a good deal of attention in order to get them finished before the summer holidays. So the real beginning in Swatow has been within the last three months, during which time I have been trying to get my teeth into it. It reminds me of the suspended apple that we try to bite into on Hallowe'en -- the problems are some-elusive and refuse to be solved without time and patience.

I wonder if you can imagine what a hospital is like without any nursing service ? One of the difficulties of getting it started is that the patients expect to bring their relatives -- and they cannot believe that we really are prepared to do everything for them -- sometimes they are willing to go if their homes are not far away, but more often they want to stay -- they make no bones about lying on the same bed, or on the floor for that matter, and why should we worry if they don't take up an extra bed - especially as they do all sorts of things for the patient, which we would much rather they wouldn't -- and provide her with food which she shouldn't have -- and make a delightful mess in the ward, which they don't mind at all -- really it is very unreasonable the way these foreigners run things, however, as they have got the goods we want, we don't get in their way any more than necessary!

And what is still more to the point -- they are beginning to learn that their attentions are not necessary and in the 2 wards in which we have been chiefly working, we are getting more and more patients without their relatives and that is encouraging.

We have taken over some of the work downstairs too -- but that is a different story. The cases there do not need nursing -- they just need their wounds dressed -- they only stay in hospital because they come from such very long distances -- they are really out-patients using the hospital as a hotel. It is rather disconcerting the way they walk in and help themselves to a bed without saying 'by your leave' -- and then when they think they are well, or when they take it upon themselves to decide that we can't cure them, they melt into the landscape without any previous intimation. We do manage to keep a little more order in the wards where we are working even downstairs -- and when we want to remind ourselves that this is so, we take a stroll around one of the wards that we have not yet taken over.

We are beginning to take over some work in the Out-Patient Department. Hitherto the former type of 'students' have been in attendance there, but they have been gradually dropping off, and soon there will be none left. We expect to take in a new class of nurses shortly, and then gradually we will get things going more satisfactorily.

On Sunday afternoons we have a ward service for the patients who cannot go to the chapel services -- the walking patients come to it too to swell the numbers. The Bible Women come regularly and teach the patients to read hymns and short prayers. Another method is the use of a series of lessons written in large characters and pinned up in sight of the whole ward -- each lesson consists of a few short sentences which they quickly learn by heart, and when they can repeat them from memory they are rewarded with a small coloured slip with the same characters printed on it. When most people in the ward know one lesson we change it for another. We only have big sheets of the first six lessons, and the constant change of patients involves going over these again and again, but patients who stay for a long time learn the more advanced lessons from the small slips. The aim is to teach them the elementary truths of the gospel, and if they stay long enogh to learn the first six, this makes a very good foundation.

Fortunately the Swatow girls manage to pick up Amoy words rather quicker than I do the local dialect, so we manage to get along together all right. Things are progressing slowly and surely, and we have every reason to be hope-ful of seeing a good nurse's training school before very long, and all the wards looking spick and span, and all the patients well-cared for. When Miss Martin gets working alongside at the end of the year, then we will soon get it up to the perfect standard we are aiming at.

M. Murray Simpson

Statistics Swatow Mission Hospital.

1930 - 1931.

1. Medical Missionaries	2.
British Nurses	2.
Business Manager	1.
3. Chinese Assistants	5.
4. Chinese Nurses	6.
Midwifery Students	1.
Dispensers, Dressers etc	12.
6.7. In-patients	2910.
8.9. Out-patients	11374.
16. Total attendances, Ist and return visits	92319.
18. Operations	1847
19. Eye Operations	1495.
	3342
23. Operations under General Anaesthesia	735.
Dental extractions. (Womens Block only)	741.
25. Hospital Beds	272.

Women's side only...Out-calls.....501.

Total visits... 1306.

Midwifery & Gynae cases.. 274.

Injections.............. 800.

Swatow Hospital
1932 – 1933

天下無難事
惟要有心人

Under heaven there is no thing impossible.
All you need is a man with a heart.

A Chinese Proverb.

E. H. SCOTT.
ENGLISH PRESBYTERIAN MISSION
SWATOW, S. CHINA

REPORT OF THE SWATOW MISSION HOSPITAL - OCTOBER 1932/SEPT. 1933.

There is so much to comment upon in the work of the Swatow Hospital during the year that we will just pick out the most noticeable features of a very full twelve months.

THE EVANGELISTIC WORK. There can be no doubt that this work has improved in quality. The preacher appointed by the Presbytery is a much more "live" man than many of his predecessors and can more effectively frame his message to fit and hold the interest of his audiences. His efforts have been supported by a blind Hakka preacher and he has also had gratuitous assistance, almost daily, from a familiar figure on the Swatow streets - a free lance evangelist. He comes into the Hospital and addresses the crowd of out-patients as they wait at the Registration Office. He always carries a large stock of pamphlets etc. and manages to dispose of quite a number of them. The Bible-women have carried on their unobtrusive work in the women's wards. In these wards also, under the direction of Miss Martin, the evangelistic work has been coordinated. Each Sunday all the patients receive a text picture which is later expounded at the ward service. Before each service the nurses lead in singing hymns and they have helped considerably in teaching the patients, particularly children, to read and sing. By confining the hymns to a few simple ones, the singing has improved and many patients go home with the message of a hymn indelibly impressed on their minds. Large posters on the walls with a daily simply text is another avenue methodically used.

A devotional society for the whole staff and run by the Chinese members has been formed and aids in developing the spirit of unity and service among the staff without which other evangelistic work would be less effective.

On Christmas Eve we showed in the wards a film depicting the life of Christ and it was a deeply moving experience to hear the young nurses, as they stood by the bedsides, explaining the pictures to the patients.

Each day starts with prayers with the staff and we hope, as time goes on, that the staff will take more and more advantage of their opportunities for evangelistic work among the patients.

THE NURSING SERVICE. It is with profound thankfulness that we report continued progress in this development. The total staff of nurses qualified and in training is now 16. The great event of the year was the graduation ceremony of the first 3 nurses to complete their course in the Hospital. Two of them went back to Chuanchow to assist in the inauguration of nursing there.

The efficiency of the new service is steadily increasing. For much of the success of this venture we gladly acknowledge our indebtedness to Miss Macpherson who contended so valiantly with the initial difficulties (and how many there were!) of introducing nursing into the Hospital. For all that she did and hoped to do (much of which is now accomplished) we give a hearty thank you and wish for her great happiness in her new sphere of service at home.

LEPROSY. This year has been a record in the number of cases treated, many of which have been particularly interesting and encouraging.

We have extended our scope in this branch of work by getting doctors in other places interested who have since taken up the treatment of leprosy on the same lines as we follow here.

Dr. Fraser has now been asked to undertake some research work into the action of certain drugs on lepers and is now making these special investigations.

PLANS FOR THE NEW HOSPITAL. We have spent many evening hours during the year discussing and drawing plans for the new Hospital which we hope to build WHEN we are able to sell the present Compound This proved to be fascinating work. It meant the pooling of ideas and there is cause for thankfulness in the fact that we were finally able to produce tentative plans acceptable to all concerned.

Subsequent land negociations necessitated modification of the plan. Other improvements and amendments may be necessary before the final plans are completed but in the meantime we are greatly encouraged to know that the general "lay-out" of the proposed new Hospital has been approved by the Home Board.

ALTERATIONS AND IMPROVEMENTS TO THE PRESENT HOSPITAL.

The general trade depression in China and the uncertainty of the political situation made it obvious that an immediate sale of the Compound could not be looked for, so delaying the prospect of a completely new Hospital. We therefore turned our minds to the possibility of improving our facilities in the present buildings. In this connection we were greatly stimulated by the recommendation of the Field Board and the subsequent sanction given by the Home Board that we should be allowed to spend up to $10,000. An account of the alterations made properly belongs to the report of the current year's work but much of the preliminary thought on the most urgent improvements needed was given in the year under review. Briefly our chief decisions allow for the reconstruction in concrete of a wooden and tile verandah which had become dangerous; the conversion of two large public wards into nursing wards; the erection of new kitchens for the nursing section of the Hospital and for the nursing staff; improving the bathroom and lavatory accommodation; reconstructing one old block, making of it a building to serve as an out-patient department for the whole Hospital (this building is the sole remaining block of Dr. Gauld's new Hospital built 54 years ago). All these plans have been subjected to most careful examination. The first two items have been completed i.e. the verandah and the conversion of two wards and we are thoroughly pleased with the improvements which have thus been made. We remainder of the work is now proceeding.

ENGAGEMENT OF DR. CHENG. Another important decision taken during the year was to invite Dr. C.S. Cheng to join the staff. Dr. Cheng graduated at St. John's College, Shanghai, and then did two years' post-graduate work at the Pekin Union Medical College before taking an appointment with the American Baptist Mission Hospital at Kityang, where he has served two years. He has the name of being

K. H. SCOTT.
ENGLISH PRESBYTERIAN MISSION
SWATOW, S. CHINA

3.

a clever doctor and surgeon and he combines his abilities with a very pleasing personality. He is obviously an earnest Christian man and it is worth recording that he has accepted our offer of $150 a month in spite of opportunity to stay at Kityang at $200 a month. We are hoping great things from his help.

His engagement has necessitated considerable alterations in the Hospital organization and readjustments among the staff. It is a matter of considerable satisfaction to us that, speaking generally, the staff are entering into all the plans of reconstruction and reorganization in a spirit of loyalty and enthusisam. We feel that the spirit pervading the Hospital is better than it has been for several years.

FINANCE. In some respects the year has been a difficult one in view of the trade depression in Swatow and two of our main sources of income show a heavy decline, viz: ward rents and donations from Chinese friends. Our staff made strenuous efforts to collect the usual donations despite much discouragement. On the other hand the unusually generous support of the foreign community in the port was very encouraging. We feel that on the whole we did fairly well by finishing the year with a debit balance of only $15 after borrowing $1000 from a special fund.

For this current year we have instituted a small charge for the treatment given to all in-patients from which we shall derive a substantial increase to our income. The reconstructions now in hand will also result in some economy in administration expenses and although part of the increased income will be swallowed up by Dr. Cheng's comparatively large salary we anticipate that the financial position will show an improvement at the end of this current year.

GENERAL. Among other developments should be mentioned our participation in an epidemiological survey being undertaken by the Research section of the Chinese Medical Association. This involves supplying the Chinese Medical Association with a detailed record of every patient seen - both in-patients and out-patients. Although this means considerable additional work for our Doctors results are justifying the labour. We receive in return for our information a classified record of all our cases but the main advantage is the useful survey that is thus being made of the [redacted] of various diseases in different parts of China.

Dr. Worth went home in June for a well earned rest.

We would take this annual opportunity of saying, "Thank you" to the many friends who by donations, parcels of goods, and in other ways have helped and encouraged us during the year.

Whilst we are very conscious of many shortcomings in our work we give thanks to God for all that has been achieved. At times during the year it almost seemed that the many problems facing us were too involved for satisfactory solution but some of the difficulties we anticipated never arose and others vanished before goodwill and a determination to overcome them. Step by step the way has opened up before us and we have been conscious of guidance when it was most needed. For all things we give thanks.

REPORT OF THE SWATOW MISSION HOSPITAL : 1934/1935.

This year has been mainly one of consolidating the internal organization of the hospital after the extensive reconstruction and alterations of last year and so there is, comparatively, little of striking interest to report.

Several changes have taken place in the personel of the staff, the tone and quality of which is perhaps better than it has been for many years. One of the most important decisions taken during the year was to invite C.S.Cheng M.D. to remain on the staff for a period of 5 years. His association with us during the last two years has been entirely happy and he has proved himself to be a capable physician and surgeon. Furthermore despite the fact that his previous experience had accustomed him to a thoroughly modern plant and nursing service he has shown himself adaptable to the difficulties of work in our present buildings and both patient and resourceful in carrying on his work without the aid of skilled nursing. We believe that he will prove to be an increasingly useful member of the staff.

We have already reported in detail on the financial situation for the year. Suffice it then to say that our keen disappointment ~~was~~ at once more ~~we were~~ being unable to close the books without a debit balance gave place to a profound thankfulness for the anonymous donation of $ 2250 received in October which wiped out the debit balance on the year's working. There are signs that the worst of the financial depression in Swatow is over. The last six months of the year under review shewed a steadily increasing income, and the results for the first quarter of the current year are equally encouraging. There is therefore ground for cautious optimism. This improvement has been reflected in the substantial increase in the number of patients coming during the year compared with the preceding year. In-Patients totalled 1748 against 1662 whilst Out-Patient visits jumped from 45,500 to 77,000. totals

The latter months of the year were characterised by a severe and prolonged epidemic of typhoid fever. For months our medical wards were full of patients suffering from this disease.

The evangelistic work has been faithfully maintained during the year and rather more follow up work has been done, although we still have ~~xxx~~ much to do in this direction. As is usual most of this work is done without visible results but we can record at least two instances of patients who have found a new spiritual life during their stay in hospital. One was mentioned in last year's report as having found a new meaning and joy in life. She came back to the hospital this year introducing a neighbour from her own village who needed treatment. During the few days we was with us she proved herself an effective evangelist never ceasing to tell the other patients of her own experience in hospital. Her face certainly revealed that "something had happened". The second case is that of a girl who was in hospital for 18 months. When she arrived she was dull, listless and rather disagreeable, but during her stay she learnt to read the Bible and Hymn book. The listlessness and bad temper gradually disappeared and she left us with protestations of thanks and gratitude for the physical and spiritual good she had found with us and with the expressed intention of joining up with the church nearest to her home. A special letter ~~txxthx~~ was sent to the preacher of that church commending her to his care.

During the year we have extended the scope of our surgical work by undertaking surgical treatment of tuberculosis and by operations for other conditions which have hitherto never been performed in our hospital. The news of such developments spreads through the district rapidly and so we anticipate a wider range of surgical work in the future.

The leprosy clinics at Swatow and the village clinic opened last year at Iam Tsau have continued. The numbers have been well maintained although the natives of Iam Tsau are beginning to express concern of the weekly congregation there of lepers from the surrounding district. Fears and lack of enthusiasm of the people at Tsang-im have made it impracticable to open the second village clinic there as was planned.

Mention should be made of the fact that our two trained Chinese Sisters have assumed responsibility for the Matron's duties during Miss Martin's absence on furlough. During the last three months they have proved their quality.

This report is written just as we are discussing some further important advances along the road towards modernising our service. Thanks largely to the enthusiasm of the headmistress of our girls' school we seem to have reached the point where further progress need not be delayed because of shortage of nurses of the right education standard. During the next three weeks we expect to receive six or seven probationer nurses and with their advent to open the first nursing service ward for male patients. We anticipate a further four nurses in the autumn which will permit the opening of a second male ward under nursing service.

We have also come to the conclusion that the time has now arrived to take the last step in the union of the Men's and Women's hospitals by uniting the two Operating Theatres under nursing service. A scheme for reconstruction to this end is now under consideration.

Another important advance urged upon us by many of our Chinese friends, and in line with our own desires, is the provision of more and better private wards with full nursing attention to which the more wealthy constituency in Swatow will be attracted and from whom we can hope for substantial additional income, besides enlarging our field of influence to include this type of patient. We have decided to adopt this policy by making some adjustments in our public ward accommodation which will increase our private wards in the nursing department from six to twelve, we are providing attractive furniture, beds and general equipment for these special wards at a cost of $ 2000.

When all these plans are carried through we shall have a total of 70 beds under full nursing service. We may, at a later date, be able to add a small children's ward to this number but 80 beds under nursing seems to be the maximum our buildings will allow. Even so the facilities will be very much in the nature of "makeshifts". However 80 beds under a full nursing service by the end of this year is a very encouraging development to have taken place within the space of five years. At the end of 1930 there was no nursing in the Swatow hospital - one of the oldest and largest Mission hospitals in China; and we are profoundly thankful that the road has gradually but steadily opened for us to effect the changes. Furthermore 80 beds will give us a safe nucleus for that happy day when we shall have a completely new hospital of 100/110 beds all under modern conditions and nursing service.

We are also discussing with the Directors of the Presbytery's Middle school the possibility of providing the 550 students there with complete and thorough medical supervision and treatment, including care in hospital when necessary, during the whole of their school careers. If this scheme can be put into operation we s. 'l have added another very important and valuable field of service to our work.

And so we give thanks for a year of steady work, during which a substantially increase number of patients have been treated and we look forward to a year which will hold new advances and new opportunities.

ENGLISH PRESBYTERIAN MISSION HOSPITAL, SWATOW.

ANNUAL REPORT FOR THE YEAR 1937.

The past year has, for the hospital, been a period of extremes. During the first few months we began to benefit from the alterations and re-organisation of the previous years, and at the same time the end of the trade depression, and return to better economic conditions had a very beneficial effect on the running of the hospital. We seemed to be in for a period of prosperity such as we had not seen for many years. The Hospital was working on a definite balanced budget, private patients were coming in increasing numbers and willing to pay "Nursing Home" fees, thereby enabling us to give a great deal of free treatment to the poor patients in our Public Wards. On an average, half the patients treated in these wards paid nothing at all for food or treatment, and the remaining half paid up to one seventh of the cost of treatment, with the exception of a minority who were able to pay something towards the cost of expensive injections, operations or X-Rays. Unsolicited donations came in well, and altogether we felt that the corner had been turned, and that whatever difficulties and problems might lie ahead, we had our feet definitely planted on the upward path.

So marked was the feeling that prosperous times were on the way, that we felt justified in planning an early appeal to the Chinese Community here for funds to rebuild the hospital, and had begun to make tentative arrangements to collect money for a new X-Ray plant and a much needed motor ambulance.

The development of the school of nursing was going ahead, and Government regulations made it necessary for us to contemplate - as well as the prospective nursing needs of Swabue and Wukingfu - the early establishment of a large "Joint School of Nursing", with its own management and plant. This was a formidable undertaking, needing much careful thought and planning, but the encouraging response from the local Chinese Community to the very tentative enquiries which had already been made, made us hope that we should be able to go ahead comparatively soon and comparatively smoothly. The comment of one of the prominent Chinese ladies of Swatow on being told of the size and difficulty of the task is illuminating:- "Just leave it to the ladies of Swatow"

The reconstructed Private wards were coming up to expectation, and in addition to wealthy Chinese patients, we were able to take in European patients with both medical and surgical conditions, and provide treatment and comfort of which we felt no need to be ashamed.

Almost all departments of hospital administration had been re-organised during the year 1936, and we were feeling the benefits of this in increased efficiency and economy.

It is no exaggeration to say that in July of this last year the hospital was at one of its highest peaks of prosperity for the past many years

In July fighting between Japanese and Chinese troops broke out in North China. On August 12th the Japanese Consul left Swatow with all Japanese residents. On August 13th fighting began in the vicinity of Shanghai. It soon became clear that this was to be a struggle of a much more serious nature than that of five years ago, and it was anticipated that Swatow would probably have to put up at least with attacks from the air, and possibly with bombardments from the sea. The wealthier members of the local population soon began to leave for safer parts, and the Chinese authorities began to encourage women, children and the aged to leave the port for safer places inland. Air-raid practices were carried out, and a certain amount of minor street fortification was begun. Trade immediately fell off, and the imposition of the blockade added a further hindrance to the free passage of goods. The Government proclaimed a moratorium to prevent the flow of money out of China, and "Froze" all money deposited with Chinese banks. It very soon became clear that even if hostilities never touched Swatow, the hospital was going to have an exceedingly difficult time financially. Our private wards emptied rapidly, and we were soon left with a fair number of poor patients who could pay nothing, but very few private cases to help out expenses. Inevitably prices began to go up, and in spite of Government efforts to prevent profiteering, the cost of living, and the cost of drugs increased enormously.

The state of our buildings made them most unsuitable for use as a hospital should there be any risk of high explosives falling anywhere in the vicinity. It would not require a direct hit to bring our flimsy structures toppling. We hoped, however, that by providing Identification marks in the way of large flags painted on the roofs, and in the absence of military objectives in the neighbourhood, we should be able to carry on. Unfortunately the Chinese military authorities mounted high angle anti-aircraft machine guns of fairly heavy calibre on buildings adjoining and opposite to the hospital, and all our efforts to get these removed were unavailing. In the first week of September, Swatow suffered a series of air-raids and a naval bombardment. As we had feared, the guns surrounding the Public Ward blocks of the hospital became a target for the raiders. The air-men obviously attempted to attack only military objectives, and ran considerable risks, diving exceedingly low, to ensure accuracy of aim, and at first only machine-gunned the buildings next to the hospital. This did not silence the guns, and so bombs were dropped, one of which scored a direct hit on the fire station adjoining the hospital, others falling in the road in front of the fire-station. The hospital buildings were badly shaken, and some minor damage was done. The Chinese staff had been getting more and more alarmed, and threatened to desert. By transferring the hospital to temporary quarters at

Kak-Chieh across the harbour, we were able to preserve one third of our total staff, the rest fleeing to the interior. Owing to the excellent air-raid precautions maintained by the police, casualties were few, amounting to some ten killed and twenty wounded, all of whom were treated in our hospital.

During the past year relations between the hospital and the municipality and Public Health departments have been increasingly cordial, and the mission doctors have been consulted on all major matters affecting the health and medical welfare of the town. At the beginning of the war a special committee of doctors was formed to discuss air-raid precautions. The hospital was represented on this committee, which submitted proposals to the municipal authorities. One proposal was that the authorities should contribute towards the expense of caring for casualties, and approximately 25% of the cost of treating the wounded in our hospital was borne by the municipality.

The writer has been appointed adviser to the Chinese committee on air-raid and emergency medical measures.

It will be seen that the outlook for the hospital has in the space of a very short time swung from the extreme of hopefulness and prosperity to that of complete uncertainty, and a new set of problems have had to be faced and met. The present situation postpones indefinitely any consideration of rebuilding, or expansion of the school of nursing. On the other hand we have to realise that the need for the hospital may at any moment become greater than ever before. We have to face the fact that any attempt to carry on an approach to normal peace-time work would in a very short time cripple our finances, but at the same time we must be prepared at any moment to cope with large numbers of casualties, and in the event of land operations in this vicinity these would be enormous. We have to realise that while for war relief work, funds and supplies are available, and can be readily obtained; for ordinary civil running of the hospital, we cannot obtain funds from private patients, since these have largely left the district, nor can we obtain much in the way of local donations, since every available cent is going to swell war funds, either through donations to war relief, or through semi-forced levies in the way of increased taxation and purchase of National Salvation Bonds, which in view of the business depression, are already becoming a burden on the population. In addition we realise that we must make every effort to avoid the necessity of calling upon the Foreign Missions Committee for additional financial assistance for the ordinary running of the hospital at the present time. Furthermore, we must not allow ourselves to be so blinded by the present emergency that we cannot look to the future, however uncertain that may be. We must be ready when the war is over, to return as speedily as possible to normal civil hospital practice, again if possible, without throwing a heavier burden either on the local population or the Home Church, and realising that if we have to go through a period of Japanese occupation, we must be as ready as possible to meet the stringent demands which the new government will make of us. This, then, has been our problem, to cut down and economise so as to be able to carry on for a further year on available resources in the happy event of there being no hostilities in this area, while at the same time being ready to expand at once to deal with large numbers of casualties in emergency, and being ready at any moment to begin to return to normal working conditions should hostilities cease, all, if possible, without throwing any additional burden upon the Foreign Missions Committee.

This we have been able to accomplish, provided that no land hostilities occur here, but only air-raids or naval bombardments. As has been pointed out above, our staff reduced itself by some two thirds, although most of those who ran away were either unpaid or lowly paid workers, so that a considerable though not a commensurate saving in salaries has been effected. The temporary buildings in which the hospital is now housed are very much more economical to run than our own plant. Stringent economy in the prescription of drugs is being carried out, and we have cut down considerably on the most expensive and least vital part of our hospital work, namely the out-patient department. A number of beds are kept permanently empty, reserved for possible wounded, and we have made arrangement for emergency treatment of up to 150 wounded.

The recent threat of an attack on South China has changed our problem, and though the attack has not materialised, general opinion is that it is inevitable sooner or later. If this comes we must be prepared for much more war work than is likely at present, and plans are under consideration for meeting this situation.

One thing the war has shown up clearly, and that is that we must adapt our preconceived ideas of conduct in an emergency to the attitude of our Chinese staff. This problem has cropped up all over China. The Chinese staff are not able to carry on, yet at least, under war conditions. If we insist on our standards of conduct, we are faced with complete breakdown of work, just when it is most vital to keep it going. We must therefore devise ways of meeting the Chinese view-point, so as to be able to carry on. We have been trying to find some plan whereby we can move our hospital back to its own buildings, where we can have room to cater for greater numbers of patients in an emergency. Our Chinese staff are willing to go, but make it quite clear that in the event of trouble they will not be able to stay, and at present we are considering whether or no it is possible to provide safeguards which will make them feel able to stay on whatever happens.

During the year Dr Milne has gone on furlough, and Dr. S. L. Strange has arrived from home for the first time. We hope the former will have a restful furlough, and return to better times, and we extend a very hearty welcome to the latter. It has been a great disappointment that his introduction to China should have had to be at such a time of distress and abnormality, making his start here more difficult than it should have been.

Mr. Scott arrived back from furlough, but went almost immediately to Hankow to help Dr. J. L. Maxwell organise a branch of the International Red Cross. To lose the services of Mr. Scott at such a time as this was a great blow, but we are proud that out of all China, and from the smallest medical mission in China, it was felt that only Mr. Scott could do the work required in Hankow, and reports from there indicate that he is doing that work exceedingly well.

Of our Chinese staff mention must be made of Dr. Cheng, who has been a tower of strength not only during the prosperous months but even more during these recent troubled times. His tact and wisdom in helping to handle a multitude of problems have been invaluable.

It is inevitable that this report should omit a great many details normally to be found there, and the whole year appear to be overshadowed by the present tragedy being worked out in China, but we make no apology for that. We have tried to paint a true and proportioned picture of the working of the hospital during the past twelve months, and hope and pray that next year we may have better news to give.

(Signed) Harold R. Worth.

Report 39/24

Stencilled 8/2/40
for Feb. ZMB

E. P. Mission Hospital Swatow.

Annual Report 1939.

Our second complete year of war conditions has closed, and we are able to report that the hospital and school of nursing are still carrying on, and have been able to effect much useful work.

In October 1938, with the occupation of Canton, we experienced a few days of uncertainty, with naval bombardments outside the port, and air-raids, confined to military objectives and causing no civilian casualties, on the town. Thereafter things settled down to the usual war-time routine of frequent air-raid alarms, and planes passing over, but for a time no further bombs were dropped.

Hospital work was confined to patients seriously ill, and large numbers of out-patients. Those suffering from diseases they did not consider urgent preferred not to come to hospital as in-patients for fear of air-raids. Our Chinese staff was further depleted until we were left with only two Chinese doctors on our staff as compared with the five we had at the outbreak of hostilities. Private patients were few and far between owing to the fact that so many of the wealthier Chinese had left the town.

In the Spring of 1939, new road communications were opened up between Chao-Chow-Fu and Shiuchow on the Canton-Hankow railway, and fleets of motor lorries operated on these roads. Freight rates made the service expensive, but we received large numbers of requests from inland hospitals from as far away as Northern Hunan both to forward medical supplies purchased elsewhere, and to purchase and forward from Swatow. Sometimes doctors would bring their lorries down with them, and have large orders for supplies which had to be rushed through in less than twenty-four hours, and at other times we had to try to beg space on commercial lorries going inland. Air-raid alarms were being sounded every few days, and on March 1st., bombing raids on Swatow began again.

Rumours began to come from the Interior, to the effect that an attack on Swatow might be expected before long. By the end of March, sea-planes had begun to machine-gun motor launches and sampans in the river, as well as dropping bombs. The Chinese Authorities began a systematic voluntary evacuation of the ~~city~~ civilian population, and persuaded about 30,000 people to leave, roughly half the population at that time. Air-raids slacked off during April, but began again about the end of the month. During May we experienced the most extensive bombing of the war. Instead of the regular objectives which people had come to know and avoid, bombs were dropped in many new places, and casualties began to come in. Most of the attacks were of the Dive-bombing character, and the planes clearly had what appeared to them good targets, but it was often difficult for us to recognise any military objective in the areas bombed. Subsequent events have led us to believe that these raids were intended as an adjunct to the blockade, with the purpose of stopping trade.

During this series of attacks, a number of demolition bombs were dropped all round the mission compound, eight of them falling within fifty yards of our boundaries on three sides. As a precaution, we moved our public ward patients away from their quarters on our extreme western boundary, over to the Sok-Tek school buildings. This was accomplished at great speed between two morning raids. Our hospital staff behaved well under trying circumstances.

On Sunday May 7th., a natural disaster added to the distress which the people of Swatow were already suffering. Each morning thousands were in the habit of crossing the harbour to Kak-Chieh to avoid possible air-raids, returning in the late afternoon. On this day, just as the harbour was crowded with sampans bringing these refugees back, a sudden squall reaching gale force struck Swatow. Many sampans capsized. Hundreds of people were thrown into the sea. A British Destroyer and a British merchant ship saved a great number of lives. We never found out the exact death roll.

In June, in addition to bombing raids there was a great deal of aerial reconnaissance over Swatow. On June 21st., the air-raid alarm sounded at 4-45 a.m. for the last time. About 10-0 a.m., a flotilla of Japanese destroyers steamed up the harbour. There was a certain amount of shelling from small calibre naval guns and pom-poms. Some twelve shells fell in our mission compound, and one in the hospital, Three refugees in the compound were slightly wounded. Four of our mission houses were hit by shell splinters, but no serious damage was done. Planes flew overhead all day, bombing the outskirts of the town. It was a trying and tiring day, but the hospital staff behaved well. By the evening, things seemed quieter, when at about 8-o p.m. we saw a red glow in the sky very near the hospital, and found that the retreating Chinese police had set fire to their quarters behind the fire-station, immediately adjoining our hospital wards and operating theatre. Two other fires, one a large one, had been started elsewhere in Swatow. There was no piped water supply, and no fire-engine available, so the hospital staff had to do the best it could with a chain of buckets, and the tearing down of wooden shutters to prevent the spread of fire to our buildings. A number of wounded were lying in our casualty clearing station close to the fire, and these were rapidly transported to a safer place. As the hospital coolies were all fire-fighting, the mission staff, including the ladies, acted as stretcher-bearers. Fortunately the fire burnt itself out in an hour or so, and the hospital was saved.

About 11-o p.m., we received a telephone call from the retreating Chinese Authorities to say that the road for civilian evacuation was open. We persuaded a fair number of refugees to set out on this road. How many got through safely, we do not know. One batch returned an hour later saying they had had to turn back as Chinese soldiers had opened fire on them with machine-guns in the dark. On the way back they had run into a detachment of Japanese soldiers, who told them to go quietly to their homes and stay there, that they had nothing to be afraid of.

The night was quiet. About 3-o a.m. the first detachment of Japanese soldiers marched along the Kialat road past the hospital. Soon after daylight, several hundred soldiers bivouacked outside the hospital on the road. They appeared weary but in good spirits, and handed out free food tickets and cigarettes to the Chinese they saw. An officer called at the hospital with an interpreter with a request for water for his men, and gave permission for our coolies to go out and bring in wounded. Notices rapidly appeared proclaiming the new government, and everywhere the Japanese and the old Chinese Imperial flags began to appear side by side.

For two months we kept a large receptacle filled with boiled water just outside the hospital gate. It proved a boon to Chinese ricsha coolies and others, but so far as we could ascertain was not used by the Japanese soldiers.

3.

Everything remained quiet except for occasional bursts of machine-gun fire. Planes flew constantly over the town very low, but the occupation was carried out quickly and quietly, with little disturbance in the town. This was largely due to the fact that a mobile unit of Japanese troops reached Am-Pou, North of Swatow, before Swatow itself was occupied, thus forcing the Chinese troops to withdraw, and avoiding any heavy fighting near Swatow.

We found we had roughly 120 patients in hospital, practically all bomb and machine-gun wounds. 40% were women and children. There was no electricity or water. Our wells were brackish, but we had a certain amount of rain water in our storage tanks. The wells were chlorinated as soon as possible, but not soon enough to avoid a small outbreak of amoebic dysentery amongst patients and staff. This was rapidly controlled. No other epidemics occurred.

During the next few weeks the hospital received constant visits from Japanese Naval and Military medical units. All were eager to obtain information as to the state of health of the port, and to enquire as to what epidemics might be expected. All were extremely courteous. The work of the hospital was not interfered with in any way. We received a courtesy call from the senior medical officer for Swatow, and later ~~from~~ the senior medical officer for the whole Kwangtung expeditionary force visited the hospital and was shown round. He paid us, indirectly, a high compliment by sending round his subordinates in Swatow, a few days later, with orders to ask us to allow them to copy some of our home-made equipment, especially the operating theatre light.

Two recent additions to our equipment reduced the difficulties of the first weeks of the occupation greatly. The first was a refrigerator which Dr. Strange bought with funds donated to him, and the second was a portable X-Ray machine with a small electric generator, which were supplied by the British Fund for Relief in China. Both were received only a few days before the occupation, and have proved invaluable. We were able to keep large stocks of serum through the hot weather, and were able to carry on X-Ray work and run the operating theatre lights from the beginning. The Japanese army had a limited supply of electricity within a month, for its own use. Although practically all other wires were cut, the hospital was allowed to retain its electric supply. No charge was made for this supply for two months until it was handed over to a Japanese company to run. Then our wires were immediately cut, but on making private representations to the company, the hospital light was immediately restored. We have not yet obtained electricity for our own houses, but the hospital was recognised as a "Public Utility", and not only given light, but no restriction has been placed upon the amount of light we consume, except that of expense.

Water supply in limited form was also available fairly soon. It remains limited owing to lack of pressure, but we obtain sufficient for our needs.

Food was a big problem, and remains so. The Chinese Authorities in preparation for the occupation of Swatow, gave the hospital a ~~large~~ supply of rice, which lasted for nearly three months, and tided us over the period when it was impossible to buy the large quantities we require. Food and fuel continue to be one of our most difficult problems. Fuel is scarce and rice is expensive. In the past six months the cost of living has almost trebled. We have not increased our charges to patients, and those members of the staff who

4.

feed themselves are allowed food from the hospital kitchen at the old price. ~~Nearly~~ More than half our in-patients pay nothing whatever for food or treatment. To try to meet the increased cost of our service to the poor we have doubled the ward rents for private patients.

For two years we had been accumulating stocks of medical supplies, assisted by the British Fund for Relief in China. This accumulation has stood us in good stead. We had not realised that after the occupation Swatow would be entirely closed to trade, as it has been, but we have been able to carry on for six months, with more than the usual number of patients, without any great scarcity in medical supplies. Some of these are xxx beginning to run short, but it is possible now to obtain special permits to import medical supplies for hospital use, although a long weary process is involved, and owing to the infrequency of ships calling here, ixxix permits are apt to have expired before one's cargo arrives.

Owing to shortage of work, and the increased cost of living, there has been a good deal of under-nourishment amongst the poorer classes of Chinese, though there has been little actual starvation. The under-nourishment has led to an epidemic of septic leg ulcers. These were desvribed years ago by Dr. Gauld in one of his early reports and associated by him with periods of hardship and under-nutrition. The patients respond well to treatment, probvided their food can be supplemented, and we have found the simplest way of doing this was to issue rations of cod-liver oil to all such patients. We have used up two very large drums of cod-liver oil in the past six months, and are now looking round for more.

Another trouble which we attribute largely to under-nourishment is a severe epidemic of malaria, mostly of the sub-tertian variety, which has broken out this autumn in the districts surrounding Swatow. Many have died as a result, for the Chinese normally have a high resistance to malaria, which they know well, and as a result they have often come for medical aid too late. A year's supply of quinine lasted us just two months.

One other minor epidemic has been noteworthy, since we have been unable so far to diagnose it. For many years a condition of prolonged low fever, affecting especially Europeans, has been recognised in Swatow. This year both Europeans and Chinese have been affected inx large numbers. The patient feels much worse than his low fever would appear to warrant, but in adults most patients do not need to take to their beds. The condition may persist for months, and is relieved when the cold weather comes. In small children the disease occasionally assumes a serious form, with high fever and xxxx delirium. We have received reports that the fever has been found all along the South China coast this year, from Amoy to Canton. It is colloquially known on the coast as "Swatow Fever". We hope eventually to be able to track down this disease. So far no treatment has been found which is of any use.

A factor of the year's work has again been the way in which European and American patients have been making use of the hospital. At practically no time have we been without at least one European patient in our Private Wards. In this way the hospital is becoming more intimately known to the Foreign community, and we reap much more xxxx benefit from this than the not inconsiderable financial return would indicate.

During the year valuable help has been given to the hospital by non-medical members of the mission, particularly by Misses Mulcock and Richards who have turned their hands to many and varied pieces of work, from secretarial to dressing septic wounds, and doing personal work amongst the patients

Most of our wounded have now left hospital, and ■ for the first time since hostilities began in 1937, we are beginning to receive in hospital what we may call normal medical and surgical cases in something approaching the old numbers. We hope that conditions may rapidly improve so that this part of our work may be restored and ■ increased.

The School of Nursing has been able to carry on, and new nurses have been admitted. It has not been possible to maintain the complete co-operation with Wukingfu which we planned, but so soon as conditions allow, this will be recommenced. At present the staff of the Wukingfu Hospital is carrying a heavy burden of giving lectures to those nurses who should normally have returned to Swatow, but who under present circumstances are unable to do so. This means that Wukingfu is having to teach the subjects of not one but two years of the nursing syllabus, whilst Swatow is again having to teach all three years for the time being. In spite of interruptions, classes have been carried on.

Now that the buildings of the Sok-Tek school have been given over to the hospital, it is planned to make them into a College of Nursing, to fit in with the Joint Nursing Scheme. Nurses based on this college will be available for work in both Wukingfu and Swabue hospitals (should they so desire), which will be as much associated with the School of Nursing as is the Swatow hospital. The Swatow hospital is accepting the entire cost of the necessary alterations which the School buildings will require to fit them for this purpose. When once the nurses are established in their new home it is hoped as soon as possible to place their organisation on its own separate budget.

Evangelistic work in the hospital has been carried on throughout the year, with daily out-patient services, ward and staff prayers, and a Sunday ward service. The hospital staff runs its own Young People's Fellowship.

Our relations with the Chinese Church grow closer year by year. The war has, not unnaturally, helped the prestige of the hospital considerably, but it has been touching to see the way in which in spite of recent hardships, small churches all over the country-side have sent in thier contributions to hospital funds. Amongst the non-Christian Chinese community the hospital enjoys an excellent reputation, as is shown not only by donations, but by the way rich and poor alike come to us for treatment.

In spite of hostilities and financial stringency, we have been able to carry out the essential repairs needed to keep our old buildings serviceable, and in addition, have been able carry out a certain amount of painting and colour-washing, to make them more cheerful to live in. By demolishing certain old dividing walls between what used to be men's and women's hospitals, we have been able to improve the general appearance of the hospital.

It is difficult to forecast the future. The coming year will inevitably be a difficult one, possibly the most difficult in some directions we have yet been called upon to face. The outbreak of war in Europe has meant an immediate large increase in prices of drugs, which is heightened by the increased cost of living and trade restrictions in Swatow. Our plans for gradually bringing our bed-strength up to standard has had to be postponed during the past two years, but we must make an effort as soon as possible to place more wards under nursing. The plan to rebuild the hospital would appear to be indefinitely postponed, and we must seek out ways of carrying on effectively in our present buildings without heavy expenditure of money.

Although he was not directly associated with the hospital, Dr. C. H. Brangwin had always been very friendly with the mission and the hospital. We owed him a great deal for help, advice, and treatment. His sudden death in January 1939 was keenly felt by all of us.

STATISTICS YEAR ENDING Sept. 30th., 1939.

In-Patients,

men	596	Of these roughly 60% were treated and fed completely free.
women	378	
children	116	
Total	1090	

Out-Patients

First Attendance,	8,507
Return Visits	11,090
Dressings	14,452
Eyes	9,477
Total Attendances	43,526

Wounded. Of the In-Patients treated during the year, 311 were suffering from bomb or machine-gun bullet wounds, or crushed by falling buildings. During May 1939, Swatow suffered 58 killed and 160 wounded in air-raids. Of these, 143 were admitted to our hospital during that month.

During the six months, January 1st., to June 30th., 1939, Swatow experienced 108 air-raid alarms, and on 26 occasions bombs were dropped in Swatow.

Staff,

Doctors	European,	3
	Chinese	2
Graduate Technicians		2
Midwife		1
Graduate Nurses		10
Nurses in Training		28
Student Technicians		3

Matron, 1

E. P. MISSION HOSPITAL SWATOW.

ANNUAL REPORT
1940 - 1941

In referring to the year ahead, the report for last year closed with the words "We hope to be given strength and opportunity to carry on." Writing at the end of another year, we give thanks to God for having received the strength and been given the opportunity to carry on under conditions which seem to get increasingly difficult year by year.

A hospital report written six years ago made mention of "that happy day when we shall have a new hospital of 100/110 beds under nursing." Between the months of April and August of this year we had 120 beds under nursing, not in "a new hospital", but in our "old" reconditioned one, although this fact did not diminish our pride that this goal had been reached. Unfortunately, for financial reasons that will be explained later, the two new wards were closed again in August, but we hope that by the time the next report is written that we will be able to record the fact that these wards have been reopened. Actually, during these last months the demand for the increased accommodation has been considerably reduced by the closing of communications between occupied and unoccupied territory. Normally we receive a considerable number of patients from the unoccupied areas, but as a result of these restrictions which are still in force, they have been unable to travel to Swatow.

The obtaining of food and fuel supplies has, at intervals, caused us great anxiety, not only because of their greatly increased cost, but because of the difficulty in obtaining them. For the first half of this year we were able to get permission to buy rice at the "official" rate which greatly reduced its cost, although much energy had often to be expended in getting the permission. Unfortunately we have had to buy it in the open market lately with the consequent increased cost. During the year the price of drugs went up at a steady rate until the freezing regulations of the British and American Governments were announced, when there was a sudden jump amounting to an average increase of 70% in prices.

With the continuous rise in the cost of drugs, food and fuel, the financial running of the hospital has brought its anxieties, but we are glad to be able to report a small credit balance on the year's working. For the past year the cost of running the hospital has amounted to £8 a day, and of this sum £5 was spent on food and fuel and £1:12:0 on drugs. The financial health of the hospital, like that of very many people in Swatow, is greatly dependent on the drawnthread work industry, which has now been brought to a standstill by the freezing regulations. In recent years we have received large sums in donations from drawnthread work firms. In addition, many of our private patients are connected with drawnthread work, while the ability of a not inconsiderable number of public ward patients to pay towards the cost of their food and treatment depends on employment in this industry. In view of the likelihood of a very big reduction in this source of income, we most reluctantly decided to close two public wards in addition to introducing other drastic economies. This amounted to a reduction in our public ward beds from 104 to 80, which is the same number as was available last year. This hospital is very proud of its tradition of treating patients irrespective of their ability to pay and there are very few Mission hospitals in China that are privileged to do such a high proportion of free work. During the last six months we have had an average of 100 in-patients each day in the hospital and of these an average of 54 a day have been treated and fed free of charge. We have been very concerned about our ability to continue this large amount of free work and so we were greatly cheered when we received a donation of $15,000 one week ago. By reason of this gift we are enabled for the time ~~mix~~ being to continue with our present amount of free work. This very generous donation was given to us by a Committee in Shanghai which is administering funds collected by the Christian Churches of the United States and in addition to this grant to the hospital, they have already provided large sums for relief work in the Swatow district.

Modern methods of treatment often involve great expense. During the summer an elderly man came to hospital with an extremely septic wound of his hand that he had received ten days earlier. The extensive infection was causing severe haemorrhage due to erosion of blood vessels and in addition it had produced tetanus, which was an even more serious complication. It was decided that the amputation of the hand held the best hopes of recovery and both before and after operation he received large doses of anti-tetanus serum. We were naturally very pleased when he was able to leave hospital ten days later completely well, although without his left hand. The serum which he had received cost us £10 and he was not able to pay anything towards its cost or the cost of his operation and food while in hospital. Unfortunately the end results are not always as happy as in this case and in spite of very expensive treatment the patient may die, but when the need arises we can do no other than meet it to the best of our ability.

During the year we have received valuable gifts of money and medical supplies. The Chinese Medical Association, through its Hospital Fund, has given us sufficient money to endow a bed for one year and three of our Chinese friends in Swatow have given donations sufficient to endow one bed each for a similar period. Hospital Sunday was observed throughout the Presbytery last May and a very substantial sum of money was given to the hospital as a result. From the American Red Cross we have received a large gift of medical supplies and also a quantity of powdered milk. This latter has enabled us to start a daily free milk clinic for children suffering from malnutrition and it has been very gratifying to see the improvement that has taken place in many of these children. When they come to us their bodies are either swollen or very thin and it is the ones with generalised swelling that are the most difficult to cure. In time, the reasonably early cases get well again when they are given a good diet, but where the condition is advanced no treatment that we have yet tried has had any effect.

One of our problems during the year has been to avoid becoming an orphanage as well as a hospital. For the past two years we have had a couple of baby girls who were deposited at the hospital gate by their parents because of the shortage of food in the families. During the last year this has become a more common practice because of the worsening economic conditions. At one time we had six of these small girls and if a close watch had not been kept, many more would have been left with us. Fortunately we have been able to trace the families of two and persuade them to take them back again, but we still have four on our hands. In normal times it would be possible to get families to adopt them but at present because of poverty and the uncertain political outlook, it is extremely difficult to find such people. Our unwillingness to receive them is not only due to the cost of feeding and looking after them, but also because if it were generally known that we accepted unwanted children, they would be brought along in alarming numbers.

Swatow continues to remain remarkably free from all epidemic diseases except typhoid and this is due to the energetic efforts made by the Japanese authorities and the Local Chinese Government in cholera inoculation and vaccination against small-pox. Unfortunately no similar efforts have been made to reduce the large amount of typhoid that occurs in the summer months. This year many of the typhoid cases were of exceptional severity and in these severe cases our efforts usually failed to avoid a fatal termination. It was very distressing to us all when, in spite of being inoculated, one of our nurses contracted this severe type of infection and died. During the course of the year diseases of malnutrition have accounted for a big proportion of our patients and the poor physical condition of so many people due to insufficient or poor food has been responsible for an even larger proportion of illness

During the year a heartening development has taken place in our evangelistic work. As in recent years, addresses are given each morning in the Men's and Women's Out Patient Departments and on Sunday afternoons a service is held in rotation in the different wards, when those patients from the other wards who can either walk or be carried are also present. Members of the Swatow Church have formed an evangelistic band which has taken responsibility for the Out Patient Department work and for conducting two of the ward services each month. In addition to these activities, visits are made to the ward patients during the afternoons and many of them are also visited in their homes after they have returned from hospital. Opportunities in hospital for evangelism are very great and we are much indebted to these members of the Swatow Church for helping us in this work.

Several changes have taken place in our staff during the year. Dr. Ang Tsak-liang, who has served the hospital most faithfully for over ten years and taken a prominent part in the evangelistic work, has resigned and taken up medical practice in the interior. His position has been taken by Dr. Moses Chang, who has rejoined the hospital staff. In February Dr. Worth left on furlough after a strenuous term of six years as hospital superintendent During most of this period he has had to act as business manager as well and for the last three year war conditions with their difficult and worrying problems have increased this burden. It was a great source of pleasure and satisfaction to us all when Dr. Cheng signed a contract last January agreeing to stay with us for three more years. Dr. Cheng joined the hospital staff in 1933 and during this period the hospital owes a lot to ~~Dr.xxChung~~ him, not only for his work as a doctor, but for his wise advice and tactful handling of many a difficult situation. In addition to these activities he has collected large sums of money in donations for the hospital during the past two years.

It goes without saying that next year will probably be even more difficult than the ones that have passed, but, looking back on the path we have travelled, our faith would indeed be poor if we did not go ahead with courage and hope in this day of opportunity.

STATISTICS.

1940 - 1941.

Medical Missionaries			3
Foreign Nurses			1
National Doctors			2
National Nurses			49
Midwife / Anaesthetist			1
Technicians			9
Preacher / Assistant Business Manager			1
Clerk			1
Almoner			1
In-patients,	male	454)	
	female	628)	1337
	children	255)	
Out-patients	First attendances		20315
	Total "		78243
Maternity Department	Confinements in hospital		92
	" " homes		93
Operations			314
Laboratory	Pathological examinations		9733.
BEDS			95

J. L. Strang

Lingtung School of Nursing Report. October 1940 - September 1941.

At the beginning of this year we had in our school, besides the Assistant Matron, 9 graduate nurses, and 42 nurses in training, five of whom were about to graduate. We were looking forward to having sufficient graduates to staff all departments in the hospital, and possibly have one free to do Private Nursing, for which there is a growing demand amongst the wealthier Chinese now in Swatow. It was, therefore, with mixed feelings we found that five of them had planned to go to West China to serve their country with the Red Cross. Eventually only three went, one of the other two joined the Staff of an up-country hospital belonging to the American Baptist Mission, the other is now working with a doctor of some standing in Shanghai. While we were sorry to lose them, we were glad for them to open the way to a wider field of service for themselves and our future graduate nurses. Incidently their going has been a stimulus to more junior nurses who had to step up to fill their places.

During this year we have completed 10 years since the opening of the Nursing School, and have passed the 100th mark in the number of nurses accepted for training.

Since the union with Yukingfu Hospital ; the change over of nurses each year has brought it's own difficulty in travelling, and this year was no exception. The change over was delayed for a month owing to Chinese being restricted from going in and out of Swatow, due to some people being discovered smuggling goods into unoccupied territory.

During the year 9 nurses entered our Church, 2 of whom received Baptism. One had been a non-Christian but was already a hearer when she came into hosptial, the other was a daughter of a Baptist father and a non-Christian mother, and has owned since that she was frankly sceptical when she came in as a pupil, but during her time of training she has found the Truth. Following on this, she was anxious that her younger sister should come in for training also, which she did in March of this year. Her service was of short duration, for, though we took the usual precautions, she contracted typhoid of a very virulent type towards the end of June and passed away about three weeks later. We were afraid of the reaction on her class mates, who had so recently come into training, but some were heard to say they intended to put more into their nursing of the patients because of her passing. The dignity with which her older sister carried herself during those trying days, when it was impossible to get in touch with her family, made a great impression on more than one of us.

One of our graduates has been granted temporary leave of absence to take a course in Institutional Nursing in the Nursing School of the Peking Union Medical College Hospital. She is doing this at her own expense, apart from the grant which that School allows to selected candidates.

In 1936 our School was registered with the Nurses' Association of China. That year our finishing class took the examination set by them. The following year the N.A.C. registered with the Chinese Government, who were to set the examination for all registered Schools, however that year and since, it has been impossible for them to do so. This year the N.A.C. are again taking up this work. When we sent up our registration this year , we were told that our Joint School did not comply with their regulations. We are still in correspondence with them on this matter. In the meantime we are holding our own Final Examination for the Nurses. We had some difficulty in getting the nurses to see the wisdom of our decision, but in the end all have promised to take the examination.

During the coming Year Sister Wu, who has been with us now for nearly 10 years, will take charge of the nursing in my absence.

I cannot close this report without mentioning the fact that during this year we have taken over the supervision of the technicians' work in the Mens Out Patient Department, a thing which would have been completely impossible a few years ago!

Maud L. Martin.

ENGLISH PRESBYTERIAN MISSION HOSPITAL
SWATOW
SOUTH CHINA
汕頭福音醫院

REPORT FOR YEAR 1st October 1947 - 30th September 1948.

During the year under review the process of re-establishing the Hospital, which began in August 1946 when it was re-opened with 33 beds, has continued and the in-patient accomodation has been increased from 71 to 107 beds. This increase has been made possible as a result of the larger and more experienced nursing staff that has been trained and THE gifts of beds received during the year.

This expansion of our work has taken place against a difficult economic background. There are two rice harvests in the year and in 1947 the first was badly damaged by flooding while the second was destroyed by a tidal wave which accompanied a typhoon, and flooded the rice fields with sea water. This tidal wave flooded the Hospital to a depth of 2½ feet and furious efforts were required that [illegible] by the hospital staff in a race against the steadily rising water level until patients, food and medicine stores had been moved upstairs to safety. In 1948 drought caused the failure of the first rice harvest but we are thankful that at the time of writing the second harvest is promising well. The result of the failure of all these harvests has been to cause rice to soar in price with consequent effects on all other items, and farmers, who form a considerable proportion of our patients, are in great economic distress. Side by side with the increase in the cost of living due to the failure of rice harvests in this area has gone the inflation of the currency from other causes. In October 1947, one and a third lb. of rice - the daily requirement of an adult man - cost $3,300 while in September 1948 it cost $980,000. The corresponding figures for the monthly expenditure of the hospital at these dates were 130 million dollars and 25,000 million dollars. Fortunately our income and gifts kept pace with expenditure but ward rents in the latter part of the year under review had usually to be increased weekly and sometimes more often. When money was received, the only wise policy was to spend it immediately on buying supplies before it decreased further in value. The bulk of the money was so great that a large rice bag was required to contain the staff salaries for half a month. The new currency was introduced in August and prices remained stable for six weeks, but since then the cost of living has increased by 150% and we fear the melancholy process is starting all over again.

During the year, police from an inland village came to Swatow, arrested our hospital secretary, and detained him in this village under very trying conditions for five weeks. Interested parties had made a false charge of murder against him in order to divert attention from the real murderer, and very strenuous efforts were required before his release was secured.

The Hospital sustained a grievous loss during the year in the resignation of Dr. H. R. Worth, the Medical Superintendent, who joined the staff in 1927 and became Superintendent in 1935. During his time as superintendent great changes took place in modernising the hospital. Some wards were already under modern nursing care, but the process continued until in 1938 all the patients were looked after by nurses instead of partly by their relations. The Lingtung School of

Page 2

ENGLISH PRESBYTERIAN MISSION HOSPITAL
SWATOW
SOUTH CHINA
院 醫 音 福 頭 汕

Nursing was established to train Nurses to meet the needs of Swatow, Wukingfu and Swabue Hospitals. But his greatest achievement was in 1946 when, four months after returning to Swatow to find the hospital buildings delapidated and stripped of all the furnishings and medical equipment they had contained, he succeeded in re-opening the hospital with 33 beds. Miss Wu, our Matron, who worked with Dr. Worth in the preparations for re-opening, said recently in an address to ministers and preachers who were visiting the hospital, how during that preparatory period, time and again she felt that it was impossible to open so soon because of the lack of supplies and equipment of all sorts but that Dr. Worth's energy and faith sustained them all in what so often seemed an impossible task. Previous reports have told of the great numbers of patients in those early days when Dr. Worth had no other doctor to assist him for the first five months after the re-opening. We will sorely miss his guidance in the everyday problems and his vision in planning for the future. His reputation here as a doctor is an enviable one and he has earned the gratitude of very many patients and the affection of those of us who have worked under his leadership.

Fortunately we have also had gains to our staff during the year. At the end of 1947 Dr. T. Y. Cheng, the brother of Rev. Sheffield Cheng and a graduate of Peking Union Medical College, joined us as physician in charge of medical wards and under his care this part of our work has been strengthened. We have also been very glad to welcome Mr. Joop Graf who after a year of language study has commenced part-time duties as Business Manager, thus relieving a doctor of this work, and we look forward to more efficient management of this part of the hospital work. During the year Dr. H. T. Tseng, who has been with us as an interne, graduated and we are glad to welcome him as a full member of the staff.

Once again we record with gratitude some of the numerous gifts from various sources. From U.N.R.R.A. we have received many medical supplies which have included 50 beds and a mobile X-Ray unit. The latter is now in operation and we are indebted to Macksoud Importing Company of New York for the gift of accessory parts, which were not supplied with the machine but which are necessary for its operation. We can only operate the machine at night and not every night either, because of the limitations of the Swatow electricity supply and our appeals for the gift of a generator have not yet borne fruit! British Red Cross has given us 25 beds and most useful equipment and drugs, while from British United Aid to China we have received six cases of dressings and woollen clothing, some of which at least was made by members of our Home Churches. We are indebted to the International Relief Committee for transmitting many of these gifts to us. Once again the Scripture Gift Mission has given us a large number of copies of the Gospels printed in Chinese for distribution to patients. From the U.S.A. China Relief Mission we have received a gift of rice and financial grants for free in-patient treatment. Other gifts of money have included Hospital Sunday collections from Churches in this area, £600 from the Foreign Missions' Committee and donations from Chinese and from British people both here and at home. We are most ~~grateful for all these gifts, which in their several ways have so greatly assisted our work.~~

grateful for all these gifts, which in their several ways have so greatly assisted our work.

This Hospital has always treated very large numbers of out-patients, especially during the summer months. Last year the attendances averaged 1,000 new out-patients and about 3,400 "repeat visits" each month of whom 52% were treated free and a further 29% partly free. Our former out-patient department had to be demolished after the war and the present accommodation is most inadequate for the amount of work that is being done. We appealed to the U.S.A. China Relief Mission for the equivalent of £8,000 to enable us to build a new out-patient department but unfortunately correspondence on the subject was still proceeding when the Mission was wound up. With increased staff it has become possible to reorganise the work of the department. Instead of out-patients being seen four days a week and men being seen on one floor and women on another, irrespective of their complaints, we now have separate clinics for the different specialities such as medicine, surgery, women's diseases, leprosy, etc., on special days. Six days each week some of these clinics are held and there has been a gratifying response from patients in coming on the proper days, though of course many patients are seen who make their first visit on the wrong day. Dr. Milne has organised an ante-natal clinic whose size is steadily increasing as more and more women become aware of the importance of ante-natal supervision.

During the year the in-patient accommodation has been increased from 71 to 107 beds and this increase has taken place entirely in the public ward accomodation. In January the Maternity Ward was re-opened and in September another men's public ward. With the increased number of women attending the ante-natal clinic, the accomodation in the maternity ward has at times been taxed severely but we welcome normal as well as abnormal cases because of the experience they give to nurses during their midwifery training. In addition our nurses go out to deliver patients in their own homes. During the last year we had a total of 1,626 in-patients of whom 27% were fed and treated free of charge and a further 23% partly free. At our present stage of expansion we are most pressed for room for women and children and it is planned that the next ward to be opened will be for children. We get many sick children, a good number of whom are suffering from malnutrition and they require a considerable time in Hospital.

During the year fifteen private wards and four public wards have been painted and colour-washed, while two public ward verandahs have been partially enclosed to provide weather protection and increased accomodation. A staff recreation room has been decorated and furnished from gifts from Scotland and Ireland, and in addition there have been numerous repairs to the fabric, which are inevitable in buildings as old as ours. Mention has been made of the need for a new out-patient department but an even more urgent need is a house for our doctors whose present accomodation is required for other purposes, and we cannot see any way at present of accepting more internes unless we can build a new house. We hope it may be possible to build during

ENGLISH PRESBYTERIAN MISSION HOSPITAL
SWATOW
SOUTH CHINA
汕頭福音醫院

the course of this year.

The last year has been free from any serious epidemics but typhoid is always with us. During the year 1947 we admitted 161 typhoid patients of whom 32 died. 20% is a heavy mortality but many of these patients come to us in a very weak condition after being ill for several weeks. During the last year we provided free innoculations against typhoid for any who desired them and also did innoculations in a centre in the City, but in general people are not so afraid of typhoid as of cholera and small-pox for which they readily come to be innoculated, although most years far more people die of typhoid than of the latter two diseases. We co-operated with the Swatow Hygiene Bureau in vaccinations and cholera innoculations both in the hospital and in centres in the city.

During the year there have been numerous patients who xxxxxx have shown a response to the preaching of the Gospel and we have good reasons for supposing that some of these have since taken the decisive step of professing the Christian Faith. Members of the Swatow Preaching Bands, whose members are drawn from the Protestant Churches in Swatow, have assisted us by visiting in-patients, and talking to out patients as they assemble for the clinics. In-patients who show a response to the Christian message are put in touch with their nearest Church after discharge from hospital. We have come to the conclusion that to grasp the great opportunities for evangelism that are ours, we need to have a whole time well trained minister on our staff, who can meet the needs of our wide variety of patients. Having reached this conclusion, the problem is not only to find a suitable man but also accomodation for him and his family. We believe that if this is the right course, the way will open up for such an appointment to be made.

This year the Ministers and Preachers of the Swatow Presbytery, who were assembled for conference, visited the Hospital. Addresses were given outlining the work of the hospital and how we sought to meet the needs of our patients, after which an opportunity was given for questions and discussion. Other visitors ~~during the year~~ were Royal Navy Medical Officers from visiting ships and medical students who were on vacation in Swatow and attended hospital clinics during this time.

During the year we have been able to maintain our policy of placing no limit to the amount of free treatment done in the public wards, so that any patients who need in-patient treatment and for whom there is room are admitted to the public wards irrespective of their ability to pay. It has been a troubled year, with much unsettlement and disillusionment, but there has also been much to cheer and encourage us and we give thanks to God that it has been possible to continue expanding our work and also to maintain our free treatment. In November 1947 a very old lady visited the Hospital to make a donation of a million dollars (then £3.10.) Seventy years ago Dr. Gauld, the first doctor of the Hospital, did an eye operation on her father with very successful results and she wished to show her gratitude. Such a reminder from the past of the long and honourable tradition in which we serve is a stimulus to renewed endeavours.

[signature]

ENGLISH PRESBYTERIAN MISSION HOSPITAL
SWATOW
SOUTH CHINA.
汕頭福音醫院

STATISTICS.

1st Oct. 1947 - 30th Sept. 1948.

	1948.	1947.
Medical Missionaries	2	3
Foreign Nurses	0	0
Foreign Business Manager	1	0
Chinese Doctors	4	2
Internes	0	1
Graduate Nurses	13	10
Student Nurses	48	34
Dispensers	2	1
Laboratory Technician	1	1
Student Technicians	7	6
Secretary	1	1
Almoners	3	2
Caterer	1	1
Woman Evangelist	1	1
In-Patients.		
Private Wards	273	283
Public Wards	1,353	971
Total	1,626	1,254
Treated and fed free of charge	443 (27%)	328 (26%)
Paid part of cost	366 (23%)	177 (14%)
Out-Patients.		(figures cover 14 months)
First Visits	11,965	12,646
Repeat Visits	23,724	22,972
Dressings	16,966	27,596
Inoculations	914	230
Total Attendances	53,569	63,444
Free treatments (including medicine)	27,818 (52%)	18,527 (29%)
Operations.		
Major	327	250
Minor	265	326
Total	592	576
Normal Deliveries	145	No figure available.
Abnormal Deliveries	54	
Laboratory Examinations.	13,097	14,728
Beds.		
Public Wards	91	55
Private Wards	16	16
Total	107	71

ENGLISH PRESBYTERIAN MISSION HOSPITAL
SWATOW
SOUTH CHINA.
汕頭福音醫院

ANALYSIS OF OPERATIONS, OCTOBER 1947 - SEPTEMBER 1948.

Abdomen.

Appendicectomy	9.
Appendix abscess drainage	1.
Colostomy	2
Repair of traumatic colostomy	1.
Perforated gastric ulcer	1.
duodenal ulcer	1.
Gastro-enterostomy	1.
Partial Gastrecomy (carcinoma)	1.
Intussusception - reduction	4.
- resection right colon	1.
Intestinal Obstruction (adhesions)	2.
Laparotomy	3.
Volvulus pelvic colon	1.

Abdominal Wall.

Femoral hernia	2.
Inguinal hernia	15.
Strangulated inguinal hernia	5
Ruptured umbilical hernia	1.
Gun-shot wound abdominal wall	1.
Suture ruptured abdominal wound	2.
Dissection malignant glands of groins	1.
Excision fibro sarcoma groin	2.

Rectum.

Ligature haemorrhoids	6.
Rectal polypus	2.
Fistula-in-ano	2.
Rectal prolapse	1.
Ischio rectal sinus	3
Imperforate anus	2

Breast.

Simple mastectomy	2
Radical mastectomy	1
Fibro-adenoma	6
Cyst of breast (chronic mastitis)	1
Cystic hygroma of axilla	3.
Papilloma chest wall	1.
Dissection glands of axilla	1.

Ear, nose and throat.

Nasal Polypi	13.
Tonsillectomy	5.
Foreign Bodies Nose	5.
Radical Mastoid	1.
Fibroma nasal wall	1.
Plastic operation of ear	1.

Opthalmology.

Excision of eye	5.
Kronlein's operation for orbital tumour	1.
Excision oedematous conjunctiva	1.
Excision mole of eyelid	2.
Meibomian Cyst	3.
Entropian	(approx.)400

Skin.

Skin grafting	9.
Excision sebaceous cysts	15.
Burns	6.
Plastic operation neck	1.
Suture skin wounds (theatre only)	11.
Excision fibromata	11.
papillomata	3.

Gynaecology

Ovarian Cysts	32.
Dilatation & Curettage	31.
Dilatation cervix	1.
Hysterectomy - subtotal	6.
Amputation cervix	1.
Repair vesico - vaginal fistula	4.

ENGLISH PRESBYTERIAN MISSION HOSPITAL
SWATOW
SOUTH CHINA.
汕頭福音醫院

Gynaecology (ctd.)

Cervical polypi	5.
Colpo - perineorrhaphy	3.
Vaginal papillomata	1.
Haematocolpos	3.
Plastic operation on vagina	2.
Therapeutic abortion (Pulmonary Tuberculosis)	1.
Ectopic gestation	4.
Hypospadias	1.

Midwifery.

Normal deliveries	145.
Caesarean Section	3.
Placenta Praevia	8.
Forceps deliveries	17.
Breech "	12.
Transverse presentations	5.
Face presentations	3.
Eclampsia	6.

Head and Neck.

Ligature external carotid (secondary haemorrhage)	1.
Partial thyroidectomy	3.
Thyroid adenoma	1.
Mixed parotid tumours	4.
Submaxillary tumour	1.
Multiple cysts neck	1.
Branchial cyst	1.
Thyroglossal cyst	1.
Fibroma neck	1.
Stab wounds neck	1.
Cut Throat	1.
Dissection glands of neck	1.
Curettage glands of neck	1.
Osteomyelitis jaw	12.
Dental Extractions	95.
Giant cell tumour mandible	1.
Adamantinoma	1.
Fibrous epulis	1.
Fibroma tongue	1.
Papilloma tongue	2.
Ranula	1.
Hare Lip	17.
Cyst of cheek	1.
Haemangioma face	1.
Other tumours face	5.

Spine and Back.

Laminectomy (bullet)	2.
Meningocele	1.
Dermoid tumour sacrum	1.
Osteomyelitis ilium	1.
Plaster bed (T.B. spine)	2.

Urogenital.

Circumcision	15.
Hydrocele	17.
Haemotocele	1.
Rupture urethra	5.
Orchidectomy	1.
Excision scrotum (filariasis)	5.
Partial amputation penis (epithelioma)	3.
Radical amputation penis & scrotum (epithelioma)	1.
Vesical calculus	5.
Urethral calculus	3.
Stenosis urethral orifice	1.
Supra-pubic cystostomy	4.
Plastic operation on perineum	1.
Sounding of bladder	2.

Limbs.

Amputations:	Arm	4.
	Thigh.	1.
	Syme's	1.
	Fingers	4.
	Toe	1.
Foreign bodies.		6.
Bomb wound leg		1.
Ligature femoral artery & vein (traumatic aneurysm)		1.
Ligature brachial artery (secondary haemorrhage)		1.
Fibro-sarcoma arm		1.
Popliteal bursa		1.
Lipomata feet		2.
Synovioma knee		1.
Fibroma popliteal nerve		1.
Supernumary thumbs		3.
Fracture tibia & fibula		6.
Compound fracture fingers		1.
Compound dislocation ankle		2.
Club feet; manipulation and plaster		4.
Manipulation hip		1.
Insertion pin in femur		1.
Aspiration knee joint		3.
Plaster spica hip		1.
Osteomyelitis	fibula	1.
	femur	2.
	toe	1.

Blood transfusions	28.
Drainage abscesses	31.

ENGLISH PRESBYTERIAN MISSION HOSPITAL
SWATOW
SOUTH CHINA.
汕頭福音醫院

SUMMARY OF INCOME 1st October 1947 – 30th September 1948.

Chinese National Currency.

Hospital.

To, Credit Balance 1st Oct. 1947	5,558,164 . 90
China Relief Mission, U.S.A.	378,000,000
Invalid's Auxiliary £5	179,310,000
E.M.M.S. Stamp Bureau £3	107,550,000
Changing East Exhibition H.K. $21.13	47,550,000
Matthews Bed Endowment H.K. $17.70	39,750,000
Bristow Bed Endowment H.K. 19.58	44,100,000
Succourer Bed Endowment H.K. $23.57	53,040,000
Edinburgh Medical Miss Socty. H.K. $31.92	71,820,000
Birkenhead St. Paul's Girls' Aux. $3.3.0	113,100,000
Donations – Chinese	1,101,777,000
Foreign	2,259,690,000
Receipts from Patients	52,655,943,300
Sales, Bank Interest & Sundries	1,079,928,200

School of Nursing.

Liverpool Presbytery W.M.A. £16	573,690,000
Donations – Chinese	6,600,000
KITCHEN RECEIPTS	623,092,000
~~Kitchen Receipts~~, Interest, Bank Sales & Sundry Income	782,547,500
	$ 60,323,346,164 . 96.

Examined & found correct
[signature]

[signature]
Treasurer

ENGLISH PRESBYTERIAN MISSION HOSPITAL
SWATOW
SOUTH CHINA
汕頭福音醫院

LINGTUNG SCHOOL OF NURSING.

Report for year 1st October 1947 - 30th September 1948.

Since its re-opening two years ago, the rate of expansion of our Swatow Hospital has depended mainly on the number of nurses available, and this in turn has depended on the numbers under training in the Lingtung School of Nursing. We are therefore glad to be able to report that there are now 61 student and graduate nurses, compared with 44 one year ago. Although the present figure is the largest in the history of the School there was a bigger number of beds in operation prior to the outbreak of the Pacific War. The reasons for this are first that of our present total of forty-eight student nurses, twenty-nine are either probationers or in their first year so that they can only undertake very limited responsibility, and secondly a greater proportion of the time of the student nurses is now occupied attending lectures than was the case before the war. During the last year two new classes of student nurses have entered the school. As the Hospital now has an X-Ray machine in operation it was possible to X-Ray the lungs of all members of the most recent class. This is a significant advance because the incidence of Pulmonary Tuberculosis in China is very great and during the last year one of our student nurses became a patient with that disease. Two otherwise suitable applicants for the last class had to be rejected because of the X-Ray findings. During the last year three student nurses graduated and have joined our staff of graduates.

The course for student nurses is three years and four months, and after graduating, suitable people are given the opportunity of a further year of training in which they do midwifery and gain experience as staff nurses. The first four months of training is a probationary period at the end of which a decision is made as to whether they are suitable for continuing with nursing training. Probationers do not wear caps and last February, for the first time in our Nursing School, a capping ceremony was held for the successful probationers. After the significance of the ceremony had been explained, the nine probationers carrying unlighted candles lined up on the platform standing opposite nine of the senior student nurses who held lighted candles. One by one each ex-probationer had her candle lit by one of the seniors and then a cap put on her head by Miss Phang, the Principal. The Hospital Chaplain concluded the ceremony by giving a short address to the nurses. We who were present felt that this was a most impressive ceremony, but unfortunately next morning we descended to the depths with the news that twenty of the first and second year nurses had gone on strike and refused to come on duty. Strikes are not uncommon in schools in China and among the various reasons given for this one was the fact that the ex-probationers new uniforms had long sleeves, while the rest of the student nurses only had short sleeves and in cold weather wore jackets! It had been decided that in future all student nurses should have long sleeves on their uniforms and this class was the first to receive them. Fortunately patients were few after the Chinese New Year holidays and the work of the Hospital continued as usual for the thirty-six hours that elapsed before

ENGLISH PRESBYTERIAN MISSION HOSPITAL
SWATOW
SOUTH CHINA
汕頭福音醫院

the nurses resumed duty. The incident was a blot on the record of the School during the last year, but its significance should not be undul emphasised

When the last report was written it was hoped that the registration of the Nursing School would have proceeded sufficiently far for the senior class of nurses to have sat for the Government examination in July 1948, but these hopes have not been fulfilled. Nursing training comes under the Department of Education and the application for registration was forwarded to the Swatow Educational authorities in March 1948 for approval and transmission to the Provincial Educational Department in Canton, who, if approving, pass it on to Nanking. In March 1948 we were informed by the Swatow authorities that they had forwarded the application to Canton, but when no further news had been received by July, enquiries were made as to the cause of the delay. In September we received a letter from Canton that stated our application had never been received there, so we are left to assume that it has been lost. In the meantime we have been informed that Government regulations have been altered requiring changes in the financial provisions which are very difficult to meet, so that we are back to the position we were in at the end of 1947. The disappointment is great not only for the Principal and Board of Managers but also for our nurses, who are still unable to sit for the Government final examination.

In January 1948 we had the pleasure of a visit from Miss E. D. E. Silver, a British Nurse, who is working with the Special Committee on Aid to Nursing Schools of the Council on Christian Medical Work. Her visit, which was a stimulating one, was made to get acquainted with our conditions and needs. Since her visit we have received the valuable gifts of sixteen rolls of uniform cloth from Canadian Aid to China and a Chase Doll and anatomical charts from British Red Cross, while in addition we have been promised a skeleton torso and a grant of U.S. $250. The School is also most grateful for a gift of £16 from the Womens' Missionary Association of the Liverpool Presbytery

Mention was made in the last report of the loss we sustained by the resignation on health grounds of Miss E. W. Kenneth just as she was about to commence work after language study and of the consequent heavy responsibility shouldered by Miss Phang and the Hospital Matron, Miss Wu. These responsibilities have increased during the past year with the further growth of the School of Nursing and the Hospital, and we are most appreciative of their labours which have resulted in the hospital beds being extended to over a hundred. They and we are looking forward to the early appointment of a Missionary Nurse who will share their burdens. In the meantime we are very glad to welcome Mrs. Braisted who as Miss Doreen Hill was our Nurse in Wukingfu, and who has come to us as Nursing Adviser for four months while her husband is in America.

The last year has brought its disappointments, and there can be few institutions in China, whether Christian or Non-Christian, that have not experienced these, but it has also been a year of growth. As a result of the rapid growth the standard of nursing is not as high as it should be, but we give thanks for what has been achieved and for the courage and cheerfulness with which our nurses have set their hands to the tasks that confronted them

ENGLISH PRESBYTERIAN MISSION HOSPITAL
SWATOW
SOUTH CHINA
汕頭福音醫院

STATISTICS

	1948.	1947.
Graduate Nurses	13	10
Student Nurses.		
Probationers	13	8
1st Year	16	13
2nd Year	13	7
3rd Year	6	4
4th Year	0	[illegible]
Total Student Nurses	48	34

colony in the Philippines. We are much indebted to Dr. Wade for his generous encouragement and helpful advice. Our work has met with considerable success. We have been able to cure some patients and effect marked improvement in many more. Our experience has revealed some very interesting features of the apparent incidence of this affliction but still longer observation is necessary before we would venture to draw definite conclusions from our discoveries. For instance, our records reveal that 70% of the patients coming for treatment are between 11 and 30 years of age. Is this an indication that immunity from leprosy is less between those ages than at other times of life or does our experience merely prove that patients between those ages are more sensitive to the disfigurement and are therefore more willing to undergo the prolonged and somewhat painful treatment necessary for a cure? We are not yet prepared to dogmatize.*

Swatow hospital honoured. Its methods adopted as standard for China.

Dr. Fraser was invited to give a paper before the First National Conference on Leprosy organized by the Chinese Mission to Lepers as an addendum to the Annual Conference of the China Medical Association. on the treatmemt of Leprosy in an Out-Patient

* 编者注：以上无翻译。

Department, - its methods and results. Large charts shewing in graph and tabular form the incidence in age and sex groups, with the methods adopted and the results secured were prepared by the conference organizers from data supplied by Dr. Fraser and were exhibited under large title headings of "Out-Patient work at Swatow Mission Hospital". Dr. Fraser also gave practical demonstrations. These and the paper aroused great interest. At the end of the conference we had the satisfaction of knowing that our experience of the treatment used at and recommended by the Culion Leper Colony (Philippine Islands) enabled the conference to recommend it as the standard treatment throughout China for those hospitals planning to undertake the treatment of leprosy. As we go to press we have received a letter from the Chinese Mission to Lepers which contains:—

"I take great pleasure in informing you that we are in receipt of an official reply from the National Health Administration to our petition sent a week ago re the promulgation of leprosy laws the resolution of which was adopted in our National Leprosy Conference to the effect that such laws are now being drafted and that we are asked to submit our views in regard to the contents of these codes. In order to give our Government our best possible advice we are soliciting for your expert opinion on this important question........ It seems quite clear that our Conference is producing results."

Whilst we recognize that we are only touching the fringe of an appallingly complex and difficult problem we cannot help being very thankful and a little proud and encouraged at these rather startling evidences that the Swatow hospital has once more done pioneer work in China and has had its work recognized. It is very easy to get depressed at our deplorable lack of decent buildings and facilities. A casual tour of the hospital leaves that sense of depression but when we come to soberly review the results of our year's work we find much cause for thankfulness at our achievements despite our handicaps. We are stimulated to know that our reputation stands high among those who are competent to assess it.*

Another scourge and ground for encouragement.

Dr. Fraser pointed out in his paper that the toll of Tuberculosis in China is much more serious than even the terrible incidence of Leprosy. Hitherto we have been able to do practically nothing to tackle it. Any satisfactory treatment of T. B. involves patients getting open air treatment under medical supervision. This has been impossible in the past. Since nursing has been introduced we have been able to have two or three patients on a verandah for several months at a stretch with very encouraging results.

---

* 编者注：以下无翻译。

《潮汕文库》大型丛书编委会

本书编委会

潮汕文库·文献系列

汕头福音医院年度报告编译（1866—1948）

（下卷）

[英] 吴威凛（William Gauld）等著

朱文平 编译

暨南大学出版社

JINAN UNIVERSITY PRESS

中国·广州

图书在版编目（CIP）数据

汕头福音医院年度报告编译（1866—1948）（下卷）/［英］吴威凛（William Gauld）等著；朱文平编译．—广州：暨南大学出版社，2016. 8
（潮汕文库．文献系列）
ISBN 978－7－5668－1665－8

Ⅰ. ①汕…　Ⅱ. ①吴…②朱…　Ⅲ. ①医院—史料—汕头市—近代　Ⅳ. ①R199. 2

中国版本图书馆 CIP 数据核字（2015）第 263203 号

汕头福音医院年度报告编译（1866—1948）
SHANTOU FUYIN YIYUAN NIANDU BAOGAO BIANYI（1866—1948）
［英］吴威凛（William Gauld）等 **著**　朱文平 **编译**

出 版 人： 徐义雄
项目统筹： 黄圣英
责任编辑： 颜　彦　杨柳婷　龙　欣
责任校对： 王嘉涵　姚晓莉
责任印制： 汤慧君　王雅琪

出版发行： 暨南大学出版社（510630）
电　　话： 总编室（8620）85221601
营销部（8620）85225284　85228291　85228292（邮购）
传　　真：（8620）85221583（办公室）　85223774（营销部）
网　　址： http：//www. jnupress. com　http：//press. jnu. edu. cn
排　　版： 广州市天河星辰文化发展部照排中心
印　　刷： 广东信源彩色印务有限公司
开　　本： 787mm×1092mm　1/16
印　　张： 50. 75
字　　数： 1215 千
版　　次： 2016 年 8 月第 1 版
印　　次： 2016 年 8 月第 1 次
定　　价： 160. 00 元（上下卷）

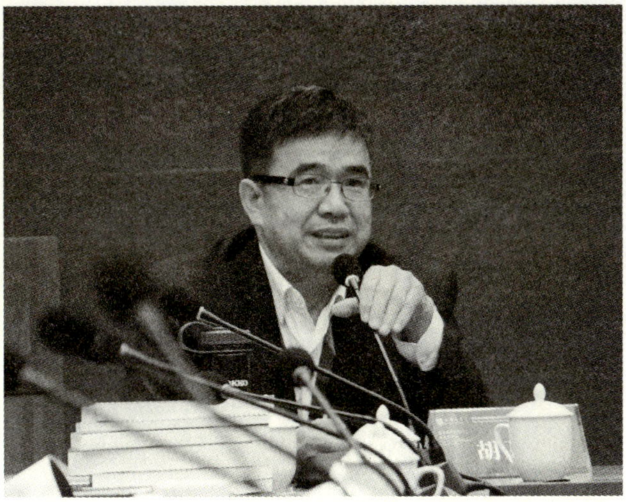

山东大学历史文化学院教授、博士生导师
胡卫清

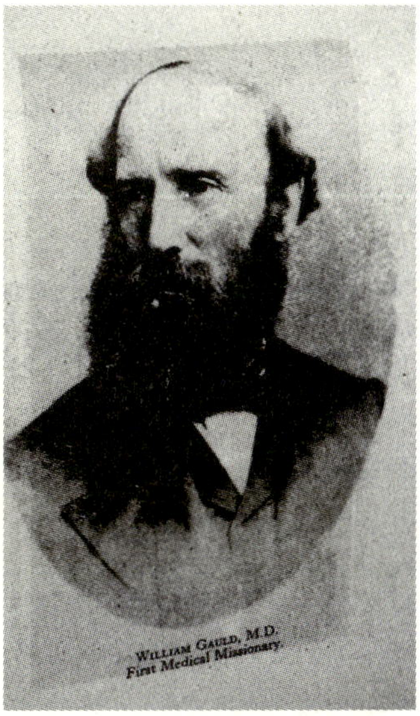

汕头福音医院创始人和首任院长吴威凛（Dr. William Gauld）（1863—1880 年任职）

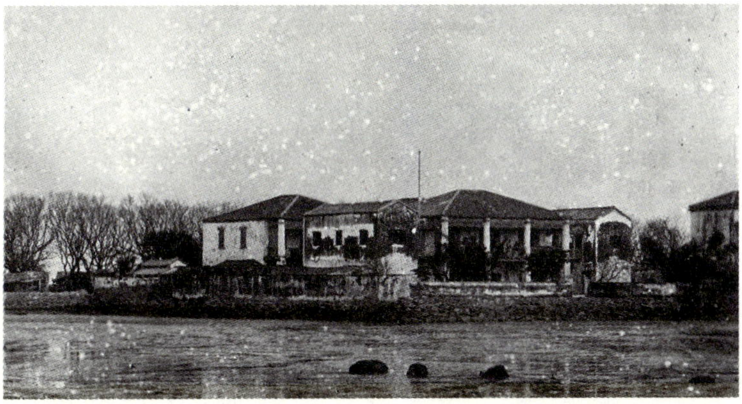

1895 年的汕头福音医院背面

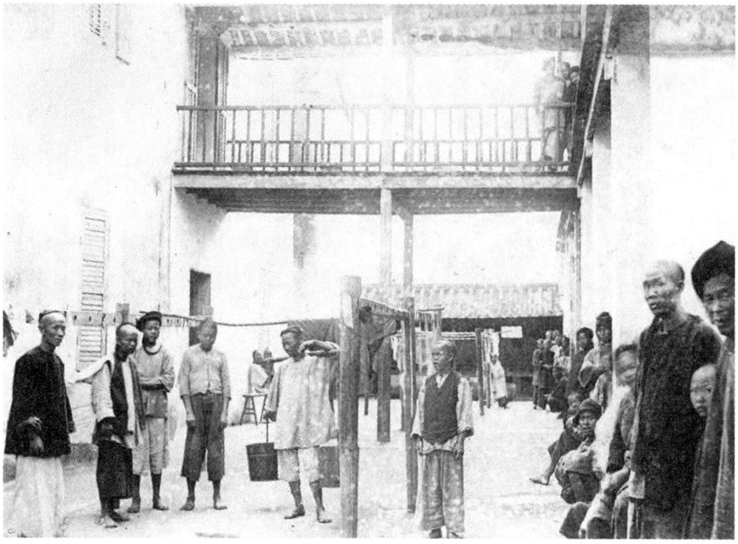

1895 年的汕头福音医院院内

1903 年 2 月 6 日（农历壬寅年正月初九）汕头福音医院之附属女医院（即福音女医院）落成，汕头富商陈雨亭行奉献礼。左一为英籍女医生雅恬娜（Dr. T. M. Alexander），左三为汕头福音医院院长来爱力（Dr. Alexander Lyall），右一为陈雨亭

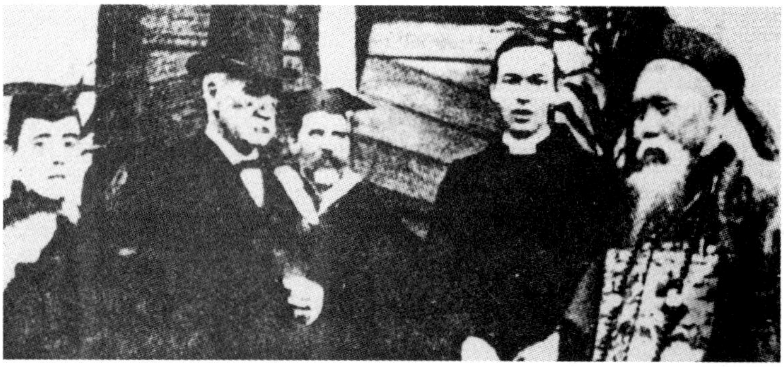

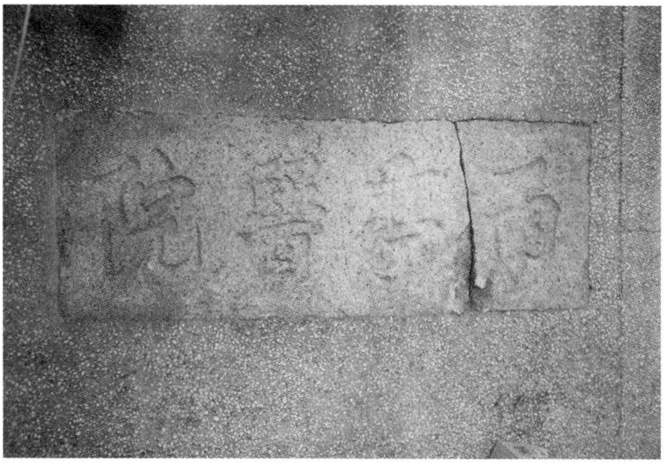

“雨亭医院”（福音女医院）石碑

1916 年，英兰长老会在汕头的传教士合影。前排左二为江克礼牧师（Rev. A. Guthrie Gamble），第二排左一为汕头福音医院院长来爱力（Dr. Alexander Lyall），后排左一为怀敦干医生（Dr. Duncan Whyte）

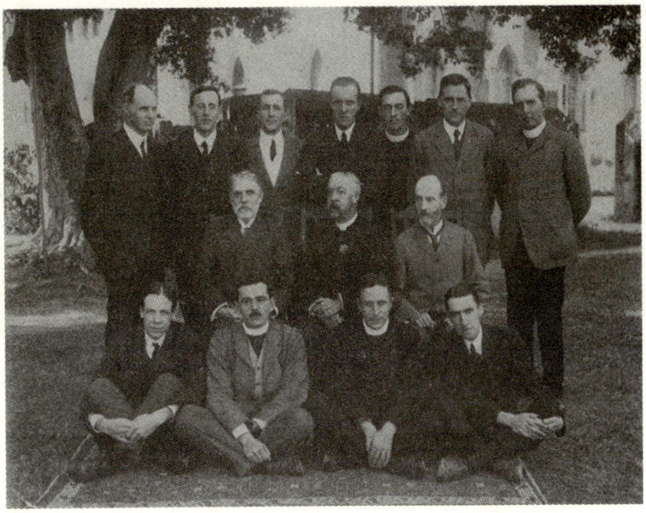

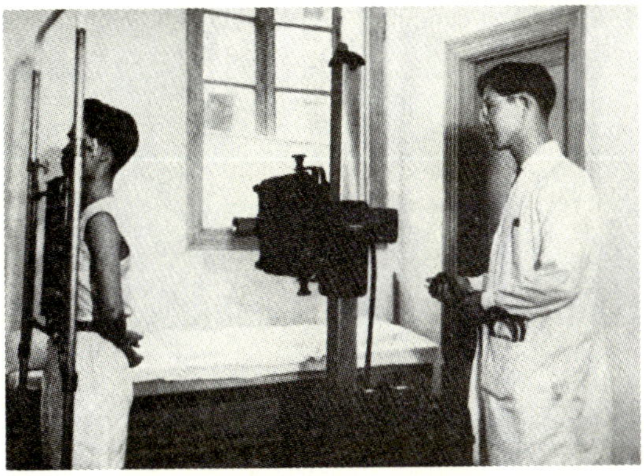

1918 年医院筹集资金从英国购买一台 X 光设备，1919 年安装完成并投入使用

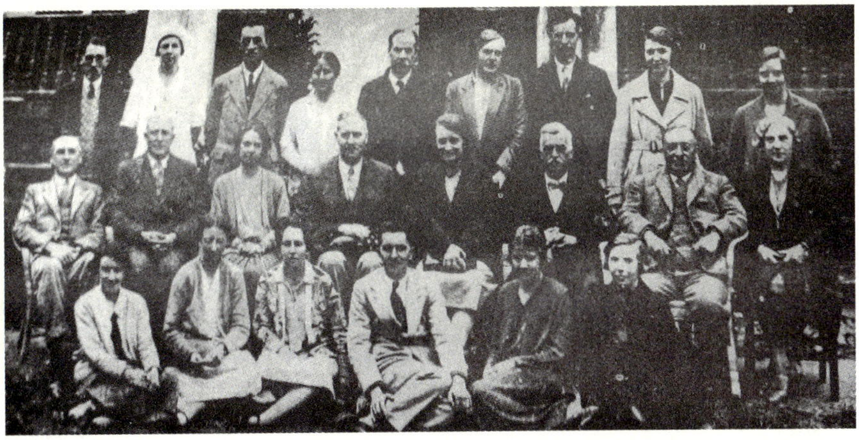

1932 年，英兰长老会在汕头的传教士合影。后排右三为汕头福音医院院长斐义礼（Dr. Neil D. Fraser），后排右二为斐义礼夫人

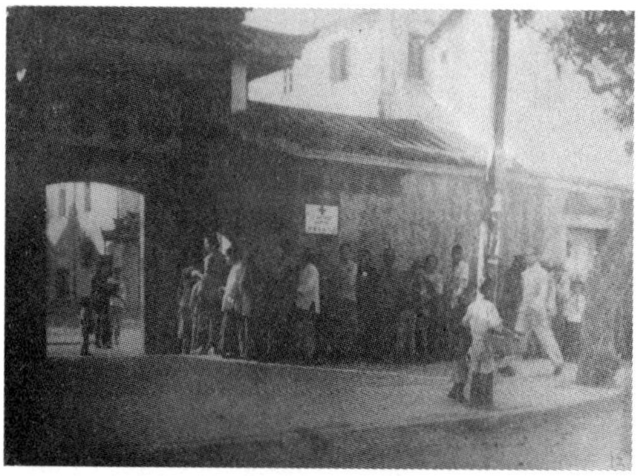

20 世纪 30 年代汕头福音医院大门

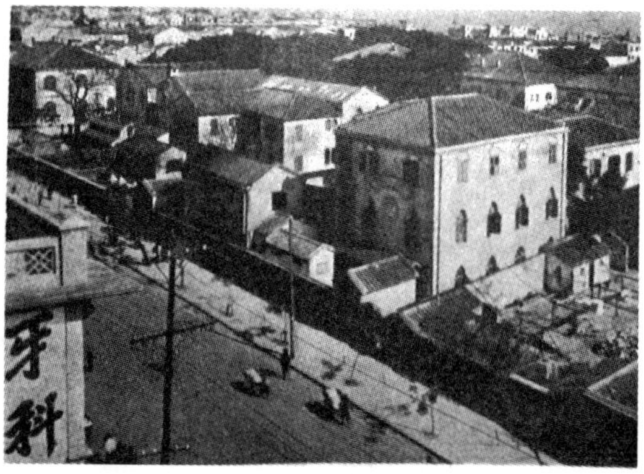

20 世纪 30 年代汕头福音医院正面全貌

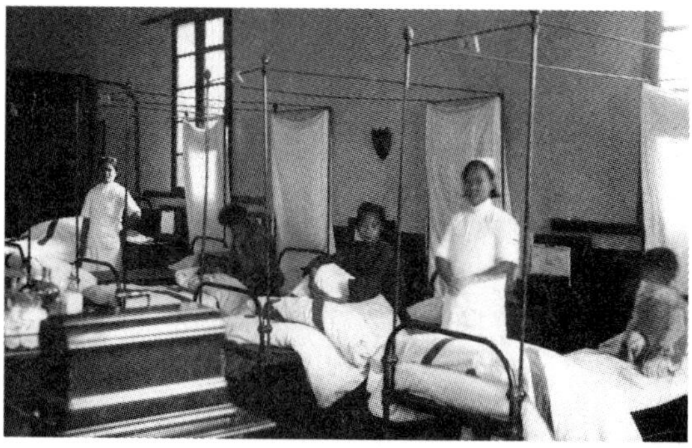

20 世纪 30 年代汕头福音医院女病房

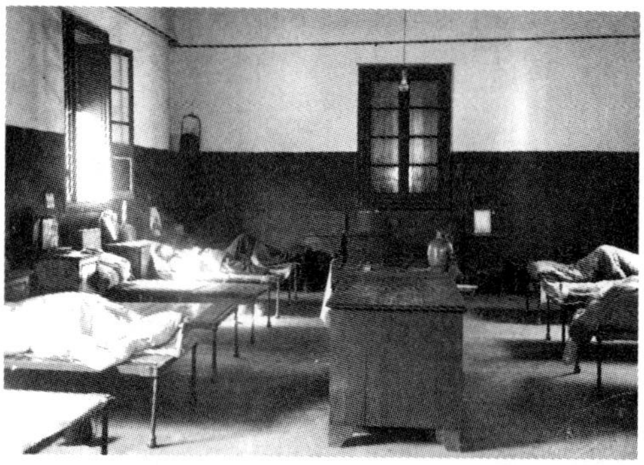

20 世纪 30 年代汕头福音医院病房

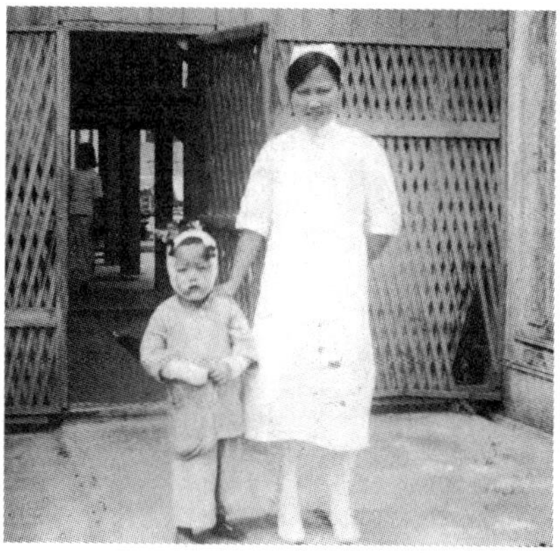

20 世纪 30 年代汕头福音医院的护士和小病人

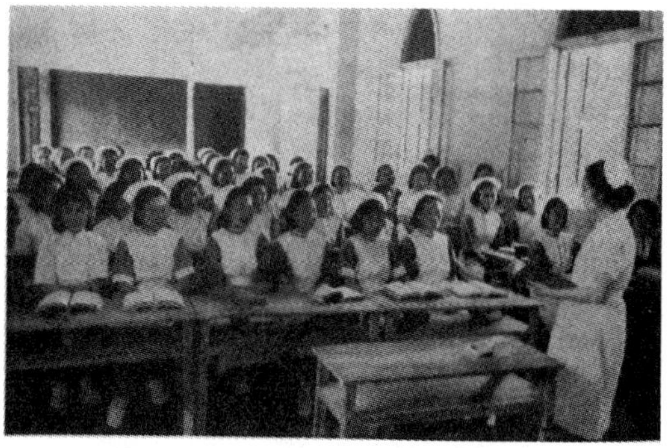

汕头福音医院护士学校学生上课

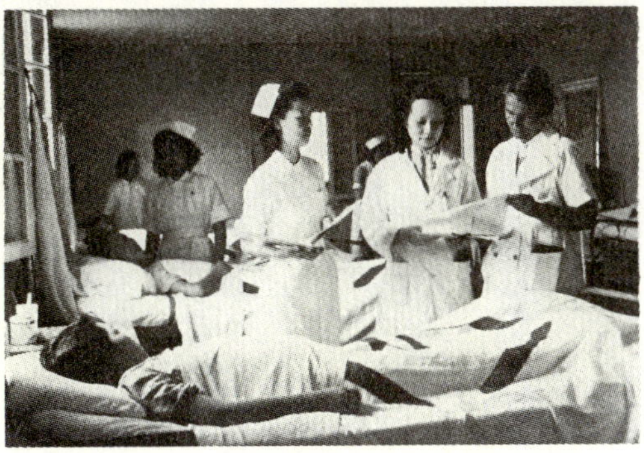

20 世纪 40 年代汕头福音医院女病房查房

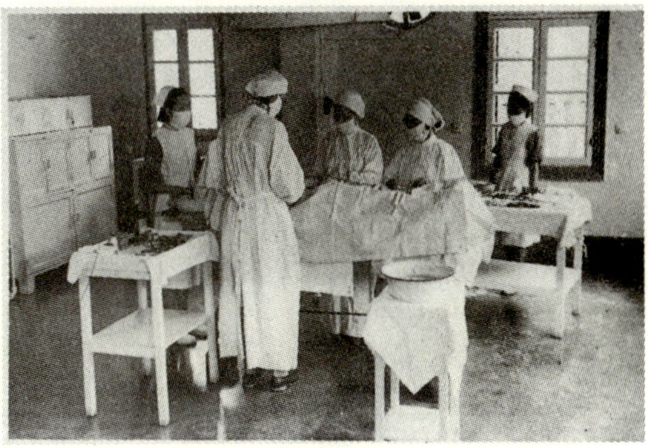

20 世纪 40 年代汕头福音医院手术室

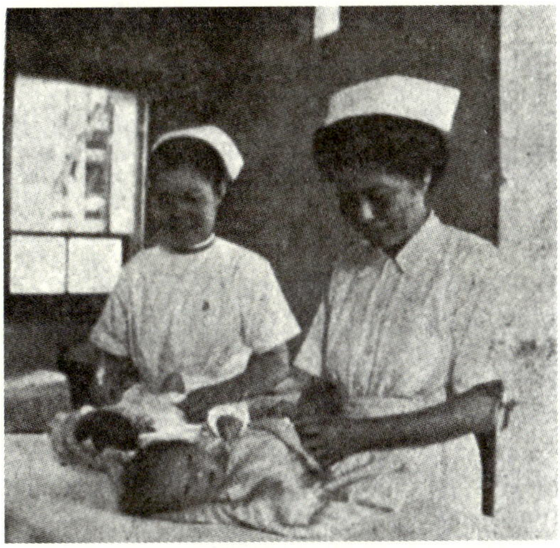

汕头福音医院婴孩室

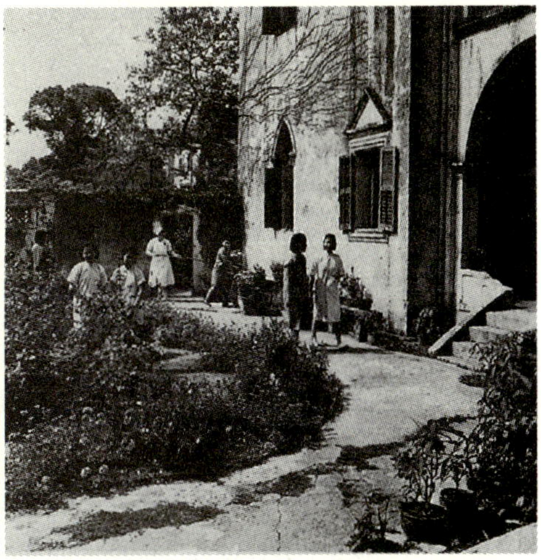

20 世纪 40 年代汕头福音医院花园

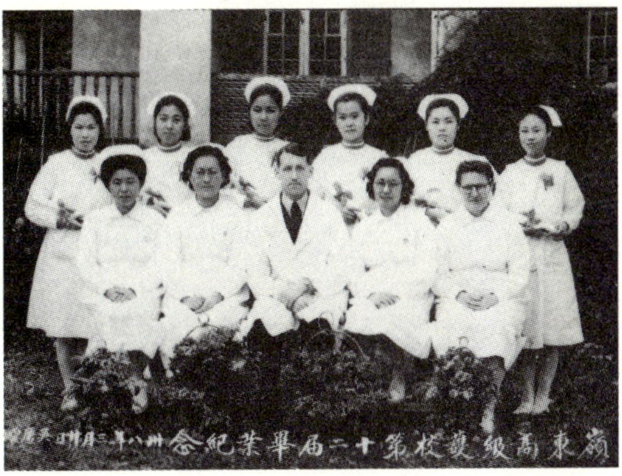

1949 年 3 月 20 日汕头福音医院院长邵志安（Dr. S. L. Strange）（前排中）等与岭东高级护士职业学校第十二届毕业生合影

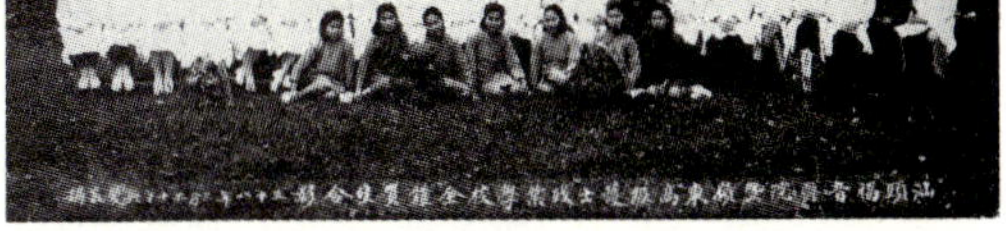

1949 年 3 月 20 日汕头福音医院暨岭东高级护士职业学校全体员生合影

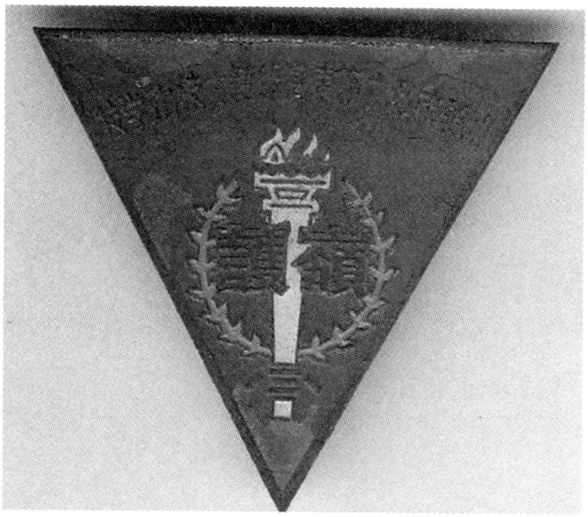

汕头市私立岭东高级护士技术学校徽章

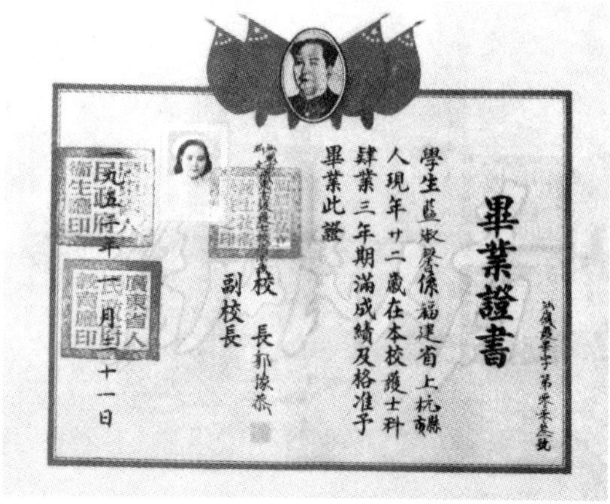

1953 年 1 月 31 日颁发的汕头市私立岭东高级护士技术学校毕业证书

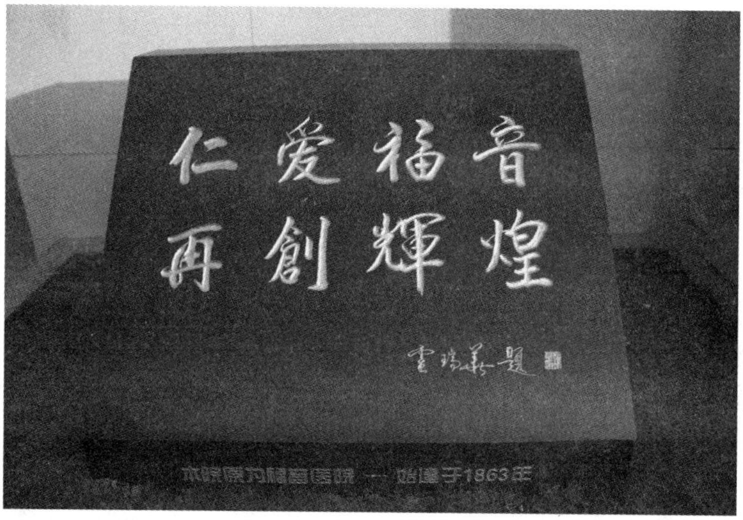

2011 年 3 月，原广东省人民政府省长卢瑞华为汕头市第二人民医院题词“仁爱福音　再创辉煌”。题词作为座右铭被篆刻在石碑上并被立在医院大门口

总　序

潮汕文化历千年久远，底蕴渊深，泱泱广袤，又伴随着潮人的迁播而兼收并蓄，独树一帜，是中华文明中的重要一脉。

秦汉之前，潮汕囿于海角一隅，与中原殆少来往；自韩愈治潮，兴学重教，风气日开，人文渐著。宋朝文教兴盛，前七贤垂范乡邦；明朝人才辈出，后八贤称显于时。明清以来，粤东地区借毗邻大海的地理优势，与域外商贸频仍，以陶朱端木之业，成中西交汇之势，造就多元开放的文化格局。饶宗颐等学界巨匠引领风骚，李嘉诚等商海翘楚造福民生，俊采星驰，郁郁称盛。

而今国家稳步发展，蓬勃兴盛，潮汕地区凭借深厚的历史积淀，务实进取，努力发展传统文化及其产业，如潮剧、潮乐、潮菜、工夫茶、陶瓷、木雕、刺绣等，保持并革新精巧特色，在世界各地广泛传播，备受青睐。更有海外潮人遍布全球，为经济文化交流引桥导路，探索共赢模式，拓宽发展空间。

为促进潮汕文化的传承与创新，进一步推动潮汕文化“走出去”，在广东省委宣传部的大力支持下，海内外学者编写《潮汕文库》大型丛书。本丛书包括文献系列和研究系列，涉及历史、文学、方言、民俗、曲艺、建筑、工艺美术等多方面，囊括影印、笺注、点校、碑铭、图文集、口述史等多种形式，始终秉承整理、抢救传统文化的原则，尊重潮汕地区的家学渊源和治学传统。以一腔丹心，在历史沿袭中为文化存证，修旧如旧，求新而不媚俗于新；以一笔质朴，在字斟句酌中为品质立言，就事论事，求全而不迷失于全；以一纸恳切，在纷扰喧嚣中为细节加冕，群策群力，求深而不盲目于深。惟愿以此丛书，提升潮汕文化品位，凝聚海内外潮人，齐心发展，助力腾飞。

在成书过程中，广东省委宣传部高度重视，协调汕头、潮州、揭阳、汕尾市委宣传部，委托潮汕历史文化研究中心、韩山师范学院、暨南大学出版社组织编写与出版。海内外潮学研究专家倾注笔墨，潮汕历史文献收藏机构及热心人士鼎力襄助，更蒙粤东籍一批著名艺术家慷慨捐赠宝贵书画作品助力出版，在此一并致谢！

《潮汕文库》大型丛书编委会

2016 年 7 月

目　录

1866 年汕头福音医院报告

（吴威凛医学博士照管下的汕头教会医院 1866 年报告）

这份报告涵盖的时间超过 15 个月，从 1865 年 9 月 20 日起到 1866 年 12 月 31 日为止。在此期间，由于诸多原因，诊所与医院的工作中断了将近 3 个月。因此，报告所包含的实际工作时间为一年多一点。

医院的运作计划与之前报告中所阐述的基本相同。在汕头，门诊一般每周对公众开放两天，时间为每周二和周五，而住院病人可以在任何时间入院，并接受每日护理。

这一年中，庵埠（Ampow）和达埠（Tathanpow）分别开设了门诊，它们是在汕头的两个相反方向的两个人口密集的城镇，距离汕头都是大约 9 英里水路。周三是庵埠诊所的开放日，周六则是达埠的。如果情况允许，我会定期去这些地方巡诊，以便鼓励这项工作继续开展下去，可能的话，甚至将其推广到其他毗邻乡镇。我们也巡诊过乡村的其他地方。

另外，许多特别重要和便利的药物已被定期派发到各个乡村传教点，它们常常供不应求。

我们的中国助理非常称职。他已经和我们共事了 3 年，虽然一开始完全没有经验，但如今已逐渐地熟悉各种我们常用的药物，能够独立配制并且巧妙使用它们。在脓肿处理和其他小型手术操作方面，他的技术非常到位，并且能够独立成功完成一些简单的眼科手术。

从下面的统计可以看出，去年我们的医疗传教工作大体上取得了一定成效。

截至 1866 年 12 月 31 日的年总病人数	2 738
其中女性病人数	465
其中住院病人数	515
就诊人次	10 854
汕头门诊开放日平均每天门诊病人数	46
最多单日诊疗人数	96

挂号的记录显示，前来就诊的病人来自 400 多个不同地方，包括潮州地区的城镇和乡村，还有一些来自福建省。

住院病人数大幅上升，无论就医疗目的还是传教目的而言，他们都是最有希望的群体，因此这种上升趋势是值得感恩和鼓舞人心的。来住院的病人通常自备食物和被褥，只有在需要的时候我们才会提供资金补助。

每天的就诊人数大概比去年的多了三分之一，这个数字很值得关注，因为它表明了每个病人的平均就诊次数。如果病人人数和每日就诊数大致相等的话，就意味着大部分病人只有单次就诊，这不会对病情带来多大好转。以此来衡量的话，面向中国人的这种纯粹的诊所业务还是不尽人意的。

部分中国人对医院的信心增强从而更愿意接受正规的治疗。

对于那些熟悉中国习俗的人来说，男性病人远远多于女性病人是再正常不过的。家离汕头远的妇女是很难出远门的。

下面是这一年来所诊治的内外科疾病的大致分类：

消化系统疾病和全身虚弱	376
呼吸系统疾病	180
风湿病	206
淋巴结核（淋巴结肿大）	23
疟疾	52
发热	42
下肢水肿	35
中风、瘫痪	28
癫痫	6
精神病	3
心脏病	10
麻风病	112
鸦片成瘾	26
眼科疾病	626
耳鼻喉疾病	22
骨科疾病	26
关节疾病	67
皮肤疾病	231
生殖器疾病	62
外伤、溃疡、脓肿	453
赘疣	40
疝气	14
肛瘘	8
痔疮	4
唇裂	1
脊柱弯曲	5
烧伤	5
脱臼	2
骨折	2
肿瘤	11

狗咬伤	4
干性坏疽	1

在所有的疾病当中，消化系统疾病是最常见且最难控制的。它的病例主要是穷人发生的消化不良和身体衰弱。这通常是常年累积造成的，因而病情十分顽固。由于疾病是由食品质量差或者供应不足引起的，这些致病因素常常影响了我们的治疗过程。此外，如果病人在医院住院一段时间，他常常比在家里吃得更少，以求能够在医院待更久。因此，提供有营养的食物而非药物更能促进治疗效果。但是，除少数特殊情况外，我们有限的经费并不允许我们这样做。这个群体的其他疾病，如痢疾、腹泻，更容易控制病情和获得良好的治疗效果。

在呼吸系统疾病中，肺结核非常值得关注。通过观察可以发现一个有意思的现象，这种疾病在极寒和极热地区很盛行，比如在北极和热带。肺结核也许在中国南方人和在格陵兰岛上的因纽特人中一样常见。

从以上的统计可以判断，心脏病在中国人身上相对少见。但是，除了已记录的病例，很多因为其他疾病接受治疗的病人到了疾病晚期也或多或少会并发心脏病。

在成为特殊观察和探究对象的 100 个麻风病例中，多达 78 例，也就是超过四分之三的人没有相识的亲属被感染；14 位患者有一到多位亲属被感染；7 位曾患过梅毒；一位病人与麻风病人在一起生活过，除此之外，不能对其疾病的根源给出其他的解释。患者年龄段在 11 岁至 67 岁。一个 17 岁的病人在免疫接种之后患病；另有一个 15 岁的病人是通过母体感染的；一位 67 岁的病人已经患病 10 年了。病人所得多为结核样型麻风。目前，麻风病的致病机制尚未明确，最有可能的应该是免疫系统的缺陷。

这一年，40 000 ~ 50 000 片药物被用于治疗鸦片成瘾者。用这些药物取得效果的实例如下：一个中年男性患者吸鸦片已 10 年，每天要吸食两德拉克马（drachma）重的鸦片提取物。他决心戒除毒瘾，开始时每天服用 10 片药片，在这期间逐步减少服药量，50 天后每天只服用两片，甚至将可以完全不服药。这是一个让人看到希望的病例。

一个发生在鸦片成瘾者身上的膀胱炎病例很特殊，因为其严重的症状迅速消退了。患者突然排出大量高黏度的血尿，伴轻度疼痛。他被嘱予使用蓖麻油、洗热水澡、使用杜佛氏散（Dover's powder）和休息治疗，一两天就好了，这让我们稍微感到惊讶，因为他的病情原来很严重。

在外科病例中，迄今为止数量最多的是眼科疾病。眼科手术列表如下：

睑内翻及倒睫症手术	64
结膜肿块切除术	5
翼状胬肉切除术	17
前房放液术	13
虹膜粘连分离术	2
虹膜切除术（人工瞳孔）	6
白内障（硬质）摘除术	11

皮质性白内障手术 …………………………………………………………… 1
葡萄肿切除术 ……………………………………………………………………… 1
泪管（粘连）分离术…………………………………………………………… 1

从结膜（眼睑和眼球间的黏膜）切除下来的肿块通常不大，而且根据因其而被妨碍功能的器官的重要性而产生相应的影响。有一个病例值得关注，其肿块附着于结膜，覆盖在眼球的角膜缘上，延伸到连接球结膜和睑结膜的反折所形成的夹角处，如榛子般大小，又圆又滑像个血凝块，但呈黑色，明显具有癌变特性，已生长了四个月，用手术刀切除并不困难。

最近，有许多从福建南部赶来看病的病人，他们下肢溃烂，伴随脾肿大，全身各系统功能下降。他们认为疾病是太平军的死尸污染水源所致。如果太平军要对这件事负责的话，更多的是因为他们荒废了周围的农田，导致食物不足，这对已在穷困中挣扎的贫苦人来说才是最大的打击。

一个女人受到腰部一个非常大的脓肿的困扰，她对它进行了奇怪的描述——脓肿聚集于身体不同的部位，使用切碎的草药制成的药膏后，脓肿会从一个地方转移到另一个地方。脓肿切开后，其病痛很快就解除了。

说到皮肤病，或许最令人关注的是几个严重硬斑病病例。通常这种病被发现是会扩散的，伴随热、痒、痛。我在农村的时候接诊过一个 20 岁的女人。她的硬斑局限在胸骨上的一处，是一颗凸起的暗红色斑点，差不多有一个大豌豆大小，可移动。其发病于两三年前，并逐渐变大。我把硬斑连同周围健康的皮肤一同切除并缝合了伤口，但是我在她痊愈之前就不得不去汕头了，或许是后来疏于照料，听说不久后疾病又复发了。另一个病例是一位 16 岁男孩，他让我看了他胸口上一块像纽扣的肿物，并希望将其切除。在检查过程中，我发现他的躯干和四肢布满大小不一的结节，呈圆形或椭圆形，具有和胸口的肿物一样的特征。切除是不可能的，只能上一些药。那个小伙子很快就离开了，因此没有机会验证其疗效。硬斑病在某些方面和癌症相似，但并不意味着它就是不治之症。

普通外科手术并没有什么需要着重提起的。除了切除脓肿与类似的手术，还有大约 50 例，包括各种肿物和息肉的切除、痔疮手术、骨病的手术、脚趾甲撕脱的手术、拇指截除、唇裂和肛瘘手术、取出子弹等。

一例烧伤致畸病例接受了手术治疗。那是一位从农村来的看起来体格强健的男病人，他的一个脚的第四、第五个趾头由于烧伤留下的瘢痕呈直角翘到了脚背上。他穿不了鞋，因此希望把畸形部分去掉。我切断瘢痕的厚凸起带，然后将其剖开至脚趾根部，把脚趾强制拉直后用夹板在脚底固定住，并用绷带紧紧绑住脚趾。手术造成了一处颇大的溃疡，好在逐渐愈合了。在夹板的纠正下，那两个脚趾也和其他脚趾处于同一平面了。脚恢复得非常好。

牛痘接种也开始推行。在去年的下半年，超过 60 名儿童接受了接种。这里的中国人对我们的这种小手术存在强烈的偏见，但一旦有了开端，接种所带来的种种好处将会被明显感受到，越来越多的人就会认同和接受它。

由于英兰长老会的慷慨解囊，加上汕头和其他地方的外国社团的大力帮助，我们得以建起一座新医院，它比我们迄今为止所拥有的任何地方都舒适和宽敞得多。这是一座大型的两层建筑，能轻松容纳超过50人住宿。一层是为病人设立的会客室，宗教服务将在这里定期举行。上面一层是诊所和传教士的休息室。整座建筑，包括买地，大概花费了4 000美元。捐助者的名字将列在这份报告的最后，我们真诚和衷心地感谢他们，在我们求助的时候他们及时而慷慨地给予了援助。中国人的捐款是通过盛鑫行（Seen Hing Hong）获得的，此外，我们真诚鸣谢莫里森船长（Captain Morrison）在他动身前往英国之前提供的热心帮助。

我们期待并祈祷着，在接下来的年度里，这所新医院对于整个潮州地区的民众意味着越来越多的身心祝福。祝愿人们来到这里最终能够获得他们想要的结果，健康得以恢复或改善，病痛被舒适安逸所取代。不仅如此，希望他们每天所听到的带给他们救赎的喜讯，引领他们去寻找那个唯一的而且永远存在的圣人——主耶稣。这是我们最伟大的工作目标，而我们的快乐在于实现这一目标。我们有理由相信在过去一年我们在这方面绝非没有成果，很多来自这个地区不同地方的病人带着对于他们所需要的“生活方式”的认识，即被上帝的精神所点燃的救赎信念回到了自己的家中。

为新医院捐款者

（略）

中国捐款者

（略）

以下的捐款被用于支付过去两三年中诊所的本地支出，它是在1864年和1865年筹来的：

（略）

（翻译：谢煊、许思婷　校译：朱文平　审校：胡卫清、余维泉、江建安　中文校正：许党泉、颜彦）

1868—1869 年汕头福音医院报告

（吴威凛医学博士照管下的英兰长老会汕头教会医院 1868—1869 年报告）

上一份关于英兰长老会对汕头地区中国人进行的医疗工作的报告已经出版两年了。如今，我们也像当初一样，很荣幸地将医院病人数量的稳步上升记录下来。医院病人数量增长如此之快，以至于两年半前建成的医院——那个我们原本以为足够收治所有病人的地方，如今有时会被病人挤满。在上一份工作报告中也提到，我们的主要照顾对象是住院病人，他们让我们无论作为医护人员还是传教士都最有成就感。据我所知，去年这里的住院病人数量比中国的任何其他医院的都多。但是，这里的门诊病人与诊所业务就非常少，不过照顾住院病人就足以占用我们所有的时间与精力了，所以我们也就不遗憾了。

在庵埠和达埠的两所乡下诊所现仍在开放，而且每周都会有当地医学助理在一两个传教士的陪同下前去拜访。

在汕头，我们的诊所仍然坚持每周开放两天，具体的运作流程大致与前一篇工作报告提到的相同。

在潮州府，这个区域的中心城市，中国人于 1868 年建立了一个公共诊所。我可以肯定地说，我们在汕头的工作很大程度上促成了这件事。它的经费由公众支持，开始时人们慷慨捐款，一切看起来十分顺利与成功，公众纷纷找那两个当地的医生看病，他们轮流上班，每个月上 9 天班。病人看完病后会拿到医生手写的处方，凭着处方就可以在一个当地的药店免费取药。但是，筹款很快变得困难，人们也开始对医生们的表现产生不满。这些所谓的“医生”当然没有受过特别的培训，他们只是识字并有足够空闲时间，可能自己阅读过一些有关处方的书籍，之后就自封为合格的医生。因为就诊病人和所需资金供应不足，这些机构如今可以说是倒闭了。这可看作是在中国成立的医疗机构的普遍历程。只有在那些子民的品格多少受基督教教义影响的国家才能保证慈善事业的长久和稳定，在这方面，中国距此还很遥远。真正的慈善事业是基督教的产物，因为对人的真爱与对上帝的爱是分不开的。

1869 年的数据是根据前 6 个月获得的数据而对全年的数据做出的合理预测。下半年的病人数目与上半年一样多，但我由于身体不适无法全勤和按时上班。大部分时间里，我的工作基本上是由 3 个本地助手完成的。很高兴的是，他们都做得很让人满意。我相信 1869 年的数据是最好的说明。

	1868 年	1869 年
病人总数①	2 950	2 500
住院病人数（包括在以上病人数中）	608	850
女病人数	486	……
汕头门诊开放日平均每天门诊病人数	52	63
汕头门诊开放日单日就诊病人数最大值	91	128

我们把一个小病房单独隔开来供女性患者使用，那里常常人满为患。

去年我们租了附近一座中式房屋来用于收治麻风病患者。有时，那里一次住了 10 个到 20 个不幸患病的人。对麻风病人的治疗方法至今仍不尽人意。听说孟买有个医生治疗麻风病十分有名，我写信给一个住在那里的医学界朋友，向他咨询这方面的信息，却失望地收到以下答复："我对他很了解，也看过他的一些病人。我个人认为，在孟买几乎所有医生都是冒牌的。"也有一些中国医生在试图治疗这种可怕的病，但至今我还没听说过一例可信的完全治愈的病例，或任何局部和暂时改善之外的进展。我们汕头的许多病例的治疗已取得这种进展了。这种疾病在这个区域很常见。依我所见，尽管它与《圣经》中提到的麻风病还是有明显的不同，但我深信不久以后这种病会成为一个致命的问题。中国人胡乱提出了多种多样无关联的麻风病病因。土壤、水源、雨水、日晒、露水、麻疹、小瘟疫，还有其他不计其数的因素被当作了病因。虽然他们认为麻风病是种遗传病，但大多数来到医院的麻风病患者都表示他们没有患麻风病的先辈，他们的麻风病也不是来自家族感染。

我们还如往常一样将诊治过的不同疾病列成表格，以下的 1868 年的清单也许能引起一些医学界朋友的兴趣：

消化系统疾病

牙疼 …… 15
消化不良 …… 281
蠕虫病 …… 19
绞痛 …… 3
腹泻 …… 12
痢疾 …… 9
—— 339

呼吸系统疾病

黏膜炎 …… 50
喉部感染 …… 11

① 这些数字只记录新病例。新旧病例一起算入的病人总数，在中国一些医学报告中为 20 000 到30 000人，可能被误记为就诊次数，即在那种算法中，一个病人来看病 6 次则算作 6 个病人。除非保存有明确的新病人登记记录，否则不可能给出这个数据。

支气管炎 …… 28
肺炎 …… 1
肺结核 …… 37
咯血 …… 16
哮喘病 …… 47

——190

风湿病 …… 169
心脏病 …… 6
淋巴结核 …… 18
弛张热 …… 25
间歇性发热 …… 56

——81

水肿 …… 10
下肢浮肿 …… 13
局部瘫痪 …… 10
偏瘫 …… 1

——11

癫痫 …… 9
精神病 …… 2
麻风病 …… 134
鸦片成瘾 …… 3
妇科疾病（白带等） …… 9
肾病 …… 7
眼疾 …… 426
耳疾 …… 9
皮肤病 …… 150
关节病 …… 37
骨病 …… 15
生殖器疾病 …… 34
外伤、溃疡、脓肿 …… 302

肿瘤

癌症 …… 14
脂肪瘤 …… 5
纤维瘤 …… 5
淀粉瘤 …… 4
胶质瘤 …… 4
血管瘤或神经瘤 …… 3
结节和疣 …… 9

——44

舌下囊肿	2
唇裂	17
腭裂（含硬腭和软腭）	1
腹股沟疝（破裂）	4
肛瘘	13
痔疮（外痔 2 例，内痔 5 例）	7
脊柱僵硬弯曲	5
破伤风（角弓反张）	1
骨折	1
狗咬伤	5
蛇咬伤	1
甲状腺肿	1
冻伤坏疽	2

1869 年间所治疗疾病的目录会与上表有点重复，只是数量稍有不同。

浏览表格，我们可以看出中国出现的疾病与在一个英格兰贫困地区巡诊时遇到的差不多。除了麻风病、象皮病、下肢浮肿，或许某种程度上还加上疟疾发热，中国的其他疾病与英格兰贫困地区出现的疾病并无差别。但是由于当地医疗技术缺乏和贫困人口众多，一些疾病在这里发展到了我们在英格兰没见过的程度。举例来说，溃疡病能蔓延到非常危险和令人恶心的状态，很多皮肤病和眼疾也是这样。

医院中不常出现急性感染性疾病病例，绝大多数是消化不良、虚弱、风湿病、胸痛、眼疾和溃疡病等慢性病。有很多病人因患病时间过长，已无法根治，如果他们能前来就医，并得到一定程度的缓解，我们将十分高兴。但是，也有一些人回去后靠引诱同乡人去治疗来赚取一些利益，让这些病人花费了大量的金钱与精力。我们曾听说有一个男人为了到四五十英里外的医院看病，把自己的一个儿子卖了换钱。

我们不时碰到一些奇怪的中医疗法。举个例子，有一个男人由于肠炎前来诊所看病。一开始他因为便秘和绞痛症状去看中医，那中医认为他应该排出体内的毒物，就给了他以下的处方！

十只西班牙苍蝇
三条蜈蚣
十条蚕虫
十只蝎子

患者要将这些东西捣弄在一起一次性吞服。不出所料，结果引起了炎症，但是，使用膏药和鸦片后该病症很快得到了缓解。

很多疾病其实是由**梅毒**或**瘰疬**引起的，尽管被归类为其他疾病。被归类为瘰疬的是只显示淋巴结核症状的病例。表现出不同症状的狼疮很常见，而中国人的狼疮常常长在鼻子上，最终这种具有毁灭性的疾病会“吃”掉整个鼻子。

一个值得注意的**脑积水**病例是庵埠的诊所接诊的一个两岁小孩。他的病情持续了一年，送来的时候他的脑袋已经大到自己无法支撑了。他的身体在其他方面没有发育失常，而且他的智力似乎也没有受到损伤。他眉毛处的头围有2英尺长，而从头顶量两边耳尖的距离是1英尺3英寸。表示有液体存在的波动感很明显，而那些形成脑壳的顶骨分离得很远，只能在头两边的较低处触摸得到。硕大的脑袋连接着这么弱小的身体使这个小孩看起来有些畸形。没有进行治疗。

很少中国人会单单为了戒除**鸦片瘾**而到医院治疗，但我们仍然会发放戒毒药片到汕头和各乡村传教点，以便给那些需要的人服用。我们观察到的下面这个病例十分有趣。患者是一位35岁的中年男人，患有哮喘病。15年前他就开始通过吸鸦片来减轻哮喘病的痛苦，但没起作用，而且染上了鸦片的毒瘾，以至于他每天要吸掉约一斤鸦片。为了戒掉毒瘾，他求助于我们的药片。一开始他每天要服用32颗药片，后来到医院的时候他已经减少到每天只需一颗药片。服用了药片之后，他就轻松地戒掉了毒瘾，但停药后他却感染了痢疾。吸食鸦片对中国人身体、心理和精神上造成的可怕后果已由几个医学传教士详述在“中国记录者”部分，而且他们的陈述也为我们所赞同。但是至今为止，对这种危害的宣传没有实际成效，这种恶习的受害者继续增加并遍布中国。像前面所说的鸦片成瘾对身心造成伤害的例子不胜枚举，只要见过鸦片成瘾者的悲惨人性，或者知道鸦片成瘾给其家人和自己带来的巨大恶果的人绝不会认为我是在夸大事实。言语无法描述鸦片的可怕。对于基督教来说，每个传教士都知道这个魔鬼多次阻碍了他们向中国人传播真理的道路。中国人能强烈地感受到这种伤害与错误，没有谁比那些瘾君子们更强烈哀叹鸦片带来的痛苦了。越来越多的事实能证明鸦片正在毒害着中国。所有人都知道这个帝国四处遍布着吸食鸦片的人，我们甚至敢说在北京，在皇宫的管辖区内，吸食鸦片之风已盛行到了危险的地步。有些人会告诉我们其他国家也有兴奋剂和镇静剂、酒精和烟草等。我们承认在一定程度上这是对的。但是中国不仅有鸦片，也有酒和烟草，而且我们通常发现一个鸦片成瘾者同时也是烟民，有时他还是个酒鬼。但是，与鸦片这个魔鬼相比起来，其他的都只是小巫见大巫。

在众多**外科手术**中，**眼科手术**的数目至今为止仍然占据首位。前来就诊的人中有不少完全失明或者痊愈无望的，但大多数通过手术都有所改善，而且效果显著，振奋人心。举个例子，有个男性患者因为被竹子刺到的伤口愈合之后一边眼皮睁不开而前来就诊，他当时的视力仅剩五分之一，用中国的一句俗语来说就是他只能看到“十份中的两份”。这是**眼睑粘连**的典型病例，它不仅可能导致失明，还可能造成脸部畸形。粘连处被切开并剥离，上眼睑的皮肤和黏膜被缝合在一起，以防止眼睑再度粘连。术后，视力恢复得很好，脸部外观也大为改善。另一位是由于眼部受到拳击，导致眼睛受到完全性伤害而前来治疗的，他一只眼睛的晶状体从囊处部分脱落，陷进眼后房，可以清楚地看到它在那里而且有浑浊和白内障。他的另一只眼睛也不幸受损。晶状体不得不切除，这不是为了恢复视力，因为恢复是不可能的，这只是为了避免造成盲眼和另一只正常的眼睛发炎。在1868年，共有142例眼部外科手术，到1869年数量达到170例。有超过半数的是由于眼睑翻转（**内翻**）和不规则生长的睫毛（**倒睫**）摩擦而损伤眼球。中国助手们通常能做这些手术和

翼状胬肉的手术（这类手术常见性紧随其后）。**斜视**的病例在这个地方的中国人中相对比较少见，虽然在过去的6年中我见过一些，但一直没有机会亲自做一例手术。

在中国，**损伤耳朵**是报复别人时偶尔使用的一种方式。有一天，有个男人前来就诊，他的两只耳朵的耳郭已经被切下来，是被一个愤怒的债主拿剪刀剪掉的。这真是一种奇怪的从欠债者处得到发泄满足的方法！另一个男人不久前因为一只耳朵被咬掉了，而后导致耳朵全部受损而前来就诊。他去找租赁者讨要田地租金时与对方发生口角并发展到打架，在打斗中耳朵被对方咬掉，真是野蛮的行径。有时候女孩子因使用了太大的耳饰而撕裂耳垂后前来就诊。这种畸形的矫正手术和唇裂类似。

骨科疾病也是常见的。有一例下巴坏死的病例，下颌骨的近一半嵌在牙龈中。通过一个非常小的切口，切除了两三块坏死的骨头后，效果非常令人满意，患者也舒适了。

象皮病，也就是下肢肿大，几乎都伴有大腿大血管上面的腹股沟淋巴结肿大。以下病例就是这样，患者是26岁的青年男子，他的两条腿在16年前就开始浮肿，随后不久就开始疼痛、僵硬。当他来到医院时，他双腿的尺寸如下：

在小腿处测量，一条腿2英尺7英寸，另一条腿2英尺3.5英寸；
在脚踝处测量，一条腿2英尺7英寸，另一条腿2英尺1英寸。

皮肤和皮下组织已经在他腿上形成厚厚的皱褶。最近，我还看到一个妇女的手肘以下的手臂也呈现与患象皮病的腿相同的症状，毫无疑问，他们所患之疾是一样的。这是我唯一一次看到这类病发生在上肢。据我所知，腿部的象皮病一般只出现在膝盖以下，相比之下，大腿一般是正常的大小。如果病情比较轻，我们会采取把肢体放高，绑上绷带，局部涂上碘，内服钾化碘的措施，至少起到缓解病情的作用；但肿胀严重、皮肤已经变形的地方，就没希望治好了。

不同种类的**肿瘤**，尺寸从豌豆大小到人头大小不等，并不少见。肿瘤切除后显著的效果、手术的安全性和术后恢复之快，都深深地震惊了中国人，使他们对于西医的外科技术产生信任。而更多的事实表明，中医由于缺乏解剖的知识，在这方面相比之下对病人没有什么帮助。如今在西方国家，解剖尸体是允许的，它可以弥补中医在手术中的缺陷。除了上海一家中国医院在一些特殊情况下会进行尸检，在广州的克尔医生（Dr. Kerr）的医院会有一些解剖的手术，中国的其他地方我还未曾听说过。在中国，在死者死于暴力或某种特别要求调查的情况时会进行官方验尸检查。坦白地说，他们的检验方式与我们的观念完全不同，我认为不能促进解剖学的发展。

脂肪肿瘤是最常见的。有一个年轻人长了颗小柚子般大小的肿瘤，像软袋般从肩胛骨上垂下来，因此影响到他的正常工作。我们很容易地就把肿瘤从它所依附的肌肉上切除了，皮肤则缝合在一起。几天后患者就伤口愈合，完全康复了。我还见过一个相同类型的但有小男孩头那么大的肿瘤，吊在脊骨上像个乞丐包袱。患者31岁，那颗肿瘤从他出生时就有了。我标记了切口线引导中国助手们并让他们进行操作，他们做手术当天我并不在场。后来手术非常成功，那个男子很快就恢复了。

在中国，**恶性肿瘤**的数量与在欧洲地区的相当。女人比男人更容易患上乳腺（乳房）

硬癌。但是，我们曾为一位男性患者切除一个牡蛎大小的乳腺肿瘤。通常癌症患者的手术切口在术后都恢复得很快。还有一个病例是患者因一边肋骨有软癌而前来做手术，由于中国医生使用了腐蚀性的药物，肿瘤的表面已经溃烂了约2英寸。切开之后，发现肿瘤由几个明显的小肿瘤组成，并且通过纤维网紧紧黏合在一起。在手术过程中我们剥离了肿瘤。在尽力清除肿瘤后，我们用碳酸洗干净粗糙的表面，并缝合皮肤。不知道疾病后来是否有复发，因为那个病人在离开医院，回到他遥远乡下的家中后，就杳无音讯了。

最大的肿瘤不总是最危险的，**血管瘤**尽管常常很小，但可怕的是它可能会由于轻微的碰撞而出血。有一个5岁的小男孩的头皮处就长了一颗这样的肿瘤。他来的时候血流不止，这种事情在之前发生过数次，这个孩子现在脸色苍白，由于体质虚弱还患上了哮喘。那颗肿瘤只有栗子般大小，通过一个小小的根部连在头上，并不比鞭绳粗。我在它的根部用了根结实的绳子勒紧它，同时把整个肿瘤都切掉，只剩一个小小的结防止绳子松开。几个月后，我在乡村的另一处地方遇到一个一模一样的病例，我用同样的方法将其治愈。上述的孩子的病例要是放在以前，不久后会由于持续地大出血无可避免地死去，但如今这种简单的手术却能拯救他的性命。

颈部纤维瘤是很常见的，有时其病情发展很快。曾有一位男性病人患结节性下垂状的颈部纤维瘤，这个长了20年的肿瘤被切除了，患者18日后就痊愈了。

有位来自府城（Foo-city）（注：潮州府）的老先生，舌下有个大肿瘤（**舌下囊肿**），妨碍了发音的清晰，而且使下巴肿起。肿瘤由一个充满状如蛋奶的半流质的厚厚皮囊构成，切开后液体就流出来了。在清理液体后，一部分皮囊被夹除，剩下的部分被注射碘酊。在病人离开之前，所有畸形的部分均被切掉，他也恢复了清晰的口齿。切除囊壁有效预防了肿瘤的再生。我之后听说这是一种永久性的治疗方式。

我们做过许多**唇裂**手术，大部分是由我们的中国助手完成的。他们通常让病人非常满意。举个实例，一个病人展示了以前一位中国人（客家人）收了两美元为他做的手术。手术效果尚可，但有一个大缺口仍留在唇上，病人非常希望能够被修复。他的愿望实现了。

在汕头西南面距离约60英里的葵潭（Kway-tham）传教站，有一个典型**破伤风**病例，伴随前弓反张（由于肌肉痉挛使脊柱向前弯曲），病人是一名9岁男孩。由于牙关紧闭，他不能张开口，只能被喂食流质。他脸色苍白，虚弱无比，醒着的时候总是流汗，四肢僵硬。病人还同时出现了痢疾和结肠的末端脱出，情况比较复杂。他在床上不能自己翻身，有时疼痛感很强烈。我只帮他诊治过一两次就不得不返回汕头。

很少有中国人能够接受截肢，无论保留着患病的肢体有多痛苦与多无用。然而，一位从海门（Hai-mung）来的患者肘部有严重溃疡和关节疾病，他的健康状况因此急剧恶化，所以同意接受**截肢手术**。来自台湾的麦斯威尔医生（Dr. Maxwell）和曼森医生（Dr. Manson）刚好在场，于是协助完成了手术。伤口大部分很快痊愈，病人也在两个星期后出院了。假肢在回家后装上了，但这位可怜的病人却在手术约一年半后死于肺病。很荣幸能让该病人蒙受主的恩典，他后来的生活也向我们和他的亲朋好友证明了他奉耶稣为救世主的虔诚之心。他去世后，应其要求，亲属刻了“耶稣的信徒”的汉字在他的墓碑上。

一位在牛庄（Newchwang）客船上工作时冻伤的中年中国男人接受了**截肢手术**，一只脚截去前半部分，另一只截去五根脚趾的前端。他来医院就医的时候，左脚所有的脚趾和前半部分都已呈黑色，坏死组织和残活的组织之间的界限非常清楚。右脚脚趾前端也受损，同左脚一样呈黑色。这是一例典型的**干性坏疽**。左脚被施予手术，距骨和脚踝没有截去，相当于保留半只脚。右脚只切除脚趾的最后一个关节。几个星期后，两只脚愈合得都非常好。即使其中一只脚还有一点跛，但病人已经能够到处行走，不需要支撑。他原本吸鸦片烟，但是住院之后戒除了吸食鸦片。之后他主动要求被洗礼，因他获得了对真理的智慧理解并虔诚追随，他的请求得到了满足。现在他已经成为我们医院的门卫，并且干得十分开心。

除了以上提及的，外科手术还包括坏死骨头切除、痔疮手术、瘘管切除、清除积液、睾丸海绵肿切除、拔牙、取出子弹以及大量的脓肿引流。

在1868年大约有160个儿童注射了**疫苗**，大多在周边农村。如今在许多分散的乡镇，母亲们都希望有教会医疗队到访，帮她们的孩子注射疫苗。

弃婴问题最近引起了中国北部和中部一些朋友的讨论，但尚未达成共识。如果那些报道当下中国国情的评论员们只叙述对自己所在区域的了解，不草率地以有限的数据给整个帝国下结论，这样对所有有关方面的利益都好。让他们代表各自所居住和熟悉的地区发言，也便于我们采集这个大国不同地区居民的不同陈述。我们所在的粤东北地区的数百万人口当中，弃婴问题是很常见的。没有一个来过这个地区的人不承认这个事实。我们在探访乡镇的过程中看见过弃婴的尸体浮在池塘上，或随着河流漂浮，或搁浅在浅滩上，旁边还有乌鸦飞落，也看见过有位父亲在一大清早将刚出生的女婴放在篮子里丢弃。甚至有些刚生下来就在母亲身边被勒死。弃婴问题如此普遍，以致他们从不对此罪行感到内疚，甚至还有理由开脱。据说在城市，情况比农村相对好些，弃婴通常会被丢在大街上，希望能被某些好心人收养或者安置在育婴堂。育婴堂原本在9个府都有设立，但现在缺乏足够的经费维持日常开支，大多已名存实亡。府城育婴堂在鼎盛时期曾收养过20到30个弃婴。每个护士最多负责照顾两个小孩，每月有2到3美元的固定收入，钱由公众捐款筹得。孩子们偶尔会被收养当作童养媳。据说弃婴问题在客家地区比较少见，这应该归功于他们的习俗，就是将女儿交由互定了娃娃亲的未来丈夫的家庭抚养。当然，客家女人都擅长干农活，这也许是她们被留了下来的另一个原因。为这项罪行开脱的理由很多。如果一个女人生养了一个女儿，那么有可能她在两三年内将不能生育；而如果她放弃哺育了，将更快有机会生育一个男孩。还有一个理由是，如果继续抚养女儿，将会妨碍到她干活补贴家用，而即使她将女儿养大之后，女儿也要嫁作人妇，相当于她之前的辛劳白费了。这是他们自己的道理。毫无疑问，贫穷是很大的原因，但是那些有能力抚养子嗣的人，却也深受生养女儿无用的传统观念的影响而选择弃婴。我曾和一个研究该课题的毕业生讨论过，据他估计，大约有百分之三的母亲为此感到内疚，但是我想恐怕几乎任何生过几个女儿的贫穷妇女都不会为此感到不安。无论如何，一个女儿的诞生都不是一件值得祝贺的事，而是正相反。所以，一旦有外籍朋友生下女儿，中国人一般不会祝贺，而如果是男孩则将给予慷慨祝贺。父母将他们的儿子当作他们晚年的依托，有多个儿子的父母被认为很有福气（养儿防老，多子多福）。

回顾过去6年在汕头的医疗传教工作，我们无比赞美仁慈的主所赐予我们的恩惠。由于他的祝福，数以千计潮州人的病痛引起我们的关注，并或多或少地得到缓解。我们特别要赞颂的是主对于病人们的救赎所表现的仁慈。在1868年的某一个月，至少有9个人在我们的医学工作中聆听真理后经过洗礼进入教会。在我们传教的很多地方，过去的病人往往在当地教会中扮演着重要角色，有一两位我们希望他们已在蒙召归天时安息主怀。除了平常与医院交流外，虽然不太可能，但我们希望能每天对很多人进行福音传播。那些在他们自己人当中宣称“对人亲善”的人们，通过神的祝福，正发挥着潜移默化的作用，准备着我们还未见过的“大业”。医疗机构对人们的有利影响不言而喻，且辐射范围很广，从教会弟兄得到的好消息不断证明这一点。他们还发现医院的好名声对于他们在嫉恨外国人的潮州地区通行有很大帮助，尤其是在陷入困境时。宗教活动的开展有时是由施饶理牧师和金护尔牧师（Rev. Messrs. Smith and Mackenzie）全权负责，这两位在各自的领域孜孜不倦地耕耘着，在神的庇佑下取得成功。当布道工作与医学工作一起执行时，后者能为前者传播福音提供特有的机会（这两个工作事实上都需要信念来支撑），我们也毫不犹豫地宣告医学工作对于传教计划有着最有价值的辅助作用。

来自爱丁堡的汤爱力医生（Dr. Thomson）适时地填补了我们不在时的空缺。

借此机会，我们高兴地向通过捐助的方式帮助我们的欧洲和中国朋友表示最衷心的感谢。名单附在报告的结尾处。

1868年与1869年捐款者

（略）

中国捐款者

（略）

*由 E. Vincent 先生和他的收账员接收。

（翻译：谢煊、朱悦阳　校译：朱文平　审校：胡卫清、余维泉、江建安　中文校正：许党泉、颜彦）

1877 年汕头福音医院报告

（吴威凛医学博士照管下的英兰长老会汕头教会医院 1877 年报告）

1878 年 5 月

尽管去年医院和诊所的日常工作都有条不紊地开展着，但我们大部分时间和精力都花在了新医院大楼的建设上，正如上一年度报告中提及过的。

多亏了道台热心协助，我们得以在海边一个合适的地点建设综合医院，正好毗邻西边的教会。在和中国官员的谈判过程中，我们有幸获得了英国代理领事福雷斯特先生（Mr. Forrest）的帮助。那块地离南面的海岸 120 英尺，离通向汕头的主要道路 180 英尺。四周很开阔，只有东面被教会建筑物稍微遮挡。

获得土地权之后，我们开始着手准备前期工作以便使其达标，并在九月份奠基。感谢上帝，新大楼在天气变暖之前及时完工交付使用，并在 4 月 18 日成为教会医院专用。彼时，在汕头的传教士和本地基督教徒，包括美国浸会的一些朋友，大家聚集在一起，进行与其有关的祈祷和赞美。传教士和本地弟兄作了有趣的发言。新医院真诚地寻求上帝对于医院建成的祝福。

医院建有 3 幢双层朝南的主楼。前面的一幢楼和后面两幢间隔 20 英尺，一楼全是布道堂或说是小教堂（大约 48 英尺 ×28 英尺），可以容纳 200 人；二楼有 5 个房间（门诊和手术室，还有助理室和私人办公室）。后面两幢则完全是为病人设立的，总共有 8 个房间（大约 18 英尺 ×38 英尺），每个房间有 10 张床。二楼相互间由一个阳台连着，从而可从这里通向前座的门诊部。在后面两幢楼的一边有一幢单层建筑是专门给女病人的，另一边也有一幢相似的建筑被分隔出四个小房间，是给那些愿意多付点钱住单间的人准备的。两边的围墙边有厨房、浴室等。这里有充足的床位供百来号病人使用。秉着“小屋模式”的原则，每个病房都是相互独立的。

建设新楼的资金来源于出售旧楼，还有来自汕头海外社团和中国人的慷慨捐款，包括道台捐助的 100 两银子，还有英兰长老会海外宣道会捐助的 100 英镑（495 美元），和由施饶理牧师（Rev. George Smith）从新西兰募集而来的 50 英镑（250 美元）。

综合医院在建的同时，我们也着手建设麻风病院。推动此项目的原因在于，逐年有越来越多的麻风病人前来就诊，而我们并不愿意将他们安置在综合医院。要不是因为麻风病人得不到救治，我们也不会想到建一所专科医院。但从我们的从医经验来看，大多数病情不严重的病患可以获得好转，甚至有些能够完全被治愈。不久前，一个经过长期治疗的病人离开后，完全没有了麻风病的症状，尽管他刚来的时候症状十分明显。在印度某地、特立尼达岛和其他地方，麻风病经过治疗过后也收到了满意的结果。迄今为止据我们观察，这种病不同于《圣经》中所说的麻风，而且似乎没有那么危险，虽然它如果没有被检查出来，还是迟早会致命。这个地区的中国人并没有将麻风病人与其他家庭成员隔离开来，除非出现极端的情况。他们对麻风病的接触传染性或感染性的看法从下面的本地谚语可以看出：

宁与癞瘸人同床，勿与生疥人对门。

我们在城外购置了一块地，它远离住宅区，但在综合医院附近。我们打算于此建一幢可以容纳20位病人的楼房。主要的建设费用由爱丁堡教会支付。用于建造综合医院和麻风病院的总费用将在报告最后的收支表中列出。

1863年到达汕头后，我们最初在一间租来的中式小民房里开展工作，租期一年。后来，我们搬到教会的一间老房子，把其中的一部分用作诊所，再租了相邻的房屋作为住院部。很快，建一座更大的医院的需求越来越明显。我们克服了很多困难，得到了一块空气流通、靠近水边的地，于是有了建于11年前的第一所医院。一切如我们所愿，我们也为越来越好的住宿条件和工作上的便利而感恩。然而，随着城镇的快速发展，现在它四面被围住，作为医院已经非常不适合，而住院病人越来越多，这促使我们建造一所更大型的医院来满足需求。麻风病人也经常被迫挤在一间小民房里，这完全背离我们的目标。现在我们的综合医院的病房数是之前的4倍，麻风病院也比之前的民房舒适得多。我们要将此记录下来，感恩上帝给予我们的所有便利，感谢所有给予我们各种帮助的汕头以及其他地方的朋友。正因为有他们的帮助，医院才得以建成。我们坚信这些更为完善的设施将激励我们为中国人的身心健康做出更大贡献。至少病人将在逐步改善的医疗条件和住院环境中受益，这会促使病人更容易痊愈。

这一年的就诊数受到夏末汕头霍乱暴发的一定影响，我认为也部分受到要抽时间监管建筑工程的影响。然而，本地的助手负责了大部分的医院工作，完成情况总体上令人满意。这一年的部分时间里，住院病人越来越多，这使我不得不限制综合医院和麻风病院的住院病人数，以防止在霍乱暴发期间环境太拥挤造成不良的后果。1877年病人数如下：

住院病人

综合医院 ………………………… 1 073

麻风病院 ………………………… 90—1 163

平均每天住院病人

综合医院 ………………………… 75

麻风病院 ………………………… 13—88

门诊病人

综合医院 ………………………… 1 104

麻风病院 ………………………… 181—1 285

平均每天门诊病人

（于每周两天的门诊开放日中） ………………………… 35

新病人总数 ………………………… 2 448

以上病人中的女病人

住院病人	115
门诊病人	197—312

迄今为止，病人主要来自汕头广大周边地区的乡镇，包括潮州府属的九个区域和惠州、嘉应州的部分地区，也有来自福建南部的。通常夏季是高峰，因为在那样的天气之下，他们不用带太多行李。下面的表格显示了去年各月份的日均病人数：

	住院病人	门诊病人（门诊开放日）
一月	116	42
二月	55	14
三月	88	33
四月	82	30
五月	130	62
六月	104	49
七月	78	26
八月	68	28
九月	102	30
十月	89	49
十一月	64	34
十二月	75	25

我们诊治过的疾病种类参见下表。由表中可以看出，眼科疾病和皮肤病占了将近一半。

常见病

发热，弛张热	21
间歇性发热	49—70
风湿病	145
麻风病	271
癌症	23
贫血	34
瘰疬（结核）性或梅毒性腺体肿大	15
衰弱	18
鸦片成瘾	3
水肿，全身水肿	10
腹水	5—15

神经系统疾病

头痛	6
瘫痪，面瘫	4
局部瘫痪	3
偏瘫	11—18
癫痫	3
局部麻痹	1
移动性共济失调	1
肌肉萎缩	1

消化系统疾病

喉咙疾病 …… 2
牙痛和龋齿 …… 5
牙瘘 …… 1
扁桃体炎 …… 1
消化不良 …… 112
呕血 …… 2
肠痛（绞痛） …… 5
蠕虫病，蛔虫 …… 26
　　蛔虫属 …… 1—27
便秘 …… 4
腹泻 …… 9
痢疾 …… 14
脾肿大 …… 12
黄疸 …… 1
直肠狭窄和溃疡 …… 8
脱肛 …… 7
肛瘘 …… 20
痔疮，外痔 …… 4
　　内痔 …… 21—25

呼吸系统疾病

失声 …… 11
黏膜炎 …… 29
支气管炎 …… 27
哮喘 …… 24
咯血 …… 4
肺结核 …… 46
肺炎 …… 2

循环系统疾病

心脏病 …… 3
大动脉瘤 …… 2

泌尿生殖系统疾病

肾病 …… 60
糖尿病 …… 1
排尿困难 …… 1
尿失禁 …… 1
遗精 …… 6
淋病和尿道炎 …… 4
腹股沟淋巴结炎 …… 1
包茎 …… 4
阴茎感染 …… 1
阴茎溃疡 …… 6
阴茎癌 …… 3
睾丸炎 …… 1
睾丸肿大 …… 3
鞘膜积液 …… 25
阴囊溃疡 …… 2
月经过多 …… 1
闭经 …… 1
白带过多 …… 3

皮肤病

湿疹 …… 16
脓疱病 …… 1
癣 …… 37
掌跖银屑病 …… 13
糠疹 …… 7
溃疡性狼疮 …… 1
象皮病，腿部 …… 24
　　阴囊 …… 8
　　混合 …… 1—33
脱发 …… 1

疥疮 …………………………………… 14
痒疹 …………………………………… 4
苔藓病 ………………………………… 1
痤疮 …………………………………… 3
湿疣 …………………………………… 2
硬斑病 ………………………………… 1
皮肤角化病 …………………………… 1
鸡眼 …………………………………… 1
疡肿 …………………………………… 8
痈 ……………………………………… 3
脓肿 …………………………………… 27
皮肤溃疡 ……………………………… 242

眼科疾病

视疲劳 ………………………………… 18
夜盲症 ………………………………… 2
结膜炎 ………………………………… 56
慢性结膜水肿 ………………………… 2
颗粒性眼炎 …………………………… 39
睑内翻 ………………………………… 98
倒睫症 ………………………………… 25
睑腺炎 ………………………………… 1
睑缘癣 ………………………………… 2
眼睑软骨瘤 …………………………… 2
黏液囊肿 ……………………………… 1
翼状胬肉 ……………………………… 30
角膜血管增生 ………………………… 12
血管翳 ………………………………… 1
角膜炎 ………………………………… 11
角膜溃疡 ……………………………… 53
角膜模糊 ……………………………… 89
角膜圆锥 ……………………………… 1
葡萄肿 ………………………………… 6
眼前房积脓 …………………………… 7
虹膜炎 ………………………………… 6
虹膜粘连 ……………………………… 9
白内障 ………………………………… 16
青光眼 ………………………………… 6
交感性眼炎 …………………………… 1
黑内障（黑蒙） ……………………… 4
肿瘤 …………………………………… 2
不可治愈的失明 ……………………… 39

耳朵疾病

耳漏 …………………………………… 3
耳聋 …………………………………… 6

鼻子疾病

感染 …………………………………… 2
鼻息肉 ………………………………… 7
鼻出血 ………………………………… 1
鼻孔异物 ……………………………… 1

骨科疾病

骨溃疡坏死 …………………………… 31
脊柱弯曲 ……………………………… 5

关节疾病

感染 …………………………………… 17
扭伤 …………………………………… 12
关节僵硬 ……………………………… 1

未分类的

肿瘤，纤维瘤 ………………………… 5
切割伤及其他 ………………………… 33

神经瘤	6	枪伤	2
脂肪瘤	5	打伤和擦伤	74
皮脂瘤	3	烧伤	3
神经节瘤	1	狗咬伤	5
疣状瘤	1	蛇咬伤	1
血管瘤	3	蜈蚣咬伤	1
腺体瘤	16	耳裂	10
骨质瘤	1	唇裂	45
卵巢瘤	1	腭裂	3
囊性肿瘤	4	瘢痕畸形	3
腹胀	1— 47	足内翻	1
脱臼	2		
骨折	2		

与往年一样，大部分病人都来自农民和工人阶层，也有一些来自当地社会的各个阶层。道台的儿子跟随父亲从潮州府来汕头拜访的时候也顺道来看病。离开之前他们也参观了教会，看到男子寄宿学校在汲约翰（Mr. Gibson）的打理之下运作得很好，道台甚感欣慰。

十月初，霍乱在汕头和周边一些较大的城镇和乡村流行起来。潮阳有一家八九口全部病亡。许多病人在死亡之前会出现疼痛和呕吐。在被收治入院的 6 人中有两人死了，一位几乎立即死亡，另一位发烧后逐渐衰竭而死。这是医院开业以来发生的第一批霍乱死亡病例。在中国的其他沿海地区的疫情明显要比汕头地区的更严重。

上一年，我记录了病房里死亡的罕见病例，这年该类病例比往年更多了。死亡的人中有一位是地方官吏的兄弟。他来医院时已经没有治愈的希望了，但他发现自己在医院住着比在家里舒服，于是选择在医院住下直到去世。

在中国分割遗产似乎并不比在犹太地区简单。一个前来就医的青年头部、脸部、手部有多处大伤口，据他说是被哥哥用一把大刀所伤，因为他（弟弟）发现父母死后的家庭财产分配方式不合理。之后，哥哥畏罪潜逃到别处。他的贪婪、不公、冷酷给他弟弟留下了终身伤害。奇怪的是在同一天，另一个来自不同地区的乡村青年也因和哥哥争吵后被刺伤小腿而来就医。

疝气在中国人中很常见，但我很少见无法复位的，更没见过因此而死的。疝气通常发生于右边。中国人很乐意买个外国制造的支架，尽管已用了木制和铁制的土工具。有个人向我展示过他自己创造发明的精巧木质支架。虽然它起到作用，但和欧洲进口的相比，显得很粗糙，并且不舒服。

做过的 299 个**眼科手术**中主要有以下几种：

去除睑内翻（睫毛倒插而摩擦眼球）	229
切除翼状胬肉（赘肉生长在眼球上）	38

虹膜切除术（做人工瞳孔）	4
切除白内障	8

有一个前来就医的女孩长了一颗几乎覆盖整个上眼睑到睫毛边缘的神经瘤。神经瘤被切除，虽然起初似乎由于皮肤缺失有导致睑缘大范围外翻的可能，但是最后伤口还是愈合了，而且几乎看不出任何畸形。

躯体手术大体上包括以下几种：

肿瘤切除术	26
坏死骨头切除术	8
子弹取出术	2
痔疮切除术	17
骨折固定术	1
唇裂手术	40
耳裂手术	9
肛瘘手术	14
包茎过长手术	3
鞘膜积液手术	25
腹腔穿刺术	1
畸形瘢痕切除术	1
	147

以上未将拔牙、切开脓肿等列入。

我们的本地助手有一天做了至少 14 个手术：8 个眼科、3 个唇裂、3 个鞘膜积液。

一个 12 岁女孩身上出现了一些**软瘤**，尽管表皮看起来平整无异样，但会引起极大痛感。用探针刺破其中最大的一个只发现里面有一些浆液。涂上碘酊，外加内服碘化钾和鱼肝油后，除了一两个出现了脓液，其他都消失了。女孩最后痊愈了。

一个老年人颈后部的一个**开放性肿瘤**被切除，肿瘤里面充满白垩质物质，部分附着于颈部。手术过程中出血很多，但通过压迫被止住了，随后其他赘生的东西也一同被腐蚀性药物清除掉了。伤口慢慢愈合了。

上一年我们特别留意了**唇裂**手术的数量，这年仍然只多不少，一度有来自各乡村的不少于 8 个唇裂病人在医院治疗。我们为两兄弟做了手术，之前他们的村庄也有一对患兔唇的父子被治愈了。之后，另外一对父子也为了手术而来。从开展手术到现在，我们做了大概 160 例手术。

有位妇女被一位当地医生以治疗所谓头部疾病为由刺破了鼓膜导致**耳聋**。她甚至被告知另一个选择是刺穿眼球！另外一例耳聋由殴打造成，殴打引起了出血，血从外耳流出，也沿着咽鼓管流入口腔。

一个男人 5 年前腿部被蛇咬后留下的伤口，如今变成了**溃疡**。另一个病例被蛇咬了手指，他的肘部以上的手臂被他的医生捆得紧紧的，造成了手臂大面积的瘢痕，留下了绷带引起的广泛性溃疡，手臂下段由于静脉循环受阻导致严重肿胀。另外一个病人在山坡上割草的时候，拇指根部被一条大蜈蚣咬伤，5 个月后才到医院就诊。被咬后，他出现发热症状，10 天后感到上臂疼痛。大概又过了 10 天到 15 天，疼痛蔓延到头部，最后侵蚀全身，像风湿关节痛那般。被蜈蚣咬伤后出现这样的症状还是不常见的。

1877 年初，从一开始便与我一起进行医疗传教的总助理离开了，开始在汕头和周边的农村独立行医。他确实是位得力的助手，在外科手术中胆大心细，经验丰富。对于他的离开我感到很遗憾。之后，另外一位年龄较大的助手取代了他，这位助手之前几年也在自己所在乡村的周边地区独立行医。他感到实际报酬与期望有差距后便欣然返回医院工作。虽然精力和勇气不及前者，但无论是在医疗工作中，还是在为病人举行宗教仪式中，他都很有帮助。

病人通过晨祷和晚祷，渐渐地被指引成为耶稣的信徒。与前几年一样，这项工作得到了我目前在这个领域的同事金护尔（Mackenzie）和汲约翰（Gibson）牧师的热情帮助。在汕头和农村的传教任务日渐繁重，以至他们每周只能负责 3 个早上。本地助理和我则负责其他的礼拜。每个星期天下午有一项针对病人的特殊服务。目前所见的结果与以往的经验没有实质上的不同。许多听过的人反应冷漠，有些已经相信基督教的真理而放弃偶像崇拜（注：拜老爷），少数已经投身成为基督徒。那些因此决定接受基督真理的人，不久便发现基督教与偶像崇拜是对立的。一个来自 12 英里开外农村的老人和另外两个病人一同接受了洗礼。一段时间后，他身体有了好转回家了，我们相信他通过耶稣拥有了永生。之后他回到医院告诉我们，他的亲戚因为听说他信了耶稣，竟然在他回家之前砸了他的房子和家具。那些耕种他的田地的农民也拒绝向他交租。因此他打算把田地卖了，但是他的亲戚不但阻止其他人购买，自己也不愿给他合理的价钱。亲戚们还说因为他放弃了对祖宗和老爷的崇拜，所以不允许他继续住在村里。老人很伤心。他曾经在新加坡待过几年，之后带着 200 美元返乡，拿出 80 美元建了一幢小住宅，剩下的钱大部分用来买田地，如今却被亲戚们剥夺了。我们建议他返回家里，采取温和的方式拿回他的财产。他照我们说的做了，之后告诉我们他从迫害他的人手中收回了几亩地，租给了他认为信得过的一个朋友。由于他的房子还是破的，我们建议他修好房子后继续住在村里，希望他通过一贯的生活，缓和他的亲戚们的敌对情绪，并向他的亲戚和乡亲逐渐介绍基督教的原理。这个地区的其他地方也发生过类似的更严重的迫害，基督教徒依靠神恩赐的支撑力量，最大限度地忍受了责骂和财物损失。必须指出，认为中国人信奉了基督教后就必然获得好处的这种想法是错误的，这只能作为一种世俗的愿望。这种情况不是没有的，但信教之后往往会受到迫害和损失。起码在农村，在没有外籍人士影响和帮助的情况下就是如此。很多信众已经做好了承受一切而不放弃真理的准备，而这源于他们身心中的一股神圣的力量。

我们欣喜地记录下我们应尽的义务，感谢慷慨贡献财物帮助建设新医院的朋友们。感谢 Schjöth 先生帮我们获取外国和本地海关的本土关员的支持，还有在德记洋行（Messrs. Bradley & Co.）和 E. 文森特洋行（Messrs. E. Vincent & Co.）工作的中国朋友帮我们收取在汕头的中国商人的捐助。同时也要感谢一些女性朋友，她们为我们提供外科敷料、住院服和病人其他用品所需要的白棉花。陈源盛行（Tang Ngwan Seng Hong）的老朋友又向我们慈善捐助了2 000张现金券和大米给贫穷的病人，总值超过50美元。他代表远方沿海城市的行业协会成员买下了老医院。他们已经把老医院改造成为商店或仓库，每年的租金作为在这片海域淹死的海员和其他人的丧葬费的基金。因此，它虽然不再是医院，但显然仍为慈善服务。

日常费用资金的捐款者

（略）

新医院建设资金的捐款者

（略）

新医院建设资金的中国捐款者

（略）

收支表

单位：美元

助手、门卫、厨师和其他人员1877年12个月工资		237.17
日常费用（包括在这里买药品）		212.10
印刷医院报告及其他费用		27.80
援助贫困患者费用		20.00
援助贫困患者现金券和大米费用		55.00
从伦敦购买药物费用		340.00
建新综合医院的费用：		
平整场地、石堤等	553.16	
建筑、粉刷等	3 879.65	
家具等	260.50	
		——4 693.31
建麻风病院的费用：		
买地、填土	210.15	
建筑、粉刷等	718.35	
家具等	23.00	
		——951.50
可用于1878年日常开支的结余款		212.84
		6 749.72

1875年5月

查核无误

金护尔（H. L. Mackenzie）

1876年结余款	867.48
日常费用捐款，如上表列	289.00
新医院建设捐款，如上表列	1 205.00
中国人捐款，如上表列	543.00
向贫困患者捐献的现金和大米票券价值	55.00
卖老医院收入	2 000.00
英兰长老会海外宣道会向综合医院拨款100英镑	495.12
爱丁堡教会向麻风病院拨款100英镑	495.12
由施饶理牧师筹集的新西兰捐款50英镑和利息	253.03
杂项	43.82
出售药品、绑带等收入	131.31
出售戒鸦片药丸收入	25.94
由爱丁堡教会支付的来自伦敦的药物价值	340.00
患者捐款（不包含在上表中）	5.90
	6 749.72

吴威凛（William Gauld）

（翻译：谢煊、朱悦阳　校译：朱文平　审校：胡卫清、余维泉、江建安　中文校正：许党泉、颜彦）

1880 年汕头福音医院报告

（吴威凛医学博士和来爱力医学学士、外科硕士照管下的
英兰长老会汕头教会医院 1880 年报告）

又到了该向汕头教会医院的朋友提交简短工作总结的时候了。1880 年的这份报告肯定比往年的要短一点、粗略一点。负责监督这项工作的吴威凛医生（Dr. Gauld），在过去的 16 年中只有一次回家作短暂休假，他的个人成就和专业上的成就对于西方医学科学的释疑和提高人们的信心有很大帮助，他在早春回家休假 3 个月，这是他应得的。他的临时继任者的语言问题一定程度上限制了其对工作的投入。

然而，医院工作的两部分——医疗和传教工作在这一年不间断地开展着。吴威凛医生训练的本地助理，积极参与医疗和传教工作，表现很令人满意。

就像前几年一样，每个星期有两天是门诊时间，有 4 天是医院工作和手术时间，这样的安排对病人和医护人员来说都很合理。

住院病人——去年住院病人数超过往年，达到 2 403 例，比前一年多了 375 例。到了夏末和秋天，总院和分院都挤满了病人，要做好所有的工作是困难的。虽然我们尝试通过尽量不让住在汕头附近的病情不严重的病人住院来减少人数，但是九月和十月的住院病人数平均仍多达 239 人，十月初更是在一个星期之内增加到 304 人。这个数字被认为是我们两所医院所能容纳的极限。大部分病人来自周边 60 ~ 80 英里范围内的许多乡镇农村，想治好他们，就必须将他们收进医院。在平时这样做绝对有好处，因为平常我们可以用一种更令人满意的方式对他们进行治疗，又有良好的环境对他们进行传教。但当疾病流行时，我们无法控制病人数，不得不去接收更多病人。

通常只有经历过的人才知道，要想让一个从 20 ~ 60 英里以外跑来汕头求医的中国人相信我们这里已经没有空房是件多么困难的事，特别是他们之前已经省吃俭用几个星期才筹出能让他在外地生存的这笔开销。有一天，6 位妇女结伴从内陆约 50 英里外一个叫棉湖的乡镇来到汕头，她们都患有眼睑内翻，正处在发病初期，只需一个小手术和几天的术后疗养便可痊愈。但医院满床了，她们被告知在另一个月才可来。于是，黄昏时分她们干脆在楼梯上铺上席子，打算晚上就在那里睡觉。在这样的情况下，我们不得不让步，为她们找到住宿，几天后她们的眼睛治好了就回家了。这种事情在那两个月经常发生。

大量病人在秋天涌入，可能是刚刚过去的夏天气候恶劣的缘故。在春天和初夏雨下得异常大而且久，大片土地被淹没了一个多月，许多地方的农作物完全被毁坏了。居民说他们在盛夏时忍受着无家可归和贫穷，生活过得很糟糕。冬种过后，我们收了很多从洪灾地区来的病人。

平均每个病人的住院天数为 23 天。

门诊病人——汕头诊所诊治的门诊病人多达 1 346 人，比前一年多了 266 人。这部分工作几乎都由两位高级助理主管。九月和十月病人数也相对增加，这两个月，平均每个门

诊开放日诊治66位病人，最多一天是117人。同时，我们也下乡施医赠药，给510位病人看了病，还做了些小手术。

下面的列表给出了每个月新增病人数量和其他方面的统计数据，能大致显示我们的工作量：

	住院病人	门诊病人	总数
一月	129	55	
二月	32	26	
三月	202	106	
四月	187	96	
五月	279	88	
六月	211	120	
七月	207	86	
八月	174	111	
九月	267	134	
十月	376	236	
十一月	129	132	
十二月	210	156	
	2 403	1 346	=3 749
下乡诊治病人数			510
			4 259

平均每天病人数：

一月至七月住院病人	124
七月至一月住院病人	183
一月至七月门诊病人	28
七月至一月门诊病人	48

以上病人数所包含的女病人数：

住院病人	465
门诊病人	286
	751

许多农村病人请求得到所需要的西药，他们因为各种原因无法到汕头来。治疗发热、痢疾、腹泻、衰弱的药物最受欢迎。我们满足了许多这种需求，并注意防止任何欺诈。

这一年的女性住院病人数很有意思，它显示出人们对医院越来越有信心。女性住院病人多达 465 人，比前一年多了 178 人，当中有相当大一部分是年轻妇女。她们通常由一位年长的女性亲属陪同前来，这位亲属通常也是医院的病人。看来很有必要单独开辟一间能容纳 20 个人住宿的大病房。但即使有额外的空间，她们的病房还是经常人满为患。一位睿智的信教老妪被指定为她们那个区域的护士长。她对女病人和女病房行使一般管理职责，并帮助包扎伤口，用一种安静的方式传教。病人们对她很友善，而她也乐于展现她的机智幽默。她只工作了 10 个星期，却在许多方面都帮上了忙。我们对于一些训练有素的本地护士的需求由来已久，希望她是个好的开端。

病人的构成和之前几年差不多。一些小官员和不同级别的文人也来门诊看病，但我们的病人主体还是乡村居民（商人和农民），他们大多很贫穷。陈源盛（Tang Nguan Seng）仍然为穷苦的病人提供大米和现金券。这一年我们总共从他那里收到价值 91 美元的捐赠，还有一位匿名捐助者提供了价值 7 美元的资助。几个病人已得到来自医院基金的一些援助。在分发大米和现金券时我们特别留意，防止有人为此在医院作不必要的逗留。

医治的病例表见附录。对于不想研究它的读者，我们提供一篇简短的摘要。

一、内科

疟疾——诊治了 41 例简单发热和 103 例间歇性发热病例，最流行的是隔日热。大多数发热病人在夏季被收入院，有许多病程已很长。患病已大约 6 个月、8 个月或 10 个月的并不少见。这种病通常还伴有贫血以及局部的水肿，有时是全身性的水肿。

在间歇发热和疟疾病人的**后遗症**中我们发现了 10 例肝脏增大、33 例脾脏增大、165 例贫血和大批的疟疾源性手足溃烂。几例肝脏肿大特别严重，肝脏扩大到骨盆边缘，其他的或多或少都有腹水。在贫血的病例中有相当数量的被中国人称为“败身”（pai sien）的病例。这种病的特质仍不能确定。其症状是全身衰弱，尿液中固体成分明显增加。中国人很害怕这种病，把它归结为许多其他疾病的根源。这种病发病前有时会发热，但其他病例没有表现出发热的历史。至少，在许多病例中，这似乎是一种疟疾源性贫血，伴随很明显的神经衰弱症状。对于这类疾病的治疗，每个低热及间歇热病例都在使用奎宁后迅速好转，一些病例的肝脾肿大迅速减轻，但其他病例，尤其那些有合并贫血和腹水的病例，没有收到任何效果。许多贫血病人的治疗效果是令人非常不满意的。这主要是由于两个原因，一是疾病的持续时间长，二是铁剂对胃肠黏膜有刺激作用，尤其是在炎热的月份。5 个最小剂量单位的着色氯化铁常导致腹泻，甚至痢疾。当给予药丸时病人更能承受药物作用。

麻风病——87 例麻风病人前来就医，但由于没有为他们提供特别的治疗——之前几年用于隔离麻风病人的一栋小楼全年都被当作普通病房使用——因此没有太多关于他们的情况报告。一些病人有规律地每隔一段时间就前来门诊看病，但大多数病人收了或者买了些能用上一两个月的药物就被送回家了。麻木型麻风比结核型麻风更为常见，我们观察到的麻木型麻风的主要症状如下：①常见在踝关节、膝盖、臀部，或在胸部和手臂的一小部分皮肤上有痛感，但没有明显的结构改变；②出现类似的斑点，由一条稍微苍白的红线包围着，将健康的和患病的皮肤明确分开；③出现红色斑点，微微凸起增厚，边缘溃疡，中心苍白麻木，从前一种发展到这种状况中间有各种过渡阶段，有些类似于常见的癣；④脚底上出现小的圆形深溃疡，像被剜掉了，周围的皮肤增厚和麻木；⑤肌肉萎缩引起手指和脚趾挛缩；⑥脚趾周围溃疡；⑦皮肤上出现有感觉缺失的褐色斑点。

毒血症——11 个毒血症病例是由于吃了病死的水牛肉而发病的。他们出现了同样的症状——腿部和手臂坏疽，看起来像脓包，一部分病例伴随出现相当程度的发热。发热很快就退了，但是有些人的恢复期却延长了。

鸦片成瘾——像我们这种大型综合医院的病房并不适合治疗此类疾病，因为需要更多的人力去照顾和监管，而我们已有过多病人。20 例申请入院治疗脱瘾，其中有 12 例能够自我控制并至少能暂时戒瘾而出院。治疗的计划是马上停止吸食鸦片，然后用奎宁和芳香兴奋剂代替。尽管一些病例症状严重，但没有病例需要重新吸食。在其他病例中，有一位已是肺结核晚期，被建议不要尝试。一个每天食用大量鸦片渣的瘦弱女人，并没有全心全意地尝试戒毒。她拒绝立马停止吸食，在急性症状缓解之后立马就离开了医院。两个来医院的男人说他们曾经戒毒，但回家后就又吸上了。他们的行为很可疑，在被要求做诚信保证后，就离开了医院。另外两个病人努力戒毒，但最终失败了。他们在住院五六天后，一般的疗效没有出现。于是我们在晚上快关闭大门时查房，发现他们不在，去汕头“买东西”了。我们向他们指出去汕头会延迟他们的治疗，最好将手头的现金交予助手，助手会找到一个值得信赖的人帮他们购物，可他们却离开了。到我们这里来的吸鸦片者每天的吸食量从 1 到 4 个德拉克马不等，显然，他们寻求治疗的主要动机是害怕不戒掉恶习将会饿死。一位因另一种病就医了几个月的高级官员每天在妻子协助下吸食价值一美元的鸦片。

消化系统疾病——这里最常见的是消化不良。各种类型的都有，最典型的一种的症状是打嗝、呕酸水、间断或周期性疼痛。大多数病例身体已受极度损害，治疗也比较困难。主要的病因有：①每餐吃过多米饭的习惯；②挨饿，食物品质差，这更常见；③还有些是痢疾引起的。第二种病因引起的最难治疗，因为住院期间这个病因也存在。这个群体中的许多人是大米和现金券的接受者，其必要性是不容置疑的。

风湿病在炎热和寒冷的月份都很常见。肌风湿病是最常见的，慢性风湿性关节炎也不罕见，留观的急性风湿病仅有一例。

呼吸系统疾病——诊治了 279 例。慢性支气管炎最常见，肺结核次之。肺结核并不罕见，各种病情阶段的都有，且病程都很长。

外因病是很常见的，其中的一些病例，以及一些红斑狼疮的病人，外貌非常令人讨厌。

死亡——这年共有 5 人死亡，其中两个不是病人。一个是年轻女乞丐，她被发现在医院的空地上奄奄一息，是被她的朋友放在那里，然后被遗弃的。她两小时后死了，医院基金出资为她举行了一个体面的葬礼。一个年轻的职业小偷，患有痢疾和贫血，在半昏迷状态下被他的朋友送到医院来，他的朋友抛下他悄悄地溜走了。他苟延残喘了几天，在此期间他的朋友们被找到了。一位中年男性患肝充血，伴随急性痢疾而致命。一个请求接受洗礼的 16 岁年轻小伙子因为贫血在我们这治疗了两个月。他的病情已经大为好转，就在他准备回家之际，又突患痢疾。他不久后又痊愈了，可是两天后，在助理不知情的情况下，他出去散步，经过小吃摊的时候买了个菠萝，吃了很大一部分，几个小时后就忽然不省人事并死去。最后一个死者是个从江西来旅游的书生，他是个瘾君子，肝肿大并伴有腹水。他的总体情况并没有多大希望康复，但他还是迫切希望被收进医院，因为他饿坏了，而且除此之外唯一的选择是流落街头很快死去，所以他被同意入院了。

二、眼科疾病和皮肤病

眼科疾病和皮肤病占了所有受诊疾病的足足三分之一，单单眼科疾病就有超过 900 例，其种类和数量很难在这份报告中一一陈述清楚。大约 70 例是单只或者双眼完全损坏的，病因一般是角膜脱落，其次是化脓性或颗粒性结膜炎，还有一些是视神经坏死的，这些我们都无能为力。另一类是顽疾和性质复杂的病例，涉及眼睛几个部位的更为常见。其中的许多病人就医了很长一段时间，按惯例来说疾病通常会得到诊治，但视力损伤或多或少还是会残留。然而大部分病例还是可以治疗的。

三、外科手术

下面是这一年来做过的外科手术：

眼科手术：

睑内翻及倒睫症手术	378
翼状胬肉手术	79
瘢痕性睑外翻手术	2
睑缘粘连手术	2
白内障手术	21
虹膜切除术	14
小管切开术	4
前房切开术	1
眼球切除术	3
肿瘤（小）切除术	3
	——507

躯体手术：

肛瘘手术	32
唇裂手术	33
耳裂手术	18
鼻孔闭合手术	2
肛门挛缩手术	2
烧伤后（疤痕）挛缩手术	1
鞘膜积液开口引流术	31
肿瘤切除术	18

阴囊象皮病切除术	3
嘴唇上皮癌切除术	2
子宫息肉切除术	1
嘴唇整形手术	1
包皮环切术	5
腹股沟疝手术	2
手指切除术	1
阴茎切除术	2
手掌切除术	1
坏死骨头切除术	15
拔牙	80
子弹取出术	3
鼻息肉切除术	12
异物取出术	2
痔疮切除术	45
窦道切开术	10
下颌关节僵硬手术	1
骨折固定	4
脱臼复位	5
尿道狭窄扩张术	3
	——335
总数	842

大部分的眼睑内翻和翼状胬肉手术以及相当数量的全身小手术都由我们的两位本地高级助理完成。长时间和高强度的工作量让他们积累了丰富的经验，手术结果也非常让人满意。许多眼睑内翻病例是顽疾，都伴随着由眼睫毛刺激引起的发炎和角膜模糊。模糊的状况在术后得到某种程度的改善，手术前患者往往只有微弱的光感，后来视力恢复了四五成。病人用他们独有的方式表达感激，向我们送来许多蛋糕等。

白内障——有 21 例白内障摘除或驱散手术。其中两例失败了，但其他的都成功了，从而使病人或多或少恢复了视力。

虹膜切除术——这种手术通常是为了治疗角膜模糊、前房粘连和青光眼的。有 3 例没有治疗效果。

唇裂——29 例单唇裂和 4 例双唇裂通过手术治愈。上述病例中有两例伴随腭裂，情况较为复杂，我们希望他们不久后也回来治疗腭裂。33 例中，只有 4 例是女性。事实上，与其说这种发育异常女性相对少见，不如说女孩的这种病很少受到中国父母关注。

阴囊象皮病——这一年有 3 例这类肿瘤被切除，预后良好。肿瘤的重量分别是 112 盎司、166 盎司、180 盎司。

子宫息肉——病人大约 35 岁，长期有带血的分泌物排出。息肉有小柚子大小，被使用绞勒器成功切除。

手掌截肢——一个从汕头周边农村来的青年男子被土糖寮中的石磨压伤了手掌，肌腱、血管、软组织严重压伤，他用一条竹丝绑住手腕后才止住血。我们对其实施了截肢手术，一块皮瓣轻微脱落，但肉芽生长使伤口很快愈合了。

鱼骨头刺进脚——一大块鱼骨头被从一位男人的脚底下剔除。这块鱼骨头在那里已经5年了，并引起了很大的痛苦。

肿瘤——这些病例中最引人注意的是长在颈部的肿瘤病例，4个此部位的大肿瘤被成功切除。有一个病例的肿瘤长到腮腺附近，牵涉到面部神经，务必切除。该病人一边面部肌肉瘫痪了。病人还是个瘾君子，但是急于切除肿瘤而否认了该事实。手术过后的那个晚上，病人毒瘾开始发作，整个人看起来就像是溺水那样呼吸困难，吸食大剂量的鸦片后他恢复了。当发现吸食鸦片不利他术后恢复时，他就戒了。

这一年来没有因为手术死亡的事件发生。中国人对于手术很配合。他们用坚忍的意志忍受疼痛，很少休克，伤口愈合得很好。很难理解为什么外科治疗很少引起负面结果。通常手术的条件并不像我们想象的那么好，但除了预计将会出现发烧，会预防性地使用几天奎宁和铁剂进行初步治疗外，患者体质很少变差，伤口也很少恶化。他们很能接受开刀，常急切恳求进行眼科手术、肿瘤切除等。但是无论情况有多危急，他们还是非常反对截肢。有几次由于病人拒绝接受手术，错过了抢救的最好时机，我们什么都做不了，只能眼巴巴地看着病人被送回家。以下是一些例子。一个从南澳岛来的大约35岁的男人被确诊患腕骨和掌骨骨疡。他的手已经患病12年，完全是无用的，必须靠一个木夹板支撑。他处在人生的盛年，但一直无法做任何工作，他的健康状况也开始变得糟糕。一个12岁男孩由于足部和踝关节功能紊乱，骨头因骨疡而完全软化，并发软组织溃疡而被父亲带来治疗。男孩患脚疾已经3年，不能行走。在这两例中，通过截肢切除病变部位的建议都未被采纳。

枪伤——只有一个最近受伤的病例。一个年轻人在枪开火时不小心挡在了前面，结果中枪了，伤得很重，在下腹壁、腹股沟、左肩和手上都有很大的伤口。后来伤口严重腐烂了，他在医院待了整整两个月才能回家。

一位17年前左脚被枪击中的老人被收治入院，由于伤口溃烂严重，差不多半只脚都没了。残端是一个大量不利健康的细菌聚集的部位，轻微的刺激便会引起出血。他拒绝截肢，其他的治疗又不起作用，他回家时身体非常虚弱。

子弹取出术——从两个病人中弹的部位可以看出，他们是躲闪不及的。其中一个被子弹射穿锁骨，锁骨一分为二，子弹留在两块碎骨之间。另一个所中子弹从大腿前面射入，穿进皮肤，正落在腿部大血管的内表面上。这两个病例的子弹都轻易地被取出了。

从医院的工作中可以一窥社会生活和人们的习惯，境况并不如意。一个男人由于大量失血休克被收入医院，他身上有个4英寸长的伤口，一边的头部和脸部上有很多割伤和擦伤。他的朋友为我们讲述了如下故事：病人在一艘买卖苦力的蒸汽轮船上当厨师，刚从新加坡回来。在返回位于一个距离汕头几英里的渔村的家途中，他遇到拦路抢劫，被人击中头部，并被抢走了30美元，这些钱是他最后这趟出行赚的。我们和其他人对他的朋友给予了帮助，希望该地区的官员能够重视这件事情，找出嫌疑人将其绳之以法。同时一个重要的法医学调查似乎将要进行，因为有另外一个相反的故事传出：病人的伤是为了骗他的债主而自残造成的。从受伤的性质和程度来看，想要证明后者那个事实成立的话，还需要更多的证据，但它充分满足了官方法规。我们遇到了一些例子说明妇女缠足的流行风俗多么邪恶，它在这里和中国其他地区很常见。一个 17 岁的漂亮而懂礼貌的女孩由于大脚趾上有个坏疽而入院。在入院前不久她开始被缠足，导致出现坏疽的状况。她的母亲是一个看起来很严厉的女人。她认为，由于她还另有 3 个女儿，她没在这个女儿出生时扼死她已有大大的功劳。她一开始对解开缠足有些反对，但最终还是同意了。解开缠足重负之后，足部健康的和坏疽的组织之间形成分界线，我们正考虑是否截肢，但这位女孩之前被许配给的曾经反对她来医院的男人要求订婚，于是她被带回了家。6 个月后，我们调查得知，她脚趾上的疮还在，而缠足继续进行着。

外伤、瘀伤等——这类病例数量很可观，包括最近的 5 个脱臼和 4 个骨折病例，还有一个是脑震荡，大多伤情不重。至于瘀伤，令人印象深刻的是许多源于邻里间和家庭内部的争吵。胸部、背部、腿部是最容易受伤的部位。这些瘀伤是由削尖的竹竿打人时其末端抽打身体造成的。表面看起来没什么事，其实这样的殴打导致严重的肌肉瘀伤，过后便会像得了风湿病那样疼，通常要持续好几年，有时会对整体健康造成伤害。胸部受伤后通常出现咯血。其他病例是因为做了违背良心的事被朋友和邻居打而受伤的。实行基督教的忏悔在许多中国农村并非易事，我们的医院工作证明了这一点。惩罚方式常是殴打和各种方式的虐待。

有几个病例是因所谓的品行不端遭受严厉惩戒的对象。如果这些惩罚不能产生守法的公民，那么伤情再严重也产生不了他们想要的结果。一例刺伤是一个外国海员酒后闹事造成的。

传教工作——宗教服务如之前几年那样进行着。在医院工作开始之前先做晨间祷告，晚间做礼拜，每天如此。卓威廉和汲约翰牧师（Rev. Messrs. Duffus and Gibson）每周负责 3 天的祷告，其他的时候由两位高级助理负责。吴威凛医生（Dr. Gauld）在年初和金护尔牧师（Rev. Mr. Mackenzie）在年底对这项工作给予了协助。修女不时来访女病房，但其他事务和流行疾病对她们的访问有较大影响。

至于传教成果，目前有众多请求进入教会的申请者，但只有一位的请求得到允许。为进一步的指导和检查，我们鼓励其他申请者出院后前往他们家附近的教堂。这些申请者中，已知有 6 人在他们的家乡继续坚持信奉上帝。一个为了参加礼拜已经放弃了他的水手职业；另一个经历了许多迫害。后者的人生经历非常坎坷，她是个中年寡妇，二月份眼睛成功进行过手术。她已故的丈夫的朋友极力反对她放弃原有的信仰，但她很坚持，所以他们对她很残暴。他们无情和残酷的对待使她终日以泪洗面，她从医院回家约 6 个月后，哭泣使她眼睛发炎，最后导致全盲。但是无论如何，她还是坚持信奉上帝。

因为许多申请者都不识字，于是我们在每天下午开办课程，教他们诵读赞美诗，又给他们释义，班级人数为 4 到 30 人。两个以前的病人在乡下的教会接受了洗礼，我们相信去年的许多申请者将一一入会。

财务——从附录中可以看到，这一年的收入有 2 023. 13 美元，支出 1 551. 20 美元，结余的 461. 93 美元可供 1881 年的前几个月使用。对此，我们衷心感谢社会各界对我们的慷慨捐助。

我们感谢 E. J. 史葛医生（Dr. E. J. Scott）一年来的多次帮助。我们也对卓威廉牧师和汲约翰牧师（Rev. Messrs. Duffus and Gibson）在口译和许多方面提供的帮助表示深深的感恩。

1880 年捐款者

（略）

收支表

单位：美元

助手等人员的工资	294.70
吴威凛博士购买药品和地图的费用	35.57
印刷医院报告、邮资费用	29.91
在中国买药的费用	161.31
从伦敦购买销售用药物的费用	114.79
从伦敦购买医院用药物的费用	530.59
援助贫困患者费用	14.95
维修、替换排水沟等费用	147.67
买猪油、油、纸张等	47.04
买布绷带	30.70
买制作搽剂、酊剂的杜松子酒	61.02
买水	44.60
杂项	38.35
结余	461.93
	2 013.13

1879 年结余款	264.03
如上表列捐款	720.27
卖地图	3.00
卖疝气绑带	27.48
卖戒鸦片药丸	10.48
卖药	385.85
卖牛奶	37.63
卖杂物	20.12
小病房租金	13.68
由爱丁堡教会支付的来自伦敦的药物费用	530.59
	2 013.13

治疗疾病目录

常见病

出痘 …… 2
低热 …… 41
间歇性发热：
日发疟 …… 20
三日疟 …… 74
四日疟 …… 3
不规则热 …… 6
慢性风湿病 …… 98
胸痛 …… 27
腰痛 …… 34
坐骨神经痛 …… 15
慢性关节风湿病和风湿性关节炎 …… 32
梅毒 …… 32
先天性梅毒 …… 5
甲状腺肿大与梅毒性腺体肿大 …… 31
溃疡性狼疮 …… 13
面部侵蚀性溃疡 …… 2
贫血 …… 165
衰弱 …… 34
毒血症 …… 11
鸦片成瘾 …… 20
肿瘤：
皮脂瘤 …… 4
脂肪瘤 …… 8
粉瘤 …… 2
腮腺瘤 …… 2
颌下腺瘤 …… 3
宫颈肿瘤 …… 34
骨质瘤 …… 2
痣 …… 2
牙龈瘤 …… 1
膀胱肉瘤 …… 2
乳腺硬癌 …… 2
乳腺腺瘤 …… 3
——64
甲状腺肿 …… 2
腹水 …… 14

神经系统疾病

移动性共济失调 …… 4
癫痫 …… 7
面瘫 …… 1
臂部瘫痪 …… 1
偏瘫 …… 6
截瘫 …… 3
中暑 …… 1
眩晕 …… 13
躁狂症 …… 1
痴呆症 …… 1
神经痛 …… 5

呼吸系统疾病

失声 …… 39
急、慢性支气管炎 …… 125
结核性肺炎 …… 69
肺气肿 …… 11
咯血 …… 21
肺炎 …… 2
喉溃疡 …… 4

耳朵疾病

耳漏 …… 12
炎症 …… 2
外耳道湿疹 …… 1
肿瘤 …… 2
损伤 …… 1
耳聋 …… 1

鼻子疾病

黏膜溃疡 …… 8
前鼻孔闭锁 …… 2
鼻出血 …… 1
鼻黏膜息肉 …… 14
鼻息肉恶变 …… 1
鼻孔异物 …… 1

循环系统疾病

心脏肥大 …… 1
瓣膜病 …… 25
静脉曲张 …… 5

消化系统疾病

唇溃疡 …… 3
唇上皮瘤 …… 3
单侧唇裂 …… 32
双侧唇裂 …… 4
齿龈溃疡 …… 2
口疮 …… 5
舌头肿大 …… 3
舌上皮瘤 …… 3
腭溃疡 …… 3
咽溃疡 …… 10
扁桃体炎 …… 6
食道狭窄 …… 5
消化不良 …… 191
绞痛 …… 18
痢疾 …… 34
腹泻 …… 30
蠕虫病 …… 25
直肠狭窄 …… 9
内痔 …… 38
外痔 …… 8
肛瘘 …… 39
直肠溃疡 …… 3
直肠脱垂 …… 3
肛门收缩 …… 2
湿疣 …… 7
肝硬化 …… 4
肝肿大 …… 10
肝充血 …… 3
黄疸病 …… 3
脾肿大 …… 33
疝气 …… 33

眼科疾病

睑内翻及倒睫症 …… 216
皮脂溢性睑板腺炎 …… 25
眼睑粘连 …… 2
睑球粘连 …… 4
眼睑脓肿 …… 2
角膜炎 …… 16
化脓性角膜炎 …… 3
角膜血管增生 …… 21
前葡萄肿 …… 8
虹膜炎 …… 7

睑腺炎	3
眼睑淀粉样肿瘤	3
眼睑挛缩	2
泪囊化脓	2
眼睑瘘管	2
眼眶凹陷	1
泪点和鼻泪管阻塞	25
翼状胬肉	57
颗粒性结膜炎	117
脓疱性结膜炎	2
化脓性结膜炎	8
卡他性结膜炎	50
角膜混浊	65
角膜溃疡	85
角膜脱落	5
单眼损毁	46
双眼损毁	28
虹膜炎粘连	22
虹膜脱出	29
白内障（硬）	42
白内障（软）	6
虹膜脉络膜炎	2
眼前房积脓	5
虹膜震颤	1
青光眼	7
视神经炎	4
视神经萎缩	13
黑内障（黑蒙）	3
色素性视网膜炎	3
视网膜色素变性	1
夜盲症	2
眼癌	3
眼眶肿瘤	3
眼外伤	2

泌尿生殖系统疾病

鞘膜积液	39
精索鞘膜积液	1
阴囊溃疡	10
阴囊窦道	4
睾丸炎	4
睾丸肿物	3
阴囊积液（丝虫病）	4
阴囊象皮病	19
遗精	26
淋病	13
淋病疣	3
腹股沟淋巴结炎	11
硬下疳	7
包茎	5
包茎嵌顿	2
阴茎癌	3
阴茎损毁	2
阴茎溃疡	10
尿道破裂	2
尿道瘘	1
尿道狭窄	3
尿失禁	3
膀胱炎	3
血尿	1
慢性蛋白尿	3
白带过多	16
闭经	4
月经过多	2
子宫出血	3
痛经	1
尿道息肉	1
外阴炎	3
卵巢肿瘤	2

皮肤病

病名	例数
肢体象皮病	29
背部象皮病	1
头皮湿疹	15
头皮黄癣	7
断发毛菌癣	6
体癣	89
叠瓦癣	8
湿疹	22
花斑癣	2
银屑病	5
疥疮	25
痤疮	1
脓肿	19
脓疱疹	5
白斑病	2
疤痕	1
黄褐斑	3
印度痘（雅司病）	4
腋臭	2
缺真皮病	2
甲床炎	1
坏疽	1
甲沟炎	2
疖痈	12
溃疡	260

骨科疾病

病名	例数
骨溃疡坏死	69
脊柱弯曲	14

关节疾病

病名	例数
感染	33
扭伤	14
关节僵硬	8

未分类的

病名	例数
脱臼	8
骨折	7
肌腱和瘢痕挛缩	9
肌肉萎缩	3
畸形	2
皮裂伤	33
枪伤	4
子弹埋入	3
烧伤和烫伤	7
狗咬伤	4
蛇咬伤	1
脸颊窦口	2
鱼骨头刺入脚	1
铁刺刺入手臂	1
耳撕裂伤	18
打伤和瘀伤	11
胸部损伤（因负重和殴打）	62
脑震荡	1

（翻译：谢煊、朱悦阳　校译：朱文平　审校：胡卫清、余维泉、江建安　中文校正：许党泉、颜彦）

1882 年汕头福音医院报告

（来爱力医学学士、外科硕士照管下的英兰长老会汕头教会医院 1882 年报告）

我年初因为医学传教工作出差了几个星期，而且春季的工作任务也比往常更繁重，这些妨碍了我早些递交一份简短回顾过去一年汕头教会医院工作的报告。这份工作报告可以为支持医院工作的或想知道工作进展的朋友们提供信息。

报告中的这些内容可能与大众利益关系不大，但我们的工作能在某种程度上缓解了许多没人关心的贫苦老百姓和为了治疗而求助于我们的人的痛苦和病情，我们很有成就感。

我有两次因为身体虚弱的原因不得不离开我的岗位几个星期，但本地助理能在我缺席期间继续工作。在我第二次请假时，他们得到了我们教会客家分会的列威廉牧师（Rev. Dr. Riddel）的指导。

我们的本地助理当中，除了门卫等，共有 6 男 1 女，其中的一个男生是学生，没有工资。他们除了负责医院的日常工作，还担负着病人术后的照料工作，他们用一种愉快和满足的态度工作着。两位高级助理甚至能够提供更有价值的帮助，除了积极参与医院里的传教工作外，还用正规的方法做了许多小手术，并能治疗被诊断出来的常见病，效果令人满意。年中，还有另外两名助理被准予为病人做某些手术，第一次执手术刀就看起来让人很放心。因此，我们经常有幸指挥着 4 位本地年轻人同时做手术。

病人数——虽然去年某些情况的发生，特别是十月份汕头霍乱流行，可能让病人数目有所减少，但最后总数比前年多出 189 人。要不是霍乱的出现和我的短暂离开，病人数和手术量会更多。我们的病房出现过几个霍乱病人，但丝毫没有影响到其他病人，因为我们费好大劲送走了几个病人去腾出一两间空病房。然而，我们有好几个星期中止接收从远方来的病人，因为怕他们会经过疫区。

1882 年的病人数如下：

住院病人	2 738
门诊病人	1 405
总数	4 143

其中女性病人数如下：

住院病人	385
门诊病人	238
总数	623

这一年平均每日住院和门诊病人数如下：

	住院病人	门诊病人
一月	174	26
二月	97	22
三月	115	25
四月	141	32
五月	233	45
六月	248	47
七月	232	44
八月	181	42
九月	233	59
十月	212	57
十一月	122	35
十二月	162	29

平均每个住院病人的住院天数是16天。

我们每周只在星期二和星期五这两天看门诊病人，但是在其他时间我们从未拒绝为任何急诊病人看病。门诊人次数多达4 021，平均每个病人看病将近3次。有很大部分的人来自离汕头较远的地方，但这些人大都是船夫，其他人则是因为生意上的事来汕头的。

我们去了农村传教站好几趟，为几百个村民看病和开药方，但没有保存准确的数量记录。

患者的籍贯如下表，将它与去年的报告中记录的当年年度患者来自的城镇和村庄的数量相比较，可能会引起将医院作为传教机构的人的兴趣。

来自澄海	571
来自潮阳	996
来自揭阳	778
来自普宁	361
来自饶平	479
来自惠来	237
来自海阳	403
来自丰顺	52
来自大埔	13
来自南澳岛	54
来自陆丰和海丰	32
来自嘉应州	13

来自福建省 …………………………………………………………………………… 144
来自其他省 …………………………………………………………………………… 10

秋天，方将军（General Fang）在汕头开了一家公共诊所，并由来自香港东华（Tung Wah）医院的两位当地医生照管。本地的商人一直为这家诊所提供资金，据说住院部不久将会开始建设。据我们所知，在治疗的过程中他们所用的药物和设备都来自本地。有趣的是病人道德上的健康没有被其忽略。每天内科医生和外科医生照料病人时都会向他们宣读“圣谕”。这些特点看起来有点像在对抗我们的关照下的传教工作。然而这家诊所的开业并没有减少反而是增加了我们的病人。去年年底的两个月，我们的工作比往年同期还要繁重。这种情况不是第一次出现，之前几年在这个地区的两个大城市也有公共诊所出现，不过持续的时间都不长。

我们非常欢迎中国人他们自己为了缓解同胞的病痛所做的一切努力，这方面的努力还很少，但恐怕在中国人的性格和习俗能有实质性的改变之后，他们才能进行一项真正的慈善工作，最终收到好的成效。本地医院的医药知识和技术尚不能对当前的流行病造成多大影响。

我们还要提到汕头的另一项慈善项目，即已经设立的女乞丐收容所。然而，这只是一间简陋的供住宿的屋子，不提供食物和钱给居住者。我们参观过几次，到目前为止我们没有发现令人不快的地方。

传教工作——病人每天早晨和晚间的礼拜由被任命的同事或者由本地高级助理带领。李洁小姐（Miss Ricketts）经常探访女病房，并多次指引那些申请受洗的女病人。参加这些活动的病人都很多，许多住院病人对教义感兴趣，人数之多着实可喜。一年中，有超过140名男女报名要求入教。关于基督教礼仪和基本知识的课堂基本上会在下午定期开放，许多人已对基督教基本教义有了较多认识。每周日下午他们会集结一个钟头左右，在一起接受考试，通常由我们的传教士主持，汕头会众的本地长者也会给予协助。在大量的申请人当中只有几个接受了洗礼，因为我们通常会要求他们在接受神圣的仪式之前，回到家里在亲戚和邻居当中展示他们对信仰的真诚并表明自己是基督徒。有些离开了医院的病人很难在家附近找到教堂，这使得他们很难继续维持信仰。还有一些，如我们所料，回家后没有宣布自己为基督教徒。不过，也有一些人会在很严重的迫害之下坚持下来。

可以预料，有的宣称将成为信徒的人，尽管接受了医院的好处，但回家后仍然会重走老路。解除身体痛苦后的感恩之情可能会使人对我们所宣传的宗教有好感，但是让一个人在充满敌意的社区里仍坚持其信仰还需要比感恩更重要的东西。虽然这种情况是令人失望的，但有时可以通过他们把真理的知识带给其身为异教徒的熟人或亲戚。我们的一位同事注意到两个这类事例。第一个与吴威凛医生（Dr. Gauld）13年前的一个病人有关。他那时获赠了一本赞美诗集，但他完全没有兴趣，回家后便把它丢在一旁。去年他的一个兄弟偶然见到那本书，读后，他对书中所讲的真理很感兴趣，去了京冈（Kia-kng）的一个教会，希望得到指引。现在，他和一个朋友都接受了洗礼，他们与几个对此也感兴趣的男女一起租了一间房子，夜间用来做祈祷。他们当中的一个现在是基督徒的男人曾是一个臭名昭著的小偷和赌徒，他的乡亲们看到他现在的变化很是感动，说他们现在晚上终于可以待在家里，不用像以前那样到农田里看守以防东西被盗了。

另一例是一个来自京冈邻近村庄的男人，他年初在治病期间申请接受洗礼。后来我们到他家乡造访他两次，第一次就在他出院后不久，而第二次在6个月后，那时他已经放弃了信仰。但他的两个朋友，或许是受到我们的病人对他们讲述教义的指引，也或许是聆听过我们在上述的两次探访中的布道而受到启发，因此产生了兴趣，以后很有可能会接受洗礼。

或许上述提到的例子不是很普遍，但我们能由此联系起其他例子，一些虔诚的信徒带动周围的亲戚和邻居也成为教徒。我们说说其中的几个事例。一个1881年接受洗礼的来自惠来（Huei-lai）的赵（Thiau）姓男人，带着他的母亲和弟弟，长途跋涉3天来到汕头，就为了得到基督教的指引。他母亲来到汕头几天后就得了霍乱，不过恢复健康了。现在他母亲和弟弟都申请入教。一个从潮阳的大村庄和平（Hua-pheng）来的颜（Hien）姓男人，1881年1月1日接受了洗礼，他已经影响了一些朋友去相信福音，他的兄弟几次来汕头接受教诲，并已接受了洗礼。一个从潮阳沙陇（Sua-leng）来的去年接受了洗礼的蔡（Tsoi）姓女人，已经能够为邻居们讲解真理，最近她遭受了一种令人难以忍受的迫害。一个秦（Chhim）姓的汕头理发师，因为要动手术入院治疗了3个星期。从那时开始，他便由他的两个朋友陪伴，定期参加礼拜，他们几个现在都在接受洗礼的候选名单中。他的生意伙伴不同意他星期天不工作，于是他离开了他们，在城里的另一个地方和他两个教友自立门户。

去年，在与我们教会有关的接受洗礼的148个成人中，有17或18个人是在医院接受治疗的过程中第一次听到并接受了福音。

我们不得不提及，福音传播工作有可能出现这样的结果：一些病人放弃了以前的信仰，但没有信奉基督教。每年我们都注意到一些这样的例子。另外，其他在医院时没有表现出信仰的，有时几个月甚至几年后在农村传教站聚了起来。这些人在他们住院时就开始偷偷崇拜上帝。

我们引述的这些事例说明，医院正如所宣称的那样，是一所教会医院。不过医疗宣教不需要辩护者，因为其在解除病痛和传播福音方面都是非常有用的。医学艺术自然地成为教会的侍女，我们相信西方医学不会损失什么，而会在传播真正宗教来引导异教人们方面收获颇丰。无论如何，它足以让我们中的一些人了解基督教斗士的使命是“治愈疾病，并指明神的国近了”。

“神的国来到，不是眼所能见的。”基督教在整个汕头地区已经缓慢地、悄无声息地，但毋庸置疑地慢慢渗透到民众中去，兄弟之间互相告知好消息，朋友之间互相传递好消息，有时在我们认为没有一个信徒的乡村都有真正的上帝信徒被发现。我们恭敬地感谢我们照管的医院促进了而且还在促进我们向着美好的目标前进。

所诊治过的疾病的表格将随后附上。我们尽可能准确地列出这张去年治疗过的疾病的表格，但一些疾病的数量大大超出了所列出的。皮肤病，比如藓、糠疹、疥疮可能有好几百例。

医疗

麻疹——四月份，一波小型的麻疹热出现在教会学校的男童身上，症状较轻，大概只有 10 个人感染。中国人对于这种病很不在意，孩子在出疹的症状消失后就可以到处跑。

霍乱——十月份，霍乱于汕头和周边地区大规模流行。它是由从马尼拉经过厦门返回的归侨传入的。最初有多个死亡病例出现，幸运的是没有传入农村，之后很快就消失了。我们医院收治过 10 个病例，死了 4 人，其他都痊愈了。最早的两个病例出现在小医院（麻风病院），可能的感染源头是只有几码远的一间小房子，那里居住着很多麻风病人。霍乱在医院出现的四天前，一位住在这间屋子的病人因为这个病死去，他的尸体在下葬前曾在这间屋子旁边停放两天。我们的这两个病人（一对夫妻）痊愈了。之后小医院再也没有出现病例，但一个星期后，一位在大医院治疗双脚糜烂的小伙子被感染到了，并在几天后去世。这个病人住院很久了，而且被严格要求卧床，至少有 3 个月没有出过病房。几天后，又有两个病人感染后死亡。这些病例均发生在我到中国北方出差期间，而就在我回来的前一天，又有一个病人感染了，我去看她时是她病得最严重的时候，不过她最后痊愈了。之后，又有另外 4 位染病患者，其中 3 位也痊愈了。

那时大约有 240 个住院病人，但是霍乱没有在病房蔓延的势头，在同一个病房里有两人同患霍乱的只出现过两例。急性腹泻和痢疾在医院以及汕头和周边乡村也很普遍。在让三四十个病人出院后，我们得以将霍乱和腹泻病人分隔开来，安置在两间大病房里。我们还采取了预防措施，每天 3 次检查所有接受治疗的病人的病情，出现稀便即马上检测、隔离，并进行严格对症治疗。

几乎每天都有汕头人来到我们的诊所替感染霍乱的朋友寻求治疗药物，常常出现的请求是要一种保证病人能够活命直到回到家乡的药。这种现象可能会导致霍乱的进一步传播。令人惊讶的是，在一个聚集了许多人口密集、卫生条件极差的村庄的地区，并没有更多的霍乱病例发生。更令人不可思议的，就是一旦这种病暴发，其传播范围不超出港口市镇 30 英里。中国人并不采取任何预防措施，他们只竖起许多长竹竿，白天挂小红旗，夜间挂灯笼，用于赶走疾病，但卫生问题却留给猪和狗去处理。

鸦片吸食者——这一年中有 128 名男性和 1 名女性到医院来寻求治疗以戒除毒瘾。其中有 3 个患有严重得无法治愈的肺结核，只能被遣送回家；4 个是门诊病人，只被诊断过一次；其他的（122 人）都是住院病人，接受了时间长短不一的治疗。下面我们给出一些统计数据以供参考，包括吸鸦片烟剂量、鸦片烟龄和病人的年龄，该统计数据并不十分完整。

每日剂量

0.5 钱或更少	15	3 钱	4
1 钱或多于 0.5 钱	29	5 钱	1
1.5 钱或多于 1 钱	30	6 钱	2
2 钱	12	8 钱	1
2.5 钱	6		

鸦片烟龄

2 年或更短	9	10 年	11

3 年	9	11 年	2
4 年	7	12 年	2
5 年	4	15～20 年	5
6 年	2	28 年	2
7 年	1	45 年	1
8 年	6		

未列入上表的占有更大比例的病例的鸦片烟龄少于 10 年。

病人年龄

20～25 岁	13	40～50 岁	19
25～30 岁	26	50～60 岁	12
30～35 岁	23	60～70 岁	1
35～40 岁	22	75 岁以上	1

每个病例都曾吸食过外国鸦片。据我们所知，潮州地区没有种植罂粟花，也没有使用本地毒品。1 钱精制的外国鸦片就要吸鸦片者花费 90 文或 8 美分。几乎所有的病人都有每天喝些酒的习惯，并且也抽烟。

在 1881 年的报告中我们预测过吸食鸦片的人占了农村总人数的约 4%。今年我们从范围更广的调查中所获得的数据为平均占 3.25%。因此说农村地区有约 3% 的人口吸食鸦片也许并不离谱。汕头的人口约为 20 000 人，我们知道的鸦片烟馆有 73 间。吸鸦片烟在走私设施比比皆是的地方更流行。

食用鸦片在这个地区绝非无人知道。我们的许多病人对鸦片是又吃又吸。许多吸鸦片的挑夫、轿夫、船夫在工作时有一个习惯，就是每间隔一段时间吞下一颗鸦片小丸，用以减轻欲望。囊中羞涩的烟鬼为了满足自己的欲望，还要吃鸦片烟管中的烟灰。尽管专业的和业余的理论家都断言，吸也好吃也好，鸦片对身体的影响都是一样的，当然程度上会有所不同，但我们通过医学观察更倾向于相信两者之间程度的不同并没有通常所认为的那么大。

有时会遇到一种脚趾和手指出现的坏疽，这明显是持续吸食鸦片的后果。这是一种干性或慢性坏疽，会导致脚趾和手指慢慢因为脱皮损毁。该疾病会让体质轻度下降。去年我们收治了两个病例，他们治疗了 8 个或 10 个星期。每年都有几个这样的病例，这些患者都是鸦片吸食者。

一个 75 岁的老人说他的鸦片烟龄已达 45 年，最近两三年更是每天要消费掉一盎司。他的身体状况很好，也希望戒除毒瘾，但他在入院后第 3 天就被他的朋友从医院带走了。这样的例子是特例。至少在劳动阶层，染上鸦片瘾对身心无疑都有很大伤害。

另外一个男人借助吸鸦片来治疗间歇热，吸食了两年，但是病情依旧没有好转。他出现了脾重度增大，严重贫血，非常虚弱。他在第 4 天就离开了医院。在过去 3 年，我们向病人、当地医生和其他人询问了关于鸦片有利于预防疟疾热的猜想，但没有得到任何确切的证据来证实或否定这种理论。然而，一个懒惰的吸鸦片者每天花几个小时吸鸦片，而另一个男人也许从天亮到天黑在田里干活，暴露在烈日下，而且忍受着变化无常的天气，两者容易发热的程度不太可能一样。

在吸鸦片者的治疗过程中，我们绝对不会给予鸦片或者任何替代品，病人也要自备食物。一旦开始治疗，大约三分之一的病人会在治疗引起的痛苦症状出现后跑掉了。其他的病人坚持了或长或短的时间，戒掉了毒瘾后欣然出院。

这一年中治疗了 1 079 例眼科疾病和 726 例皮肤病。

外科手术

下面是一年来施行的外科手术：

眼科手术：

睑内翻及倒睫症手术	361
翼状胬肉手术	92
白内障手术	7
睑球粘连手术	3
虹膜疝手术	5
上睑下垂手术	1
眼睑外翻手术	3
泪小管分离术	12
眼眶恶性肿瘤切除术	1
眼皮小肿瘤切除术	2
眼球切除术	3
前房葡萄肿切除术	1
前房穿刺术	5
虹膜切除术	31
角膜碎片清除术	3
滑膜切除术	2
	=532

躯体手术：

唇裂手术	37
肛瘘手术	53
耳裂手术	31
包皮（过长）环切术	10
鼻窦炎手术	12
腱鞘囊肿手术	2
蹼指手术	1

涎腺瘘手术	1
睾丸海绵肿手术	1
下颌骨囊性肿瘤切除术	1
肿瘤切除术	35
乳腺硬癌切除术	4
皮脂囊肿切除术	2
阴唇象皮病切除术	1
阴囊象皮病切除术	1
淋巴阴囊切除术	1
扁桃体切除术	2
外痔切除术	7
湿疣切除术	1
肉赘切除术	1
足茧切除术	7
龈瘤切除术	2
瘢痕瘤切除术	1
睾丸瘤切除术	1
皮肤上皮瘤切除术	4
嘴唇上皮细胞瘤切除术	1
拔牙	127
坏死骨头切除术	26
从鼻孔中取出种子	1
竹碎片取出术	2
拔针	1
子弹取出术	3
鼻息肉切除术	6
尿道结石取出术	1
拇指切除术	1
手指切除术	5
脚趾切除术	2
阴茎（上皮瘤）切除术	3
碎石术	1
囊性肿物切开术	2
鞘膜积液引流和注射术	22
内痔结扎术	25
残耳整形手术	2
鼻孔裂缝整形手术	1
脓肿、甲沟炎、痈切开术	75

烧灼术	4
遗精烧灼术	2
尿道狭窄扩张术	8
脱臼复位术	5
骨折固定术	3
	=546
总数	1 078

这一年没有任何手术死亡病例。

睑内翻及倒睫症——为了治疗这种疾病所做的361例手术取得了令人满意的效果。这种非常常见的眼睑疾病是由长时间的颗粒状结膜炎和被忽视的结膜黏液脓性炎症所致的。在很多病例中，双眼的上眼睑都感染了，有几个病例出现双眼上下眼睑睫毛全部内翻的情况。接受了手术的大约有220位病人。一些慢性病例的眼裂也被缩短了，同时切了外眼角来补救。

睑外翻并不是常见的疾病，而且相比睑内翻也难处理得多，有3位患这种病的病人做了手术。有两例是由结膜炎症增厚引起的，第三例是上眼睑瘢痕挛缩引起的。后者需要做整形手术，于是瘢痕被切除，额头上的一小片健康的皮肤被移植到此处，对于病人和手术者来说，结果都是令人满意的。

虹膜切除术——有30个病例因为角膜混浊而实施了该手术，只有三四例没有好转。3个几乎完全失明的病人在术前只能看见微弱的光，术后的视力足够让他们不用辅助就能自行走路。一例青光眼病例也做了同样的手术，病人的痛苦得到缓解，视力也稍有改善。

眼球摘除术——中国人强烈反对眼球摘除术，不管摘除的必要性多急迫。然而，由于有导致健康的那只眼睛交感性眼炎的巨大危险，有3个病例同意我们切除带来痛苦的无用眼睛。

肛瘘这种病很常见，就像在英国一样，有的致病原因和肺病有关。大多数是由肠周围的蜂窝组织脓肿引起的。患这种病的大多是农民，他们在为水稻田整地时，需要赤脚泡在水中几个小时，这可能与脓肿有因果关系。此病患者的总体健康状况通常低于一般水平。治疗的方法是用刀把瘘管切开，做过的53例效果都很满意。

鞘膜积液是另一种常见的疾病。去年总共治疗了22例，数量比往年少了。治疗时扩张的囊被切开，然后注入1.5德拉克马的浓碘酊。有时这种治疗并不能完全使其治愈。

阴唇象皮病——一名46岁的女人的阴唇上生长了两个带蒂生长的包块，约一个柚子大小，结构类似象皮病肿瘤，我们用绞勒的方法成功摘除。

淋巴阴囊——偶尔也会碰到这种罕见的疾病。患病部位增厚，但是摸起来很软，表面由于存在许多囊泡而变得粗糙，挑破会流出大量澄清的液体。这种疾病与象皮病密切相关，一些当地的医生甚至认为它会逐渐转变成象皮病。这一年共有4例，其中一例除了淋巴阴囊还有腿上象皮病。4例中只有一个病人同意接受手术。治疗很轻松地完成了，而且术后恢复得很好，伤口部分第一期愈合，部分肉芽愈合。

阴囊象皮病——我们为一个32岁的惠来男人实施了手术。他患病一年多，阴囊肿胀之前有频繁的寒战发作，腹股沟的淋巴结也肿大。一个重3磅的肿瘤被切除了，恢复的过程中没有不良的症状。

两个有巨大阴囊肿瘤的病人前来就诊，不过他们拒绝做手术。

尿路结石——一个病例的结石被粉碎 4 次，在尿中排出超过一盎司的碎石。在我不得不离开汕头那段时间，还有一两个小碎石待排出，而病人在我回来之前已离开医院。

尿道结石——一个病人前来取一个小结石。结石嵌在尿道附近的三角韧带处，我们的一位本地助理沿结石的位置切下，取出结石。几天后伤口就愈合了，病人也完全康复。

眼眶恶性肿瘤——这个 42 岁的妇女病了两年，她把发病的原因归结于上眼眶所受的伤。眼睛肿了起来，患者也用了很久的刺激性药物。肉瘤从眼眶中突出，摸起来很软，足足有一个橙子那么大，把眼球向上挤到了眼睑的下方，眼睑被撑开。

病人很愿意接受任何能缓解病情的手术，即使只是暂时的。她被用氯仿麻醉，然后整个眼眶的内容物被取出。为了使病变的所有残留部分能够被彻底清除，眼腔的顶部和底部被热烧灼过。眼眶的部分骨质顶部也被腐蚀过，用手指一触摸就变成了碎片。这些骨碎片被小心清除，脑膜因此露了出来。

病人术后恢复得很好，在摆脱了难看和令人痛苦的肿块后非常高兴地出院了。

女性乳腺硬癌——切除了 4 例这样的肿瘤，除了一例其他的伤口都第一期愈合了。有两例在手术的过程中顺便切除了腋下增大的淋巴结。手术是在严格的无菌预防措施下实施的。

上皮瘤——数量可观的病人因为这个病被施予手术，使用了开刀或者热烧灼的方法。这些病例中较为令人感兴趣的是：①口角上皮瘤，很小程度地涉及双唇，并短距离地延伸到牙齿的颊线，瘤体切除后留下的空隙由健康的皮瓣填充，皮瓣从两个切口取得，一处向下至颌下区，另一处向上至脸颊；②颏上皮瘤，这个病例还接受了整形手术；③阴茎上皮瘤，有 3 个患该病的病例被使用通常的方法将器官切除。

残耳修复术——对于一些反社会的罪行，如通奸，中国的村民都习惯于运用他们自己手中的法律，给罪犯一个稍显野蛮的惩罚。偶尔会有病人耳朵被整个或部分割下，或眼睛被利器刺穿而完全毁掉，他们很希望外国医生能够帮他们修复。这样的情况我们也常常帮不了忙，但是有个病例只是耳朵的上半部分被割下，残余部分状况良好，我们进行了整形手术后病人很满意，因为在一定程度上恢复了他耳朵的听力。手术分两阶段进行，先取下耳后一块皮肤黏合到耳朵残余的部分上去。几个星期之后，切断该皮瓣与头皮的连接处，又从太阳穴处取下另一块皮肤，并应用到第一次手术不被覆盖的地方。病人回家几个星期后，我们又接诊了另外一个男人，这是他的邻居，他一只耳朵被整个割下，希望接受像前一位病人一样的治疗。

外伤等——多数的损伤、外伤等都比较轻，但也有几个危及生命的病例。最严重的病例是一位 45 岁的船上苦力，他从桅杆顶端摔到雨篷上，脸着地，右侧对应犬牙部位的下颌骨折，鼻骨粉碎，眼眶边缘上方的骨头也断裂了，脸上和额头上的皮肤严重擦伤。病人抽烟，而且每天要食用多达两钱的鸦片灰。经过漫长而反复的治疗后，他最终康复出院了。

下颌脱位——曾有一个男人间隔几个月两次来诊，两次都是因为打哈欠的时候嘴巴张得太大造成的。

财务——从附录中可以看出，年度收入是 2 237.23 美元，支出是 1 903.80 美元，结余 333.43 美元。

陈源盛（Tang Nguan Seng）行继续为我们的贫穷患者提供大米和现金券，总共价值 120 美元，已在这一年收到。

最后，我们必须衷心鸣谢来自汕头外国社团和其他人的慷慨捐助。波洛克医生（Dr. Pollock）热心帮忙募集了大量捐赠物品；一台李斯特思（Listers）牌蒸汽喷射器（消毒机）由牧师 J. C. 吉普森硕士（Rev. J. C. Gibson，M. A.）赠送，该设备被用于伤口的无菌治疗；我的老师，爱丁堡大学的辛普森（Simpson）教授赠送一台热烧灼器。在此一并致谢。

（附上一份客家医院工作的简短报告，该医院使用的药物由汕头医院供给）

1882 年客家医疗工作报告

牧师雷德尔医生（Rev. Dr. Riddel）记录：自从 1881 年 12 月份以来，客家地区的医疗工作开展得断断续续。在访问传道站期间我一直带着药篮。访问期间的工作成效因种种原因根本就比不上医院的。病人知道医生在这里的工作是短期的，因此诊查疑难病例时通常非常匆忙，这是不可能有令人满意的效果的。并且药品供应有限，外科器械缺乏，此外，也很少有为任何病人第二次看病和开药的机会。

1882 年初，我在五云洞（Ng-yun-thung）逗留，为期几个星期，因此能够给病人更多的照料，我希望效果更好。在这个区域有大约 500 个病例接受了治疗。之后我们在五经富（Ng-kang-phu）逗留时接诊了超过 300 个病例，8 月份在大埔（Ta-pu）期间有超过 200 个病例。

我发现从 1881 年 12 月至 1882 年末有超过 1 100 位新病人，这些病人中有超过 200 位回来重新开药一次或两次。

由于还没有购买场地作为诊所，所以仅做了几个小手术，如眼睑内翻和耳裂伤手术，这些当属明智的尝试。

1882 年捐款

（略）

收支表

单位：美元

助手和门卫工资	359.00
印刷医院报告费用、邮资	30.33
地租、房屋保险	25.00
病房的修复和刷白	55.48
买猪油、油	66.98
买布绷带、药棉	57.91
买制作搽剂、酊剂的杜松子酒和精馏酒	124.02

买纸、蜡、煤油、木炭	11.50
买杂物	61.70
买水	44.45
援助贫困患者费用	102.71
在中国购买外国与本国药物费用	162.27
买外科器械	53.27
来自伦敦的药物、外科敷料、牛奶及其运费和保险费	129.18
来自伦敦的由爱丁堡教会支付的药物等费用（大约）	500.00
大米和现金券（大约）	120.00
结余	333.43
	2 237.23

1881年结余	293.80
如上文所示的捐款	1 150.17
卖疝气绑带	28.98
卖厕所用品	29.18
卖杂物	4.13
卖药（利润）	95.03
小病房租金	15.85
大米和现金券（大约）	120.00
来自伦敦的由爱丁堡教会支付的药物费用（大约）	500.00
	2 237.23

治疗疾病目录

常见病

低热	34
间歇性发热	131
慢性关节风湿病	43
肌肉风湿病	93
肌肉性腰痛	32
肌肉性胸痛	9
风湿性关节炎	1
淋病性风湿病	2
梅毒	30
先天性梅毒	4
肿瘤：脂肪瘤	9
皮脂瘤	8
纤维瘤	10
格兰内瘤	5
恶性肿瘤	17
乳腺硬癌	5
囊性肿瘤	6
痣	1
粉瘤	1
神经节瘤	2
未分类肿瘤	7

梅毒性腺体肿大与甲状腺
肿大 …… 30
甲状腺瘤 …… 5
麻风 …… 150
贫血 …… 139
衰弱 …… 69
鸦片成瘾 …… 129
甲状腺肿大 …… 7
饥饿 …… 2
坏疽性口炎（走马疳） …… 1
麻疹 …… 11
霍乱 …… 10
丹毒 …… 2
坏疽 …… 3
毒血症 …… 1
腹水 …… 6
全身性水肿 …… 1
局部水肿 …… 3

消化系统疾病

唇溃疡 …… 6
唇上皮瘤 …… 4
唇裂 …… 41
齿龈溃疡 …… 2
龋齿 …… 11
牙龈（纤维）瘤 …… 3
舌头肿大 …… 2
涎瘘 …… 1
牙龈、口腔或咽喉溃疡 …… 21
舌上皮瘤 …… 1
悬雍垂过长 …… 1
咽喉肿瘤 …… 3
扁桃体炎 …… 5
腭裂 …… 2
食道狭窄 …… 8
消化不良 …… 239
酒精性消化不良 …… 2
绞痛 …… 28
痢疾 …… 25
腹泻 …… 27
蛔虫病 …… 33
呃逆（?） …… 1
便秘 …… 1
直肠狭窄 …… 10
内痔 …… 36
外痔 …… 14
肛瘘 …… 60
直肠溃疡或瘘 …… 7
直肠脱垂 …… 2
肛门溃疡（鸡奸） …… 17
肛门闭锁 …… 1
疝气 …… 34
脾肿大 …… 33
肝肿大 …… 5

耳朵疾病

耳聋 …… 8
耳漏 …… 7
炎症 …… 1
战争堆积物进入外耳道 …… 1
湿疹 …… 1
耳损伤 …… 1
耳瘘 …… 1
耳垂残缺 …… 4
创伤 …… 2
外耳道瘢痕挛缩闭锁 …… 1

循环系统疾病

心脏瓣膜病	7	腘窝动脉瘤	1
静脉曲张	5		

呼吸系统疾病

喉溃疡	4	结核性肺炎	72
失声	14	肺气肿	7
支气管炎	133	咯血	9
肺炎	2		

鼻部疾病

鼻溃疡(狼疮和梅毒性)	23	鼻裂	2
黏膜溃疡	6	鼻息肉恶变	1
鼻外伤	1	鼻息肉	11

眼科疾病

睑内翻及倒睫症	217	角膜糜烂	18
眼睑外翻	6	角膜模糊	86
上睑下垂	1	角膜老年环	1
睑腺炎	2	角膜碎裂	2
眼睑软骨肥厚	2	角膜损坏	1
眼睑小肿瘤	7	虹膜炎	14
眼睑痣	1	虹膜炎粘连	35
颗粒性眼炎	210	虹膜脱出	16
化脓性眼炎	16	眼前房积脓	4
卡他性眼炎	63	前葡萄肿	15
脓疱性眼炎	2	白内障	28
淋病性眼炎	1	晶状体异物	2
苔丝性眼炎	29	青光眼	9
翼状胬肉	74	一只或两只眼睛损毁	53
泪点或鼻泪管梗阻	15	虹膜震颤	1
泪腺脓肿	5	视神经炎	2
睑球粘连	3	视神经萎缩	3
睑缘粘连	3	黑内障（黑蒙）	4
角膜炎	11	夜盲症	3
角膜血管增生	10	外渗血进入视网膜	1
角膜溃疡	99	眼眶恶性肿瘤	4

关节疾病

髋关节结核 …… 10
膝关节结核 …… 4
肩关节结核 …… 2
肘关节结核 …… 1
髋关节炎（急性或慢性） …… 11
滑囊炎 …… 1
踝关节炎 …… 15
髋关节僵硬 …… 6
踝关节僵硬 …… 2
肘关节僵硬 …… 1
指关节僵硬 …… 2

神经系统疾病

偏瘫 …… 5
截瘫 …… 3
臂部瘫痪 …… 4
面瘫 …… 2
癫痫 …… 9
移动性共济失调 …… 1
局部麻痹 …… 18
躁狂症 …… 2
痴呆症 …… 3
神经痛 …… 9
坐骨神经痛 …… 16
癔症 …… 1
眩晕 …… 3
脊柱疾病 …… 1

皮肤病

体癣 …… 108
断发毛菌癣 …… 10
须癣 …… 14
黄癣 …… 4
花斑癣 …… 8
疥疮 …… 20
痒疹 …… 5
湿疹 …… 32
头部湿疹 …… 5
银屑病 …… 10
天疱疮 …… 2
鱼鳞病 …… 4
脓疱疹 …… 7
秃头 …… 2
白斑病 …… 2
痤疮 …… 6
苔藓病 …… 1
带状疱疹 …… 1
荨麻疹 …… 1
瘢痕瘤 …… 3
腿部象皮病 …… 35
鸡眼 …… 4
疼痛性疤痕 …… 2
上皮瘤 …… 7
系统性红斑狼疮 …… 3
尖锐湿疣 …… 8
疣 …… 1
甲沟炎 …… 12
疖痈 …… 6
炎症 …… 17
脓肿 …… 56
溃疡 …… 301
窦道 …… 28
裂伤或裂隙伤 …… 9

泌尿生殖系统疾病

阴囊溃疡或窦道 …………………… 9
阴囊湿疹 ……………………………… 7
阴囊积液 ……………………………… 4
阴囊象皮病 ………………………… 11
阴囊上皮瘤 ………………………… 1
阴茎下疳和溃疡 ………………… 16
阴茎上皮瘤 ………………………… 6
阴茎小肿瘤 ………………………… 1
包茎 ……………………………………… 9
包茎嵌顿 ……………………………… 1
淋病 …………………………………… 20
尿道狭窄 …………………………… 11
尿道损伤 ……………………………… 3
尿道瘘 ………………………………… 2
尿道结石 ……………………………… 1
遗精 …………………………………… 27
睾丸炎 ………………………………… 1
鞘膜积液 …………………………… 24
睾丸海绵肿 ………………………… 1
膀胱炎 ………………………………… 1
膀胱结石 ……………………………… 2
乳糜尿 ………………………………… 1
尿潴留 ………………………………… 1
尿失禁 ………………………………… 2
阳痿 ……………………………………… 1
慢性蛋白尿 ………………………… 2
生殖器发育不良 ………………… 1
腹股沟淋巴结炎 ………………… 6
白带过多 ……………………………… 5
月经过多 ……………………………… 1
月经不调 ……………………………… 1
女阴象皮病 ………………………… 1
子宫肌瘤 ……………………………… 2
子宫癌 ………………………………… 1
卵巢肿瘤 ……………………………… 2
肿瘤（未分类） …………………… 3

骨科疾病

骨溃疡坏死 ………………………… 61
骨膜炎 ………………………………… 1
脊柱弯曲 …………………………… 10

外伤、损伤及其他

下颌脱臼 ……………………………… 2
肩脱臼 ………………………………… 3
肘脱臼 ………………………………… 1
手指脱臼 ……………………………… 2
髋关节脱臼 ………………………… 5
桡骨骨折 ……………………………… 4
腓骨骨折 ……………………………… 1
下颌骨、鼻骨骨折和旋后肌
上颌骨眶突 ………………………… 1
肱骨复合骨折 ……………………… 1
大脚趾复合骨折 ………………… 2
枪伤 ……………………………………… 4
耳裂 …………………………………… 27
跌打损伤 …………………………… 53
胸部损伤（由于负重和殴打） … 65
扭伤 …………………………………… 27
外伤 …………………………………… 32
烧伤和烫伤 ………………………… 14
手中竹片残留 ……………………… 1
大腿竹片残留 ……………………… 1
手中针残留 ………………………… 1
子弹残留 ……………………………… 3
狗咬伤 ………………………………… 5
猪咬伤 ………………………………… 2

未分类的

腿部淋巴管炎	1	腹股沟淋巴结肿大（象皮病）	7
手臂发育不良	1	肌腱挛缩	4
不由自主的肌肉抽搐	1	赘生拇指	1
		鸦片中毒	1

（翻译：谢煊、朱悦阳　校译：朱文平　审校：胡卫清、余维泉、江建安　中文校正：许党泉、颜彦）

1883 年汕头福音医院报告

（1883 年来爱力医学学士、外科硕士照管下的英兰长老会汕头教会医院报告
暨牧师列威廉医学学士、外科硕士照管下的客家乡村医疗传教工作报告）

过去一年，本地区公众健康状况相当不好。疾病流行的春季刚过，紧接着就来了一个漫长、炎热、异常难熬的夏季。夏初，一场严重的霍乱在汕头暴发，蔓延至潮州府更广大的地区，在人群中引起了大浩劫。随着年关将至，天花流行起来，导致了相当高的死亡率。

因此，总的来说，过去一年汕头教会医院的工作显得异常繁重和令人担忧。

在霍乱流行期间，本地的助手工作表现良好，在被要求照顾院外病例时也很热心。医院工作人员中只有一名助手受到该病传染，他在相当严重的病情折磨下最终得到良好恢复，我们对此心怀感激。

病人数量——接受治疗的病人总数如下：

住院病人	2 838	
门诊病人	1 597	—4 435
乡村看诊及开药病人		1 150
总数		5 585

当与中国其他一些门诊病人较多的医院比较时，我院的病人总数看起来可能较少，但住院病人占这么大的比例，工作量之大可想而知。

也许以下两个表格会对已完成的工作量有更好的展示。

（1）该年度每月初诊病人数。

	住院病人	门诊病人
一月	234	131
二月	56	25
三月	267	114
四月	276	145
五月	502	279
六月	277	178
七月	208	144

八月	64	67
九月	194	140
十月	333	135
十一月	178	101
十二月	249	138
	2 838	1 597

（2）该年度日均住院病人数和门诊病人数。

	住院病人	门诊病人
一月	192	35
二月	79	14
三月	157	24
四月	195	31
五月	328	51
六月	285	47
七月	183	38
八月	98	22
九月	119	32
十月	204	48
十一月	168	30
十二月	162	30

住院病人——在我们照管的医疗机构里，住院病人数大于门诊病人数，我们深信这种情况在中国是绝无仅有的。我们已有 2 838 名住院病人，其中 379 名是女性。这一年中，我们多次发现医院住院楼太小，以至于难以容纳所有申请住院的病人。因此，我们不得不把一些病人在得到妥善照顾前送走。五月份的日平均住院人数达到 328。

由于霍乱流行，夏末住院人数大量地减少，所以到了八月份，我们日均住院病人只有约 100 名。在某段时间内，由于害怕病人穿过传染区域，我们暂停接受长途跋涉的病人就医。

整个夏天，虽然只是几码之外就有大量死于该病的患者，但是大医院的病房没有出现一宗霍乱病例。然而，小医院就没有那么幸运了。在院外照顾病例的高级助理感染了该病，接下来两三个星期内，感染病例增加了 8 个，于是我们把其他病人尽快送走，一度封闭了该住院楼。

年底前出现了两个天花病例，其中一名是助理。他们被隔离了，该疾病没有进一步蔓延开来。

去年，医院的死亡人数比往年增加了，总计 18 人，但其中一些是被遗弃在我们手上的穷困且无亲无故的人士。一个将近 18 个月大的失明婴儿由她父亲带来治病，他们来到医院时已近傍晚，助理让他在病房待到第二天早上来见我，然而，他趁夜独自离开，把小孩留给我们。这个孩子几个月后死于痢疾。另一个贫穷而瘦弱的人由于饥饿和痢疾横卧在广东公会后面，被一些本地的基督徒发现而带过来。我们应他们请求收留他，但他第二天就去世了。据说他是当地一个富商的儿子，由于惹上官司而不得不紧急逃亡，以保住自己的脑袋。这个失败的吊儿郎当的小伙子已经被父亲抛弃了。有两个男人从国外回来，被从轮船上带来时已奄奄一息，到医院几个小时后就死了。另一个病人是自杀。这个人来自陆丰，其颗粒性黏膜炎已经被治好，当被要求回家时，他服毒自杀了。有 3 位病人死于霍乱。

医学传教士对于在中国进行医疗传教的最佳方法有不同的见解。有些人喜欢花更多的精力在门诊病人上，只开一间较严重的病患才能够得到更细心的医治的小医院。虽然这种方法最为省力，但这种工作的价值可能会受到质疑。

在汕头这样的小地方，患者绝大多数来自方圆 80 英里或 100 英里的周边地区。若要得到治疗，让他们住院是非常有必要的。但即使不考虑我们的特殊环境因素，我们也完全相信医院比门诊具有更高的价值。从一些经验看，我倾向于认为门诊完成的工作是不能令人满意的。一个病人拿了药回去后，要他按照我们指定的方式去服药的可能性很小，因为中国与西方的服药方式有很大的不同。住院虽然不能完全达到理想的效果，但至少在医护人员的照料之下，通过每天一次、两次甚至更多次的巡视，我们能够根据病情修改或改变治疗方案。当然，必须承认的是，实行这一计划要接收一些严格地说并不适合住院的病例，但对于教会医院来说，这利大于弊，因为这样做会使福音工作更容易进行，在病情不严重或不痛苦的患者中推广也许会更成功。医学传教士也许对一个只看一次病的门诊病人影响不大，但他能更接近那些他负责照顾的住院病人。他慢慢了解病人们，而更重要的可能是病人们也能慢慢了解他。在这样的环境下，传教士能给其所负责的病人带来更大的个人影响。

因此我们认为，医学传教士想要在中国人中真正做好工作，必须有一幢好的大房子供病人暂住，他们在那里可以尽可能地把时间和精力投入到病人身上。

我们不希望看到门诊病人的数量增加，但看到住院的病人多起来我们会很高兴。

住院病人和我们在一起的时候食物自理，但不用支付医药费用。

门诊病人——在 1 597 个门诊病人中有 229 位妇女，病人每周只能在两个门诊开放日即星期二和星期五接受诊疗。在这一年中，相当多的汕头人在自己的家里接受出诊服务。

下乡诊疗——大约在春节的时候，我在同事陪同下花了一个月的时间访问了远在西边和西南边的客家和闽南地区的传教站，秋季的时候在潮阳平原地区的村庄待了两个星期。在这些行程中约有 1 150 人接受诊治和开药。

传教工作

布道的工作迄今为止有序进行着，每一天工作开始前我们都将病人集中起来读上帝之道并向他们讲解，日落时分他们再次聚集在教堂里，举行一个较短的仪式，一般由一个本地的助手负责。一周有几天的晨祷由传教士和施饶理夫人（Mrs. Smith）主持。李洁小姐（Miss Ricketts）和她带领的妇女传道员在妇女中的工作开展得很好。

这一年间有12位病人接受洗礼，还有更多的人希望进入教会。一个专为这些人举办的特殊集会定期在星期日下午举行。我们发现，除了那些申请洗礼的人，许多其他的人对真理有了清晰认知。我们应该期望在未来的日子里，其中有些人会诚心追随他们某种程度上已经了解的真理。

通过苏格兰国家圣经协会的慷慨协助，现在有一位卖《圣经》的小贩和医院联系上了。上述协会已答应给予补助，每年向这名代理人支付12英镑的薪酬。一名目前在汕头学习的学生被派来负责这项工作，他将在春节后开始履行他的职责。他将到原来在医院申请洗礼的人的家中进行访问，并利用这个机会尽可能地进行布道，销售宗教书籍及小册子。

在潮州府的福音传播中，医院已经发挥了有益的作用。它给人们提供的认识福音的机会是特别有利的，因为现在平均每天有近200名来自各个周边农村的住院患者。此外，平均每一个病人的住院时间大约是3周，在此期间他们每天都有接受宗教教育的机会。

下表列出了患者来自的不同地区的城镇和村庄数量，以及每个区域的患者的数量。

可以看出，患者共来自1 439个城镇和村庄。这本身就表明了医院作为一个福音机构的价值。

	村庄数	病人数
潮州府：		
澄海	79	552
潮阳	279	1 139
揭阳	270	698
惠来	88	232
饶平	200	629
普宁	168	361
海阳	157	380
丰顺	34	91
大埔	12	27
南澳岛	12	65
嘉应州	19	31
陆丰和海丰	14	36
福建省	102	181
其他州和省	5	13
	1 439	4 435

以下是所治疗疾病的列表：

常见病

低热	48
间歇热：	
日发疟	8
三日疟	23
四日疟	224
不规则热	7
麻风病	218
贫血	128
全身虚弱	61
梅毒并甲状腺肿大	27
梅毒	23
慢性风湿性关节炎	41
先天性梅毒	1
肌肉风湿病	8
腰痛	2
胸痛	2
梅毒风湿病	1
风湿性关节炎	
霍乱	8
天花	
斑疹伤寒	
丹毒	
糖尿病	
坏疽	
饥饿	
吸鸦片烟（接受治疗）	11

消化系统疾病

唇裂	27
嘴唇溃疡	3
唇上皮瘤	2
齿龈溃疡	1
齿瘘	2
龋齿	2
腭裂	3
腭溃疡	1
腭上皮瘤	2
舌炎	1
咽喉溃疡	8
慢性扁桃体炎	16
咽喉乳头状肿物	1
食道狭窄	3
消化不良	280
酗酒后消化不良	1
胃癌	1
绞痛	47
便秘	
腹泻	2
痢疾	2
呕血	
肝肿大	
肝癌肝肿大并黄疸	
脾肿大	4
直肠狭窄	
直肠裂伤	
直肠息肉	
直肠下垂	
肛门溃疡（鸡奸）	1
直肠创伤	
肛瘘	5
内痔	4
外痔	
疝气	3
腹水	

胃肠炎 …… 1
蠕虫病 …… 24
单纯腹壁瘘 ……

淋巴系统疾病

腹股沟腺体肿大并发热 …… 8
腿象皮肿 …… 42
阴囊淋巴肿 ……
阴囊象皮肿 …… 1

呼吸系统疾病

喉阻塞 …… 2
支气管炎 …… 130
肺结核 …… 92
哮喘 …… 1
咯血 …… 1
肺气肿 ……

眼部疾病

睑内翻及倒睫症 …… 204
眼睑外翻 …… 1
眼睑梅毒性溃疡 …… 2
眼睑创伤 …… 1
眼睑不自主抽搐 …… 1
眼睑脓肿 …… 1
眼睑肿瘤（小） …… 4
眼睑肿瘤（恶性） …… 2
眼睑疣（恶性） …… 1
软骨关节增厚 …… 3
眼睑软骨囊肿 …… 1
上睑下垂 …… 2
睑腺炎 …… 2
睑缘粘连 …… 6
睑球粘连 …… 8
苔丝样眼炎 …… 9
卡他性眼炎 …… 71
脓疱性眼炎 …… 4
化脓性眼炎 …… 6
颗粒状眼炎 …… 349
淋病性眼炎 …… 4
翼状胬肉 …… 58
角膜混浊 …… 66
角膜溃疡 …… 47
角膜脱落 …… 14
角膜创伤 …… 3
结膜下纤维增生 …… 2
角膜翳 …… 5
角膜炎 …… 15
虹膜角膜炎 …… 2
前葡萄肿 …… 23
虹膜炎 …… 19
虹膜突出 …… 8
慢性虹膜粘连 …… 37
眼前房积脓 …… 7
青光眼 …… 9
视神经萎缩 …… 4
黑蒙症 …… 10
近视 …… 1
夜盲症 …… 2
白内障 …… 22
角膜和晶状体创伤 …… 2
一只或两只眼睛损毁 …… 56
眼球恶性肿瘤 …… 2
眼眶恶性肿瘤 …… 5
泪点或鼻泪管梗阻 …… 18
泪液溢出 …… 3
泪囊瘘 …… 3
石灰烧伤 …… 1

鼻部疾病

鼻息肉 …… 10
恶性鼻息肉 …… 1
黏膜溃疡 …… 8
鼻和唇溃疡 …… 9
鼻骨病 …… 1
鼻出血 …… 2
鼻炎 …… 2
鼻损伤 …… 1
鼻挫伤 …… 1
鼻孔和口（部分）闭合 …… 1
果核卡在鼻腔内 …… 1

生殖泌尿系统疾病

白蛋白尿 …… 8
膀胱结石 …… 3
遗精 …… 31
淋病 …… 23
尿道狭窄 …… 9
尿外渗 …… 1
尿瘘 …… 2
包茎 …… 13
阴茎溃疡 …… 25
包皮龟头粘连 …… 1
阴茎上皮瘤 …… 6
包皮过长 …… 1
阴茎损伤（狗咬伤） …… 1
阴囊溃疡 …… 6
阴囊湿疹 …… 3
阴囊癣 …… 4
睾丸海绵肿 …… 2
阴囊积水 …… 28
阴囊肿瘤 …… 1
阳痿 …… 1
腹股沟淋巴结炎 …… 7
子宫肿瘤 …… 1
白带过多 …… 4
闭经 …… 2
痛经 …… 1
外阴瘙痒 …… 1
外阴肿瘤 …… 2

耳朵疾病

耳聋 …… 8
耳液溢 …… 8
外耳息肉 …… 1
耳垢 …… 2
耳部恶性肿瘤 …… 2
耳裂 …… 19
耳垂囊肿 …… 1
耳痛 …… 1

皮肤病

疥疮 …… 22
体癣 …… 110
黄癣 …… 8
发癣 …… 8
湿疹 …… 40
牛皮癣 …… 9
鱼鳞癣 …… 4
溃疡 …… 264
上皮癌 …… 8
狼疮 …… 2
甲床炎 …… 2
蛎壳疹 …… 5

天疱疮	1	梅毒性结节	4
痤疮	7	梅毒瘤	1
蛇皮癣	6	湿疣	2
痱子	1	钉胼	9
带状疱疹	1	疖痈	12
白癜风	1	疣	2
瘢痕瘤	1	裂伤	4
痒疹	2	窦道	16
深脓疱	8	脓肿	48

肿瘤

痣	5	腺体瘤	7
龈瘤	4	恶性肿瘤	15
粉瘤	1	下巴恶性肿瘤	5
甲状腺肿	2	女性乳房恶性肿瘤	3
舌下囊肿	1	囊肿	7
腱鞘瘤	3	下颌囊肿	2
脂肪瘤	12	未归类的	6
纤维瘤	11		
淀粉样瘤	7		

神经系统疾病

癫痫	9	面瘫	2
坐骨神经痛	26	截瘫	3
神经痛	11	偏瘫	2
局部麻痹	13	手臂瘫痪	2
眩晕	7	弱智	1
慢性脑积水	1	口齿不清	1
中风	1	脊髓疾病（未分类的）	1
运动性共济失调	3		

血管系统疾病

主动脉瘤	1	心脏肥大	1
心瓣膜病	7	静脉曲张	7

骨科疾病

骨疡和骨坏死	64	脊柱弯曲	8
骨膜炎	8		

关节疾病

甲状腺肿髋关节病	16	小趾跖趾关节滑膜炎	1
甲状腺肿膝关节病	5	踝关节僵硬	1
甲状腺肿肘关节病	1	膝关节僵硬	6
甲状腺肿肩关节病	1	髋关节僵硬	2
膝关节滑膜炎	7	肘关节僵硬	2
踝关节滑膜炎	17	滑囊炎	1
肩关节滑膜炎	1	关节挫伤	8
腕关节滑膜炎	1	膝外翻	1

外伤、损伤及其他

肩关节脱位	2	扭伤	20
肘关节脱位	1	烧伤和烫伤	5
踝关节脱位	1	猪咬伤	2
脚趾脱位	1	猫咬伤	1
胫骨骨折	2	狗咬伤	6
股骨骨折	1	女人咬伤	1
脚趾骨折	1	子弹嵌入	1
桡骨骨折	1	竹片残留在脚上	1
外伤	50	鱼骨卡在食道	1
跌打损伤	48	针残留在手腕	1
胸部损伤(由于负重和殴打)	45	玻璃碎片残留在脚上	1

未分类的

烧伤和溃疡后挛缩	4	助产	2
肌肉抽筋	1	刎颈	2
		曼陀罗中毒	1

霍乱——去年夏天这种病的流行已到了可怕的程度。老居民说这种病是自从汕头成为一个通商口岸以来最致命的传染病。这种病目前据说是由于打开两名在轮船上死于这个病的中国船员的棺材而引起的，但这不大可能。1882 年秋天出现大量的霍乱病例，我认为冬季这个病会在汕头流行。

炎热的天气一到来，人群中急性腹泻和痢疾便很普遍，许多人死亡，尤其是儿童。

霍乱典型病例直到六月末才开始出现，一旦暴发后，就迅速蔓延到农村各地。无法准确预估死亡率，但应该很高。光是在潮州府，据说死亡人数就有 4 000 至5 000 人。

中国朋友告诉了我们许多这种疾病在几个小时内致命的例子，其中的许多病例很少或没有腹泻或呕吐。我们听到很多令人悲伤的故事，例如，府城有一个家庭失去了 11 位成员中的 9 位。

到医院受到照料的病例大多数都得到了相当恰当的治疗，尤其是处于早期的患者。准确的治疗人数没有记录，但在我们有记录的 83 个病例中，完全康复的占四分之三。

霍乱合剂被送到很多与汕头基督教会相关的传教站，一些中国人购买了大量这种合剂在贫困人群中发放，或再次出售。我们后来听说，通过这些方式，许多病例成功康复。

许多不同的治疗方法都试过了，总体来说我们发现一个由等量的鸦片酊、辣椒、大黄、薄荷精和樟脑制成的合剂在这种疾病的早期阶段也许是最有用的。当霍乱病情正盛时，著名的印度“霍乱滴剂”是最好的治疗药物。病情到了衰竭阶段，或当患者开始出现衰竭症状时，我们给予皮下注射醚或白兰地。除了药物治疗，热水瓶、芥子泥等被给予病人使用，按摩也被用以解除痉挛性疼痛。对于呕吐不严重的病例，在很短的间隔中小心喂食稀释的牛奶。

对一个病例在病情第二阶段开始时用吗啡皮下注射有明显的效果。

我们得到 3 例用石炭酸治疗成功的病例报告。一位中国绅士从医院买了大量石炭酸溶液用于消毒，他把一些给了一个有霍乱病人的家庭，用来给排泄物及其他用品消毒。这个家庭误解了他的意思，把它当作药物喝了一些。他们在开始使用后不久就查出了病，但很快恢复了。

疟疾——间歇性发热病例的数量与前几年相比显著增加，这是本季节不健康状况的另一个标志。在这一年中有 282 例间歇性发热病例和 48 例简单发热病例，1882 年前者只有 131 例，后者只有 34 例。除了这些，在因为其他疾病接受治疗的病人中有约 280 个简单发热病例出现。

治疗间歇性发热我们通常首选奎宁和三氧化二砷。通过这种疗法疗效能更快显现。许多病例病程较长，间歇性发热中四日疟是最常见的。

奎宁的唯一缺点是价格非常昂贵。我们已经测试了相当数量的奎宁替代品的药用效果，其中在印度大量用于治疗穷人的金鸡纳退热药，也许是最好的一种。它比奎宁的使用剂量大一点，而且比奎宁对胃多一点刺激性，但使用它能得到非常好的效果。因为它比奎宁便宜多了，我们打算在今后更广泛地使用金鸡纳退热药。如果从印度送到中国的是金鸡纳退热药而不是鸦片，这对中国人民将是一大幸事。

吸食鸦片者——我们给出一些这类患者的统计信息，供那些对吸食鸦片这个主题感兴趣的人参考。

有 111 位吸鸦片烟者入院，但其中的一些在尝试戒除烟瘾两三天后离开了医院。

像以前一样，在治疗中没有使用任何鸦片替代品。在一年中我们遇到了相当数量的老病人，我们有理由相信，这些人大多数都没有复吸。这些人中有两三位已获准入教。

每日剂量

0.5 钱或更少	15
1 钱或多于 0.5 钱	32
1.5 钱或多于 1 钱	24
2 钱	16
2.5 钱	5
3 钱	10
4 钱	2
5 钱	4

鸦片烟龄

1 年或更短	6
2 年	9
3 年	7
4 年	10
5 年	5
6 年	5
7 年	2
8 年	2
9 年	1
10 年	17
11 年	1
12 年	3
13 年	1
14 年	2
16 年	1
17 年	2
18 年	1
20 年	6
25 年	2
30 年	2
34 年	1

吸鸦片者年龄

20~25 岁	11
25~30 岁	15
30~35 岁	24
35~40 岁	21
40~45 岁	18
45~50 岁	9
50~60 岁	9
70 岁以上	2

眼科疾病——我们经手的眼科疾病患者超过 1 120 人。

外科手术

这一年做了以下外科手术：

眼科手术：

睑内翻及倒睫症手术	326
翼状胬肉手术	51
眼睑外翻手术	1

睑缘粘连手术 …… 5
睑球粘连手术 …… 1
白内障手术 …… 7
前房葡萄肿切除术 …… 3
虹膜疝手术 …… 4
眼前房积脓手术 …… 4
上眼睑裂缝重塑手术 …… 1
人工瞳孔虹膜切除术 …… 29
眼球切除术 …… 2
结膜纤维切除术 …… 3
眼皮小肿瘤切除术 …… 8
眼皮恶性肿瘤切除术 …… 2
睑疣切除术 …… 1
眼眶恶性肿瘤切除术 …… 1
眼睑脓肿切开术 …… 1

=450

躯体手术：

唇裂手术 …… 26
肛瘘手术 …… 47
耳裂手术 …… 21
包皮（过长）环切术 …… 14
神经节手术 …… 8
痣手术 …… 1
直肠溃疡手术 …… 1
尿外渗手术 …… 1
骨疡手术 …… 8
肿瘤切除术 …… 46
外痔切除术 …… 14
肩关节切除术 …… 1
肘关节切除术 …… 1
扁桃体切除术 …… 2
牙龈瘤切除术 …… 4
乳腺硬癌切除术 …… 2
下颌部分切除术 …… 1
粉瘤切除术 …… 1
皮肤上皮瘤切除术 …… 2
包皮肥大切除术 …… 2

阴囊象皮病切除术	3
阴蒂和小阴唇象皮病切除术	1
钉胼切除术	9
舌下囊肿切除术	1
直肠息肉切除术	1
唇伤口整形手术	1
唇畸形整形手术	1
鼻孔和口（部分）闭合整形手术	1
外耳道闭合整形手术	1
碎石术	1
鼻窦切开术	8
下颌下腺区囊性肿瘤切开术	2
睾丸鞘膜积液抽吸和注射术	24
睾丸鞘膜积液切开术	1
内痔结扎术	46
阴茎（上皮瘤）截断术	4
坏死骨头剔除术	27
拔牙	67
鼻息肉摘除术	16
子弹取出术	1
从鼻孔取出种子术	1
指甲拔除术	2
竹碎片取出术	1
玻璃片取出术	1
针取出术	1
甲沟炎、脓肿等切开术	49
尿道狭窄扩张术	5
脱臼复位术	2
	=482[①]
	932

这一年没有任何手术死亡病例。

结石——这个病人是一个5岁左右的小男孩，已经患病约两年。他的健康状况相当好。经过几天的治疗准备后，我们通过横切的方法进行取石，一枚小母鸡鸡蛋大小的结石被取出。小病人恢复良好，术后16天左右便可以出院了。

鼻孔和口挛缩闭合——病人的鼻孔是完全闭合的，进入口腔的入口直径不足半英寸，这是由以前的溃疡所造成的。

① 相加应为481，但原文如此，此种情况下文不一一说明。

我们做了两次手术。第一次手术切开两侧鼻孔，然后置入银管，银管前面通过狭窄的中间物件连接，两头分别插入鼻孔，以防止鼻孔再次闭塞。这些管通过绳子来保持其位置，绳子一头固定管子，另一头绕过头部的两侧绑在脑后。同时，在口的两侧的脸颊上开孔，置入小银条并系好。几个星期后进行第二次手术，切开口中间的皮肤和现已经显露的孔。结果是令人满意的。

下颌骨部分切除术——病人是一位年轻男性，患有下颌骨囊性肿瘤，位于颞下颌关节和下颌角中间。1882 年间，我为病人切除肿瘤，将其清理干净，再用高浓度的氯化锌溶液擦洗残腔，几个月之后肿瘤复发。这一次肿瘤生长的这片下颌骨被切除。伤口经过了很长时间才愈合，但是效果非常好。

阴囊象皮肿——我们做了 3 例手术，切除的肿瘤的重量分别为 76 盎司、160 盎司和 100 盎司，病人恢复良好。

阴唇象皮肿——一个中年妇女阴唇长了两个象皮肿，一个重达 10 磅，另一个重 1 磅，我们从阴蒂和小阴唇的中间将肿瘤从颈部切除，由于用一条弹力带紧紧绑住肿瘤的颈部，手术过程中出血很少，病人恢复良好。

关节切除术——一个年轻男人的肩关节和一个男孩的肘关节因为骨疡和关节结构破坏而被切除。两个都是长期发病的老病例，病人的健康状况很不好。手术需要切除大块的骨头，而结果不是很令人满意。

肿瘤切除术——大量的各种类型的肿瘤从身体的各个部位被切除。他们中有许多是很有趣的病例，但在这份报告中不可能进行记述。有几个是大尺寸的：一个从臀部切除的脂肪瘤重 81 盎司；另一个类似象皮肿，重 2.5 磅，从髂骨的区域被切除。

财务

从附表可以看到，这一年收入达 2 320.94 美元，支出 2 201.40 美元，结余 119.54 美元。我们还附上一个捐款者的列表，对他们的慷慨捐赠我们表示衷心感谢。我们相信，我们的医疗机构是值得他们支持的。

这一年内陈源盛（Tan Nguan Seng）给出价值 100 美元的大米和现金券分发给贫穷患者。他的慷慨帮助到现在已持续了几年，很让人感激，它使我们能够留住许多贫穷的病人直到他们完全治愈。

1883 年捐款

（略）

收支表

单位：美元

助手和门卫工资	370.00
印刷医院报告费用、邮资	30.50
地租、房屋保险	25.00
病房的粉刷、修复和涂漆	83.02

买猪油、油、纸、蜡、木炭	94.60
买布绷带、药棉	70.48
买制作搽剂、酊剂的杜松子酒和精馏酒	130.19
买水	48.20
买新病床、仪器和杂物	139.10
援助贫困患者费用	135.79
在中国和加尔各答购药	170.63
来自伦敦的药物、外科敷料及其运费、保险费和起岸费	293.89
来自伦敦的由爱丁堡教会支付的药物等费用（大约）	510.00
大米和现金券（大约）	100.00
结余	119.54
	2 320.94

1882年结余款	333.23
如前列捐款	1 179.76
卖疝气绑带	17.00
卖厕所用品	28.55
卖杂物	20.44
卖药	121.20
小病房租金	10.76
来自伦敦的由爱丁堡教会支付的药物费用（大约）	510.00
大米和现金券	100.00
	2 320.94

1883年客家地区医疗工作报告

在提交我在客家地区第二年进行的医疗工作的短篇报告时，我觉得从医学的角度看令人感兴趣的内容较少。尽管如此，我们有理由相信，许多患者的病痛已经解除或减轻，从而间接地通过其精神的实践展示颂扬了福音。

自年初我与丰约翰医生（Dr. MacPhun）一起工作，他同时主要将精力用于提高他的语言能力，但打算不久以后就全力进行医学工作。我们在五经富（Ng-kang-phu）的中心固定工作了约200天，那时我们独留一人或两人一起驻扎在那里。此外，我们带着一批药品访问了几次分站，访问时间从几天到两三个星期不等。丰约翰医生是与纪多纳牧师（Rev. D. Mac-Iver）一起访问的，包括在今年年初对顶埔（Thai-pu）地区的一次重要访问。

大部分在五经富的工作已经完成了，并在那里的教堂继续进行着。这年年末一间房子被抵押用作医院，但因为它必须进行大修，新的一年里，我们仍然要在教堂看诊，这对医生和传教士来说都极为不便。在这样的情况下，我们今年没有公开接收住院病人。还好我们不时想出某种方法为少数急症病人提供几天住处，我们希望对他们有好处。

我们的医院现在差不多做好了准备，它包含一间相当大的男性病房、一间女性病房、一间手术间和一间传教的房间，还有两间可使用于各种用途的小候诊室，这样我们将能接收约 20 位住院病人。我们早已觉得非常需要这样一个地方。我们建议一些病人去汕头接受更好的治疗，但很少有人去，原因显而易见，他们中的大多数人很穷，难以承担这样的旅费。我们似乎很难让一些人明白病情的真实状况。他们似乎认为，建议去其他地方治疗就是暗示他们无法被治愈，或者说我们是因为某些原因不愿意为了他们而给自己找麻烦。几个月前，两位男人患尿结石而来诊。我们煞费苦心地向他们解释其所患疾病的特点，指出靠"吃药"是没用的，并说明去汕头医院治疗几乎肯定能获得的好处，但很明显他们很不愿意接受我们的建议。

治疗这样的疾病伴随的危险性，使我们在一段时间内不宜在这里尝试治疗。的确，把五经富的小医院的设备升级是值得的，至少到目前为止还是经常有病人必须被送往汕头。对于许多不太严重的手术，我们希望很快能进行并获得满意的治疗结果。我们已经有了一个开端，年内进行的手术操作列表将证明这一点。我们确信这样的工作是值得做的。我们有一位在汕头培训的本土配药师，不久他将为我们配药，并包扎伤口，现在这些工作是由我们自己在做，耗费了大量的时间。

我们保存了五经富来诊病人数的准确记录，共记录了 1 024 个病例。其中不少是两次、三次或更多次来诊，但对这些复诊情况没有保存准确的记录。病人大多数是客家人，但有一部分是主要来自棉湖（Miow）附近的闽南人。我们的病人来自南面的新田（Sin-thyen）至北面的汤坑（Thong-hang），还有两三位病人是专程从崇乐（Chong-lok）来的。

经粗略估计，我们访问偏远农村期间诊治的病人大约有 576 人，如果加上丰约翰医生在顶埔、汤坑、河婆（Hopho）和其他地方诊治的病人数，在外诊治的大约有 1 000 人，因此这一年的病人总数应有 2 000 人以上。

我们的病人中从一开始便有一定比例的女性患者，主要希望医治眼疾或消化不良、风湿病、慢性咳嗽等普通疾病。在五经富治疗的 1 024 个病例中有 340 个（约三分之一）是女性患者。

在五经富，我们固定十一点到一点为看病时间，平均每天的新病例在 5 例左右。虽然我们的目标是通过医学技术传播福音，但是由于每天病人人数少，以及缺乏可在规定时间与其进行礼拜的住院病人，我们无法像所期望的那样定期向病人布道。当病人较多时，我们会派一名学生向他们布道，其他时间我们会简单地向他们讲述教义并邀请他们到教堂来了解更多。

我们的药物一直由来爱力医生（Dr. Lyall）提供，我们感谢一直以来援助汕头医院的朋友们。我们的朋友应该知道农村患者使用了大量药物，也许就所占病人比例来看比在医院更多。可以说，医院的主要工作是做手术，而我们的主要工作是配药。为了有效率地工作，我们需要充足的药品供应。迄今为止我们都是免费配发药品，仅有少数人从我们这里批量买药。

从附表可以看出我们在五经富被祈求治疗的疾病的种类及病例数，末尾还有我们对内外科疾病的评论。

内科病例

消化不良、**疟疾**、**慢性支气管炎**和**肌肉风湿病**病例是最常见的。

秋收以后田地干涸时，**疟疾**最常见。奎宁的疗效在这里的每一个地方都是众所周知的，如果我们使用其他药物，我们总会被提醒“白色的药”是最好的。对症状较轻的病例，先服一剂奎宁，即两或三格令，接着使用一个疗程的铁剂和砷剂往往足以治愈该病。

我们所见到的类似疟疾的病例可能也是因**贫血**和**乏力**而引起的，我们仅在一些病例中能够采集到疟疾的病史。治疗疟疾的药物同样对这些病例起作用，奎宁加铁剂，或铁剂加砷剂能显著增进疗效。

对于儿童的疾病，我们发现对很多病例很难做出满意的诊断。大多数是缺乏照料导致的慢性病例，为了给它们一个更好的病名，我们将其分类为**婴儿衰弱**。

其中有一些只是简单的**蛔虫**病例。其他的则是因急性疾病治疗不当而衰弱，有的病例也许最初就有甲状腺肿的趋势。有几个孩子非常瘦弱，手脚肿胀，眼睛紧闭着。当我们费很大劲使他们的眼睛睁开后，就发现双眼都无可救药了，角膜脱落、虹膜凸出。这个地区的人将这些婴儿疾病称为“疳积”（Kam-tsit）。大多数但不是所有病例都是蛔虫病例，使用散道宁病情几乎能立即得到显著改善。对于一些极度严重的病例，除了尝试使用瑞士炼奶没有更好的方法了。我们发现这种做法很好。这些人显然不懂得护理技术。一个孩子若进食普通食物那就好办，但如果不吃，他们就不知道要准备什么更容易消化的食物了。

我们有许多**吸鸦片烟者**申请得到“戒鸦片药丸”，我们一概拒绝。我们坚信，如果给予他们这些，只会使那些希望从中受益的人产生误解，更不必说有的申请者可能和我们一样知道“戒鸦片药丸”含什么成分。我们通常建议他们去汕头医院，并马上戒除这种习惯。

外科病例

眼部疾病病例最多的是**颗粒性结膜炎**。一些病人是多次就诊才治愈的，但是另一些病人不能常来就得不到最好的治疗效果。

许多病例来时流眼泪而且眼睛不舒服，但无炎症或产生颗粒，显然这是由于烟尘不断刺激引起的，且容易发展成颗粒性疾病。使用一种低浓度的硫酸锌溶液是我们通常的治疗方法，其现在名声大振，我们发现很难使我们的病人相信这种药不可以用于所有的疾病。

我们所做的共15例眼睑内翻手术中大约有10例获得成功。

对于其他外科病例我们仅对以下进行详述：

下颌骨骨折和头皮裂伤——一个11岁的男孩的头被压在甘蔗榨糖厂的梁柱之间。一块约5英寸长的大皮瓣向着耳朵撕裂，大部分为覆盖在颞窝上的头皮，几乎与头部断离。下颌骨在离下巴中间线一英寸处骨折，嘴因为后面的骨碎片向内凹陷而歪斜。所有伤口已用一些植物制剂涂抹用于止血，但他的父母同意将这些清除掉，并进行伤口清洗。一些容易脱落的组织被用剪刀去除，皮裂伤两边被缝了几针以保持在适当的位置。下巴很容易就固定了，没有使用任何绷带来保持它的位置，应该几乎是立刻就接合了，因为几天之后男孩就能很轻松地使用他的下巴。后来伤口化脓，小皮瓣脱落，但随着时间的推移，加上每天的照料，它愈合得非常令人满意。

唇裂——这种先天性畸形的手术有 4 例。第一例是一个双侧唇裂的重度病例，这是一名 7 岁的男孩，他的父母都是教会的成员。来爱力医生年初到五经富访问时完成该手术。孩子很难控制，我们使用了手头最好的银丝线，还是不足以固定手术部位，尽管如此，情况还是非常好。

其他病例的手术是八月份在访问崇乐的巴塞尔（Basel）传教站期间完成的。其中一例 11 岁，一例 4 岁，还有一例 9 个月，所有的手术情况都很好。

肿瘤（纤维瘤）切除——在崇乐访问期间，有一位病人因为靠近腋下的肋骨部位长有一个靠外蒂悬挂的大肿瘤而来诊。我们用一个粗木夹夹住肿瘤的蒂，临时凑合着用刀切断肿瘤。病人的背部和胸部还有许多其他肿瘤，但没有比小鸡蛋大的，而被切除的这个肿瘤足有两磅重。

以下是这一年中完成的手术的准确列表：

唇裂	4
睑内翻（上睑 11 例，下睑 4 例）	15
翼状胬肉	3
耳裂	4
下唇裂	1
拔牙	6
骨折固定	5
肿瘤（纤维瘤）切除	1
上颌囊性肿瘤切开	1
下颌囊性肿瘤切开	1
鼻息肉摘除	1
脓肿切开	5
内痔结扎	1
肛瘘	1
	49

所治疗的疾病总表

常见病	263
消化系统疾病	119
循环系统疾病	9
呼吸系统疾病	72
神经系统疾病	22
生殖泌尿系统疾病	6
耳部和鼻部疾病	9
眼部疾病	160
关节疾病	4

骨头疾病	2
皮肤病	115
外伤、损伤及其他	44
未分类的	199
总数	1 024

（翻译：谢煊、郑庭凯　校译：朱文平　审校：胡卫清、余维泉、江建安　中文校正：许党泉、颜彦）

1886 年汕头福音医院报告

（1886 年度高仕兰医学学士、外科硕士和麦克方医学学士、外科硕士照管下的英兰长老会汕头和五经富教会医院报告）

1886 年的病人数如下。因对收治吸食鸦片者有了新规定，申请戒毒治疗的病人数量减少了，所以这一年的病人数比起前一年稍有减少。在夏季的几个月里，米价上涨也导致就诊病人数持续大幅度下降。

个体病人的数量如下：

住院病人	3 592
门诊病人	1 944
合计	5 536
以上包括女性病人	842

此外，还有大量患者在非门诊时间接受了高级助理的诊治。这些病例主要是一些小事故和轻症病人，那些病人或多或少与教会有关。

平均每日病人数：各个月的平均每日住院病人数及门诊病人数如下：

	住院病人	门诊病人
一月	172	27
二月	66	18
三月	169	41
四月	162	32
五月	263	46
六月	196	53
七月	184	43
八月	201	46
九月	263	58
十月	278	63
十一月	164	41
十二月	170	40

门诊如常于星期二及星期五向病人开放，但也会在星期一、星期四及星期六接诊那些需要住院的病人。手术则是在星期三及星期六进行。

汕头是一个比较小的地方，而且完全商业化了。只有很少家庭居住在这里。不可思议的是这里极度缺乏提供给旅行者的住所。这里只有几间旅馆，且收费非常昂贵。所以，从远方来的病人除非在这个城镇里有一些认识的人能够收留他们，否则他们只能住在医院里。这就导致医院有时会过分拥挤。在夏天炎热的晚上，教堂及走廊经常会被占用。

去年夏天有两批女病人不得不住在教堂中。她们花了一些时间积攒现金，希望来医治眼疾或者缓解消化不良症状，我们很难把她们打发走。

医院的建筑物由 3 幢两层高的楼房组成。其中一幢是行政楼，另外两幢楼各有 4 个大病房——两个在楼上，两个在楼下。另外还有一些小病房用作特殊病房、私人病房和学生房间，还有一间以前的麻风病医院。后者只需步行几分钟即可到达。总共可以容纳 150 位住院病人。

其中一间病房专为鸦片吸食者保留。以前是不向这些病人收取费用的，然而由于这个措施成效不令人满意，去年设立了一项新规定，向这些病人收取 1 美元的费用作为诚信担保。这项规定减少了超过一半的病人数，但前来的患者得到了更好的治疗。

我要非常感谢李洁小姐（Miss Ricketts）的礼物，她为我们提供了一部连接医务人员的住处与医院的电话，这在各个方面都为我们带来了很大的帮助。

病人的地区分布

	病人数
潮州地区：	
澄海	655
潮阳	1 345
揭阳	979
海阳	686
饶平	554
普宁	492
惠来	331
丰顺	69
大埔	15
南澳岛	90
惠州地区：	
陆丰	34
海丰	6
嘉应州	26
福建省：	
来自诏安地区	226
其他地区	12
其他省份	16
	5 536

教育

这一年里有一个6人组成的班级接受教育。课程包括药物学、解剖学及生理学。克尔医生和奥斯古德医生（Drs. Kerr and Osgood）的著作被用作教科书。一架有关节连接的骨骼模型是最主要的解剖学教学辅助工具。在伦敦的J. T. 莫尔顿先生（Mr. J. T. Morton）的好心帮助下，今年学生在复习解剖学知识方面将会获益良多，因为他们可以借助Dr. Auzoux装配的人体模型。

每半年一次的考试能够非常直接地表明学生们对学科知识的掌握情况。

传教工作——传教方法没有什么改变。每天的晨祷和晚祷，以及每周日下午的答疑解惑聚会都如常举行。

医院没有专属的传教士。两位高级助理主持礼拜仪式，而我的牧师同事每人每周负责一次晨祷。神学院的学生上学时在小医院举行晚祷。早上所有的病人都集中在大医院教堂里。之前几年在门诊病人中的传道工作没有显著的成效，但在大多数住院病人中的工作获得了一些成果，他们中有20人，其中有7位女士及13位男士，被接收入教会。还有一位男士获准洗礼，但他在仪式进行之前就去世了。有一些被接收的人还是在去年首次听到他们的名字。许多人都是申请了很久的，直到他们在家里公开表明信奉基督教以证明他们的诚意，才得以接受洗礼。这是非常必要的，因为在医院没有办法测试他们的态度是否真诚。

外科手术

眼科：

睑内翻及倒睫症手术：	
上眼睑	313
下眼睑	188—501
睑球粘连手术	4
睑缘粘连手术	1
翼状胬肉手术	55
结膜黄斑手术	1
结膜囊肿手术	2
结膜肥大手术	2
角膜缘球结膜环状切开术	1
虹膜切除术	11
晶状体取出术（白内障）	13
不透明囊切开术	5
前房打孔术	1
前房积脓手术	11
眼睑裂伤修复手术	1
眼球切除术	3
	612

躯体手术：

小腿截肢术	1
手指切除术	2
赘生拇指切除术	2
阴茎切除术（上皮癌）	5
良性肿瘤切除术	21
恶性肿瘤切除术	13
囊性肿瘤切除术	15
血管瘤切除术	1
旋后肌肉瘤最大部分切除术	2
皮脂腺囊肿切除术	12
动脉瘤切除术	1
嵌入子弹取出术	1
扁桃体肿大切除术（切除器）	2
唇裂手术	39
鼻孔疤痕闭锁手术	2
下唇上皮瘤手术	1
舌下囊肿手术	3
耳垂裂口修补术	42
上唇修补术	1
鼻裂伤修补术	1
阴囊撕裂伤修补术	1
肛瘘手术	52
外痔手术	26
内痔手术（结扎）	42
包皮环切术	10
阴囊象皮病手术	4
咽部腺体增生手术	1
脓胸手术	1
先天性无直肠畸形手术	1
神经节手术	5
股骨粉碎性骨折手术	1
手指矫直手术	1
疤痕电切术	3
痣电切术	3
膀胱抽吸术	1
肝脓肿抽吸术	1
脓胸抽吸术	3

坐骨神经痛针刺术	1
鞘膜积液抽液注射术	27
囊性甲状腺肿抽液注射术	3
会阴切开术（尿道破裂）	1
鼻中果核取出术	1
咽喉中鱼骨取出术	3
死骨剔除术	20
鼻息肉切除术	8
耳息肉切除术	1
痣皮下结扎术	1
痣结扎术	1
脚趾甲拔除术	2
手术总数	1 004
拔牙	115

此外，还有切开脓肿和瘘管、脱臼复位、导管术等未包含在上表中。

睑内翻及倒睫症——可能汕头外科工作最有特色的是大量的睑内翻及倒睫症手术，去年达到501例。各种严重程度的病例都能看到，从轻微的倒睫症，到完全的睑内翻，上下眼睑的睫毛整个平贴在角膜上。有许多患者就诊得太迟。角膜布满血管的，溃疡状的，云雾状的，已经穿孔的，或多或少伴有虹膜炎性脱垂的都有。奇怪的是有时睑内翻所致的痛苦很小，人们还能每天干活，似乎睫毛并没有结成束摩擦到他们角膜上的溃疡。女性患此病的比例比男性大。去年男性病人中有120位，即2.5%的人患睑内翻，而女性患者中有119位，即14%的人患此病。患颗粒状眼炎的男人有290位，占6%，而女人有86位，占10%。

丰约翰医生（Dr. MacPhun）告诉我，客家人很少患沙眼及睑内翻，他在五经富诊治的大部分是闽南人。即使是在这两种人混居的边界地区，也是闽南人患病。虽然女性病例有很大的不同，因为客家女人不缠脚，而且经常帮助男人干农活，然而男性病例没有任何区别。至于烟雾、强光和泥垢，任何人都无法逃脱这些因素。我不知道用什么理由去解释这种病在汕头如此令人讨厌地高发。我不认为这里的人与广州人和福建居民在生活方式上有什么不同，可以解释这种疾病在此地区的闽南人中更流行。

腹部瘘——患者是一个11岁小女孩，病程3个月，位置在肚脐眼下方一点，受伤的原因是被水牛角顶伤。粪便一部分经瘘管排出，一部分经肛门排出。尝试通过将黏膜连续内翻缝合，同时缝接皮肤的方法闭合伤口，但失败了。之后对伤口进行了两次烧灼治疗，第二次终于成功地使之闭合了。

脓胸——病程5个月，左胸腔明显扩张，尤其向后扩张。心脏右移。患者是一个瘦弱的年轻男人。我一个星期内为其抽胸液3次，共抽出210盎司的液体，其中四分之一是脓液。由于病情只得到暂时性缓解，所以为其做了开胸引流，用Hey氏锯及骨钳切去病人第八根肋骨1英寸。应用可卡因实行了局部麻醉。由于天气影响了吸引器的印度橡胶管，在最后一次抽液时，空气被不幸吸入，手术过程也没能做到严格消毒。不久之后表示肠道淀粉样变性的腹泻开始出现。应患者的强烈要求，他在手术后两个月就回家了。由于持续腹泻，排脓并没有减少，痊愈希望是极低的。假如他能早些来就诊，结果或许会不一样。

一个女孩的**上唇修复**。她上唇中心的大半部分和鼻中隔的一部分在患天花后溃烂。在皮瓣能被调整之前需要在每边开3个切口，即：①通过鼻翼外侧向上切口；②从相同的起点到脸颊与唇平行切口；③从嘴角向外平行切口。唇部相关手术的结果令人非常满意，而鼻子部分还有待改进。

疤痕及痣电切术——能够被追踪到的病例效果都很令人满意。

阴囊象皮病——4例。重量分别为2.5、2、21和20磅。第二个病例有理由去怀疑是阴茎上皮癌细胞转移所导致的，在手术过程中诊断得以明确，病变部位被切除。这一年唯一一例手术死亡病例发生在一名来自福建的男人身上。切除后排干液体肿瘤重达20磅。病人两条腿也因象皮病而肿大。死亡原因是休克。以后对于腿部受到严重感染的病例的手术我要非常谨慎。

肝脓肿抽吸术——记录这个病例，是因为这是我第一次在中国人身上遇到这种情况。这个病例病程两个月，肝脏肿大至乳头线肋缘下3英寸。实施的抽吸术是诊断性的，抽出1盎司多一点的脓液。这个病人无法住院，所以无法对他实施进一步治疗。

本地的虫肠——（阿拉特斯飞蛾幼虫的吐丝器官）在这一年被使用到一些手术中。我发现它作为缝线非常好用，但缝扎血管用这种线就太硬了，而且不能溶解。这种线非常便宜。

一些被治疗的疾病列表

常见疾病

间歇发热：

日发疟	9
间日疟	12
三日疟	189
不规则的	8
脾肿大（疟疾）	19
麻风病（90%有斑点）	270
脚气病	10
甲状腺肿	6
吸鸦片者的治疗	306

神经系统

痴呆症	4
产褥期痴呆症	1
癫痫	7

消化系统

食管恶性狭窄	4
直肠溃疡及狭窄	31
腹股沟疝（右边占7成）	42

循环系统

心脏瓣膜病变	16

眼部

颗粒性眼炎	376	睑内翻及倒睫症	239

淋巴系统

右小腿象皮病	14	阴囊的象皮病	18
左小腿象皮病	10	淋巴阴囊	10
右小腿及阴囊象皮病	2	腹股沟淋巴结肿大	3
双小腿及阴囊象皮病	2		
双小腿象皮病	1		
未记录哪一侧的象皮病	10		

泌尿生殖系统

膀胱结石	2
助产	3

脚气病——在汕头教会男子中学和女子学校暴发过一次萎缩型脚气病。

男子学校在新年假期之后的三月初开学，女子学校在春节期间没有放假。第一批病例大约在五月初发现，几个本在治疗消化不良的男孩开始反映腹部及小腿的皮肤麻木，一次小调查探查出这些普通症状。不久有 7 位男孩患了此病，因为没有办法控制病情，他们被送往 60 英里外的内陆山区客家农村，在五经富由丰约翰医生（Dr. McPhun）照管。这天是 5 月 26 日。3 天之后，因为又有 7 位男孩及当地的老师受到感染，学校就放假了，男孩们被送回家。

6 月 2 日有一位女孩患病，6 月 11 日又有一位，6 月 17 日再有两位。由于还有五六个人有轻微的先兆症状，学校提前停课放暑假了。

患者的症状不同，但差异很小。首先是在患病的部位有风湿病的感觉，许多患者有胃炎的迹象。接下来会出现前胫骨及股骨区域麻木，然后延伸到腹部，上至脐部。同时，这些区域的肌肉开始僵硬及疼痛。疼痛部位据说会发热、发痒、抽筋，有一些病人会痛得睡不着觉。接下来的几天受感染的肌肉会明显感到软弱和乏力。一些回家休养的男孩由此产生局部麻痹，他们的腿会忽然发软。这使他们不得不躺在床上。膝盖也会感受到疼痛，如果腿伸直会加重疼痛。有些病人的局部麻痹甚至会延伸到前臂，除一个可疑病例外，没有病人会延伸到唇部。

麻痹的区域在所有的患者中并不相同。有一个男孩大腿部位没有麻木。其他人则从小腿及大腿后面直到大腿前面都麻木。

踝阵挛及膝反射消失。遗憾的是，我没有留下皮肤反射的记录。最后患病的那批男孩最突出的症状是膝关节及踝关节后方的跟腱疼痛。在男子学校最严重的病例中，呼吸困难现象非常明显。只有两个病例出现水肿。有一例是脚踝轻度水肿。他的二尖瓣听诊区可闻及收缩期杂音，在应用了洋地黄后水肿在几天后便消失了。另外一个男孩的脸部有轻度浮肿，在他的主动脉瓣听诊区及肺动脉瓣听诊区可闻及第二心音的分裂。这两个病例呼吸困难最明显，对其他患者的听诊显示仅有轻度心律失常。所有男孩的上胸椎都有不同程度的叩击痛，这种情况没有在女孩中出现。

排泄物则很正常。

两位女孩腿部疼痛发作得相当突然。其中一位在教室里发病，号叫着被抬到楼上。总体来说，女孩患病比男孩少。在女子学校放假之前，那些患有脚气病的病例已能够小步曳脚而行。病情不像另一所学校那样进一步恶化。五六个女孩一些天有轻微的前驱症状，但这些症状并未发展为其他疾病。

那些被送往五经富的男孩中，有 4 位很快就痊愈并被送回家。其他的 3 人则在五经富多住了一个半月。其中一个现在仍在家里，另外两个于 1886 年和 1887 年交接的冬天回到学校并接受小腿肌肉僵硬及萎缩的治疗。其他直接被送回家的患者经过两三个星期疗程的治疗痊愈。我想说，无论强壮或虚弱，年老或年轻，均会患此病。3 个最严重的病例中，两人之前身体很健康，另一个则曾经因为慢性风湿性关节炎卧床一个月。

没有发现任何药物治疗有作用，但从感染场所迁走产生的医疗效果是最显著的。对于后遗症，鳕鱼肝油、士的宁、电疗有一定的作用，而禁止那些受感染的病人食用大米没有收到明显疗效。

直到男子学校停课，我才诊断出脚气病的病因。教科书上的脚气病描述相当符合干性表现。值得庆幸的是，我读到西蒙医生（Dr. Simmon）发表在《1879—1880 年海关医学报告》上的文章，它消除了我对这次脚气病发病性质的所有疑惑。

至于暴发的原因，还难以得到一个满意的结论。

传教站和贝理神学院与受影响的学校在同一个院子，毗邻医院，但没有学校外的人受到疾病的侵袭。食物可能是一种特殊毒物的传播媒介，尤其有人曾指出有可疑的细菌孢子附着于大米上，而如今大量的大米来自中国中部、日本及泰国。如果是那样的话，在这混住的院子、在汕头，事实上甚至在全国各地的中国人当中，应该会有一些病例，然而我一个都没有听说，而且经询问发现学校并没有使用这些大米。为什么脚气病在这两所秩序良好、干净、通风的学校暴发还是个有待解决的问题，它们和其他教会建筑一样最近才修建，位于围海造地的陆地上，两所学校相互之间没有交流。在其所处地区到目前为止脚气病还不被人们认知，在周围的所有中国人中又没有听说过此病。值得注意的是，这时的气候特别干燥。在 1884 年夏天男子学校有一个单独病例，我认为那应是一个脚气病病例。

上述的脚气病暴发后，有 10 位患者已在医院治疗。其中两位来自邻近的海阳地区，我有点怀疑他们是干性脚气病。其他病人 7 位来自新加坡，1 位来自槟城，他们全部都是水肿型的。据他们所说，这段水路有一个明显的益处，上船前水肿还很明显。当他们到达汕头的时候全身性水肿几乎都消退了。他们的肌肉萎缩和麻木和干性脚气病病例发生在同样的部位。此外还会呼吸困难，在肺动脉听诊区可听到收缩期杂音，伴有便秘。受感染的肌肉恢复肌力非常缓慢。

最近在马来西亚的调查表明脚气病可能会感染到一个地区。这种病在学校的出现是否与从海峡殖民地来的这些病例的不断输入有某些关系呢？

助产——最严重的一个病例是一个胎儿横位的产妇。该产妇产前已经阵痛 3 天。在第二天，助产士已把胎儿的前臂拉出来。胎儿被紧紧卡住了，胎位不能动，直至整个被掏出。胎儿脑积水，而当我尝试去剥离胎盘的时候，我发现子宫在胎头挤压的地方有严重的裂伤。她最终在30小时后死亡。

1886年的捐款

（捐款名单略）

1885年，陈源盛（Tan Nguan-seng）继续为我们提供大米和现金券，总数为6 000张的现金券价值191.36美元，这给贫困的病人提供了3 000顿饭。

另外，曾阿喜（Tsan A Hi）捐献了200张现金券，总值13.18美元，另一位朋友贡献了106张现金券，价值6.26美元。

依靠这些现金券，我得以让许多慢性病人保持治疗直到产生疗效，他们本来没有能力支付足够长时间的治疗费用。

收支表

单位：美元

欧洲人的捐款	853.56
中国人的捐款	198.24
卖药、绷带	634.01
卖牛奶给病人	191.95
向吸鸦片者收费	138.84
私人病房的租金	21.32
各种各样的收入	58.97
爱丁堡教会提供的药物费用	681.10
	2 777.99

上年度赤字	36.58
工资及旅行费用	364.96
出版医院报告	31.00
两年的火灾保险费	40.00
从伦敦购买牛奶	229.41
在汕头买药	64.01
从香港及印度购买药物及酒精	353.00
从英格兰等地购买药物	258.38
购买猪油	23.17
修理费	54.75
油费	104.03
羊毛费	48.57

水费	49.08
洗涤费	9.82
帮助贫困病人及丧葬的费用	44.46
各种费用：布、纸等	96.88
爱丁堡教会提供的药物费用	681.10
结余	288.79
	2 777.99

1886 年客家五经富地区的医学传教工作报告

在这一整年中，医院及诊所的工作几乎一直在进行。

八月份曾中止工作大约两周。去年就诊病人数只是稍有增加，而且他们的就诊次数与田里的工作量成反比。

医院的工作对客家人的影响多半局限于五经富地区。部分原因与客家地区的地理因素和自然因素有关。客家人生活在山区，而且住在河流的上游，这条河流流经闽南人居住的平原地区。

这个区域被分成多个小地区，此处居民与下游闽南人的交流比起与邻近地区的客家同胞的交流更多，而且更便利。缺少方便的水路交通极大地限制了医院能影响的地区，因为很少有病人愿意走一段长距离的陆路来医院。

我们附近的一些闽南人来这里接受治疗，而且接近一半的住院病人是闽南人。

四月和五月间，大米价格非常贵，这毫无疑问会让许多悲惨的需要治病的贫苦人留在家里。大部分人非常穷，以至于米价的一点上升都会令他们非常痛苦。我们的一个传教士告诉我，他所在地区有 300 个家庭，估计只有约 20 个家庭能够吃得饱。

从附表看，在就诊病人中，只有相当小部分的病人接受手术，约占十分之一。客家人特别不愿意接受需要切割的手术，即使是肿瘤或脓肿，他们也希望能够通过吃药或敷药来消除它们。

一些人越来越认识到西药的疗效，不少人来到医院开药，要求开奎宁、散道宁、碘剂等。

今年的治疗病例数如下：

新的门诊病人数	2 225
新的住院病人数	315
以上包括女病人数：	
住院病人数	40
门诊病人数	451
12 岁以下的小孩	350

除了以上病人，到乡村巡诊期间还看了许多病人。

这一年有一部分下午时间用来向助理们教授解剖学及生理学要领。

传教工作——早晨及夜晚的祈祷每天都在医院进行。除了规定的仪式以外，福音传教者还尽量与每个人交流。这样做很有用，但并不是表现在揭露他们随意信仰神明的愚蠢上，而是在消除他们关于信仰上帝的许多错误想法方面。那些愿意接受教诲的人学习诵读十戒律、主祷文和赞美诗，这些成为许多人甚至教会成员的主要神学读物。很少人可以诵读《圣经》，所以挑选一些段落以有利于记忆。有许多病人在医院时表示对这方面很有兴趣，当他离开时对教义已经有相当的了解，其中有两三个人我们认为他们的心已受到感化而去侍奉真神。

在这一年里德尔医生（Dr. Riddel）和我花了很多时间拜访乡村传教站与新的教区。在以传播福音为主要目的的行程中，我们由一位当地传教士陪同，得到了大量传道机会。从医学的观点来看，这并不等同于医院工作，然而这对打破偏见，开辟新教区的道路是最重要的。通过这种方式，福音在许多新村庄得到宣扬，我们将诚挚地请求得到上帝子民的祷告，希望这样的播种会有福报。

先天性肛门缺失——一个两天大的新生儿因为这个病被抱来诊治。切入超过1英寸后没有发现肠管，我当时就不再进一步进行手术了。孩子的父亲当天把他抱回家，说他会在第二天早晨回来，然而他没有回来。

外伤性坏疽——病人是一个男孩，他跌倒摔断了颈部桡骨。他的臂膀被一个当地医生用绷带绑得太紧。10天之后入院时他的整个前臂已坏死了，死皮分界线向上推进，且上臂炎症渗出很严重，体温为103华氏度。肘关节处形成了分界线，几天后手术只将尺切保留，邻近的组织几乎全部切除了。因为他父亲不愿意做任何进一步的手术，于是留下表面粗糙而且已经愈合的残肢。

已治疗的疾病列表

常见疾病

疟疾	45	麻风病	63
贫血	19	鸦片吸食者（为了治疗）	53
贫血合并脾大	4	淋巴结	12
全身衰弱	62	斑疹伤	1
婴儿衰弱	31	梅毒	5
丹毒	3	全身水肿	8
低热	13		

神经系统疾病

神经痛	3	脑积水	1
神经麻痹（面部）	3	斜颈	1
局部麻痹（腿伸肌面）	3	躁狂症	2

偏瘫	1	癔症	3
麻痹（区域性）	5	眩晕	14
癫痫	4	脑肿瘤	1
抽搐（婴儿）	1	未分类的	6
坐骨神经痛	7		

循环系统疾病

动脉瘤	1	心脏瓣膜病	3
痣	1	心律失常	9
静脉曲张	3		

呼吸系统疾病

哮喘	20	支气管炎	80
喉炎	2	肺结核	11
鼻炎	15	咯血	2
胸膜炎	1		

消化系统疾病

唇裂	1	口疮	5
口腔及咽喉溃疡	8	腮腺炎	4
牙龈肥厚	2	蠕虫病	4
扁桃体炎	2	黄疸	7
牙齿不规整	4	蛔虫病	25
龋齿	36	便秘	2
咽部溃疡	2	呕血	3
吞咽困难	1	内痔	3
食管狭窄	1	外痔	2
消化不良	164	脐瘘	14
腹泻	28	肛门溃疡	5
肠绞痛	6	先天性肛门缺失	1
痢疾	3	直肠脱垂	6
腹水	3	未分类的	7
腹股沟疝	5		

蜂窝组织疾病

脓肿及窦道	82	炎症	51
疖及痈	31		

泌尿生殖系统疾病

包茎	3	遗精	9
包茎嵌顿	1	尿潴留	1
龟头炎	5	血尿	1
尿道炎	3	闭经	1
硬下疳	9	白带异常	3
淋病	2	月经过多	3
尿道狭窄	5	膀胱炎	1
尿道结石	2	子宫脱垂	1
鞘膜积液	1		

皮肤疾病

痤疮	1	疥疮	13
湿疹	96	痛性疤痕	3
癣	115	痒疹	5
白癣	1	牛皮癣	1
疣	5	脓疱疹	4
色素斑点	1	蛎壳疹	1
钉胼	3	未分类的	5
红斑	2	溃疡	122
苔藓	5		

运动器官的疾病

风湿痛（肌肉和关节）	115	滑膜炎	10
腰痛	8	腿浮肿	3
骨溃疡和坏死	16	腿象皮病	1
骨膜炎	2	髋关节病	3
黏膜囊炎	1	脊柱后凸	2
		前臂创伤性坏疽	1

眼部疾病

上睑下垂	1	角膜溃疡	9
睑腺炎	1	星状角膜炎	5
下眼睑肥厚	1	角膜白斑	14
睑内翻及倒睫症	41	葡萄肿	11
卡他性眼炎	108	虹膜炎	8
颗粒状眼炎	98	白内障	7

化脓性眼炎	12	夜盲症	3
疱性眼炎	9	黑蒙	2
脓性黏液溢	5	虹膜后粘连	4
结膜黄斑	1	晶状体脱位	1
翼状胬肉	15	眼球运动混乱（一只或两只）	9
角膜炎	11	角膜异物	1
角膜炎伴前房积脓	4	未分类的	5
瞳孔闭塞	1		

耳部疾病

耳瘘	4	外耳道湿疹	1
耳垂裂口	6	未分类的	2

鼻部疾病

鼻息肉	4	鼻黏膜溃疡	5
鼻出血	3		

肿瘤

囊性肿瘤	18	恶性肿瘤	6
脂肪瘤	2	神经节瘤	3
纤维瘤	2	未分类的	9

外伤

擦伤	30	狗咬伤	5
扭伤	19	异物残留	5
创伤	38	骨折	4
烧伤	6	脱臼	11

手术

睑内翻及倒睫症手术	44
翼状胬肉手术	8
虹膜切除术（人工瞳孔）	2
唇裂手术	1
肛瘘手术	1
肿瘤切除术	11
鼻息肉切除术	1
外痔切除术	1
疣切除术	3
钉胼切除术	1
坏死骨剔除术	1

尿路结石取出术	2
拔牙	41
异物取出术	5
耳垂裂口修复术	5
包皮纵切术	4
脓肿切开术	26
牙龈粒状组织切除术	3
窦道切开术	10
创伤缝合术	7
内痔结扎术	1
神经节打开术	3
脱臼复位术	1
尿道口收缩手术	2
肛门闭锁手术	1
疤痕挛缩分离术	1
囊肿抽吸术	1
脚趾头截除术	1
创伤性坏疽病人尺骨头切除术	1

（翻译：刘慧翔、许思婷、谢煊　校译：朱文平　审校：胡卫清、余维泉、江建安　中文校正：许党泉、杨柳婷）

1887 年汕头福音医院报告

（1887 年度高仕兰医学学士、外科硕士照管下的英兰长老会汕头教会医院报告）

过去一年医院的工作像往常一样持续开展，没有哪天例外，入院病人的数量也没有减少。自从要求鸦片吸食者支付入院费用后，由于这类病人的减少，病人总数有所减少。普通病人数比以往要多，尤其是女性病人数增长明显。近年来，女性病人的比例有所增加，虽然她们中有许多人来自较远的农村，必须乘船到来。

统计数据

个体病人数：

住院病人	3 242
门诊病人	2 130
合计	5 372
以上包括女性病人	933
诊疗时间以外主要由高级助理处理的病例	2 000
平均每天住院病人数	174
门诊开放日平均每天门诊病人数	53
手术数	863

工作方式没有改变。门诊病人在星期二及星期五就诊，星期三及星期六被用作手术时间。病人们被要求自备食物及木炭，他们自己在医院的厨房里烹调，但药物是免费提供的。要支付费用的只有鸦片吸食者——他们要支付 1 美元。

一些中国商人帮了很大的忙，他们向我提供大米券和现金券，这些券都可以在他们的商店里进行兑换，一种能换成米，另一种每张能换 25 文钱去买肉及蔬菜。依靠这些方法，我能为那些看上去最贫穷的病人提供丰盛的食物，而且能保证许多病人留院直至疾病治愈，否则他们不得不回家去，而且情况比他们来的时候好不了多少。去年提供了 6 900 份饭。这些现金券的主要捐赠人——陈源盛行（Tan-nguan-seng hong）的老板今年提供了更多的福利，为那些在医院花光钱的病人提供回家的路费，并为那些太穷而无法为自己买适合的瓶子的病人捐赠了 700 个玻璃瓶。这些捐赠是非常少见且令人欣喜的，因为富有的中国人一般都不与外国机构有所交涉。

英瑞公司（Anglo-Swiss Co.）提供大批炼乳供病人们食用。病人们抗拒“生”牛奶，但他们对这些炼乳并没有偏见，事实上他们把这些罐装的牛奶当成一种药物，而且他们非常偏爱它的甜味。由于有营养且容易吸收的食物与药物都极其需要，我们手头常备这样的牛奶，并鼓励病人食用。不用说，他们要花钱购买炼乳，但相当一部分提供给了那些太穷而无法买的人。在手术治疗的初期及后期，这些牛奶非常有用，而酒精几乎没被用于辅助治疗。医院的格言应该是“要牛奶，不要酒精”。

中国人说，在一些地区炼乳一般是富有阶层食用的，在许多婴儿不适宜的米食中添加它也许就能使他们远离失明或死亡的威胁。然而，可惜的是，他们可以很容易地获得自己的水牛及奶牛的奶，却要去购买炼乳。

一个病人展示了有点极端的戒赌治疗结果。他一定是个赌桌上根深蒂固的幽魂，他的妻子很可能发现用温和的方法劝告没有用，就用斧头砍断了他小腿前方的肌肉，使他变跛了。这种形式的惩罚一直被官府用于暴徒身上，他们被从邻近地区的城市带过来处理。然而因为惩罚时只是瞎打一通，所以没有造成什么永久性的损伤。

教育

一个星期有 4 个下午用来教授初级助理及学生，一共 7 人。其中有 3 人固定在医院学习，学制 3 年，他们的父母支付他们的全部费用；第 4 位是以前的学生，他的 3 年学习期已满，我们支持他再学一年以完成课程；其他的都是有报酬的助理，其中一个在培训期间还陪同我去了潮州府。

学习的课程包括内科和外科实践、皮肤及眼科疾病，以及临床教学。在年底有两个年轻人离开了，他们分别和我们相处了 6 年及 4 年的时光。他们将会减轻人们的许多痛苦，如果他们好好利用机会，还能对他们所居住城市福音事业的进步有很大帮助。

卓威廉牧师（Rev. Wm. Duffus）在去年有一段时间为学生们开办了一门《圣经》的课程。

中国人对人体解剖模型非常感兴趣，有许多人要求允许他们看一下。当他们看到模型被一点一点地拆成部件时的惊奇和快乐是最有趣的。想到他们对人体解剖学及生理学的荒唐想法会因此发生多少改变，我有一种满足感。

传教工作

从传教的角度来看，医院工作的成果不是非常明显，但我们从不缺少在病人中传播基督教信义的鼓励。在周日下午的问询者会议上，经常有人声称他们放弃异教而接受了基督教，去年至少有 3 个男人和 3 个女人被允许进入教会。此外，值得说明的是，在去年被传教士洗礼的那些人中，有一些是由于其朋友或亲戚首先在医院里听讲而转变了宗教信仰，所以他们的转变是因为受到医院的间接影响。大多数问询者失去了联系，因为我们没有足够的方法去追踪他们，但一些人很可能还会聚集到各个传道站。传教的结果无法单从申请入教会的人数来判定，因为我们的代理人经过农村地区时经常会遇到一些以前的病人，他们在医院没有显示出被启示的迹象，但他们记住了他们在医院里所听到的，并已经在自己的异教家庭里根据他们的领悟追寻对上帝的信仰。

通过展现基督教慈善事业，医院在消除人们的憎恶和偏见方面有着明显的作用，除此以外，医院的福音布道在推翻中国人的偶像崇拜和其他有辱人格的迷信上也产生了有力的影响。很少住院患者在出院时不对他们原来的信仰产生严重的怀疑，有许多人甚至放弃了原先的信仰。我们的工作影响再加上上帝启示的传播，应该能够在整个汕头地区发酵，为基督事业在汕头的最终胜利做准备，我们有更大的慰藉去相信，年复一年，将有更多人得到救赎。

值得注意的是，我们的工作影响所到达的地方，即病人所属的乡村和城镇等约为1 800个。

外科手术

眼睛方面的手术：

睑内翻及倒睫症手术：

上眼睑	281
下眼睑	129—410
翼状胬肉手术	46
结膜肿瘤手术	4
睑板腺囊肿手术	1
虹膜切除术（人工瞳孔）	6
晶状体取出术（白内障）	11
不透明囊切开术	6
前房抽吸术	1
前房积脓手术	2
内眼角黑色素瘤切除术	1
	488

身体常见外科手术：

髋关节切除术（死于休克）	1
前臂切除术	1
足截肢术（赛姆氏术式——Syme's）	1
足截肢术（肖帕尔氏术式——Chopart's）	1
脚趾切除术	3
手指切除术	4
阴茎切除术（上皮癌）	2
脂肪瘤切除术	5
肘部及大腿对称的纤维瘤切除术	3
皮样囊肿切除术	1
乳房肿瘤切除术	5
脂肪囊肿切除术	11
其他肿瘤切除术	20
硬结切除术	7
嵌入子弹取出术	2
扁桃体肿大切除术	3
唇裂手术	32
鼻孔疤痕闭锁手术	2
唇成形术	3

舌下囊肿手术	3
耳部囊肿手术	2
耳垂裂口修补术	41
鼻裂修补术	1
上颌窦囊肿手术	1
瘢痕手术	4
肛瘘手术	58
外痔手术	19
内痔手术	38
包皮环切术	13
阴囊象皮肿手术	8
包皮象皮肿手术	1
尿道口狭窄手术	1
人造肛门手术	1
神经节手术	4
痣电切术	4
疤痕电切术	1
痣结扎术	3
腹部（腰部）囊肿抽吸术	1
坐骨神经痛针刺术	1
淋巴囊肿开放术	1
鞘膜积液抽液注射术	16
鼻中果核取出术	1
窦道开放术	6
探查手术	3
后鼻孔填塞术	1
巨大脓肿切开术	6
咽后脓肿切开术	1
骨疾病烧灼术	1
死骨剔除术	5
鼻息肉切除术	16
耳息肉切除术	2
角状物、肉赘等切除术	5
手术总数	863
拔牙	117

以上手术总数不包括大量小手术，如脓肿切开术、游离死骨片剔除术、导管插入术、骨折矫正术等。

一些被治疗的疾病列表

常见病

间歇性发热:
- 日发疟 …… 12
- 间日疟 …… 12
- 三日疟 …… 117
- 复三日疟 …… 2
- 四日疟 …… 1

脾肿大 …… 7
麻风病 …… 244
脚气病 …… 9
甲状腺肿 …… 5
梅毒 …… 207
吸鸦片者的治疗 …… 94

眼部

颗粒性眼炎 …… 430
睑内翻及倒睫症 …… 270
其他眼病 …… 528

淋巴系统

右小腿象皮肿 …… 13
左小腿象皮肿 …… 11
左小腿和阴囊象皮肿 …… 1
双小腿及阴囊象皮肿 …… 2
两小腿象皮肿 …… 2
未记载哪一边的象皮肿 …… 3
包皮象皮肿 …… 1
阴囊象皮肿 …… 21
淋巴阴囊 …… 2

泌尿生殖系统

膀胱结石 …… 6
阴茎结石 …… 1

脚气病——8 位归侨在新加坡患上了脚气病。其中 3 位是干性，其他的患水肿者在来汕头的途中消失了。奇怪的是这些患者中有一位已经回家 8 年，可是每年都有一次疾病复发。症状最初发生在四五月份，直到十一月份消失。我没有见过类似的病例，因为病人回家后似乎病就会好了。因为这个年轻人的家乡在低洼地区，我建议他搬去海拔较高的地方。1887 年女子学校再次发现有人患上脚气病，结果学校不得不关闭。虽然前年脚气病在男子学校有一次致命的暴发，但奇怪的是，去年没有一位男孩患上脚气病。

饮酒——1 709 位成年男性的饮酒习惯调查结果显示，57% 的人说当他们能接触酒时偶尔饮用，36% 的人否认他们饮用，7% 承认他们每天都饮用。最后一类被调查者平均每日饮酒 11 盎司，数量从 2 盎司到毫无节制的 32 盎司。饮用的酒一般是廉价米酒，而且晚上饮酒似乎已经成为一种习惯。然而很少见到中国人酗酒，我也从没遇到一例真正的慢性酒精中毒病例，尽管每年总会有一位（医生）被叫去治疗一些由于习惯性饮酒而带来痛苦的病人，这可能是因为当地的酒使用了不纯的原料。不幸的是我并不知道有没有人对其进行分析，以及分析的结果是什么。

这些统计资料也许会被指责说有误导性，因为如果饮酒的后果是有伤害的，那么比起在普通人群中随机抽取的类似统计数量的成年男性来说，酗酒者在病人中应该会占更大的比例。我并不那么认为，因为许多人说之前他们习惯饮酒，但自从他们患了现在的疾病后就戒了酒。尤其是对于患有眼疾的人来说，饮酒会加重炎症。所以我相信真实的统计数据应该远远高于而不是低于这里所说的。

我无意依据这些统计资料做任何评论，我只是单纯地想把它们作为一个项目中确定的信息展示出来，所有那些为了使中国人生活得好而努力的人都应注意到它们的重要性。

14%的成年男性患者去过国外，多数去过新加坡，其他的去过槟城、暹罗、安南，他们在国外的平均逗留时间为5年。不幸的是他们很少因去过国外而在身心上受益，其中患梅毒及因淋病性眼炎或多或少导致失明的病人的比例相当高。

P. B. 高仕兰

注：关于结余的590美元，必须声明其将全部用于几个星期后的医院建筑的维修和行政大楼的扩建。

来爱力医生（Dr. Lyall）从国内休假回来，现在重新主持汕头的医疗工作。

1887年捐款

（略）

收支表

单位：美元

去年结余	329.46
欧洲人的捐款	873.00
中国人的捐款	271.89
卖药给欧洲人及中国人	552.80
卖牛奶给欧洲人及中国人	202.46
卖杂物	81.21
卖疝气绑带	61.50
对吸鸦片者收费	92.00
私人病房的租金	11.00
海外宣道会拨款	620.00
	3 095.32

工资	355.33
一般费用	163.56
帮助贫穷病人	33.32
维修费	56.44
从伦敦购买牛奶	274.18
在汕头买药	44.04
在香港买药	156.84

从英格兰等地买药	477.45
海外宣道会买药	620.00
丧葬费	28.89
油费	95.45
猪油费	24.32
羊毛费	63.09
水费	46.87
买布	43.40
买纸	10.93
清洗病房	10.82
结余	590.39
	3 095.32

（翻译：刘慧翔、许思婷、谢煊　校译：朱文平　审校：胡卫清、佘维泉、江建安　中文校正：许党泉、杨柳婷）

1888 年汕头福音医院报告

（1888 年度来爱力医学学士、外科硕士照管下的英兰长老会汕头教会医院报告）

在这一年接近尾声的时候，依照以往的习惯，我们为支持汕头福音医院的朋友和捐赠者提交一份简短的年度工作摘要。简单地说，不管是在医疗方面还是在传教方面，我们在各个工作分支都获得了一定的成功。下面提供的统计数据，以及被治疗的疾病清单，都可以说明这一年我们确实做了许多辛苦的工作。高仕兰医生（Dr. Cousland）在我休假期间负责管理医院，并继续帮助了我们几个月，直到他去潮州府。他在门诊开放日给病人看病，这让我多了点闲暇时间处理医院工作——这令我非常感激。非常遗憾的是，九月份我们的社区医生去世了，经同事们同意，我们承担起港口卫生干事的职责。这些工作我们都持续进行着，因为这些是必要的，当然我们并没有忽略自己的正职。

统计数据

个体病人数：	
住院病人	2 719
门诊病人	2 397
合计	5 116
以上包括女性病人	807
诊疗时间以外主要由当地高级助理诊疗的病例	1 500
到中国病人家中出诊次数	137
平均每天住院病人数	160
门诊开放日平均每天门诊病人数	45
门诊开放日门诊病人总数	7 500
手术数	853

此外，我们对大量的住在教会里面的中国人提供了医疗照料，如小学生、助理、仆人等。

去年夏天对潮州当地的民众来说是一个不健康的季节。春季降雨量较以往大且持续时间较以往更长，而且接下来就是长时间的干热天气。5 月份，霍乱开始出现在汕头及其他小镇，但只要潮湿的天气持续下去，霍乱就不会大范围扩散。7 月初，天气开始变得干热，接着疾病就开始在整个农村流行开来。此次霍乱并不是最致命的那种类型，但一些大城市的死亡率相当高。只要是我们发现的疾病我们就有责任去治疗，大约 75% 的患者被治愈了。汕头的疫情严重，但在 1883 年曾暴发过传染病的邻近大村落却幸免于此。而且令人惊奇的是，不管是 1883 年还是去年，霍乱都没有侵袭西面山区的客家村落。丰约翰医生（Dr. McPhun）并没有看到或听说五经富及其附近出现病例，虽然这个疾病在只有几英里外的揭阳河边的村庄非常流行。

由于霍乱的流行，我们的住院病人数在七八月份大大减少。有几个星期几乎没有远道而来的病人，因为他们怕旅途中经过被传染的地区。人们经过那些霍乱高发区须冒着可能被传染的危险。医院发现的许多病例显然是在他们来汕头的途中被传染上的。在汕头，我们照料了不少来自农村、打算坐轮船出国的人。没有一个医院助理或服务人员被传染，即使医院里发现这样的病例，也没有出现传播开来的迹象。

春季，脚气病再次在教会学校暴发，但没有很严重的病例，而且患者在被遣送回家后都很快痊愈了。这个疾病似乎每年都变得更为流行。在汕头，没有一种病像脚气病一样流行，但我们想很快会有了。在医院治疗的病例中，有一些是从没去过国外的。我们虽然没有这种疾病的死亡病例，但有一些病例是很严重的。一个男人有两个多月无法走路，甚至无人搀扶就无法站立。这个男人是潮阳的当地居民，他从 1887 年底就在我院治疗鸦片毒瘾，回家数月后就患上了脚气病。

在汕头的医学大事中有两个事件值得注意，虽然事件与工作回顾都没有直接的联系。11 月，高仕兰医生（Dr. Cousland）在潮州府开了一个门诊，我们相信这项刚刚起步的工作会给当地及邻近居民带来很大的益处。从第一周开始，来看病的病人就非常多，以至于有必要限制每日诊治的病人数。目前，这间房子很不适合为医疗目的使用，但无疑不久将会有一个更加舒适的场所。

另外一个事件是汕头的当地商人提出建议，根据当地的原则建设一所大医院，并由从上海或香港来的中国内科医师负责管理。这个医院在福音医院附近，地基已经打好了。令人高兴的是，中国人自己开始致力于建立慈善机构以救济贫苦的病人。在像潮州府这样人口众多的地区必须有这样的医院，因为位于汕头的医院无法顾及那里大量的病患。这个地区的其他许多城镇都非常需要建医院，我们相信当地富有的商人的善举是不会仅限于这个城镇的。

今年年初，手头有 500 美元的结余，我扩建了大医院前面的两幢小楼，增加了 6 个小房间。但今年许多月份都是超员的，增加这几个小房间完全不足以满足需求。在历年的年度报告上总有评论说，我们医院的大部分病人来自远方，我们如果要治好他们的病，就必须为他们提供住处。汕头几乎没有好的旅馆。提供给外地人的旅馆非常昂贵，超过了许多病人的支付能力。如果是女病人，在汕头几乎没有能过夜的地方。我的目标是，当我有足够的资金后，要对原先那个小的麻风病院进行扩建，将其改造成一个实用的旅馆，让它能轻松容纳至少 120 人，以使我能够严格地控制大医院的病人数。这种安排将让我摆脱许多麻烦和担心，而且能够提供一个理想的福音传播场所。

传教工作

已有评论认为，医学传教士与牧师有所不同：人们主动来找前者，而后者必须去找人们传教。我们在汕头的经历证实了这种评论。我们去年的病人来自潮州、惠州、嘉应州和福建省南部共 1 663 个不同的城镇和乡村，在教区所附近有一所大医院有一个优势——

位传教士认为这是不小的优势，即所有的传教士都能参与对病人的传教工作。汕头医院的许多成功皆缘于此。

乡村的数量

潮州地区：	
澄海	115
潮阳	339
揭阳	289
惠来	130
饶平	170
普宁	190
海阳	224
丰顺	26
达埠	19
来自惠州地区	15
来自嘉应州地区	47
来自福建省	80
来自其他地区	19
合计	1 663

在我的请求下，我的夫人写了大量的福音著作。她现在正在计划把当地的女基督教徒组织起来，安排她们在女病人当中做工作，这是一个很有价值的计划，期待将来能得到许多成果。在这一年经过洗礼进入教会的新增人员中，有 21 个是在他们住院的时候首次接触基督教并接受了福音的。这些人中有许多是前几年接受过治疗的。来爱力夫人（Mrs. Lyall）这样写道：以前，我们做了许多努力，以便能给病人带来基督教教义的知识。每天早晨及晚上的祈祷，还有星期天下午的特别问询会就像以前一样进行，并由传教士、学院学生及两个当地的高级助理主持。教会的女人们做了特别的努力，使每个出院的女病人都了解到充足的基督教知识，一旦她们渴望某些东西，她们会发现这些东西比偶像崇拜（注：拜老爷，即拜神，下同）更好，迟早会引导她们成为基督教信徒。这种努力不仅仅出现在女传教士身上。6 名或更多年轻的基督教女信徒——她们当中有许多之前是女子学校的学生——现在已经结婚了并居住在汕头。她们表示愿意每个星期花一个小时去拜访女性病房，去帮助病人更清楚地了解福音的知识。除了普通的帮助，如学习阅读赞美诗，还专门为那些希望能读到白话版本的妇女、女孩、男孩开设了一个班级，这些白话版本的书本大都是由教会准备的。开设这个班只是个实验，我们担心大部分病人在短暂的住院期间并不能从中获得很大的益处。结果却是令人振奋的，有 28 人成为长期或短期的班级成员，其中 9 人已经诵读得相当好，这些人离开医院后只需做点练习就能诵读我们的任何拉丁文的书籍。

我们用各种可能的方式宣传基督教真义，毫无疑问这些努力得到了好的结果。这一年，有超过100位病人申请受洗，其中仅有一些被接受了。对于大部分没有受洗的人，我们没有理由怀疑他们的真诚，但要接受一个还没有回家，没有在自己家过一段基督教徒生活来测试其真诚的人作为教徒，这是有违我们的惯例的。出于各种原因，大部分住在远离教堂的村落的人们不会再有任何消息，因为极少人（可能是医院以前的病人，也可能是医院咨询者）要求洗礼，我们几乎不拜访任何一个乡村工作点。

在这些事例中要谈谈丁海芯（Teng-haisim）。她8年前第一次在医院听教义，当她回家的时候，她放弃了原有的信仰，但没有马上成为一个基督教徒。她牢记她所听到的，而且被自己的罪恶所困扰，并感到很不快乐。两年前，她再次来到医院，得到了进一步的指引，回家的时候，她觉得受益良多，开始暗地里信奉基督教。由于害怕她的丈夫，她不敢承认自己是基督教徒，但她用各种理由拒绝参加盲目崇拜习俗的活动。今年她必须再来医院治疗，在离家前，她鼓起勇气告诉丈夫，她决定成为基督教徒。在她到达后的第一个星期天，她提交了申请。因为她的村子离一个乡村工作点不远，于是她被建议在那里申请。她这么做了，于是在金护尔先生（Mr. Mackenzie）对这个站点最近的一次访问中，她接受了洗礼。

在一个最远的站点有一个接受了洗礼的男人，他10年前在医院听教义，并从此成为主的信奉者。由于他住的地方离最近的教堂有30英里，所以他很少能去做礼拜，然而他在家里设了安息日。多年后的今天，他已申请并获准进入教会。

孙好（Sun-ho）是今年接受洗礼的另一个病人，两年前为了带他儿子就诊而来到医院。他被他当时所听到的教义深深打动，当他回家的时候，他不仅成了一个热心的崇拜者，而且满怀激情，诚挚地向其他人普及福音知识，这给他带来了痛苦和烦扰。在此之前，他在这个村子有些影响力，经常被叫去帮助调解小纠纷，现在他却到处被辱骂、被嘲笑，甚至遭受粗暴地反对他的新信仰的妻子拳打脚踢的侮辱。但他很耐心地忍受着所有这些，现在他上中学的儿子及他年老失明的父亲均申请接受洗礼。

病人们住院的时候非常容易表现出对基督教的兴趣，但当他们回到乡下，又是另外一回事了。契婶（Koi sim），一位以前的病人，今年再次来到医院。她告诉我们去年回到家时，她向家里人宣布她要成为基督教徒。她作为一家之主的儿子本来是不反对的，直到听见邻居的嘲笑。他们说："我们村子超过4 000人，至今没有一个人抛弃我们的老宗教去接受新教义，但现在有一人这么做了，这个人就是你的母亲。"这是她的儿子无法忍受的。他感到受辱和气愤，于是把母亲打至重伤，使她10天都无法走路，从此之后，他再也没有与她说话。这只是这个可怜的女人所忍受的一小部分事情而已。当听到她的故事时，有的人会说："是的，契婶，你受苦了，为何不放弃基督教，回归原来的信仰？""不，"她回答，"我想在死了之后去到耶稣所在的地方，不再诞生在这个世界上。"（一种佛教观念）

今年在一个乡村工作站的申请人中有一位盲人。若干年前他曾来到医院，希望能恢复他的视力，但这是不可能的。然而，他逗留了10天左右，学习了教义，然后回到家，创立了家庭礼拜以及安息日仪式。他的妻子也成了基督教徒。这次他申请洗礼，本应被接受的，但最后被拒绝了，因为他仍在给崇拜偶像的活动（注：拜老爷）凑钱。他之所以这样做，是因为他的乡亲威胁他，扬言若他不这样做就要把他赶出村子。

偶尔会遇到有些曾经听过教义的人，来医院不为别的，就只是为了了解更多的基督教知识。今年有这样一个实例，两个女人来自离小教堂很远的村庄，在若干年前已经从一个被派去乡村访问医院老病人的圣女那里听取了基督教的教义，其中一个很感动，为了得到进一步的指导，她对婆婆借口说患了慢性眼炎来到医院。她回到家时受到了许多迫害，她都忍受下来，一直坚定不移，今年她和她的朋友来申请进入教会。她们说，在周日会有6名或8名妇女聚集在一起做礼拜，包括读赞美诗、做祈祷，那些会读一些赞美诗的人教其他人读。这些妇女被带进教授读拉丁文白话版本的赞美诗的班级。6个星期过后，其中一位可以读得相当好了，希望她们回家后可以读一部分拉丁文白话版本的《圣经》，当她们周日相聚的时候，可以教授其他妇女。这些话可能不算不合时宜，若考虑到反对用拉丁文课本教授中国皈依者的那些人，要这些妇女学会读汉字的福音书籍，也许要花费数月甚至数年。

外科手术

眼部：

睑内翻及倒睫症手术	298
翼状胬肉手术	50
睑缘粘连手术	1
虹膜脱出手术	2
前葡萄肿（脱落）手术	2
眼前房积脓手术	2
白内障切除术	19
白内障切除术（外伤性的）	1
角膜异物切除术	1
白内障切除后针刺术	2
人工瞳孔虹膜切除术	10
抗青光眼虹膜切除术	1
疤痕性睑外翻塑形手术	1
眼睑囊肿组织切除术	11
结膜赘生物切除术	4
眼球切除术	3
眼眶肉瘤切除术	1
血管翳球结膜环状切开术	2
	411

躯体：

兔唇手术	33
包茎环切术	10
肛瘘手术	58
耳朵裂伤手术	54
肛门闭锁手术	2
短舌系带手术	1

骨溃疡手术 …… 6
神经节手术 …… 7
舌下囊肿手术 …… 3
包茎手术 …… 2
侧面切石术 …… 3
会阴切除术 …… 1
剖腹手术 …… 1
疝气根治术（Wood's） …… 1
手指切除术 …… 5
前臂截肢术 …… 1
手臂截肢术 …… 1
小腿（通过膝关节）截肢术 …… 1
多余的拇指切除术 …… 1
阴茎（上皮瘤）切除术 …… 2
阴囊象皮病切除术 …… 2
骈胝切除术 …… 17
唇上皮瘤切除术 …… 1
皮肤上皮瘤切除术 …… 1
粉瘤切除术 …… 3
牙龈瘤切除术 …… 3
脂肪瘤切除术 …… 8
囊肿切除术 …… 4
纤维瘤切除术 …… 4
腺瘤切除术 …… 1
大纤维瘤（纤维软疣）切除术 …… 1
肉瘤切除术 …… 4
乳腺肿瘤切除术 …… 2
下巴部分切除术 …… 1
睾丸切除术 …… 1
睾丸海绵肿切除术 …… 1
皮脂腺囊肿切除术 …… 16
扁桃体肿大切除术 …… 5
舌系带息肉切除术 …… 1
直肠息肉切除术 …… 1
女性尿道息肉切除术 …… 1
包皮乳头状瘤切除术 …… 1
外痔切除术 …… 22
副耳郭？切除术 …… 2

足部骨瘤切除术	1
跟骨和距骨（骨溃疡）切除术	1
第一跖骨和中间的楔形骨（骨溃疡）切除术	1
直肠脱垂切除术（用热烧灼）	3
鼻息肉摘除术	22
尿道结石取出术	1
竹刺、针取出术	6
从膝盖骨取出子弹	1
死骨取出术	22
阴囊积水穿刺术	2
阴囊积水穿刺和注射术	22
淋巴囊肿穿刺和注射术	1
囊肿穿刺术	2
内痔结扎术	34
阴茎先天畸形塑形手术	1
大脓肿切开术	9
直肠裂伤修补术	1
鼻窦成形术	6
髋关节切开术	1
疤痕电灼术	2
痣电灼术	1
疣电灼术	2
膀胱抽吸术	2
坐骨神经痛针刺术	1
脊柱疾病烧灼术	1
合计	442
拔牙	191

此外还有脓肿切开、脱臼包扎固定、骨折复位、尿路扩张手术等等。

白内障——19 例高龄白内障患者接受手术，结果如下：18 例痊愈，没有不良症状且视力良好，1 例术后第四天并发虹膜炎。这例手术刚好是在东北季风来临之际进行的，气温的急剧下降使病人忽然发高烧，过了两天就得了虹膜炎，这位病人的另一只眼睛在数周前成功进行了手术。有一个病例角膜、虹膜、晶状体受到损害，我们尝试通过摘除晶状体来挽救受损的眼睛，但失败了。

这类手术要么使用改良的线性摘除术，要么是切开 3 毫米的瓣，配合适合个体情况的虹膜切除术。17 例手术的切口在角膜上缘。有好几次我用注射器将角膜物质冲洗出前房，但这种方法的效果不见得优于轻柔手法。彻底消毒在白内障手术的应用是一个很大的进步，使用的消毒剂是一种硼酸饱和溶液。

有一个没有进行虹膜切除术的病例有点反常，晶状体的囊壁在没有被破坏的情况下排出。眼睛是小的，可能切口相对比平常的要大。不管怎么样，当我刚想将虹膜钳放进去时，患者转动了他的眼睛，然后晶状体就排出来了。晶状体囊是坚韧的，而里面的内容物是柔软且几乎是液态的，手术结果令人满意，病人视力也得到了恢复。

针刺手术只进行过两次。一些其他眼疾需要进行这项治疗，由几根细线像手一样张开穿过瞳孔，但我发现中国人很少愿意进行这项手术。他们满足于已经获得的视力，而不想对眼睛进行更多的干预。

疤痕性睑外翻的塑形性手术——患者上眼睑翘起并向外翻，露出发炎的眼睛。疤痕性皮肤延伸到整个前额和睑部边缘，因此从这些地方无法得到健康的皮瓣。眼睑及睑部边缘的疤痕组织被去除，并在前臂取下皮瓣，用于原眼睑及睑部的表面。因为知道中国人对疼痛及不适有巨大承受能力，我取下依附于臂膀的皮瓣，牢固地附着在睑部边缘。这个患者忍受了这种不适长达36小时或更久。手术效果非常满意，病人获得了一个性状良好的眼睑。

眼球切除术——每年都有眼球疼痛萎缩以及前葡萄肿患者要求治疗。早些年我经常建议这些患者摘除眼球，但很少人同意这样的治疗。中国人似乎不容易得交感性眼炎，所以在前葡萄肿病例中，我不采取这样的治疗，通常只是切除眼球的突出部分。在过去的几个月中，有两个人要求我摘除他们患病的眼球，并放置一个玻璃球取而代之。因为手头上没有人造的眼球，我无法同意他们的要求。但是应他们的迫切恳求，我从英国订了一些玻璃眼睛，由他们付费。他们在下一年就可以回来做手术了。有一个接近适婚年龄的女孩，她父亲毫无疑问是想她嫁个好人家才带她来做手术。也许不久之后，如果本地能够提供人造肢体的话，会有人来要求截去病痛的肢体。

主要的截肢——今年做了3例成功的手术。一例是前臂，一例是肘关节以上的胳膊，一例是包含有膝关节的小腿。最后那位病人是一个虚弱的男人，患了踝部大肉瘤，仍在治疗中。长前皮瓣部分脱落，延迟了他的恢复。

横向截石术——有5人得了膀胱结石，但只有3人接受手术治疗。在所有的病例中，采用横向截石术均取得了成功。第一位病人是一个3岁的小男孩，从他膀胱里取出了120格令重的结石。第二位是一个7岁的男孩，结石重80格令。第三位病人是一个41岁的男人，是最有趣的一个病例。检查发现有一块巨大的结石充满了他的膀胱的顶部。碎石器进入膀胱尽力去压碎它，结果发现这块结石很脆，碎石器叶片只用了最轻的力度。然后进行侧面的取石术，发现膀胱后壁大部分覆盖了厚厚的钙质沉积物。用勺子和手指伸进去便可刮去，去除了大约2盎司的沉积物。切口保持开放两周，每天坚持用消毒剂冲洗膀胱。患者恢复得非常好，4个月以后，他回来告诉医院自己很健康，不再受膀胱疾病的困扰。

尿道结石——从病人阴茎头的尿道里取出一个弹珠大小的结石，这个结石已经有10年之久了。

大纤维瘤——病人是个46岁的女性。她的右后背肩胛骨下方长了一个带蒂的大瘤子，巨大的肿瘤延伸到臀部附近，最宽处周长达2.5英尺。瘤体很重，以至于患者坐下时，常常失去平衡，往后倒到地上。这个肿瘤从6年前就开始生长了。甲状腺峡部及右叶也有肿大，导致有轻微的压迫症状。但身体的其他地方并没有发现纤维小结及肿瘤。患者的总体状况良好，但精神状态比较差。切除的肿瘤重 23 磅。患者很倔强，术后几天她就无法待在床上。不过，手术伤口很大程度上得到了一期愈合。过了两个星期，患者恢复得很好，能够走出医院和丈夫在路上跑步了。这类肿瘤在中国的这个地区不罕见，背部是最常发的部位。其他种类的纤维软疣也碰到过。

剖腹手术——手术在一例大肠的慢性肠套叠病例上进行。病人是一个 7 岁的男孩，已经病了 4 个月，手术前两个月我们一直在照料他。我们用空气使他的肠管扩张，肠套叠看起来消失了。他的病情有很大的改善，回家后的一个月都很健康。后来症状又出现了，第二次入院时孩子病得很重。开腹之后，我们发现在左边有一大块肠套叠，我们无法复原它，因为它紧紧地粘连了。做了人工肛门，但孩子在手术后 13 个小时就死了。

部分下巴切除术——一个 18 岁的年轻男人下巴得了骨肿瘤，位于左边且与骨头融合在一起。它位于骨内，并向骨外板及内板延伸，整个肿瘤的大小就像中等大小的橘子。在下巴的边缘做了切口，切开软组织，肿瘤一侧的骨头被分离，然后肿物切除了，患者恢复良好。

会阴切开——为了治疗外伤性尿道狭窄而做了这个手术。病人数年前跌落时撞伤会阴。一号探条有两次机会通过（尿道），第二次用器械打开通道时，由于病人完全性尿潴留引起的尿路（感染）发热而受到严重影响。膀胱（尿液）被抽取了若干次，但因为持续发热，病人变得非常虚弱，所以我切开了会阴，没有仪器能够通过尿道。过了很长一段时间，病人康复了，尿道很容易就被一条大的探条通过。任何尝试通过仪器扩大创伤性狭窄都很容易导致尿路（感染）发热，与淋病引起的狭窄相比只是严重或不严重而已。我发现在这一方面让中国人接受手术治疗很困难。

男性乳腺肿瘤——有两个乳腺肿瘤病例被切除乳腺。一例是 17 岁的少年，肿瘤是肉瘤而且非常大，周长 18 英寸。另外一个病例是乳腺肥大。

阴囊象皮病——今年只做了两例手术。病变组织分别重 25 磅 10 盎司和 9.33 磅。两个病例的伤口都一期愈合。

副耳郭（?）——两个病例都是耳郭前方长了一块小的先天性增生组织，构造与耳朵相似，被手术切除了。多拇指和多指畸形很常见，然而这类先天性畸形我则是第一次遇见。

肛门闭锁——有一个病例的手术并不成功。无法找到肠管，这个小孩大便经尿道排泄。

跗骨和跖骨切除手术——3 例手术中有两例治疗效果良好，另一个病例中跟骨和距骨中的病变（骨溃疡）在其他骨头复发，这个病人还在接受治疗。

一系列意外事件——严重的外伤并不常见，然而在去年 10 月份，我们遇到了一些病例，具体如下。这样的经历在中国医院工作中是比较少的。

从 10 月 13 日到 27 日我们遇到了以下病例：

殴打所致眼球损伤——眼外伤。

两个肱骨断裂的病例。

脊柱的断裂——当这个病人以蜷缩的姿势坐在船板上时被一根倒下的桅杆砸到。一个月后出院时，下肢仍是无力的。

头盖骨的断裂——伤者在数小时内就死亡了。

压碎的足骨——足背部及侧面的软组织被撕裂或撕脱，几块骨头粉碎性骨折。患者拒绝截肢，最终足部约 2/3 脱落了。

腹壁损伤合并肠道脱垂——一个 6 岁大的男孩被水牛顶伤，伤口在左侧接近肋骨的地方。肠管破裂了，排泄物因此通过人工肛门排出。

肩膀脱臼。

伤口和严重膝关节损伤——从屋顶掉下来所导致。

脱臼——臀部股骨的向后移位是我们最常被叫作复位的脱臼。在一个因为不幸的事件发生而致伤的病例中我们尝试这样做。一个 8 岁的男孩被从猪背上抛下，他的臀部向后移位了。两个月后他被带到了医院，经过处理相对容易地把脱臼的骨头复位了。3 个月后这个男孩因为同样的脱臼又被带到了医院，原因和之前是一样的。因为受伤才几天，预计站立没有什么困难。首先是尝试通过操作使股骨头向下移动，它碰到髋臼的边缘。在尝试完成复位（并未用力过大）时股骨断成两半。

手腕背部的脱臼——遇到了这种典型的损伤病例。肱骨也断裂了。

缠足——一个 9 岁的女孩被确认在缠足期间遭受了有些残酷的对待。她妈妈希望她的女儿能有双很小的脚，于是锤打她的脚趾和脚以便“使骨头变得柔软”，然后把它们缠得紧紧的，导致一只脚的前半部分脱落，留下肉芽组织的表面，这样的脚估计要截肢。

我们经常被中国人（例如在潮州府）中非常罕见的先天性足部畸形所震撼。畸形足的通常种类甚至很少见到，有可能是因为人们认为不值得因为这样的疾病带他们的孩子来治疗，然而在汕头和乡村的人群当中，我也很少见到有人有先天性马蹄足或者其他足部畸形。

中国女人缠足，据说有至少 1 000 年的历史了，因此我们自然地想到：这种漫长而持续的损毁的结果，会使形状和大小各异的畸形脚很常见。但中国人看来有着与他们的身高成比例的脚，脚的大小与那些不知道缠足这一残酷习俗的人们相比较没有差别。据说犹太民族的包皮环切术并没有使包皮缩短，所以我觉得缠足也不会使中国人的脚永远地变短。

疾病列表

常见病

间歇性发热：	
日发疟	9
三日疟	15
四日疟	99
不规则的	12
低热及简单的持续发热	88
伤寒	1
霍乱	140
丹毒	1
瘰疬	46
佝偻病（?）	1
风湿病	240
贫血	55
贫血伴脾肿大	20
一般的和疟疾性的衰弱	109
脚气病	25
酒精中毒	2
甲状腺肿	3

病名	例数
梅毒	221
先天性梅毒	9
麻风病	251
绝食	1
治疗鸦片吸食者	81
吞鸦片自杀者	3
手淫	5

呼吸系统疾病

病名	例数
鼻炎	2
喉炎	5
哮喘	17
肺气肿	5
支气管炎	114
肺结核	101
急性肺炎	2
咯血	5

泌尿生殖系统疾病

病名	例数
慢性尿路炎	5
血尿	2
闭尿	1
尿失禁	3
尿潴留	1
膀胱结石	5
尿道结石	1
前列腺肥大	1
包茎	13
包茎嵌顿	4
阴茎上皮瘤	9
硬下疳及阴茎、阴囊梅毒性溃疡	34
尿道狭窄	9
尿瘘	3
创伤性的尿道狭窄	1
淋病、慢性尿道炎	35
遗精	18
龟头炎	1
睾丸炎	3
阴囊积液	37
精索静脉曲张	3
梅毒性睾丸肿大	3
睾丸肿物	1
睾丸海绵肿	5
包皮疣、乳头状瘤包皮	2
生殖器先天畸形	1

病名	例数
白带	8
闭经	5
痛经	2
月经过多	3
月经紊乱	2
子宫息肉	1
卵巢肿瘤	1
外阴硬性下疳	2
外阴尖锐湿疣	1
外阴瘙痒	2
淋病	2
直肠阴道瘘	1
尿道息肉	1
阴道癌	1

淋巴系统疾病

病名	例数
阴囊象皮肿	15
腹股沟淋巴结肿大(象皮肿的)	4

小腿象皮肿	32	淋巴腺瘤	2
小腿及阴囊象皮肿	3	腹股沟淋巴结炎	3
阴囊淋巴积液	4		

消化系统疾病

唇上皮瘤	1	便秘	3
齿龈脓肿	4	呕血	1
齿瘘	3	蠕虫病	21
牙龈溃疡	5	腹股沟疝	38
口腔炎	1	上腹部疝	1
舌乳头肿大	2	脐疝	2
舌系带过短	1	粪瘘	1
上颚裂	5	肛门直肠溃疡（鸡奸）	37
唇裂	34	肛门上皮瘤	2
咽喉阻塞	9	肛瘘	72
颗粒状咽炎	9	内痔	50
咽喉溃疡	11	外痔	16
慢性扁桃体炎	10	直肠狭窄	6
食管狭窄	4	直肠脱垂	6
消化不良	379	直肠息肉	1
胃胀	1	直肠裂开	3
绞痛	6	肝病——未分类的	9
痢疾	34	腹水	5
腹泻	22		

皮肤疾病

硬结	17	天疱疮	2
上皮瘤	5	疤痕	3
溃疡	186	带状疱疹	2
湿疣	7	疥疮	24
脓疱疹	5	皮脂溢	1
湿疹	76	间擦疹	1
体癣	148	黑皮病	1
黄癣	4	痱子	1
叠瓦癣	7	软疣	1
糠疹	15	甲床炎	5

牛皮廯	19	瘙痒症	6
苔藓	21	梅毒疹	45
白斑病	5	侵蚀性溃疡	1
痤疮	3	秃头	2
狼疮	7		

神经系统疾病

一侧面瘫	4	精神错乱	9
一侧上肢瘫痪	3	低能儿	2
偏瘫	11	聋哑	3
截瘫	1	假性肥大性麻痹	1
神经痛	19	运动性共济失调	1
癫痫	8	未分类的脊椎病	2
神经炎	3	局部麻痹	20
癔症（?）	1		

循环系统疾病

心脏瓣膜病	15	痣	1
未分类的心脏病变	4	静脉曲张	5
动脉瘤	2		

肿瘤

皮脂腺囊肿	11	神经节瘤	10
皮样成本	2	乳头状瘤	7
纤维瘤	10	海绵状淋巴管瘤	1
囊肿	8	纤维软疣	4
舌下囊肿	4	乳腺过度生长	1
腺瘤	4	未分类的未知肿瘤	5
软骨瘤	1	先天性的肿瘤	1
骨瘤	4	肉瘤	19
脂肪瘤	10	癌	11
龈瘤	2	女性乳腺癌	5
粉瘤	2	未分类的恶性肿瘤	25

眼部疾病

卡他性结膜炎	62	全眼球炎	4
化脓性结膜炎	25	眼球伤口、损伤	8
泡性结膜炎	7	视神经萎缩	3

颗粒性结膜炎	476	黑蒙	15
翼状胬肉	53	视网膜出血	1
结膜增生	3	夜盲症	4
角膜溃疡	24	外直肌麻痹	1
角膜剥落	6	近视	2
角膜脓肿	2	睑球粘连	2
角膜白斑	39	睑缘粘连	1
粘连性角膜白斑	47	睑外翻及倒睫症	215
角膜异物	1	睑外翻	4
前葡萄肿	24	皮脂溢性睑板腺炎	14
虹膜疝	16	上眼睑下垂	2
角膜炎	13	眼睑及眉毛处囊肿、肿瘤	9
非化脓性淋巴结炎	7	下眼睑上皮瘤	2
虹膜炎	8	眼眶恶性肿瘤	6
虹膜脉络膜炎	1	眼睑脓肿	1
角膜虹膜炎	8	眼睑烧伤	1
瞳孔闭塞	15	眼睑外伤	4
眼前房积脓	6	眼睑水肿	1
白内障	33	睑腺炎	1
创伤性白内障	2	睑板腺囊肿	2
晶状体浑浊	3	睑板腺软骨肥大	1
慢性青光眼…	15	鼻泪管狭窄	6
一只眼或两只眼损坏	49		

耳朵疾病

耳垂裂口	42	外耳道耵聍	1
耳窦道	3	耳郭脓肿	1
耳漏	12	耳郭囊肿	2
非化脓性卡他性中耳炎	4	副耳	2
耳聋	4	先天性耳郭畸形	1
外耳道炎	1		

结缔组织系统疾病

甲沟炎	11	窦道	20
炎症	21	疖、痈	22
脓肿	64	梅毒瘤	6

鼻部疾病

臭鼻症 …… 7
鼻出血 …… 2
鼻息肉 …… 19
纤维性息肉 …… 1
前鼻孔闭锁 …… 1
鼻溃疡 …… 16
鼻黏膜溃疡 …… 9
鼻黏膜肥大 …… 1
鼻中隔偏曲 …… 1

运动系统疾病

骨膜炎 …… 5
骨炎 …… 11
骨溃疡 …… 28
坏疽 …… 41
脊柱弯曲 …… 8
滑膜炎 …… 27
黏液囊炎 …… 1
髋关节的腺疾病 …… 12
其他关节的腺疾病 …… 6
关节僵硬 …… 5
脚趾头和手指坏疽 …… 7
腿坏疽 …… 1

局部外伤

受伤 …… 74
枪击伤 …… 2
腹部外伤伴肠脱垂 …… 1
擦伤、挫伤 …… 61
扭伤 …… 36
烫烧伤 …… 9
碎片、针残留 …… 6
子弹残留 …… 2
咬伤 …… 19
脱臼 …… 12
骨折 …… 10

未分类的

助产 …… 3
拇指多指畸形 …… 1
肌肉抽搐 …… 4
肌肉挛缩 …… 2

以上列表只是大致准确，表明病人来医院后摆脱了什么样的病痛，比起统计治疗每个病种的实际数量更有意义。许多疾病的病例数量比我们所报告的要多得多，像体癣、疥疮这样的皮肤病数量更是达到几百例。此外，至少 70% 的颗粒状结膜炎会并发其他眼科疾病，如角膜炎、角膜溃疡、血管翳、虹膜疝、倒睫症等等。

伤寒——一个典型病例正在接受治疗。汕头很少见到伤寒。我的当地高级助理偶然识别出了一例这种疾病，这在这个地区很少见。中国乡村时兴的开放型排水系统对于外国人的嗅觉神经来说是令人讨厌的，但至少预防了像伤寒这样的发热性疾病的发展。

财务状况

就如我们在报告里提到的，我们承担了外国人社区的医疗保健工作接近 3 个月。收入是973.46美元，花费了102.37美元（5个船员和人力车苦力的工资），手头结余是871.09美元。其中370.07美元我交给了高仕兰医生（Dr. Cousland），剩下的500.12美元我记人医院账务的贷方。我们衷心感谢所有给予医院支持的朋友。

1888年的捐款

（略）

收支表

单位：美元

工资	327.00
一般费用	156.53
建设新楼及修葺	639.33
从汕头及香港购买的药物	272.12
从伦敦购买的药物	191.15
由爱丁堡教会支付的药物	864.23
帮助贫穷的病人	32.94
丧葬费用	14.09
买油	84.20
买猪油	23.60
买棉花	57.63
买水	42.22
买布	32.81
买纸	46.23
清洗病房	10.03
结余	764.18
	3 558.29

去年结余	590.93
外国人的捐款和报酬	1 447.10
中国人的捐款和报酬	217.43
向鸦片吸食者收取的费用	68.00
小病房租金	12.85
卖药、疝气绑带、牛奶、低值与低消费物品	358.29
爱丁堡传教委员会的拨款	864.23
	3 558.29

P. B. 高仕兰医学学士、外科硕士照管下的潮州府医学传教所

我们终于在这座城市有了临时场所，还进行了必要的修理和配备，1888 年 11 月 18 日开了一个诊所。从那时起，直到年末，诊治了 1 660 个病人，其中有一些是去病人家里诊治的。

诊所每天都开放，我们尽可能在短时间内多看病人。值得一提的是，那些最先到来的病人已从某些渠道知道了汕头医院。一些人去过那里，其他的是有朋友去过那里，更多的人是听说的。这样我们便有了一个好的开始，而且不久之后，其他人从那些来看过病的人那里听说了我们，于是过来看病，这说明他们对医院有信心。

有一个好的特点是有很多妇女来看病，登记在册的有 500 人，占病人总数的近 1/3，这确实体现出病人对我们和我们的方法有信心。

每天早晨由一名当地的传教士召集病人进行传教，然后，他利用这个机会开始与那些人在等候室交谈。

统计数据

个体病人	1 660
包括的住院病人	20
包括的女病人	500
复诊的门诊病人	721
手术总数	55

此外，有超过 300 个病人是在春季到访这座城市时来看病的。

手术

睑内翻及倒睫症手术	27
针刺治疗先天性白内障	2
翼状胬肉手术	1
鼻泪管狭窄手术	1
鼻息肉手术	4
兔唇手术	3
耳垂裂口手术	9
包皮过长手术	3
粉瘤手术	1
足底胼胝手术	1
从食道取出硬币	1
腿部慢性脓肿切开术	1
背部脂肪瘤切除术（重 12 磅 12 盎司）	1

菲利普 · B. 高仕兰

（翻译：刘慧翔、许思婷　校译：朱文平　审校：胡卫清、余维泉、江建安　中文校正：许党泉、杨柳婷）

1890 年汕头福音医院报告

（1890 年度来爱力医学学士、外科硕士照管下的英兰长老会汕头教会医院报告）

因为各种原因，我没能及早提交去年汕头教会医院的工作报告。个中缘由不必细说，下面的统计数据说明我们完成了大量的工作，整体来说是成功的一年。

统计数据

个体病人数：	
住院病人	2 958
门诊病人	2 926
合计	5 884
以上包括女病人	1 017
到中国病人家中出诊次数	227
平均每天住院病人数	180
门诊开放日平均每天门诊病人数	55
门诊病人总数（不完全统计）	8 913
外科手术数	1 026

亨利·莱恩医生（Dr. Henry Layng）全年定期在外科工作中提供了大力帮助，当高仕兰医生（Dr. Cousland）在潮州府的传教工作不忙碌时，也多次提供了帮助。

汕头有一位中国商人多年以来对医院深感兴趣，他的妻子以前也接受过我的治疗。他要求我建一些女病房，与总医院的男病房完全分开，而且他为此提供了 1 000 美元的资助。教会接受了他的资助。从那以后他又筹集了 2 000 多美元，据我所知，这些钱被存在银行，在我开始动工时他就会马上拿出来给我。他所提出的唯一条件是提供一些小病房租给富有阶层的妇女，这样她们就不需要和各式各样的人混杂在一起。至今，我仍然没能够建设（他想要的病房），因为在现在的医院附近找到额外的土地很困难。此外，我也希望能获得一笔更大的资金，用以变更各种行政部门，使我的管理工作更容易。

外国人社区的慷慨捐献，让我在年终手头能有一笔可观的结余。对于他们以及中国捐赠者的好心帮助我表示感谢。

在我的同事的同意下，我设想从日常资金中拿出 500 美元用于设立“女医院”基金。这些资金本来是为外国人社区提供医疗服务得来的，被我记入医院账务的贷方。

借这个机会我要感谢陈源盛（Tan-nguan-seng），他每年捐献大米和现金券以发放给贫穷的病人。去年收到的这些捐赠价值超过 100 美元，许多贫穷的病人因此能够继续住在医院，直到完成治疗。

传教工作

施饶理牧师（Rev. George Smith）于年终去世，医院失去了一位真诚的好朋友。在汕头，无论何时，他都不允许任何事情干扰他在病人中的传教工作，他孜孜不倦地教导那些对福音有兴趣的人。

除了传教士和当地助理的日常服务之外，这一年，木荫庐姑娘和侯玛利姑娘（Misses Black and Harkness）主要负责为妇女及男孩开设班级。这些努力取得了相当大的成功。值得关注的是，人们转信基督教的事被发表在《中国医学传教士杂志》上。

外科手术

眼部：

睑内翻及倒睫症手术	357
倒睫症手术（电解法）	42
睑内翻手术	4
虹膜脱出手术	3
眼前房积脓手术	1
睑球粘连手术	1
上眼睑的疤痕挛缩手术	1
翼状胬肉手术	58
血管翳球结膜环形切开术	4
白内障——吸出术	17
白内障——吸出后针刺术	2
白内障——虹膜切开术	2
虹膜切除术	14
结膜下增生切除术	5
眼睑皮脂腺囊肿、皮样囊肿等切除术	9
眼球摘除术	1
前葡萄肿切除术	3
睑板腺囊肿切除术	3
泪小管切开术	2
	529

躯体：

横向截石术	2
女孩膀胱结石取出术	1
会阴切开术	4
兔唇手术	31
肛瘘手术	77
包皮环切术	18

骨溃疡手术 …… 4
耳裂口修补术 …… 27
神经节手术 …… 8
鼻窦炎手术 …… 7
肛门狭窄手术 …… 1
尿道下裂手术 …… 1
腹股沟淋巴结炎手术 …… 3
直肠裂开手术 …… 1
鼻孔瘢痕闭锁手术 …… 1
阴道瘢痕闭锁手术 …… 2
肱骨骨折移位手术 …… 1
上颌窦囊肿手术 …… 1
甲状腺囊肿 …… 1
耳朵塑形手术 …… 2
鼻子塑形手术 …… 1
腿截肢术 …… 1
足截肢术（肖帕尔氏术式——Chopart's） …… 1
足截肢术（赛姆氏术式——Syme's） …… 1
阴茎截除术 …… 3
前臂截肢术 …… 1
手指切除术 …… 3
拇指多指畸形切除术 …… 1
脚趾切除术 …… 3
阴囊象皮肿切除术 …… 4
鼻息肉切除术 …… 14
死骨剔除术 …… 30
竹碎片等取出术 …… 3
食管鱼骨取出术 …… 1
膝关节截除术 …… 1
关节积液抽液术 …… 1
卵巢囊肿抽液术 …… 1
鞘膜积液抽液和注射术 …… 37
内痔结扎术 …… 46
探查性切开术 …… 1
大脓肿切开术 …… 6
胼胝切除术 …… 11
外痔切除术 …… 19
脸部瘢痕切除术 …… 2

皮肤上皮瘤切除术	1
包皮上皮瘤切除术	1
唇上皮瘤切除术	1
楔状骨及第二、第三跖骨切除术	1
湿疣切除术	4
龈瘤切除术	2
软纤维瘤切除术	1
纤维瘤切除术	1
腺体肿瘤切除术	4
脂肪瘤切除术	8
肉瘤样肿瘤切除术	3
皮脂腺囊肿切除术等	19
皮样囊肿切除术	1
肉芽肿切除术	4
直肠乳头状瘤切除术	1
扁桃体乳头状瘤切除术	1
直肠息肉切除术	3
囊性肿瘤切除术	3
舌头囊性肿瘤切除术（先天性）	1
颈导管囊肿切除术	2
女性乳房硬癌切除术	3
女性乳房肉瘤切除术	3
女性乳房复发性肿瘤切除术	1
腮腺瘤切除术	1
外阴软纤维瘤切除术	2
肿瘤（未分类的）切除术	4
疤痕电解术	3
痣电解术	2
各式各样的小手术	30
	497
拔牙	138

以上的清单大体上显示了手术日（星期三和星期六）完成的外科工作。很多小手术，如脓肿切开、伤口缝合、植皮手术、尿道及直肠狭窄扩张、骨折固定、脱臼复位等都是在非手术日完成的，但这些工作没有保留记录。这一年有两个手术后死亡病例。①一个病例19年前难产后完全性阴道闭塞。这是手术病例中病情相当严重的一例，接着发展成盆腔腹膜炎。手术后两周，病人在垂死状态下被送出医院，然后很快就死了。②病人死于手外伤前臂截肢手术后的破伤风。病人的手被一枚小炸弹几乎炸成了碎片，进行了前臂截肢手

术，伤口逐渐愈合了，除了一个曾用来置入引流管的小口，第11天开始出现肌肉强直性收缩。这些“玩具”小炸弹有时被中国人用来炸乡村池塘里的鱼，去年有至少4例这种病人前来接受治疗，都是因为使用炸弹不慎而导致了严重的手部外伤。

内痔——从1880年开始我们已经手术治疗了415例内痔，大多数是结扎术。我已经尝试了其他各种各样的治疗方法，但最终还是回归结扎术，在我的经验中这种方法与其他方法一样成功。我记得到目前为止，这个手术除了一个短暂的尿潴留并没有其他的并发症。

膀胱结石——3例。①一位6岁的小男孩，通过横向截石术取出重85格令的结石。②一位26岁的年轻男人，他从3岁开始就一直有泌尿系统病征。我通过用碎石钳压碎了结石，但在手术当中带有黏性的碎屑堵塞了吸引管。三四天后行了横向截石术，膀胱最终被清理干净了，虽然过程有点困难。病人恢复良好，但一条会阴造瘘管残留了3个月，最终也痊愈了。结石重2盎司4.5打兰。③一位8岁的小女孩，尿道被稍微切开，然后扩张，取出了一颗重280格令的结石。没有发生尿失禁。

大肿瘤——成功切除了以下大肿瘤：

阴囊象皮肿 ……………… 12磅
阴囊象皮肿 ……………… 7磅2盎司
阴囊象皮肿 ……………… 4磅13.5盎司
阴囊象皮肿 ……………… 2.5磅
女性乳房包囊性肿瘤 ……………… 约12.33磅
腮腺肿瘤 ……………… 2磅5盎司
腹股沟软纤维瘤 ……………… 2.5磅
阴唇软纤维瘤 ……………… 5磅13.5盎司

白内障——17例。有一例手术中一些玻璃体漏出，第三天便发生了虹膜炎。病人的眼睛做了两次虹膜切开术，获得了好的结果。另有一例手术失败了，其他15例手术结果都很满意。

1890年捐款

（略）

收支表

单位：美元

去年结余 ……………… 1 014.74
欧洲人的捐赠 ……………… 960.65
中国人的捐赠 ……………… 219.60
爱丁堡宣教委员会的拨款（药物） ……………… 406.00
向鸦片吸食者收取的费用 ……………… 62.94
病房租金 ……………… 33.87

出售药品、疝气绑带	948.28
	3 646.08

查核无误。

纪多纳（D. MACIVER）

单位：美元

工资	326.11
一般费用	148.10
建筑修缮	24.51
救助穷病人及丧葬费	112.94
买布、油、猪油、木材及其他物品	284.84
买水	131.94
在中国购买的药物、精馏酒精	477.65
来自伦敦的药物、外科敷料、器械等	1 230.15
结余	909.84
	3 646.08

（翻译：刘慧翔、许思婷　校译：朱文平　审校：胡卫清、余维泉、江建安　中文校正：许党泉、杨柳婷）

1891 年汕头福音医院报告

（1891 年度来爱力医学学士、外科硕士照管下的英兰长老会汕头教会医院报告）

我在汕头生活的这么多年里，1891 年是汕头健康状况最糟的一年。然而，统计数据显示教会医院就诊总病人数有轻微的下降。这是因为夏天霍乱的流行，几乎阻止了来自外地的病人正常前来就诊。因此，相比在往年工作较为繁重的九月份和十月份，这一年却比较轻松。前面所说的霍乱疫情虽然在汕头流行了两三个月之久，但没有在医院内流行。一些霍乱病人被送进医院，感染了几位患者，但病情没有在医院大范围扩散。

我必须衷心感谢外国人社区和很多中国朋友为支持我们工作的慷慨捐助，也非常感谢亨利·莱恩医生（Dr. Henry Layng）的友好帮助，他有规律地每周两次来外科帮忙。约翰·郎医生（Dr. John Lang）在七月间承担了医院的工作。我们还要感谢所有在对病人的定期传教活动中提供帮助的人们，也要感谢陈源盛行（Tang-Nguan-Seng hong）给贫困患者提供的大米和现金。

在去年的报告中，我提及有意建立一所女医院。然而我很遗憾地告知大家，由于没有合适的地址，这件事没有如愿取得进展。那处和医院相邻的地方我本已看中，却被道台大人拒绝了，所以我们将会去别处寻找理想的地方。

下面，我给出了本年度的统计数据，让数据来说话。

个体病人数：	
住院病人	2 670
门诊病人	2 991
合计	5 661
以上包括女病人	847
到中国病人家中出诊次数	300
平均每天住院病人数	172
门诊开放日平均每天门诊病人数	55
到诊所就诊的门诊病人总数（不完全统计）	10 106
外科手术	845

外科手术

眼部：

睑内翻及倒睫症手术	221
倒睫症手术（电解法）	54
翼状胬肉手术	30

睑球粘连手术 …… 1
虹膜疝手术 …… 3
前葡萄肿切除术 …… 7
眼睑软骨肥厚手术 …… 5
角膜翳角膜缘球结膜环状切开术 …… 1
人工瞳孔虹膜切除术 …… 33
青光眼虹膜切除术等 …… 6
白内障摘除术 …… 7
结膜下增生切除术 …… 2
眼睑囊肿切除术 …… 1
睑板腺囊肿切开术 …… 4
眦成形术 …… 4
上、下眼睑整形术 …… 1
泪小管切开术 …… 1
上睑菜花样肿瘤切除术 …… 1
眼部恶性肿瘤切除术 …… 1
角膜异物剔出术 …… 2

385

躯体：

耻骨上切开取石术 …… 1
横向切开取石术 …… 1
尿道结石存留取出术 …… 2
会阴部尿道切开术 …… 2
兔唇手术 …… 24
耳裂 …… 24
肛瘘手术 …… 99
包皮环切术 …… 16
直肠阴道瘘手术 …… 1
阴道瘢痕闭塞手术 …… 2
鼻孔瘢痕闭塞手术 …… 1
膝关节瘢痕挛缩手术 …… 1
髋关节瘢痕挛缩手术 …… 1
肛门闭锁手术 …… 1
涎腺瘘手术 …… 1
上颌窦囊肿手术 …… 1
肱骨骨折移位手术 …… 1
鼻窦手术 …… 17
腱鞘囊肿手术 …… 5

舌下囊肿手术	1
腿部复合性骨折手术	1
复合性手指关节脱位手术	1
舌外伤手术	1
直肠裂伤手术	1
胼胝切除术	12
外痔切除术	24
睾丸切除术	2
先天性牙龈增生切除术	1
直肠息肉切除术	1
肿瘤切除术——脂肪瘤	7
皮脂腺囊肿	7
肉芽瘤	3
牙龈瘤	4
纤维瘤	1
腮腺瘤	4
膀胱肿瘤	5
腭肿瘤	1
女性乳腺恶性肿瘤	3
男性乳腺恶性肿瘤	1
肉瘤	2
未分类的肿瘤	6
复合掌侧神经节切除术	1
神经节切除术	1
睾丸海绵肿切除术	1
下颌下腺切除术	2
截肢术——手指	3
脚趾	2
大腿	1
腿下 1/3	1
阴茎（上皮瘤）	3
阴囊象皮肿	4
腿	1
鼻息肉摘除术	7
死骨剔除术	30
食道鱼骨取出术	1
卵巢囊肿抽液术	1
关节积液抽液术	1

睾丸鞘膜积液抽液注射术 …… 22
膝关节抽吸术 …… 3
内痔结扎术 …… 47
巨大急性脓肿切开术 …… 7
髋关节疾病——扩大窦道和引流术 …… 1
痣电灼术 …… 2
各式各样的小手术 …… 27

460

拔牙（不完全统计） …… 191

1891 年捐款

（略）

收支表

单位：美元

工资 …… 377.00
一般费用 …… 137.20
建筑修缮 …… 169.33
在中国购买的药物 …… 384.82
来自伦敦的药物、外科敷料、器械等 …… 919.11
由爱丁堡宣教委员会支付药物费用 …… 493.75
资助贫困患者 …… 32.84
丧葬费用 …… 57.29
棉花、羊毛制品、绷带布 …… 139.79
医院的水 …… 129.90
猪油、蜡和油 …… 129.10
纸张 …… 15.61
转账至新大楼基金 …… 500.00
结余 …… 17.46

3 503.20

1890 年所示结余 …… 909.84
上表所示的捐赠 …… 865.03
劳特（Lauts）和黑斯卢普（Haesloop）先生捐助病人 …… 9.25
出售药品 …… 999.98
出售疝气绑带、瓶子和杂物 …… 124.45

收取鸦片吸食者的费用	84.00
私人病房租金	16.90
爱丁堡宣教委员会拨款	493.75
	3 503.20

查核无误。

纪多纳（D. MACIVER）

新大楼账目

单位：美元

伦敦史葛（Scott）小姐捐助	19.20
从医院资金转账	500.00
	519.20

查核无误。

纪多纳（D. MACIVER）

（翻译：陈坚龙、许思婷　校译：朱文平　审校：胡卫清、余维泉、江建安　中文校正：许党泉、杨柳婷）

1892—1893 年汕头福音医院报告

（1892—1893 年度来爱力医学学士、外科硕士照管下的英兰长老会汕头教会医院报告）

由于 1892 年没有写报告，因此在这份报告中仅记录了 1892 年和 1893 年的统计数据、捐赠者姓名和收支明细。这两年的工作相当繁重，虽然中国南方的教会医院比较灵活，且中国病人对于病房空间的要求不高，但在某些季节申请住院的人数的确超出了医院的收容量。这就解释了为什么病人这么多，而住院病人数量却没有相应地增加的情形。我很高兴现在手头上有充足的资金去建立一所独立的女医院，但仍需要找到合适的地址。现有大楼西边的浅滩能满足大部分要求，但地方当局拒绝将此地租给我们。在英国，在筹集资金建设新医院的过程中，我得到了木荫庐小姐（Miss Black）的热情帮助。在此我要对她表示衷心的感谢，也请相信在她善意的支持下，我们会好好利用这些资金。

统计数据

个体病人数：

	1 892	1 893
住院病人	2 544	2 766
门诊病人	4 115	4 586
总数	6 659	7 352
以上包含女病人	1 209	1 317
到中国病人家中出诊	325	371
平均每天住院病人数	157	176
门诊开放日平均每天门诊病人数	67	73
到诊所就诊的门诊病人总数（不完全统计）	11 872	13 237
外科手术	984	1 118

最近，我们新聘了一名卖《圣经》的本地小贩和一名女传道员作为我们的员工。大约 10 年前，我们曾雇了一个卖《圣经》的小贩来随访老病人。但他并未完成工作。我们专门聘请他流访各地乡村，但医院的老病人却不认得他，因此他未能起到连接医院与老病人的桥梁作用。这一次我们将尝试另一个计划，大家建议让小贩大部分时间在医院内工作——卖书、教授病人（单独地或在班级里）、读福音短文和赞美诗集。偶尔，他也需要前往农村拜访老病人，尤其是那些对福音真理有兴趣的人和接受他传教的新传教士。我们希望他由此被

确认为医院的员工，也希望他拜访的人像朋友一样待他。B. and F. 圣经协会已同意支付他一半的工资。

女传教士的工作由教会中的一位女士来完成任务。女传教士的主要职责有两方面。其中一方面是教那些较聪明的病人阅读简单的短文和赞美诗集，或者让她们在有限的住院时间里尽可能学得更多。从事这项工作，女传教士得牺牲下午的时间，而早晨的时间则用来照顾病房里那些不能起身的患者，包括老年人、智障者、盲人及部分失聪患者。希望她的诚心工作能使女性患者在出院时对福音知识基本上了解。这位女传教士本身就是医院的一个成果。约6年前，她作为一个非基督教徒到医院，经过几个月的体验，她已从理智上相信了福音的真理，直至心灵被感化，自从那时候开始，她在才智和灵性知识上取得了相当大的进步。她毛遂自荐，认为自己适合做这份工作。这几年中，与福音传教工作相关的传教班由 W. M. A. 的代理人维持进行，其他女士基本上都常来到女性病房看望，也为传教工作贡献良多。

前几年，亨利·莱恩医生（Dr. Henry Layng）一直协助外科工作，而1893年在我去日本的两个月期间，他帮我管理了医院，事无巨细，尽心尽责。高仕兰医生（Dr. P. B. Cousland）在潮州府闲暇时也偶尔过来帮忙。

对于医院基金的捐赠者，我们表示衷心的感谢。陈源盛行（Tang-Nguan-Seng hong）连续为贫困患者送来大米和银票等礼物，每年的价值达100美元。每当银票用完他们又会及时送来，他们的慷慨资助真是不可估量。不必说，那些受惠的病人会对这样的恩惠心存感激，我自己也是如此。

因为3月初休假，我不在期间医院将由高仕兰医生（Dr. P. B. Cousland）负责。

1892 年捐款

（略）

1892 年收支表

单位：美元

工资	397.69
一般费用	79.42
建筑修缮	261.12
在中国购买的药物	214.25
来自伦敦的药物、外科敷料和仪器	719.94
由爱丁堡宣教委员会支付的药物、外科敷料和仪器	648.00
水	140.14
棉花、羊毛、绷带	150.69
猪油、蜡和油	118.08
纸张和杂物	40.80
资助贫困患者	48.22
丧葬费用	38.70
	2 857.05

1891 年结余	17.46
上表所示的捐款	876.12
出售药品	963.24
疝气绑带、瓶子和杂物卖出	113.46
吸毒患者支付	85.00
私人病房租金	16.95
爱丁堡宣教委员会拨款	648.00
赤字	136.82
	2 857.05

新大楼账户

现金	519.02

查核无误。

J. 斯蒂尔（J. STEELE）

1893 年捐款

（略）

1893 年收支表

单位：美元

1892 年超支	136.82
工资	421.98
一般费用	124.99
建筑修缮	49.59
在中国购买的药物	191.32
来自伦敦的药物、外科敷料和仪器	392.54
由爱丁堡宣教委员会支付的药物、外科敷料和仪器	744.00
丧葬费用	48.17
水	131.97
猪油、蜡和油	174.54
棉花、羊毛、绷带	202.07
精馏酒精	248.26
纸张和杂物	55.36
资助贫困患者	30.47
结余	174.51
	3 126.59
上表所示的捐款	1 213.05

出售药品	935.82
出售疝气绑带、瓶子和杂物	162.77
吸毒患者支付	51.00
私人病房租金	19.95
爱丁堡宣教委员会拨款	744.00
	3 126.59

新大楼账户

现金	519.02

查核无误。

J. 斯蒂尔（J. STEELE）

1892 年外科手术

眼部：

睑内翻及倒睫症手术	272
倒睫症手术（电解法）	43
翼状胬肉手术	44
虹膜疝手术	3
白内障（晶状体）摘除手术	26
人工瞳孔虹膜切除术	27
青光眼虹膜切除术	2
角膜翳角膜缘球结膜环状切开术	1
结膜下增生切除术	3
眼睑囊肿等切除术	7
前葡萄肿切除术	1
眼睑整形术	3
角膜异物取出术	4
睑板腺囊肿切开术	5
	441

躯体：

正中切开取石术	1
横向切开取石术	2
尿道结石存留取出术	2
卵巢切除术	1
尿道外切开术	5
尿道内切开术	1
死骨剔除术	42

唇裂手术	20
肛瘘手术	84
耳裂修复术	33
尿道口瘢痕挛缩手术	1
鼻孔瘢痕挛缩手术	1
肛门瘢痕挛缩手术	2
上唇上皮瘤手术	1
皮肤上皮瘤手术	1
手指上皮瘤手术	1
腕上皮瘤手术	1
膝上皮瘤手术	1
肛门闭锁手术	1
耳朵息肉手术	2
耳瘘手术	1
眼睑挛缩手术	2
包皮过长环切术	18
包皮过长切开裂口术	1
舌下囊肿手术	3
鼻窦手术	14
阴囊血肿手术	3
直肠脱垂手术	2
截肢术——手指	7
手（部分）	1
前臂	2
拇指	1
阴茎（上皮瘤）	3
腿	2
脚趾	1
阴囊象皮肿	7
胼胝切除术	19
外痔切除术	15
睾丸切除术	1
肿瘤切除术——皮脂腺囊肿	26
黏液囊肿	3
颈导管水囊肿	1
皮样囊肿	1
黏液囊肿	3
女性乳腺囊肿	1

血管瘤	2
血肿	2
扁桃体肿大	3
牙龈瘤	3
直肠息肉	2
脂肪瘤	3
乳头状瘤	1
肉瘤	4
肉芽瘤	2
腮腺瘤	4
纤维瘤	4
颈部颗粒物	1
股骨头切除术	1
鼻息肉摘除术	23
巨大鼻咽息肉摘除术	1
体内子弹取出术	4
碎片、针取出术	9
食道鱼骨取出术	2
内痔结扎术	50
睾丸鞘膜积液切开放液注射术	15
囊性甲状腺肿切开放液注射术	1
前额成形术	1
鼻子成形术	1
口唇成形术	1
耳朵成形术	1
麻风病尺神经拉伸术	1
各种各样的小手术	60
	543
拔牙（不完全统计）	224

1893 年外科手术

眼部：

睑内翻及倒睫症手术	229
睑外翻手术	1
翼状胬肉手术	47
睑球粘连手术	5
白内障（晶状体）摘除手术	52

白内障二次手术	1
虹膜切除术	88
眼眶囊肿切除术	1
眼睑囊肿切除术	7
角膜先天性增生切除术	1
眼眶恶性肿瘤切除术	1
前葡萄肿切除术	3
角膜翳角膜缘球结膜环状切开术	1
眦成形术	2
上睑整形术	1
未分类的小手术	6
	490

躯体：

内痔结扎术	48
睾丸鞘膜积液切开放液注射术	38
甲状腺肿切开放液注射术	1
腹水切开放液术	1
急性膝关节滑膜炎切开放液术	1
死骨剔除术	40
尿道外切开术	6
横向切开取石术	3
卵巢切除术	1
剖腹手术	2
瘢痕瘤电解术	3
耳朵成形术	1
膝关节切除术	1
上腭成形术	1
截肢术——臂	1
手指和脚趾	3
腿下1/3	2
足（部分为先天性增生）	1
多指	1
多趾	1
阴囊象皮病切除术	7
阴囊淋巴肿切除术	1
龈瘤切除术	3
第一、二跖骨舟状骨和距骨切除术	1
男性乳腺增生切除术	1

血管瘤切除术	1
神经瘤切除术	1
痈切开术	1
硬结切除术	26
外痔切除术	25
皮脂腺囊肿切除术	33
血肿切开术	2
脂肪瘤切除术	3
包皮上皮瘤切除术	2
甲状腺囊肿切除术	3
软骨囊肿切除术	2
腮腺瘤切除术	2
纤维瘤切除术	4
肉瘤切除术	5
肉芽瘤切除术	3
舌下腺囊肿切除术	2
睾丸肉瘤切除术	2
腺肿瘤切除术	3
未分类的肿瘤切除术	8
肘关节切除术	1
肛瘘手术	103
包皮环切术	18
包皮过长切开裂口术	1
唇裂手术	30
耳裂修复术	38
骨疡手术	8
鼻窦手术	9
肛门瘢痕挛缩手术	2
外耳道瘢痕闭塞手术	1
鼻孔瘢痕闭塞手术	2
膝踝瘢痕挛缩手术	1
先天性小肛门手术	1
髂关节病引流术	5
鼻息肉摘除术	18
针、碎片取出术	5
食道鱼骨取出术	1
各种各样的小手术	92
	628
拔牙	240

卵巢切除术——在已进行的两例手术中，一例成功，另一例在术后第 27 天死亡。成功的病例肿瘤与子宫粘连处多，手术难度较大。而第二例死亡的原因仍不明确，可能是死于大肠的感染性并发症。虽然粘连比较少，但肿瘤与子宫粘连固定，且大肠的下半部分明显扩张。在切除卵巢肿物时发现肿块几乎填满了整个盆腔。患者在术后很快出现发热症状，紧接着是腹泻，伴有疼痛及降结肠线上的小硬结。两个星期后，已经一期愈合的腹部切口的最上缘出现了轻微的肿胀。最终证明为瘘管。很明显，扩张的结肠下段在某种程度上受损。该病人在术后第 27 天死于衰竭。除了肠道并发症，莱恩医生（Dr. Layng）和我都找不到关于这些症状的其他解释。

（翻译：陈坚龙、许思婷　校译：朱文平　审校：胡卫清、余维泉、江建安　中文校正：许党泉、杨柳婷）

1894年汕头福音医院报告

（1894年度高仕兰医学学士、外科硕士照管下的英兰长老会汕头教会医院报告）

对潮州人民来说，1894年是艰难的一年。继1893年收成不好之后，这一年由于干旱之后又是洪水，夏天大米的收成也不好，而且有一段时间从北方引进大米的渠道也中止了，因此食物的价格被抬高，给人们造成了很大的困难。这种困况在10月份达到了极点，一场大米骚动眼看就要暴发。所幸运粮轮船的及时到达缓解了紧张的局势。一看到轮船进入港口，汕头大街小巷的人几乎都高兴得跳起来。

由于食物的稀缺，一些病人放弃来医院就诊，住院的病人也不会长时间留院。关于香港外籍医生治疗鼠疫患者的方法令人可怖可怕的谣言，以及道听途说的中国或许正与某个国家打仗的消息，都对就诊人数产生了一些影响。

在我负责管理医院期间，住院病人很多，以至于门诊病人都尽量被限定到了常规门诊出诊的时间，即周二、周五前来就诊。因此引起了住院病人的减少。

来爱力医生（Dr. Lyall）的健康状况迫使他在3月初休假，于是我离开潮州府过来担任医院的主管。大量的外科工作，如此多需要照料的住院病人，门诊部、学校、学会、外国传教机构的医疗保健工作，以及日常教会的一部分工作，这些对于一个人而言实在太繁重，不过，令人欣慰的是，宣教委员会答应再派一名医务人员来汕头。

早些年亨利・莱恩医生（Dr. H. Layng）给予我们很多帮助，我们还要对外国及中国热心团体表示最衷心的感谢，在他们的帮助下，我们得以为病人带来健康与慰藉。陈源盛行（Tang-Nguan-Seng hong）的领头给了我们价值364美元的票券，相当于为贫困患者提供15 000次有质量膳食。他给每个病人一日量的大米用来庆祝中国的新年，97位留在医院的患者中有94人收到了他的礼物。

这一年医院在建设上唯一重要的改变，就是花费了89美元建了一个崭新的系统有所改良的公共厕所。

这一年有3个初级助理和4个学生接受教育，学习科目是解剖学、化学和生理学，并练习了读写拉丁文处方。

统计数据

个体病人数：	
住院病人	2 317
门诊病人	2 746
合计	5 063
以上包括女病人	994
到中国病人家中出诊次数	173

平均每天住院病人数 ………………………………………………… 151
门诊开放日平均每天就诊病人数 ……………………………………… 62
到诊所就诊的门诊病人总数 ………………………………………… 10 583
外科手术 ……………………………………………………………… 920

这些数据只表明常规工作时间的工作量。另外，利用高级助理们还在业余时间看了大约2 000 例的小病。

传教工作

我们教导病人如何正确看待病痛——但还有比身体康复更重要的事情，这可以从下表中了解：

上午 8:30——医院教堂的早间服务——由传教士或者高级助理负责。

上午 9:15——为女性患者短暂的服务——由木荫庐小姐（Miss Black）或者女传教士负责。

下午 2:00—3:00——妇女阅读课——由侯玛利小姐（Miss Harkness）或者女传教士负责。

下午 3:00—4:00——妇女阅读课——由女传教士负责。

下午 2:00—3:00——男孩阅读课——由木荫庐小姐和一位基督徒年轻人负责。

晚上 7:00——教堂的晚间服务——由高级助手承担。

在病房，由医院卖宗教书的小贩和木荫庐小姐的助理与男性患者对话并教他们阅读。

在病房，由女传教士、差会女士和本地一些女信徒与女性患者对话并教她们阅读。

由小贩销售四福音书和短文。

礼拜日下午 3:00——为测试和指导洗礼的申请人而集会，由传教士进行观察。

对于那些年轻聪明而且延长住院时间的患者，通过让其阅读《圣经 · 新约》大部分内容、短文及教堂月报，来学习拉丁语。而对其他患者，则通过口头讲授《赞美诗集》与《十诫》的方式，使不能阅读的患者能或多或少记住部分内容。

与 10 年前我担任院长工作的情况相比，现在的教学内容要多得多。不管有没有成为基督教徒，患者们在离院时都对基督教教义有了更清晰的认识，而且他们还带走了有用的书籍和短文，里面的内容他们也基本上有所了解。我不知道那些明确拒绝信仰基督的人与加入教会的人在数量上会有多大的差距。这些课堂和病房工作是对早间和晚间礼拜的补充。而且我们足够有理由心怀感激，因为我们有两个既热心又能干的福音传教士作为高级助理。在过去的 20 年里，这两个人在当地传播基督教所带来的影响是深远的。

3 月份阅读《圣经》并贩卖宗教书的商贩开始履行职责，他被几次派往两三个社区寻访以前的病人。他将大部分时间花在医院病房和男性患者的教室，出售短文和四福音书给门诊病人。他在医院内的推销比出去寻访更成功。

这一年大约有 100 人申请接受洗礼。其中一些人我们怀疑不够真诚，另外一些人我们担心他们回家后会屈服于村里的舆论的压力，但对于一些人我们有理由相信他们是真诚的，而且他们会坚定信念，抵抗所有迫害。

很多老病号在乡村教堂接受洗礼，有两三位在医院接受洗礼。其中一些人并没有在这里申请洗礼，但他们回家后就毁掉了他们的崇拜物，并在最近的教堂参加宗教仪式，这是非常鼓舞人心的。一位教会女士在拜访了一个乡村服务站后给我们写了一封信，从摘录的一段可以说明医院的影响力是如何被扩大的："一个接受洗礼的妇女在医院陪她截足的儿子期间听说了那些教条，他们回家后，（她的）丈夫也非常乐意聆听，他和一个小儿子也成了申请者。我丈夫并没有让这个小儿子洗礼。他（我丈夫）非常乐意接受这个有丈夫、妻子、长子和小婴儿的家庭，以及另外一个年轻人。我们希望在没有基督教徒的乡村，这个家庭的做法可以带动许多人崇信基督教。"

在皈依者中偶尔有一些人虽然是教会成员的亲戚，但并没有在家庭影响下成为基督教徒，反而在医院更集中持续的基督传教影响和布道之下觉醒而做出了决定。

病房里有 9 个死亡病例：①年轻男性，因胫骨坏疽接受治疗。出现恶性疟发热。心力衰竭而死。②肺结核患者。突发致命性大咯血。③从新加坡回来的男性患者。嗜酒成性，出现衰弱及心力衰竭。④年轻男性，因沙眼接受治疗。出现发热、便秘，随后一两天出现严重绞痛，之后疼痛缓解。无呕吐、腹胀或腹肌紧张，但脉搏持续减弱直至死亡。⑤年轻男性，患脚气病（?）、神经炎（?），心力衰竭而死。⑥年老男性，鸦片吸食者。跌倒致使尿道破裂及阴囊尿瘘。没有愈合能力，阴囊糜烂，褥疮，哪里受压最轻哪里就长痂，营养、鸦片及酒精都没有效。因脓毒性发热而死亡。⑦年老男性，患慢性痢疾。夜间在病房跌倒，早晨被发现死亡。心力衰竭而死。⑧老年女性，患严重痢疾。⑨鸦片吸食者。摔倒后被一袋糖压住，鼻子及左耳出血。第三天好转逃跑。两天后被带回，体温高达 105°（译者注：华氏度，相当于 40.6 摄氏度），谵妄而死亡。没有术后死亡病例。

腺型鼠疫——尽管有通过水路和陆路从香港及广东来的病患，汕头及周边地区幸运地躲过了鼠疫侵袭。

继长时间干旱之后，连绵大雨来临。我们尽最大努力做好大部分的防疫工作，对所有来自受感染港口的轮船进行检查。轮船由莱恩医生（Dr. H. Layng）检查，所有可疑病例都被送到一个由商业机构建起的棚子医院里，由中国当局指派一位本地内科医生照料。这个计划成效很好，那个本地医生是一个很好共事的人，他的出现防止了谣言的兴起。在外来的 11 个病例中，有两例恢复了。其中一个在被转送上岸时从船上跳下，从外国人手中逃离厄运，他恢复了。

尽管做足了预防措施，汕头还是出现了几个病例。甚至到 8 月底，我还被叫去看望电报局的一个职员，他当时正饱受此病的折磨。

流行性感冒——在今年前几个月和后两个月都有流行。年末的发病情况并不太严重。与年初暴发的流行性感冒有所不同的是，扁桃体炎作为早期症状，发病率较低，背痛和其他疼痛症状相对少见。片状肺充血以及咳嗽时痰少而难咳出，这些特点与平时一样。但没有像之前一样导致器官衰竭。

秋季整个辖区广泛流行**急性卡他性结膜炎**，儿童尤其易受感染。所有来院观察的病例都没有留下严重后遗症。

典型的**血友病**病例是一个 6 岁的男孩，他因为头部划伤出血而被带来治疗。在这个小伤口愈合之前还几次出血，而且当他的肢体被抓住时上面会出现瘀斑。他有经常出血的病史，包括呕血。他已故的兄弟也有一样的病情，然而没有人了解遗传病史。

最悲惨的是有一个病人因为自己的罪过而使整个家庭受牵连。他因为淋病性眼炎来诊治些许时日，但回家时仍有一侧眼球患有全眼球炎。两个月后他带着他的父亲和兄弟返回，父亲已经失去了双眼，兄弟则失去了一只眼睛，我们只能抢救他的另一只眼。他说他的母亲也失明了，家里所有人都遭受到他眼疾的传染。

两个**脊柱病例**恢复情况出人意料。第一个为 52 岁男性，他从高处跌落，伤及背部。没有感觉到有病变，但有完全性截瘫，括约肌也失去了控制。第五天，他的大腿有了恢复力量的迹象。第八天他出院了，已经可以下地行走，括约肌也可以控制了。他被诊断为一个出血病例用麦角碱及 K. I. 进行治疗。

第二个病例的病史如下：他是一位 40 岁的男性，在入院前 4 个月出现了发热病状，紧接着下肢瘫痪，而且病情发展时间长达两个星期，随后开始逐渐改善。入院时他不能站立，但他的括约肌没有完全失控。麻木感也已经消失了。病人没有梅毒病史。各种各样的救治方案也尝试了。K. I. 总是导致受影响肌肉的阵挛，但会延长 Hydr. Perchlor. 的作用过程，使用麦角碱和莨菪碱则会有明显的改善。他自己也体验到治疗时所使用的药方的效果。6 个月后他可以不用拐杖走路了。这里我们有一个病例证据显示为充血，而且有硬化的倾向。

这一年所遇到的罕见的疾病如下：

白血病，男孩，白细胞与红细胞比例为 1∶5。

雷诺病，年轻男性，双足趾尖发病，持续 5 个月。

尿崩症，16 岁男孩，尿比重 1 000（克/升），24 小时尿量 320 盎司，持续 6 年，无有效治疗方法。

急性糖尿病，中年男性。

慢性糖尿病，老年矮胖男性，去年在本院诊治，这次因糖尿病性神经炎来诊，应用水杨酸钠（Sod. Salicyl.）后缓解。

癔症，一例，年轻妇女。

直肠和肛管多发腺瘤。直肠内远处上方能够感觉到的由小肿瘤形成的一个肿块。

膀胱异位及尿道下裂，8 岁男孩。

虹膜缺损（下方）	1	圆锥形角膜	1
麻风病	162	鼠疫	1
哮喘	25	鸡奸所致梅毒	75
运动性共济失调	1	膀胱结石	5
帕金森氏病	1	阴茎结石	2
癫痫	12	大腿象皮病	36

脚气病	1	阴囊象皮病	18
甲状腺肿	7	大腿阴囊象皮病	2
淋巴腺瘤	1	纤维软疣	1

有一个大腿象皮肿的病例，感染集中于股内收肌侧；而有一个阴囊象皮肿的病例，是阴囊淋巴肿向象皮肿的转变的典型案例。

在过去的两年中，皮下注射的吗啡在本辖区被广泛应用，表面上是为了治疗鸦片成瘾。有一段时间这种做法非常流行，因为在计划突然戒断毒瘾的过程中，这种疗法痛苦小，见效快。但当人们发现吗啡的剂量不能减少时，这个方法遭人诟病，一些病例的管理员日子也非常不好过。我没有听说过哪怕一例染毒者治愈的消息，但很多受害者来医院接受我们的疗法。他们的手臂有的脓疱满布，有的疤痕累累。这很明显是因为没有注意药剂或注射器的清洁问题。但仍有很多人使用这种疗法，结果是发现重新拿起烟管不能使他们感觉像注射吗啡一样过瘾。

1894 年外科手术

眼部：

睑内翻及倒睫症手术，上睑	206
睑内翻及倒睫症手术，下睑	96
睑外翻手术	1
翼状胬肉手术	50
上睑下垂手术	1
白内障晶状体摘除手术	17
白内障二次手术	2
虹膜切除术	40
虹膜切开术	2
角膜侵蚀性溃疡烧灼术	2
结膜增生切除和刮除术	3
眼眶肿瘤切除术	1
恶性肿瘤眼球摘除术	1
睑板腺囊肿手术	3
内眦血管瘤电解术	1
多方面的手术	2
	428

躯体：

外痔切除术	27
内痔结扎术	55
阴囊积水抽液注射术	33

淋巴囊肿抽液注射术	1
甲状腺肿抽液术	3
腹水抽液术	1
死骨剔除术	29
尿道外切开术	3
膀胱横向切开取石术	2
扁桃体部分切除术	1
骨疡、狼疮、溃疡、腺体等刮除术	38
肛瘘切开术	3
儿童脐带息肉结扎术	1
耳郭部分修复塑形术	1
鼻梁修复塑形术	2
截肢术前臂骨疡（环切）（A）	1
手指截除术	2
腿部骨疡截肢术（大块后皮瓣）	1
足部骨疡截肢术（赛姆氏——Syme's）	1
足趾及先天性肿瘤截肢术	1
拇指多指畸形切除术	4
拇趾切除术（B）	4
阴囊象皮肿切除术（C）	7
阴囊淋巴肿切除术	1
龈瘤及部分下巴切除术	2
头皮血管瘤切除术	1
直肠腺瘤切除术	3
胼胝切除术	10
皮脂腺囊肿切除术	18
其他囊肿切除术	3
脂肪瘤切除术（D）	3
上皮瘤切除术	1
结节性腺体切除术	1
瘢痕瘤切除术	2
外生骨疣切除术（E）	2
纤维瘤切除术（F）	3
肉瘤切除术（G）	6
腱鞘囊肿切除术	2
小肿瘤切除术	10
未分类的恶性肿瘤切除术	4
下腭腺体切除术（麻风病患者）	1

胫骨切除术	1
肱骨头切除术	1
肛瘘手术	51
包皮过长环切术	14
包皮过长切开裂口术	3
唇裂手术	25
慢性巨大脓肿手术	2
耳垂裂开手术	30
跗骨骨疡手术	1
窦道手术	3
先天性肛门闭锁手术	1
阴囊血肿切开填塞术	2
膝关节僵硬矫正术	3
髋、肩、下巴脱位复位术	3
鼻息肉摘除术	8
耳息肉圈断术	1
针、碎片取出术	3
各种各样的小手术	46
	492
助产术	3
（一例侧前置胎盘病例行宫内倒转术，胎儿死亡，母亲康复）	
拔牙	201

上表中并没有包括在病房或非工作时间进行的大量小型的外科手术。

外科工作日记

虹膜切除术——这个手术绝大部分是为了人工瞳孔进行的。其他病例则是为了治疗青光眼、侵蚀性角膜溃疡，以及前粘连所致的虹膜炎。对于之前的粘连病例，我们经常很难决定是否进行此项手术。一些病例如果不进行手术治疗效果也很好。其中一个做了手术的病例结果令人非常满意，感应性完全消失了。

尿道外切开术——在3例创伤性尿道破裂并尿瘘的病例中进行。破裂的位置被切开，将一条导管插入膀胱并固定。这种情况很常见。其他几个病例进行治疗时，他们不需要手术就可以将导管插入。其中一个最后死亡了，这在死亡病例中已经提到过。

截石术——横向切口。结石分别重达14德拉克马和3.5盎司。

第一个病例说明了灌肠在痢疾中的效果。术后一个星期一切情况都很好，后来他的体温升至104华氏度，到了第11天，病情朝非典型痢病症发展。大便中不带血，有时候看起来一半像腹泻，一半像痢疾。常规的口服治疗并不能制止或减轻病情。第15天时他的情况非常糟糕，上午体温达到 101.8 华氏度，下午为 104 华氏度，几乎摸不到脉搏，患者神志不清。医生不断给予氨和酒精刺激，皮下注射洋地黄达 70 毫克，（这些措施）在这一天的病程中都不起作用。晚上予大肠内灌入 3 品脱 0.5% 的克勒奥林（Creolin）溶液。第 16 天，早上体温 98.6 华氏度，大汗，脉搏较前有力。这一天患者进食不少牛奶，但应尽量减少刺激。再次接受灌肠，下午体温 100.2 华氏度，大便 4 次。第 18 天，体温早上及下午均为 98 华氏度，大便 3 次。

当遇到病人的反对，或者每当其体温开始升高，大便变得更频繁时，我们都得停止灌肠。再次灌肠后病情有了明显的改善。第 33 天，患者第一次排出成形的大便。会阴的窦道在闭合前不得不烧灼 3 次。病人是一位 41 岁的军官，体格相当强壮。

①一个非常灵活的老人，伤口穿过上臂中部。第 3 天下楼，导致伤口二次出血。最终伤口很快愈合。②均为年轻女性。缠足导致局部坏死，拇趾严重溃烂。使用 Amp.（腺嘌呤核糖核苷酸?）是最好的治疗方式。伤口很快愈合。③最小 1.375 磅，最大 4.5 磅。每个病例都有游离小皮瓣覆盖睾丸。④肩胛处 8 磅，肩膀处二又八分之五磅。⑤一例有蒂，菜花状，在股骨干下末端。另一例为第二跖骨。两个重量均为 2 盎司。⑥乳腺纤维瘤，19 盎司，老年女性。一个男性肩膀处 1.5 磅。⑦囊性，年轻女性大腿，5 磅。乳腺梭形细胞，年长男性，曾两次切除。女性乳腺肉瘤。

一例割喉自杀未遂的病例来院观察。对喉部伤口进行缝合，但病人是精神病患者，几天后就离开了。

一个男孩因急性化脓性骨膜炎致整个胫骨骨坏死被送来治疗，这种病在这里罕见。患者骨头被移除，上达骨骺，术后病人整体病情得到明显改善，但新骨生长缓慢，5 个月后新骨仍然很脆弱，因而不能使用新骨骺。

氯仿麻醉只使用了 80 次，因为闽南人或者讲潮州方言的人极少有疼痛的感觉。

1894 年捐款

（略）

1893 年收支表

单位：美元

工资	477.24
一般费用	94.10
来自伦敦的药物等	907.86
来自宣教委员会药物等	876.00
来自中国及香港药物等	207.84
灵酊剂及其他	186.99
猪油、蜡和油	135.96
棉花、羊毛、绷带布	190.77
资助贫困患者	63.35
建筑修缮	114.47

新公共厕所	89.00
水	112.62
纸和煤油	34.99
丧葬费用	5.14
	3 496.33

1893 年结余	174.51
捐助和捐赠	1 157.46
吸毒患者支付	59.00
私人病房租金	7.00
宣教委员会药物等拨款	876.00
销售药物等	1 051.33
结余	171.03
	3 496.33

新大楼账目

现金	519.20

（翻译：陈坚龙、许思婷　校译：朱文平　审校：胡卫清、余维泉、江建安　中文校正：许党泉、杨柳婷）

1913 年汕头福音医院报告

（1913 年度英兰长老会汕头教会医院报告）

1913 年是汕头福音医院的 50 周年大庆。

1863 年 11 月吴威凛医生（Dr. Wm. Gauld）在汕头开始了医学传教工作。当时他租了一栋中国人的房子，经过一番装修后成了门诊和医院，并且每周有三天用来接诊病人。

在他 1864 年和 1865 年的第一份报告中，吴威凛医生统计了在这个临时搭建的医院就诊的病人总数和去传教点的人数。在 1864 年一共诊治了 1 967 位病人，其中 200 名为住院病人，312 名为妇女和女孩；1865 年有 1 779 位病人，其中有 250 名住院病人，343 名妇女和女孩。这些病人来自 500 多个不同的城镇或乡村。报告结尾呼吁人们给新的医院捐款，院址已经确定了。

在这 50 年中，对建立“新医院”的呼声很高。在吴威凛医生执事期间，医院经历了 3 次搬迁。1879 年底，在他把医院交给继任者时，医院搬进一个新的大楼里，旁边连着传教点的院子，是道台为感谢他的专业服务而赠予他的。

1879 年，在他最后一份报告中，吴威凛医生统计的总病人数是 3 108 人，其中 2 028 名住院病人，466 名为妇女和女孩。门诊开放日平均每天门诊病人数是 25 人。报告还提到，这一年中有 10 位病人接受了基督教的洗礼（在 1878 年有 12 人接受洗礼），在医院也有过一次多达 10 名病人申请接受洗礼的情况。在那一年，医院一次性有超过 250 名住院病人，有的住在大点的病房，有的在小点的病房（麻风病人）。谈到这点，吴威凛医生说：“我们应该好好地记住我们在宣布汕头医学传教工作开始时的那种喜悦，16 年前，医院只有 6 位病人，那时候的医院只是普通的中式建筑。从那时候开始，工作量与日俱增，一年又一年，在耶稣的保佑下，一切有序地进行。”

住院部的扩展速度比门诊部快了很多。门诊病人数量仍然很少，一部分原因是汕头是个小城镇，病人大多数是从周边地区过来的，因为他们需要解决住宿和医治的问题，因此很需要医院和旅店相结合。直到现在，医院仍然保持这个传统，虽然情况已大有好转。但在未来，如果出现紧急情况，则需要医院有更好的设备和更高水平的专业工作，因此必须彻底抛弃这种旅店式的观念。现在不太需要旅店，因为在整个汕头地区分布有相当数量的医院。英兰长老会教会在五经府、潮州府、汕尾、三河坝都有医院，还计划于一两年内在上航（Shong-hong）再开一间医院。美国浸信会传教联盟在礐石（Kakchieh）、揭阳（Kich-yang）设有医院（注：在礐石有益世医院，在揭阳有真理医院），而且计划在潮阳（Chao-yang）、河婆（Ho-po）和黄冈（Ng-kng）再开一些医院（注：在潮阳创办潮光医院）。在嘉应市（Kia-eng city）有一个传教基地。以前这些地方的病人都要来汕头医院看病，实际上，他们现在仍然会来，但现在大部分的病人不再仅仅冲着提供住宿的医院而来，而更看重我们能够给予他们的最好的护理和治疗。

10年前，医院进行了重建，规模比以往任何一次都要大。此外，在它旁边还修建了一座女医院，由一名女医学传教士掌管。这两所医院可以为300位病人提供良好的住宿条件。

下面是截至1913年10月31日总医院和女子医院的相关数据。

今年是忙碌的一年，在夏季的3个月中，这两所医院平均每天至少治疗400名病人。

统计数据

	总医院	女医院
住院病人	2 879（男性）	
	529（女性）	1 388（妇女儿童）
门诊病人	5 716（男性）	
	2 677（女性）	2 209（妇女儿童）
到病人家出诊	402（男性）	
	395（女性）	344（妇女儿童）
总病人数	12 598	3 941
门诊病人人次	26 831	7 615
到病人家出诊人次	1 822	536（不完全统计）
助产例数	11	146
眼科手术	456	382
普通手术	907	184
产科和妇科手术	11	179
牙科手术	657	102

鼠疫疫苗接种2 990例，霍乱疫苗接种等49例。

在以上的手术中，有531例（大都是大手术）是在氯仿麻醉下进行的。

总医院

住院病人——每天收取10美分的餐费，但是药品和其他治疗是免费的。

有很多小病房提供给这些病人，因此他们不用考虑搬去普通病房。这些小病房的收费是每月4美元。这一年中他们都一直使用这些病房，所以有数百美元的纳入医院的总收入。

门诊病人——每周两天（周三和周五），病人可以过来看病，一些必需的药品和治疗都是免费的。如果有意外和紧急情况，病人也能随时得到诊治和看护，而且不收费。

如果门诊病人不在规定开放时间就诊，则需要另外支付20美分，贫困的病人可以接受免费治疗。这里不会拒绝任何一个穷人。

怀敦干医生（Dr. Duncan Whyte）2 月份因重病在家休养。当时越晏如医生（Dr. A. Wight）正要离开去休假，汕头福音教会要求他推迟一年再休假，在汕头接替怀敦干医生的工作。越晏如医生很快同意了，他的善良和帮助使我们非常感激。查默斯医生（Dr. R. Chalmers）也给了我们很大的帮助。

医院的工作仍旧进行着，月复一月，全年都未曾间断，我们忙得不可开交。边远地区的病人因经常受到流行病的困扰而前来就诊，这也使我们一直忙碌着。春天和初夏之时，鼠疫在该地区的一些地方盛行，汕头出现过一些病例。8 月和 9 月出现了很多霍乱病例，9 月份登革热开始流行，在此期间我们有 3 名医学传教士用两三天的时间与这种有些痛苦的发热病情斗争。在这些疾病流行期间，前来就诊的病人也并没有中断，席卷了广东省的“叛乱”也没有在汕头地区引起骚乱。这个 50 周年院庆也记录了到目前为止最多的病人数量。

过去，除了闽南人和客家人，要让其他中国病人留在医院住是很困难的。由于病人之间语言不通，难以交流，因此他们之间互不信任。现在这方面已经有了很大的改善。我们的病人中现在有很多是广州人，甚至有来自其他省的。我们还腾出一间病房给士兵，他们大都讲粤语或官话。这些病人大部分是来治疗性病的。在过去两年，汕头地区的梅毒和其他性病病例数量增长得很快。这是革命时期对道德约束进行扬弃而造成的一个可悲的结果。

门诊病人数量逐年增长。医院病房的紧缺在某种程度上限制了住院病人数量，但门诊病人由于没有受到这种限制，数量增多。出入汕头的更加快捷的蒸汽船和火车意味着医院能辐射到更广阔的农村地区。而在一些门诊开放日，病人数量多到难以容纳的程度。在住院病人中进行的医疗和传教工作变得更高效了，与二三十年前相比，现在门诊部为传教工作提供了更多的机会。例如，我们在一年中有很多溃疡、沙眼等病例，这些病人在很长的一段时间中定期来就诊；有些病人一周两次甚至更频繁地前来治疗他们特殊的小病况。

有件事是看起来是永远不会改变的，并且每天都在继续着，从未停止，那就是同一切污浊作斗争。

传教工作

关于传教工作，与我们之前的报告大致相同。

在过去这一年中，我们勤奋地追寻，用尽各种方法来向病人们传授福音的智慧。由教会的同事、我们的中国助手与学生协助医院的牧师黄寿亭（Ng-Siu-Teng）来主持每天早上与晚上的礼拜，而且我们开设了各种班级来教授那些愿意学习拉丁语和汉语经文的病人。

探究班是由已经申请洗礼的人组成的。在总医院中，这个班的病人数达到 78 人，而且没有算上之前已申请的人数，女医院有 96 人。

当这些申请者回到自己的家中，我们的后续工作就很难做了。我们尝试过所有方法来联系这些人，但计划最终都失败了，中国助手执行的工作更是如此。

今年我们听说有 17 名申请者参加了自己家附近教堂的礼拜。我们得到的线索并没有包括这一年全部的工作结果，也没有覆盖到所有的教堂。我觉得今年医院在传播教会精神上取得的成果与往年一样丰硕。

黄寿亭牧师的工作做得很好。他是中国教会的前任主教，在1880年夏天来医院看病接受了福音教育，他本身也是医院传教工作的一个成果。

另一名以前的病人叫陈海珍（Tau Hai-tien），后来被任命为本地教会的牧师，但他在9月份的台风灾害中由于搭乘的蒸汽船倾覆而溺水身亡。

财务状况

借此机会，我们再一次向去年所有在经济或在其他方面给予我们帮助的人们表达我们诚挚的谢意。

我们尤其感谢下列外国社团和中国朋友们的慷慨捐赠。在过去的50年里，医院总是可以收到来自汕头外国社团成员的慷慨支持，这些外国人来自很多国家，他们的帮助极大地缓解了医院工作人员的经济压力：来爱力夫人（Mrs. Lyall）从她的基金中赠与我们842美元，朱雪和（Tshu sok hua）和朱雪之（Tshu sok che）捐款250美元用于建设医院的供水系统。

当汕头开始安装电灯时，主管的工程师向一些中国朋友建议，他们可以利用这个机会为医院安装一台X光设备。我们收到郭丽州先生（Mr. Kwok lai chow）一笔297元（合262美元）的赠款，可以由我们自主决定如何使用。但是这笔钱并不够购买X光设备，与此同时，这笔钱已被列入明年账目。英兰长老会海外宣道会捐赠了140英镑用于支持我们购买这款设备以及外科敷料。

外科工作

这一年所做手术的数量在以下的数据栏中列出，但女医院的数据不完整。有很多的小型手术，例如切开脓肿手术、缝合伤口等，都是在门诊进行的，但这些记录没有被保存下来。

以下是所做手术的主要类别：

	总医院	女医院
睑内翻手术	259	333
翼状胬肉切除手术	61	15
病变虹膜切除术(人工瞳孔)	41	6
白内障摘除术	20	8
囊性肿瘤切除术	112	26
颈部腺体切除术（结核性）	10	15
阴囊象皮病切除术	5	
骨疡——骨坏死剔除术	85	15
膀胱结石手术	9	
囊性甲状腺肿手术	2	2

	总医院	女医院
包茎手术	36	
唇裂手术	24	4
鞘膜积液手术	29	
痔疮手术	95	27
尿道切开术	12	
整形手术	7	4
截肢手术	36	6
子弹取出术	21	
鼻息肉摘除术	18	4
腹股沟疝根治术	5	
卵巢切开手术		7
膀胱—阴道瘘手术		15
会阴破裂手术		3

532 例手术都是在氯仿的麻醉下完成的，氯仿是唯一常用的麻醉药。氯仿可能是目前最安全有效的麻醉药，在 50 年里这种麻醉药只造成一例死亡。死者是一名年轻男子，大约在 20 年前，当时进行的手术是治疗胫骨骨疡——骨坏死。我的前辈，吴威凛医生（Dr. Gauld）过去习惯于让外国医生注射氯仿。但从 1880 年开始，这项工作就完全由中国助理接手，他们中很多人都已能熟练进行氯仿注射。一般来说，呕吐后也几乎没有什么大碍，我也从未发现使用氯仿后出现中毒的现象。

要准确统计出过去 50 年里使用氯仿的病例总数几乎是不可能的，因为其中有 20 多年没有留下任何的数据。在过去的 10 年中，这两所医院平均每年约有 500 个病例。在之前的年份中从未出现这样的数字，但 1880 年以来，每年的病例数就变得相当大。我们可以大概推测过去 50 年中使用氯仿的病例总数为 10 000 例也是合理的。

睑内翻和倒睫症的手术数量也是不可胜数的。这种状况应该非常普遍，因为潮惠辖区现有的其他 6 家医院和诊所也可以做这种手术，此外，目前很多去做这种手术的中国人，几乎都是由于沙眼引起的。

翼状胬肉也很常见，而且病因也基本一样。

白内障——不常见。这类手术的数量每年都基本持平，最多的一年也就稍高于 40 例。

疝气——我们第一次尝试做腹股沟疝根治术是在 1888 年，那时用伍德氏（Wood's）术式进行手术。

我们的手术数量仍然较少，主要是因为我们大多数病人普遍身体好，他们对长达一个月的住院时间望而却步。

膀胱—阴道瘘——这种病例每年都持续增多，现在已经能够通过手术治愈，而在 20 年前这种病是被拒绝诊治的，因为它无法治愈。通过一两个手术就能修补好很大的“洞”，这是件很神奇的事情。

卵巢切除术——在肿瘤很小的情况下，我们很少让卵巢肿瘤患者做手术。实际上，我们所有的手术病例肿瘤都是大的，病人的身体或多或少变得虚弱，但是手术结果还是让人满意的。这一年有7个病例，其中一例有两侧卵巢的大肿瘤，做了双侧卵巢切除术。另一个病例的手术未能完成，那是一个非常大的单房囊肿，囊壁似乎已经与周围完全粘连在一起。病人的心脏情况很差，显然，如果不实施手术她的康复机会更大。所以我们没有尝试去分离她的囊肿，而是用抽液的方法，可能有效。那个病人在经历很长一段时间的疗养后，现在可以四处走动了。

医院在1888年为慢性肠套叠病人实施了第一例剖腹产手术，在1892年实施了第一例卵巢切除手术。后来，这个病人加入教会，随后结婚并生了两个孩子，年级大一点的那个孩子现在是女医院一名有前途的学生。

假脊柱裂——有两例先天尾骨生长病例成功进行了手术，一名是婴儿，另外一名是三四岁的孩子。这些肿块虽然罕见，但每年都会见到真正的脊柱裂病例。

畸形足——在汕头很少见。进行过一例足内翻和一例马蹄足手术。这些孩子因为送来医院及时，手术取得满意的结果。

腿象皮肿——我们为这种疾病尝试了很多外科手术方法。

两三年前，怀敦干医生（Dr. Whyte）和我在一些病例中尝试了汉德利（Handley）的“线”方法，但这种立竿见影的结果对我来说似乎比不上卧床休息的作用大。有一个病例出现了脓毒血症未能改善的情况。过去的10年或者12年中，我们在很多的病例中尝试了在康德黎先生（Mr. Cantlie）的诊所里首次见到的操作方法，过程如下：无论增厚组织是在腿部的内侧还是外侧，将这里的皮肤进行又长又深的楔形切开，产生一道深深的疤痕会起到抵御水肿复发的作用。尽管这个手术取得立竿见影的效果，但是我担心这种效果并非永久性的，当病人重新回去从事他平时的工作的时候，肿胀会复发。

今年我们采用康多莱昂（Kondoleon）的方法进行了一次手术，当即的效果是很好的。在大腿的外侧和内侧切开一条纵向的切口，从膝关节延伸到踝关节附近，剖开皮肤，从腿的两侧增厚的肿胀组织切下一条深达肌肉的3英寸宽的长皮瓣，然后肌肉腱膜被切除相同大小。这种方法值得进一步尝试。

脑积水———名婴儿从出生时候开始出现脑积水，头颅严重膨胀，惊厥经常复发，通过腰椎穿刺治疗。手术进行了3次，之后惊厥很快停止了。在第一次腰椎穿刺后没再出现剧烈的惊厥了。

我们最近又见到那个孩子，已经一岁大，在经历第3次也是最后一次穿刺的时候是5个月大。他现在个头很大，营养充足，没有痉挛性麻痹，但是腿软弱无力。虽然这个小孩在辨认事物方面的智力是可以的，但是他无法行走。

通过治疗，他的病情稳定了。不管怎样，惊厥是完全停止了。

收支表

单位：美元

去年结余	510.06
捐款	3 677.53

药物、疝气绑带等	923.97
病人的付款	773.01
小病房的租金	587.95
伦敦海外宣道会为木料油漆工作的拨款（15英镑）	154.37
海外宣道会的资金支持（12.1英镑）	121.96
海外宣道会拨来的药物	1 250.00
超支	97.18
	8 096.03

安得烈·越晏如、A. W. 埃德蒙兹审计。

工资	1 652.48
房屋修理、清洗等	601.01
电灯和水费	927.43
在当地买的药	1 589.28
从伦敦买的药	1 465.27
纸张、文具等	330.34
衣服、软麻布、汽油、猪油、棉花、羊毛	1 253.04
一般场地租金和保险	132.00
给贫苦病人的食物	145.18
	8 096.03

总医院厨房账户

单位：美元

收入：

病人的进款	3 885.34
来爱力夫人（Mrs. Lyall）捐款	100.00
为贫穷病人捐款	52.75
	4 038.09
借方余额	48.11
	4 086.20

支出：

食品支出等	4 086.20

捐款名单

（略）

为女医院捐款的名单

（略）

特殊捐款名单

（略）

为女医院病床捐款名单

（略）

（翻译：许思婷　校译：朱文平　审校：胡卫清、余维泉、江建安　中文校正：许党泉、杨柳婷）

1914 年汕头福音医院报告

（1914 年度英兰长老会汕头教会医院报告）

以下总结了截至 1914 年 10 月 31 日 12 个月间医院医治病人数。

	男	女
住院病人数（住在医院的病人）	2 850	567
门诊病人数（住在自己家，到医院取药或治疗）	6 018	2 730
医生到家中诊治病人数	538	505

医院医治总人数 13 217 人，其中男性 9 406 人，女性 3 811 人。
到医院医治总人次数 27 137 人次。
到病人家中诊治总人次数 2 246 人次。

与去年的数据对比，可以发现接受诊治的男性病人增加了约 400 人，女性病人增加了约 200 人。

很显然，面对如此庞大的就诊数量，若没有足够的中国助理协助欧洲医生，将无法对表格中记录的病人进行诊治。杨怀瑾（Ie Huai-kun）先生作为一名资深助理，已经在医院工作 12 年，他完全值得信赖。他与助理陈先生和官先生（Messrs. Tan & Kuan）及高年级学生的工作，确保了在上午的接诊过程中，不论有多少病人就诊，每个病人都能够得到必要的、细心的照料和彻底的检查。

助理们和高年级学生学习了官话和粤语，又会说自己的方言，这有助于对许多不熟悉潮汕话的病人进行治疗。

怀敦干医生（Dr. Duncan Whyte）休完 12 个月的病假归来后，在怀特医生休假期间协助来爱力医生（Dr. Lyall）工作的越晏如医生（Dr. Andrew Wight）回家休假了。

徐先生（Mr. Tshu）在去年成为第四个助理，现已经到黄冈（Ng-Kng）工作。

下表为去年完成手术数量，与前一年相比有很大的增加，其中，增加了 50 多例普通外科手术、90 多例眼科手术，以及 60 个需要使用全身麻醉（氯仿麻醉）的病例。

普通外科手术	954
眼科手术	549
助产例数	7
全麻下手术	435
疫苗接种	3 341

早些年，在需要麻醉手术时，另一位欧洲医生经常被要求去帮助进行麻醉，但是当一年中有400多个病人需要进行氯仿麻醉时，这样的安排就不可能了。目前，有7位中国职工能够胜任麻醉工作。

下表是这一年完成的主要的手术类别：

睑内翻手术	228
翼状胬肉手术	61
人工瞳孔虹膜切除术	56
青光眼 Elliot's 环切术	5
白内障摘除术	32
球结膜环状切开术	33
睑外翻整形手术	4
前葡萄肿切除术	8
膀胱结石手术	9
骨疽性坏死手术	92
唇裂手术	20
包茎手术	28
鞘膜积液手术	30
关节结核手术	12
囊性甲状腺肿手术	2
痔疮手术	90
肛瘘手术	68
耳垂裂口手术	18
尿路结石取石术	9
子弹取出术	9
鼻息肉摘除术	22
耳、鼻、食道、肢体异物取出术	45
截肢术	24
尿道外切开术	9
腹股沟疝根治术	5
肿瘤、囊肿等的切除术	120
颈部淋巴结结核切除术	19
舌半切除术（上皮瘤）	2
阴囊象皮肿切除术	7

除了以上记录的数据，还有一些小型外科手术没有统计，如脓肿切开术、动脉止血包扎、伤口缝合、骨折固定、穿刺抽液（如腹水）等等。

去年的工作报告主要记录了外科工作部分。人们普遍认为欧洲医生的治疗手段只能在外科手术上发挥出优势，即使是受过教育的中国人也这么认为。因此这篇报告希望能让大家注意到内科工作。

鼠疫——1914 年春季，有 3 341 人接种了预防性鼠疫疫苗。有些人会亲自到医院接种疫苗，但大多数人，比如基督教社区或者村里的老人，都会请医院派人到他们的社区或村庄进行接种。为了这个要求，工作人员在汕头东奔西走，有些时候，到达联合起来发出请求的几个社区需要两天的行程。

这是连续第四年在这个专题之下报告疫苗接种者达到几千个，这表明这种方法已经通过了实验阶段。人们要求注射预防性疫苗，不是因为外国医生建议他们这么做，而是上千的乡民亲身验证了哈夫金氏（Haffkine's）疫苗（注：霍乱及鼠疫预防疫苗）能够在一定程度上预防鼠疫。不幸的是，也有一些人直到鼠疫出现在他们城镇或者村庄才请求接种疫苗。来接种疫苗的人一些或许已经被感染，这些人可能在注射疫苗几天后成为鼠疫杆菌的牺牲品，这时疫苗都还没来得及发挥保护作用。当发生一个人在接种疫苗数天后因为鼠疫死亡这样的不幸时，邻居们就会怀疑哈夫金氏的方法，但有识之士现在已意识到，预防这种不幸的方法，就是需要在鼠疫发生在邻里之前就接种疫苗。

我们想要把来自达埠（Tat than pou）的林先生（Mr. Lim）的事迹记录下来。他每日向医院捐赠，因此我们派出一位有能力的助理跟随他。他在广大地区进行宣传，使那些渴望接受疫苗接种的穷人到他的家中免费接种。

一些樟林（Tsng-lim）的有钱商人，当鼠疫在他们家附近肆虐的时候，也会这么做。

几年前，在港口和印度医学部门（生产、销售预防用品）的欧洲医生的安排下，官献廷医生（Dr. Kuan Hien-theng）取得进行鼠疫疫苗接种的执照，但到今年年初，很明显，如果只有欧洲医生和官医生，要完成所有疫苗接种是不可能的。因此，在印度医学部门的默许下，闽南的医生利用有利条件提出一项计划，即增加合格的疫苗接种医生人数。在这个计划下，汕头、潮州医院的 24 名历届学生及助理被授权执行鼠疫疫苗接种。

霍乱——今年因为下雨等原因，霍乱没有广泛传播，这真是万幸。大约有 78 个病例使用加尔各答的伦纳德·罗杰斯（Leonard Rogers）描述的方法将盐溶液输入静脉。虽然在有些病例中，这样的操作必须重复三四次，但是大多数结果是非常令人满意的。当小孩因感染霍乱而腹泻时，要找到一条足够大的静脉来输液比较困难。在这种情况中，对于一些成年人，液体会被直接引入腹腔。这样的结果是可以预期的。病人死亡大多数是因为就诊太迟或者病人不理会医生在控制饮食等方面的指导。

除了上述提及的 78 位病人，还有很多病人稍事治疗就完全康复了。

汕头的卫生工作最迫切需要开展的是一所医治传染病的医院——一所隔离的医院。在这方面，我们再怎么强调这一观点也不为过。

我们情不自禁地表达对大峰（Tai-hong）寺（位于到教会医院的路的对面一边）那些善良和乐于助人的慈善事业的赞赏。承蒙他们的恩惠和仁慈捐赠，大多数霍乱病人得以在那些像“临终者之家”的小房间里治疗。然而如果有了传染病医院，就能够提供更多的住处，并拥有在欧洲医生指导下训练有素的员工。

这个机构有两个小小的好处。在这样的一个医院里，病人能够得到受过正规培训的服务人员更好的照顾，这好过由病人悉心但无知的亲人来照顾。此外，如果病人被集中在一个地方，医生能够更加容易、更加频繁地观察所有的病人。

一所传染病医院可以给整个社区带来极大的利益。现在，如果邻居因感染了类似鼠疫、霍乱这样的传染病而生病或死亡，人们就会时常面临被传染的危险。如果得这些病的病人能够被集中在一个地方，与他们身边的人相隔离，这样就能把风险降到最小。没有比两年前在这个港口流行的霍乱能够更好地说明这一点了。新发病例的数量每个星期都在增加，直到吴将军（General Wu）允许将（不久前修复的）旧城堡作为一所霍乱医院，所有病人马上被集中到一个地方，这样就解除了病人对家属和邻居的威胁。从那时起，传染病的病人数就开始持续快速下降。

结核病（肺结核）或许在中国的学生群体当中是最常见的死因。骨结核、关节结核是影响工人身体健康的主要因素，可以导致几个月到几年的病弱，经常导致他们永久性的畸形或者身体机能衰退。

如果说有哪个国家需要“讨伐”结核病以及随处吐痰这种常常将疾病染病给健康的人的习惯的，那就是中国。如果我们不能尽力制止该疾病的传播，当后代意识到结核病曾给人们带来那么多的痛苦和死亡，那么他们必将责备我们。为了阻止这疾病的肆虐，禁止随地吐痰是很有必要的，而且，被感染的病人必须在疾病的可能治愈阶段尽早诊治。判断病人不是感冒或者支气管炎而是结核病，毋庸置疑的证据是痰液中存在结核杆菌。有5个学生助理能够检测出痰液中存在的杆菌，这要在经过适当的染色之后，放在显微镜下观察。去年检测的148份痰液标本中，61份有结核杆菌存在。

钩虫病。过去一年里，另一种导致数百人就医的疾病就是钩虫病，近年来有很多人得这种病。这么多人前来就医是因为美国严厉打击钩虫病带虫者移民到北美。

这里不着力去详细描述在热带地区，这些体内的寄生虫怎么像传说中的吸血鬼一样，吮吸受害者的血液，使得人们身体虚弱。钩虫仅有半英寸长，不需要很多的血液来维持生命。但是一个病人身上可能藏匿了300～1 000条虫，每条钩虫在体内进行穿刺会引起长时间的渗血，很明显，钩虫可能导致大量失血。

虽然距离第一个汕头福音医院的钩虫病病人被治愈已经过去了很多年，但是仅仅在近几个月里，汕头附近的村民才发现，福音医院的治疗工作可能治好他们的贫血（当地的药物是不起作用的），把他们从钩虫造成的困乏无力的病态中解脱，让他们重新拥有生命的欢乐和工作的能力。

去年有120位钩虫病病人被治愈。其中56位来自汕尾、华坞或者邻近的村庄。剩下的分布于潮州分出的9个县中的7个地区。

怀敦干（G. D. W.）

财务状况

这一年所有来源的收入共9 061.36美元，支出共8 994.87美元，财务主管手中的结余为66.49美元。

我们衷心感谢所有通过捐献和其他方式帮助医院维持运作的人。我们也感谢每天在病人中帮助进行福音传播的那些中国人和英国人。

收支表

单位：美元

捐款、酬金及其他	5 047.79
出售药品、疝气绑带	1 044.88
病人支付费用	977.19
小病房的租金	622.50
来自海外宣道会的药物（130 英镑）	1 358.00
	9 061.36

怀敦干（G. Duncan Whyte）审计。

单位：美元

去年超支	97.18
工资	1 656.74
建筑修缮	369.37
在本地购买的药品、精馏酒精等	1 747.01
从伦敦购买的药品	2 543.11
调料油、棉花、软麻布等	1 001.49
文具、纸与杂货	335.93
一般费用（场地租金，保险）	139.46
水、电费	757.99
贫困病人的资助及食物	346.59
财务主管手中的结余	66.49
	9 061.36

来爱力（A. Lyall）——财务主管。

厨房账户

单位：美元

收入：

病人的进款	3 844.67
来自资助贫困病人的医院基金	346.69
借方余额	14.09
	4 025.35

支出：

食物、工资、煤等支出	4 025.35

捐款、酬金等列表

（略）

（翻译：汤意芝、许思婷　校译：朱文平　审校：胡卫清、余维泉、江建安　中文校正：许党泉、杨柳婷）

1915 年汕头福音医院和汕头女医院报告

（1915 年度英兰长老会汕头教会医院和汕头女医院报告）

这份报告是对 1914 年 11 月 1 日至 1915 年 10 月 31 日工作的总结。为了与英兰长老会的财务年度保持一致，医院的（年度）账务通常统计至 10 月底。

这一年的工作紧张有序。在这个时期，这片以汕头为中心的区域没有霍乱流行，鼠疫病例也少于往年。在汕头，几年来少有鼠疫病例，但在今年早春时，曾出现小规模鼠疫性肺炎的暴发，但范围仅限于一条街上，发病者主要是广东人。幸好我们采取了有效的措施，又恰逢天气转暖，使该疾病没有传播下去。

方法方式——方法方式问题已引起我们关注。几乎所有东西的价格都大幅上涨，许多常用药物的价格不仅上升明显，而且难以获得。

病人数量的增加意味着使用药物的增多及其他方面费用的增加。如何获得这些必需品的供应已经给我们带来了不少烦恼，并引起了我们的关注。我们很庆幸在年终有结余，同时衷心感谢大量的国内外朋友对医院基金的慷慨捐款。甚至有些人比平时捐得更多。我们企望来年捐助会像以往一样慷慨。

英兰长老会海外宣道会继续为我们送来价值 120 英镑的药物和 10 英镑作为医院房屋修缮的费用，为此，我们特别感谢布鲁斯·劳医生（Dr. Bruce Low）和桑德兰的圣乔治长老会教堂（St. George's Presbyterian Church，Sunderland）。

我们收到一箱来自利物浦的海沃思小姐（Miss Heyworth）的有用的物品，对此也表示衷心感谢。

汕头自来水厂公司继续以半价供应自来水，以最实际的方式帮助医院在周围患病的中国人中开展慈善救助工作。

有一段时间我们还得到了罗模康医生（Dr. M. S. Ross）的帮助，直到他前往潮州府，掌管那里的医疗传教工作。臧乐毕医生及丁沾庇医生（Drs. Chalmers and W. C. Dale）在九月份也给予我们一些帮助。

新私人病房

那些比一般病人收入或受教育程度更高的病人对私人病房的需求量很大，他们愿意为拥有自己的小病房这个优越条件而花钱。我们满足这种条件的小病房有 14 间，但仍然远远不能满足他们的需求。

去年夏天，我们的老朋友，来自永福行（Yong Hock Guan Hong）的刘长意（Low Cheang Yee）为我们提供了 2 100 美元用于增设单人病房。这是他对我们多年来向他提供的医疗服务的感谢，我们接受了他的捐赠。其他来自中国朋友的捐款总额为 5 742 元（汕头货币，合 5 443. 85 美元）。我们建起了一座 3 层的楼房，连同房间装修、电灯安装及供水工程建设一共花费 5 469. 27 美元。

在大楼的第一层及第二层共有 12 个病房，每个病房有两张床、两个给中国护士使用的房间、两个供病人使用的厨房。每个房间每周收取 2 美元的租金。在顶层，有一个房间为显微工作用房，另外有 6 个房间供医学学生们使用。为此我们向所有提供资金援助的中国朋友表示感谢，我们很高兴地告知他们，这座楼房自建成并投入使用以来，所有的病房都得到了充分的使用。

X 光设备需求

当汕头安装了电灯，主管的工程师便向一些杰出的中国商人建议，他们可以利用这个机会为医院安装一台 X 光设备。而第一步就是为了这个目标筹集资金。3 年前，郭丽州先生（Mr. Kwok Lai-Chow）将一笔总数为 297 美元（262 美元）的赠款给了我们。此后这件事没有什么进展，然而对 X 光设备的需求一年比一年迫切，不仅仅是医院，港口也很需要。而汕头尚没有 X 光设备。虽然目前并不是呼吁捐款的最佳时期，但我们希望那些想为医院和汕头的医疗事业出一份力的中国人支持这个方案。我们没有做金额需求预算，但加上现有的 262 美元，至少还需要 1 000 美元，用来购买变压器和蓄电池，这才能充分利用目前的电力。由于每年有一半的时间白天没有电力供应，所以有了蓄电池才能保持 X 光设备无论什么时间都能使用。

统计数据

以下是这一年的统计数据：

住院病人（男）	2 928
住院病人（女）	641
门诊病人（男）	6 785
门诊病人（女）	3 161
到病人家中出诊病人数	980
个体病人数	14 495
门诊病人就诊人次	42 381
到病人家中出诊次数	1 414
接种抗鼠疫疫苗	944
眼科手术	618
普通外科手术	913
产科手术	3
牙科手术	635

以上手术有 452 例（主要是大手术）是在氯仿麻醉下的手术。

治疗个体病人总数为 14 495 人，比去年增加 1 278 人。

接种抗鼠疫疫苗例数明显减少，不足去年的三分之一。部分原因在于之前大面积接种过抗鼠疫疫苗的一些地区没有暴发鼠疫。

关于这一年所要完成的主要手术的总结会在后面另行介绍。除此以外，对于大量的内科及外科工作量，本报告将不作任何描述。尽管有很多中国员工提供帮助，两位负责医疗工作的传教士并不轻松。

中国员工中，除了护士及护工，有5名助理、11名学生、1位牧师及1位《圣经》阅读者。他们承担着医院大量的日常工作，并且工作成果令人满意。

住院病人——平均每天的住院病人每个月都在变化，如2月份为119人，10月份为226人。

住院病人一天的膳食费用为11美分，药物及其他治疗免费。

正如上文所提到，对于不愿意人住普通病房的病人，目前有两种类型的付费病房。一种是每月4美元，这种病房共有14间；另一种是每周2美元，这种病房共有12间。

门诊病人——门诊开放日平均每天病人数不同，从2月份的136人上升至10月份的370人。

每周两天，周二及周五看门诊病人，这样的药物及治疗如果是必需的则免费。不在固定门诊日或在门诊时间以外来诊的病人，需要支付30分，除非很明显是穷人。我们不拒收贫困的病人。

如果有意外和紧急情况，我们会随时处理，而且不收费。

传教工作——传教工作是医院工作的一个重要方面。随着中国教会的发展，传教方法也需要变革，在过去这些年多种力量的影响之下，各种状况都发生了变化，沼涌出许多新的机会，我们要充分利用起来。但到目前为止，医院提供的机会超越了基督教传教领域。因此遗憾的是，出于许多原因，这些机会通常没有被充分利用。

这一年的大部分时间，我们没有医院的牧师。被指派到这里工作的牧师因为健康原因而不得不退休。

卖宗教读物的小贩的职责主要是上午在门诊部，下午巡访病房，与病人尤其是与那些全天卧床的病人聊天，为他们朗读基督教文献。他的工作成果令人非常满意。

汕头教会的牧师、来自学校和学院的助手、神学专业的学生和医院员工的共同组织每天早晚在小教堂的礼拜。

在侯玛利小姐（Miss Harkness）的监督下，两位女传教士在下午为了让病人受益而举办学习班。这种学习班广受欢迎，全年来上课的人数一般在30~50人之间。

由于参加这些课程学习班的人员不断发生变化，许多人要花一年的时间才能完成课程。这些班级的很多人已申请进入教堂。

申请接受洗礼及其他任何愿意来听讲的人在周日下午齐聚一堂，接受考核，听取教义。

这个班级的大部分课程主要由黄寿亭（Ng Siu-teng）主持。

这一年有5名病人被准许进入汕头教堂，但我们没有机会去查阅分散在汕头的其他40或50所教堂的记录。女传教士表示，她们曾经访问过一所农村的传教站，没有遇见那些曾经在医院听过课的妇女。

外科手术纪要

眼科手术：

睑内翻及倒睫症手术	284
倒睫症手术（电灼）	124
翼状胬肉手术	42
虹膜切除术	52
白内障手术	25
球结膜环状切开术	10
前葡萄膜肿切除术	5
眼球摘除术	4
青光眼 Elliot's 环切术	3
睑球粘连手术	4
眦成形术	3
眼睑整形手术	6
囊肿、赘生物切除术	26
鼻泪管切开术	1

普外科手术：

膀胱结石手术（大部分耻骨弓上）	12
骨疽性坏死手术	110
内痔手术	88
外痔手术	15
肛瘘手术	78
唇裂手术	15
鞘膜积液手术	24
直肠脱垂手术	1
耳垂裂口手术	22
鼻窦炎手术	45
肛门闭锁手术	3
肛门狭窄手术	2
脓胸手术	1
跟骨肥大手术	2
唇上皮瘤手术	2
象皮腿手术	1
整形手术	5
截肢术	19
腹沟股疝根治术	3

先天性疝气根治术 …… 1
股疝根治术 …… 1
枪伤剖腹术 …… 2
肠套叠剖腹术 …… 1
甲状腺囊肿摘除术 …… 1
子弹剔除术 …… 12
尿路结石取石术 …… 6
鼻息肉剔除术 …… 21
直肠息肉剔除术 …… 3
鼻、耳、食道异物等剔除术 …… 41
扁桃体切除术 …… 18
胼胝切除术 …… 11
女性乳房切除术 …… 1
男性乳房切除术 …… 1
乳腺囊肿切除术 …… 1
牙龈瘤切除术 …… 5
鳃源性囊肿切除术 …… 2
颈部脑脊膜膨出切除术 …… 1
囊肿、皮脂腺囊肿等切除术 …… 42
肿瘤切除术 …… 36
颈部腺体、肿瘤切除术 …… 33
阴囊象皮肿切除术 …… 5
腹水抽出术 …… 19
胸腔积液抽出术 …… 6
尿道外切开术 …… 2

收支表

单位：美元

去年结余 …… 66.49
捐款、酬金，减去拨款给女医院部分及美元损失 …… 6 723.87
出售药品、牛奶、疝气绑带 …… 1 608.05
病人支付费用 …… 748.94
小病房的租金 …… 599.15

9 746.50

助理及服务人员工资 …… 1 876.52
一般费用（场地租金及保险金等） …… 131.86
建筑、设备维修 …… 431.06

医院支付从英国来的药品 …………………………………………………… 328.73
从本地购买药品、精馏酒精、牛奶 ………………………………………… 4 162.24
用于敷料、棉花、油、软麻布 ……………………………………………… 1 108.43
纸、文具和杂货 ……………………………………………………………… 337.37
水、电费 ……………………………………………………………………… 786.00
资助贫困病人 ………………………………………………………………… 187.00
财务主管手中的结余 ………………………………………………………… 396.55

9 746.50

查核无误。

怀敦干（G. Duncan Whyte）

J. C. 史密斯（J. C. Smith）

总医院厨房账户

单位：美元

总收入 ………………………………………………………………………… 4 114.77
总支出 ………………………………………………………………………… 3 960.28
财务主管手中的结余 ………………………………………………………… 154.49

4 114.77

新私人病房账单

单位：美元

（捐款名单及数额略）

捐款总额 …………………………………………………………………… 5 742.00

合计：5 443.85

借方余额计入医院账目 ……………………………………………………… 25.42

合计：5 469.27

建筑成本（包括油漆） ……………………………………………………… 4 333.66
重建围墙及修缮部分庭院 …………………………………………………… 167.58
格林岛水泥 …………………………………………………………………… 82.60
病房设备 ……………………………………………………………………… 565.92
电源设备 ……………………………………………………………………… 224.31
铺设水管 ……………………………………………………………………… 33.20
纪念石碑 ……………………………………………………………………… 62.00

合计：5 469.27

捐款及酬金

（略）

女医院

统计数据

住院病人	1 532
门诊病人	2 221
医生到家中出诊次数	539
个体病人总数	4 292
门诊病人就诊人次	9 164
医生到病人家中诊治人次	667

手术

普通外科手术	226
眼科手术	356
妇科手术	44
产科手术	175
牙科手术	128
氯仿麻醉手术	164

酬金及捐款（截至1915年10月31日）

（略）

（翻译：汤意芝、许思婷　校译：朱文平　审校：胡卫清、余维泉、江建安　中文校正：许党泉、杨柳婷）

1916 年汕头福音医院和汕头女医院报告

（1916 年度英兰长老会汕头教会医院和汕头女医院报告）

财务。在进行汕头福音医院截至 1916 年 10 月 31 日的年度报告前，首先要表达我们的感谢。尽管困难重重，特别是在药品及其他医院物品供给方面遇到了困难，但是医院的正常工作依然继续进行，治疗的病人数也比以前多。尽管英国生活消费增加，我们的朋友仍然多次迫切呼吁对医院慷慨捐款，并启动海外宣道会继续为医院提供每年 130 英镑的拨款。

去年报告的特色专题涉及新的租用病房大楼，大楼是在刘长意先生（Mr. Lau Cheng Yee）的倡议下花费了超过 4 000 美元建成的。或许明年年度报告的特色专题将是正在考虑捐给医院的新 X 光设备的安装。今年记录我们的中国捐赠者为了这台新设备而无私慷慨增加捐款的行为就足够了。

一旦新病房大楼的费用被完全捐认，纪万顺先生（Mr. Kee Buan Sun）将在老实琴先生（Mr. T. M. King）的帮助下按照去年报告中提到的行动建议去做，也就是"对 X 光设备的需求一年比一年迫切"。这两位绅士已经筹集 2 000 多美元，这个加上之前手头上的现金及其他已经捐助给这台设备的金额，应该足够支付一台好的设备以及在医院为其提供足够的设备用房的费用。

事实上，去年这些额外的资金已经筹集到了，而且这并没有影响到中国人费用和用于医院运转开支的捐款的正常增长，本年度的捐款比之前的年份都要多。这些捐款中有些是作为服务补偿归还医院，但大部分是自发的慷慨捐款，是心甘情愿地做好事，不期待任何回报。

在设备准备投入使用时，所有为 X 光设备捐献的人的名字将被公布。医院日常支出的捐献者的名单将与去年账目的审计报表一起公布在报告的最后几页。与去年收支决算表的对比表明，因为出租病房大楼的建立，这一项所得到的收入几乎翻了一番。所有的病房几乎持续地使用。

病人。参照与病人有关的统计，我们发现在过去 12 个月里在医院接受医治的病人（包括男、女、儿童）超过 15 000 名。90% 的病人免费得到药品、外科绑带以及专业的建议。这么多的人能够得到免费治疗得益于捐款者对医院一如既往的慷慨行为。其中有 500 名病人需要进行大手术因而要进行全身麻醉。

大约有 3 000 人次的病人由医生到病人家中出诊。其中只有少数能够支付足够的费用，而大部分只能支付其中药品的费用，有些病人太穷，甚至连这部分费用也不能支付。

下表各条目的明细将不予列出。

统计数据

（1915 年 11 月 1 日—1916 年 10 月 31 日）

住院病人（男）数	3 112
住院病人（女）数	640
门诊病人（男）数	7 170
门诊病人（女）数	3 147
到病人家中出诊（男）次数	581
到病人家中出诊（女）次数	530
病人总数（男）	10 863
病人总数（女）	4 317
门诊病人就诊总人次数（首诊、复诊）	42 990
到病人家中出诊总人次数	2 975

手术*：

普外手术	967
产科手术	8
眼科手术	532
牙科手术	738
接种疫苗等	799
鸦片吸食者治疗	30
医院床位	252

外科手术。从专业角度来看，工作总是发展的。中国人日益增长的信赖使我们能够实施那些在几年前他们不肯同意的手术。比如：今年来爱力医生（Dr. Lyall）为一名小孩实施了一个巨大肾脏囊性肿瘤的摘除术、第一例伴有腹水的慢性腹膜炎手术、另一例是大动脉瘤的手术，同时结石、疝气（其中有两例疝气是绞窄性的）、甲状腺肿物等的手术也越来越常见。众所周知，中国人本性是好的，但是，我们每年都接收了许多例斗殴致伤的病例，今年甚至有两例出现罕见的外伤。一例是一个男人腹部被深深的地刺伤，导致内脏穿孔并从伤口处脱出。他立即被送到医院，伤口被缝合并完全治愈了。另一个男人是个本地监狱的守卫，犯人们（可能是他们每个周日听取布道的结果）在其身上重复雅亿（Jael）对西西拉（Sisera）做的事情，当来爱力医生来到病人床边的时候，他发现钉子被钉入守卫的颅骨 1.5 英寸深，最后这个病人也痊愈了。

内科。人们越来越相信西医在非手术病例中的价值，这令人十分欣慰。因心脏瓣膜病及其他心脏病到医院就诊的病人数量增加了，同时越来越多的患有胸腔积液的病人需要进行抽液，其脓胸需要引流。

* 其中有 545 例是在全麻状态下进行。

麻风。这一年有少数麻风病人听从了来自马尼拉的赫瑟医生（Dr. Heisser）建议的治疗方案。这方法会带来一定的疼痛，而且必须一周接着一周地实施治疗，持续数月。尽管有这些缺点，坚持治疗的病人都取得非常令人满意的治疗效果。治疗过程中会使用从大风子树的种子提取的一种油，这种油从很久以前就被中国的医生用于治疗麻风。最近，伦纳德·罗杰斯（Leonard Rogers）在试验一种新的制剂，从相同的原料中提取出一种叫做大风子酸钠的物质，它能够用于静脉注射，这样可以减少疼痛。在印度，在使用这种药物后，病人有了显著的疗效。所以我们从加尔各等地订购了这种药。

白喉。几年前白喉还不被汕头地区的人们所认识，但它现在作为寒冷天气的“访客”而被留意。这是双重的不幸，首先，中国医生对这个疾病没有经验，不能够诊断它；其次，他们没有一种能比得过白喉抗毒素的疗法，这种方法能够减少该病的死亡率，在欧洲的死亡率从大概33%降低到10%以下。

与汕头本地一样，在澄海、潮阳，这样的病例经常出现，那些在早期充分得到抗毒素治疗的病人有希望得到康复。

钩虫病。过去12个月中有800例钩虫病病人到医院就诊，大部分需要两三个疗程才能根除所有的钩虫。逐年增多的病例使我们发现这整个地区被这种疾病伤害的人是那么多。每个村庄大部分人被寄生虫感染，在农民中，有70%～80%的人感染钩虫病。每个个体都可能藏匿几百条这种微小的钩虫。它们通过攻击肠道的内膜，不仅吸取了病人的血液，同样严重地干扰了营养物质的吸收。毫不夸张地说，在这个地区，上千的人因为感染了这种寄生虫，本来能够干些日常工作的，却变得无力劳作，无法养家糊口。

口颊坏疽。从去年开始，我们尝试使用一种新的治疗方法——使用“606”治疗口颊坏疽。这种疾病是坏疽的溃疡从颊部开始后蔓延到脸部。它只侵害身体虚弱的儿童，并且通常是致命的。2/3的病人使用这种药物治疗后完全康复。

福音传教。医院通过5种不同的方式开展直接的传教工作。

（1）每天早晨医院的教堂都有礼拜仪式，门诊病人及那些能够下床活动的住院病人可以参加。每周二、周五（当礼拜由神学院的教师们主持，门诊病人没有紧要的病情时）出席人数往往超过300人，其他时间的礼拜由中国教堂牧师、教会的财务主管和一些外国传教士主持。

（2）上午的礼拜结束后，卖《圣经》的书贩可能花两三个小时的时间在教堂与病人不拘礼节地交谈或者在病房与卧病在床的病人交谈。这些非正式的谈话在下午同样在病房进行。

（3）在病人吃过午饭后，有些人喜欢再次在教堂聚集，有教他们阅读拉丁文的福音书，这是教中国人最简单的阅读方式，其他人用心学习比较简单的唱诗，这部分工作的监管由侯玛利小姐（Miss Harkness）负责。

（4）教堂的晚祷由一位书贩或者医院其他工作人员主持。

（5）周日下午，我们会为那些希望加入教会的人举行一个会议来考察、指导他们。许多还未申请受洗但对教会有兴趣的慕教友也会前来参加。“他们寻求上帝，或者可以揣摩而得，其实他离我们各人不远。”

外科手术纪要

眼科手术：

睑内翻及倒睫症手术	261
睑内翻电切手术	30
翼状胬肉手术	46
青光眼虹膜切除术	1
青光眼 Elliot's 手术	2
人工瞳孔虹膜切除术	53
白内障摘除术	20
皮质性白内障手术	5
继发性白内障手术	1
球结膜环切术	28
睑球粘连手术	2
前葡萄膜肿切除术	3
眼球摘除术	7
虹膜脱垂手术	5
眼前房积脓手术	5
睑外翻手术（整形）	2
泪腺囊切除术	2
眼囊肿、增生切除术	37
眼异物剔除术	5
未分类手术	17

普通外科手术：

膀胱结石手术	9
唇裂手术	37
耳垂裂口手术	12
骨疽性坏死手术	116
肛瘘手术	82
内痔手术	60
外痔手术	30
直肠脱垂手术	3
肛门闭锁手术	4
肛门狭窄手术	2
包皮过长手术	32
包茎嵌顿手术	5
鞘膜积液手术	46

尿道下裂手术 …… 2
鼻窦手术 …… 23
脓胸手术 …… 3
肝脓肿手术 …… 2
肝探查手术 …… 1
唾液腺瘘手术 …… 1
化脓膝关节炎手术 …… 2
肠套叠手术 …… 1
肠道枪伤手术 …… 1
肠道刺伤手术 …… 1
腹壁刺伤手术 …… 1
象皮腿手术 …… 1
髌骨粉碎性骨折手术 …… 1
尺神经缝合术 …… 1
耳化脓 Stacke's 手术 …… 1
跟腱割伤手术 …… 1
枪伤（大部分为骨头）手术 …… 10
关节僵硬手术 …… 7
大、冗长的大腿的股动脉瘤手术 …… 1
前臂动脉瘤手术 …… 1
股动脉大出血结扎术 …… 3
扁桃体切除术 …… 16
胼胝切除术 …… 17
阴囊象皮肿切除术 …… 4
结核性淋巴结切除术 …… 27
唇上皮瘤切除术 …… 3
舌头上皮瘤切除术 …… 1
阴茎上皮癌切除术 …… 7
肾大囊肿增生切除术 …… 1
整形手术 …… 6
截肢术 …… 21
腹股沟疝（嵌顿）手术 …… 2
腹股沟疝根治术 …… 10
外尿道切开术 …… 8
胸腔积液抽吸术 …… 14
膝关节抽液术 …… 2
腹水引流术 …… 13
尿道内结石取出术 …… 4

鼻息肉摘除术 …… 20
淋巴结摘除术 …… 2
埋入的子弹摘除术 …… 11
食道、耳、鼻等的针、碎片、异物取出术 …… 32
直肠息肉摘除术 …… 4
肿瘤切除术：
　脂肪瘤 …… 8
　牙龈瘤 …… 5
　纤维瘤 …… 4
　肉芽肿 …… 7
　骨瘤 …… 1
　足趾内生软骨瘤 …… 1
　囊肿、粉瘤等 …… 26
　舌下囊肿 …… 2
　血肿 …… 2
　腮腺囊肿 …… 3
　颈导管水囊肿 …… 3
　女性乳腺腺瘤 …… 2
　女性乳腺复发性肿瘤 …… 2
　女性乳腺癌 …… 1
　血管瘤 …… 6
　腮腺增生 …… 1
　肩膀先天性大肿瘤 …… 1
　恶性肿瘤 …… 8
　未分类肿瘤 …… 8
甲状腺囊肿摘除术 …… 1
肘关节切除术 …… 1
瘢痕电解术等 …… 14
未分类手术 …… 137

收支表

单位：美元

收入

去年结余 …… 396.55
捐款、费用——外国 …… 3 318.72
　　　　——中国 …… 5 233.74
出售药品、牛奶、绑带 …… 1 498.84
病人付款 …… 1 156.98

小病房租金	1 264.00
投资	975.07
	13 843.90

查核无误。

怀敦干（G. Duncan Whyte）

帕廷顿（Thomas Bowen Partington）

备注：除了上述收入，医院得到了英兰长老会海外宣道会一笔130英镑的拨款，用于购买药品。

支出

助理及服务人员工资	2 214.41
一般费用（场地租金及保险金等）	117.79
建筑、设备维修	1 034.05
医院修缮从英国购买药品	405.08
购买药品、精馏酒精、牛奶	6 885.65
购买手术布类、棉花、油	1 107.53
纸张、杂物	442.80
水电费	989.75
资助穷困病人	212.56
女子医院公开募捐	434.28
	13 843.90

财务主管：来爱力（A. Lyall）

总医院厨房账户

单位：美元

去年结余	154.49
收入	4 141.16
	4 295.65
支出	4 290.60
交财务主管	5.05
	4 295.65

财务主管：来爱力（A. L.）

捐款及报酬

以下名单包含自1915年11月1日—1916年10月31日捐款及报酬。其中，名字后带有“f”的表示报酬收入。

我们非常感谢那些在经济上及其他方面帮助我们的人。在此我们特别鸣谢通过van Izeren先生的善行收到的来自The Deli Planters' Vereeniging的慷慨捐款。

（捐款及报酬名单略）

女医院

统计数据

住院病人 …… 1 362
门诊病人 …… 2 518
个体病人总数 …… 3 886
就诊总人次 …… 9 258
到病人家中出诊病人数 …… 435
到病人家中出诊病人人次 …… 751

手术

普通外科手术 …… 195
眼科手术 …… 327
产科手术 …… 167
妇科手术 …… 43
牙科手术 …… 141
氯仿麻醉下手术 …… 170
小手术（不完全统计） …… 113

米尼拿（N. H. Beath）

女子医院捐款和报酬名单

（略）

（翻译：汤意芝、陈练意　校译：朱文平　审校：胡卫清、余维泉、江建安　中文校正：许党泉、杨柳婷）

1918 年汕头福音医院和汕头女医院报告

（1918 年度英兰长老会汕头教会医院和汕头女医院报告）

下面的表格摘要以最简洁的方式总结了截至 1918 年 10 月 31 日的 12 个月期间汕头福音医院的工作。

这份数据统计之后，将给出内科和外科手术情况的一些记录，最后会报告财务状况。

统计数据

住院病人（男）	2 407
住院病人（女）	539
门诊病人（男）	6 307
门诊病人（女）	2 270
到病人家中出诊（男）	602
到病人家中出诊（女）	394
总个体病人数（男）	9 316
总个体病人数（女）	3 203
总门诊就诊人次（包括首诊、复诊）	44 179
总出诊人次	2 302
普通外科手术	580
眼科手术	612
牙科手术	314
应用氯仿麻醉的手术	445
医院病床数	232

与去年的数据相对比，上述数据大部分的项目都略有下降。考虑到自 1917 年 11 月 1 日以来汕头和医院遇到的困难，这算不上异常状况。

首先，在 12 月，在护法战争中获得胜利的南方军队进入汕头，他们打劫商店、杀害警察。在这个高潮前后几个月的时间里，汕头的政治气氛动荡不安，很多患病的民众不愿意离开家门到医院来获得有益的治疗。当 12 月北方军队逃离和次年 6 月在汕头的南方军队暂时撤离的时候，医院有幸能够采取合适的措施医治撤离军队所遗留下来的受伤士兵。

中国商业公司在邻近医院的地方建起的遮棚和木场已经存在了许多年，来爱力医生（Dr. Lyall）就多次指出他们要对将医院靠近易燃建筑物造成的风险负责。1918 年 1 月他的担心变成了事实，那里发生了一场大火灾，幸亏持续时间很短，但仍严重威胁到了医院。消防队和其他许多朋友强有力的救援行动保护了医院建筑免受严重的损害，修理工作只花费了约 120 美元。我们得到保证，对方那些在火灾中烧毁的建筑不会被重建。

2 月份发生了地震。2 月 13 日及接下来的日子，我们接诊了数百号病人，但是因为楼上的一些病房不稳固，以及当时很多人害怕住在楼上，导致了病人数没有预料中那么多。

由于所有这些原因——战争、火灾、地震，以及后半年来爱力医生不在医院，使病人数比去年少变得不足为怪。但仍有 42 418* 人次到医院就诊。需要特别强调的是，这么多的病人（39 354 位）中除了 7% 之外，其他病人获得的医嘱、治疗、必需的药品、敷料和绑带都是免费的。我们对门诊病人提出的唯一的要求是他们必须按时就诊（即周二、周五上午 9 时以前），以及他们必须自己带好适当的容器用来保存药物。当然，意外事故和其他紧急病例是随时来都能得到医治的。每天都有一名资历深的中国医务人员日夜值班，为这样的病人诊治。住院病人（病人随时可以住院）每天只需花 13 美分的伙食费。如果他们能够自己准备食物，把一日三餐带到医院，那他就不需支付任何费用。

当然，如果门诊病人不能按时就诊，他们需要支付一小笔费用——大约 30 美分才能得到治疗建议和药物。同样地，住院病人如果想住私人病房，他们必须确保能够支付从每月 4 美元到每周 3 美元不等的租金。除那些无关紧要的以及使用新胂凡纳明（neo-salvarsan）或其替代药品的治疗以外，在医院的其他所有的治疗措施，包括手术，都是免费的。

在后半年，我们做了这样的安排：优先接诊儿童，不管是父亲还是母亲带来的，看完儿童，我们再看成人，这使得小家伙可以不耽误病情且早早地被带回家。

医疗记录

肺结核。长期以来我们一直认为必须为那些患肺结核的病人提供足够的住所。肺结核病人不应该与其他病人在同一个病房接受治疗，不管是内科还是外科的病人。我们不会拒绝给予病人尽可能的救治，就算对那些治愈希望渺茫病人也是如此。朝南（4 个通风的窗户均不能关闭）的小病房现在已经被准备好，可以住 5 位病人。这间病房的病人在那里的治疗效果显示了开窗通风治疗以及提供好的食物对于康复的作用。如果在疾病的最早期开始治疗，肺结核算得上是最容易治愈的疾病。不幸的是，很多病人就诊时病情已经到了晚期，不可能治愈了。

钩虫病。在我们碰到的各种疾病中，除了钩虫病，很少有疾病会表现出这么多不同的症状。有些病人腹部不适，有些感到全身乏力，有些贫血、活动后呼吸困难，更多晚期的病人可能腿部肿胀。不管他们的症状如何多变，治疗反应是一致的，当他们体内的血吸虫被驱除后都得到了康复。这一年，600 多个钩虫病病人被治愈，其中大部分人需要两三个疗程才能完全排出钩虫。

脑脊髓膜炎。1918 年春天，大量暴发型脑脊髓膜炎病例引起了我们很大的焦虑。这种病人可能早上还很健康，但傍晚就死了。大多数中国医生对这种疾病并不了解。通过腰穿排出脑脊液，减轻脑和脊髓的压力来治疗，很多病人的病情得到显著的缓解，我们被叫去治疗很多这样的病人，其中很多都痊愈了。

伤寒热病。当脑脊髓膜炎的流行结束后，伤寒热病例开始出现，整个夏天医院里该病

* 很明显，如果没有那些有能力、有经验的中国人的协助，仅凭外国医生的努力是无法应对那么多病人的。

病人不断，主要是士兵和百姓。罗希拉医生（Dr. Ross）有3周一直独自支撑着医疗工作，却不幸被严重感染，治疗了两个月才完全康复，随后离开港口。

除了这些特殊病例以外，我们已经治愈了大量的内科病人，包括在医院及到病人家中出诊的。比如，心脏瓣膜病及其他心脏病（动脉的情况不同于暂时的高血压或者晚期的动脉粥样硬化）、肺部疾病、支气管病变、胸膜病变（我们每年遇到越来越多脓胸、胸膜炎、胸积液），还有多种影响消化道的疾病，以及不同类型的布莱特氏（Bright's）病（肾小球肾炎）。即使一个人将其注意力限定在纯粹医疗工作方面，他的日常工作也是丰富多样的。

最有趣的是，从专业来讲，一个病例呈现了小脑肿瘤最典型的症状。对于被要求做的轮替动作他感到不耐烦，于是直接回家去了。

外科手术

下表是由罗希拉医生制作的，表中列出了这一年完成的手术。

手术列表

（详见上卷第374～378页，因原文已有翻译，此处不再赘述。）

这一年治疗的病人分类显示在下表。其中儿童指未满15岁者。

医治场所	总数	内科	外科	眼科	儿童
医院	12 519	32%	32%	10%	26%
病人家中	996	51%	7%	1%	41%

南澳。这部分报告不能不提及地震后在南澳开展的救灾工作。在地方官员的邀请下，一批来自医院的工作人员和童子军中的红十字会成员，以及官献廷医生和陈兆桐医生（Drs. Kwan & Tan）来到南澳，配备药品、夹板、绑带以及各种各样的医院必需品。我们在那里停留了将近一周，为病人进行骨折固定、脱臼复位、截除坏疽肢体，同时照顾其他各类伤员。

通过向香港、汕头的外国社团呼吁，我们募集到6 000多美元的资金。其中主要花费在给1 900个无家可归的家庭提供防雨帐篷。其中有不到1 000美元用于搭建一所“急救医院”。毕业于汕头医院的谢医生和陈医生（Drs. Chia & Tan），在镇周围执行约两个半月的医疗救助。

这笔救济金有少量结余，在医院捐款列表中出现的（救济金）占款项的一半，另一半给童子军。

财务状况

地震。由蔡彦士（Tshua Ngan-su）、杨寄沧（Ie Hai-lau）和谢卓权（Chia Tok-khuan）先生募集到的资金将在后面单独给出（见上卷第388页），详细记录用于地震中两所医院受损修复的支出。据此，这几位先生提出将结余的资金用于准备一个合适的地方安置X光设备。因此，总额1 000美元转移到X光设备基金。X光设备账目将在后面单独给出（见上卷第388页），我们借此机会表达对纪万顺（Kee Buan Soon）、老实琴（T. M. King）、萧少南（Siau Siau Lam）先生的感谢，感谢他们筹集的资金，使得我们能够采购一台高质量的性能良好的X光设备。

看了之前的报告，应该会对医院许多朋友慷慨解囊的行为印象深刻。两块刻有文字的石碑被嵌到医院的墙上，以纪念在上述筹集资金方面给予帮助的先生。

整体财务状况。我们必须承认，尽管从去年夏天开始，医院的募捐有非常慷慨的回应，但整个财务状况依然是入不敷出。虽然来爱力医生（Dr. Lyall）在年初保证了400美元的结余，但年终赤字为大约300美元，这显示了日常支出超过日常收入约700美元。事实上，王廷献先生（Mr. Wang Shing Hsion）援助了我们，他在香港筹集了2 000多美元，其中500美元捐献给了女医院，这项捐赠会出现在今年年终公布的账单上。尽管有这些资金的支撑，医院的财务状况还是岌岌可危。药品和外科的绑带材料的高昂价格，以及因生活花费增加引起的薪水和工资需求的大幅增加，造成了沉重的负担。

很高兴能够记录这一整年外界对医院的许多善举。据说当电灯被引进医院时，开明公司对医院每个单元收费不超过20美分。多年来，自来水公司在没有与我们这一方签订任何协议的情况下，给予我们每月的水费50%的折扣。当需要额外的水时，陈长荣（Tan Chang Yong ）先生同样慷慨地给我们半价供应。

这多年过去，病人们在每年圣诞节都能高兴得收到橘子。两果篮橘子由怡和洋行的唐宏祥先生（Mr. Tung Hong Seang）和太古洋行的陈缉尧先生（Mr. Tan Chhip Ngian）按时送到医院。唐宏祥先生还附送一盒茶叶作为礼物。

这一整年，医生们经常收到鸡蛋作为礼物，为此他们都心怀感激。医生们其实并不希望收到那么多礼物，这一点医院的朋友们知道了应该会感到欣慰。鸡蛋是很多病人需要的额外营养品，特别是对于那些肺结核病人和脚气病患者来说，是非常宝贵的。

以前医院的一个朋友会在中国新年送给每个住院病人20美分。但是最近几年没有了，这对病人来说是遗憾的。如果任何人希望在一些节日时将喜悦带给在医院的穷人，我们将很高兴作为代理人。

传教工作

在医院开展的教育、传教工作在这里不详细列举，但是这里要列出3个类别的病人。

第一类人数或许是最多的，这类人回家后减轻（或彻底打消了）对先前迷信的恐惧。第二类是许多慢性病患者，那些人来到医院前可能完全不识字，但在医院里学到了足够多的知识，从而能够独自阅读《新约》和《天路历程》等。

最后一类，在年复一年的福音感召之下，那些人迈出了极其重要的一步，从偶像崇拜转向侍奉永生的真神。对此，我们的确应该心怀感恩。

汕头女医院账目表

单位：美元

收入

中国人捐款	919.20
地震捐款（中国商人）	150.00
外国人捐款	627.25
售卖所得	303.00
病房租金	721.77
给贫穷者的床位补助金	110.00
来自学生费用的捐款	20.00
存款利息收入	6.97
来自国内（英国）的拨款	1 359.12
公共捐款分配	495.73
赤字	136.79
合计	4 849.83

支出

单位：美元

去年赤字	317.50
工资	782.21
电费	83.58
水费	42.94
药品费用	1 997.03
修理费用	437.87
医院必需品	422.05
杂项	379.29
兑换损失	95.66
牛奶	108.55
火灾保险费	37.50
场地租金（两年）	55.44
海关、货运、码头等	40.21
为供穷人饮食而向厨房提供资金	50.00
合计	4 849.83

汕头女医院统计表

1917—1918

住院病人数	993
门诊病人数	2 379
到病人家中出诊次数	538

个体病人总数 …… 3 910
就诊总人次（初诊、复诊） …… 9 555
到病人家中出诊人次 …… 989

手术

普通外科 …… 221
眼科 …… 201
妇科 …… 29
产科 …… 141
牙科 …… 144
氯仿麻醉下的手术 …… 145

米尼拿（N. H. Beath）

汕头福音医院全年进支总数

（详见上卷第385页，因原文已有翻译，此处不再赘述。）

查核无误。
越晏如（A. Wight）
江克礼（A. Guthrie Gamble）
1919年11月9日

地震捐银收整院屋之银项

（略）

易士镜之数项

（略）

福音女医院捐银与诊金诸君芳名

（略）

本院向各善士捐题者

（略）

捐助本院诸君芳名

（王少文、王廷献先生于香港经手）

（略）

各善士亲至本院捐题者

（略）

诊金一览表

（略）

（Brangwin 医生付给福音医院的诊金是为了让他的病人在 Brangwin 医生没有时间亲自诊治时，可以随时向我们求助。）

（翻译：汤意芝、许思婷、陈练意　校译：朱文平　审校：胡卫清、余维泉、江建安　中文校正：许党泉、杨柳婷）

1919 年汕头福音医院和汕头女医院报告

（1919 年度英兰长老会汕头教会医院和汕头女医院报告和
账务与捐款等列表）

杨怀瑾先生（Mr. H. C. Yang）来到福音医院已经有 18 年之久了，在今后的 8 年时间里他都是高级中国医生。他的受聘对双方都有好处：一方面医院感激他在获得出租病房“新”大楼及 X 光设备的捐赠方面的积极参与，以及其他一些不是特别起眼但是很有价值的服务——向医院提出帮助病人的新方法和在其他方面的打算。

另一方面，多年来，他与外国医生分担诊室及手术室的工作，也分担医院的管理工作，他在这里获得了丰富的医学经验，掌握了一定程度的外科技能，这些对于他的新事业将是非常宝贵的。我们祝愿镇邦街（Chin Pang Street）德和（Tek Hua）诊所的杨怀瑾医生事事如意。

1918 年 11 月 1 日—1919 年 10 月 30 日汕头福音医院报告

今年最突出的事件将概括为以下几个标题：

（1）经治病人数量的稳步增长以及所看疾病的很多专业上让人感兴趣的记述。

（2）霍乱流行。

（3）医院的朋友们继续慷慨解囊。

（4）财务状况形势严峻。

（5）X 光设备的安装。

（6）医院的传教工作。

经治病人统计在下面的表格中阐述：

病汇表

（详见上卷第 412 页，因原文已有翻译，此处不再赘述。）

医院里有 232 张病床，与去年的数据比较，住院的男性病人已经增加了 800 人，门诊病人增加了 900 人，这一年经治的成年男性及男孩超过 11 000 人。

汕头福音医院接诊各种类型的病人，除接诊男人以及男孩外，同样也乐意接诊成年女性及女孩，但是为女性病人安排的住处非常有限，隔壁就有一所条件很好的女医院，由一名英国女医生和一名有能力的中国医生照管。鉴于我们特别为女性病人提供的这些设施，使得我们在接诊病人时，先女后男的顺序显得不太合理，所以现在门诊病人会依据下面的顺序来治疗：首先是 12 岁以下儿童，无论男孩或者女孩；其次是所有的成年男性或年长的男孩；再次是愿意来我院治疗的成年女性或年长的女孩。通常我们会接诊 30 到 50 位儿童病人和超过 115 位女病人。9 月份，罗希拉医生（Dr. Ross）在接管医院的时候，门诊病人数已经超过500名。

尽管大部分病人患的都是常见病，然而也有相当一部分病人的疾病十分罕见。

医学记录

昏睡性脑炎最显著的症状是嗜睡，常伴有眼睛和/或面部的麻痹。这种疾病在1918年引起了公众的注意，当时在整个英格兰有100多人发病。现在汕头有3例确诊，其中一人有性命之忧。

脑脊髓膜炎和白喉是另外两种几年前在汕头还不为人知的疾病，但现在每年凉爽的季节都会暴发。暴发性脑膜炎病例一开始就诊断明确，腰椎穿刺是仅有的、有希望可以缓解病情的措施，即通过一根空心的针刺入脊椎引流去除一些炎症产物。自从人们知道这种方法之后，外国医生经常被要求出诊。这种治疗方法与抗脑膜炎球菌血清（我们已从香港得到）的应用相结合，已经使我们能够去挽救许多康复希望渺茫的病人。

如果诊断及时，**白喉**比脑膜炎更容易治疗和控制。不幸的是我们所看到的病人通常处于疾病晚期，需要进行气管切开术，即在喉下面的气管切开一个孔。我们现在已经拥有整套**插管**设备，借以缓解由于白喉膜阻塞咽喉引起的呼吸困难，从而不用切开。病人的父母也更赞成去做插管而不是切开气管。

以此类推，通常类似于白喉引起的呼吸道闭塞病人也可以使用这种方法。众所周知，**花生仁吸入性支气管炎**是由于小块花生（猴子坚果）意外吸入肺部造成的，最近我们就遇到一个这样的病例。这种情况在这个地区的确很常见，这里富产花生并被用来逗小孩。"花生酸"是花生的成分，它被怀疑是导致气管支气管炎病情发展的物质，"发病时与白喉有相似的症状，有时候症状非常显著，一部分病例是要应用抗毒素的"。

血栓闭塞性脉管炎的突出症状是手指及脚趾的坏疽和脱落，这种情况将会持续数年。过去人们习惯性认为发病的几乎只有俄国犹太人，但是现在已证实这种病遍及中国。我们的病房一直都有患这种病的病人，我们尝试着去减轻这些病人的痛苦。

在我们治疗过的许多病人中，有一些令人关注的**神经系统疾病**病例，不少病人在治疗下已经好转。一个快速生长的梅毒瘤压迫大脑启动左侧肢体运动的区域，因此左侧肢体瘫痪了。积极的抗梅毒治疗不但可以控制瘫痪的发展，而且实际上恢复了病人已经不能使用的肢体的肌力。

另外一位病人连续几次中风，这是由于从心脏脱落的血凝块栓塞部分脑部动脉而致病的。

有的病人其大脑中枢与语言的理解及表达相关联的区域的功能停止了一些时间。此后病人好转的过程可以分为以下几个阶段：①他能够听懂别人的话；②他可以唠叨一些话语，说话能力一天一天迅速恢复；③他既能阅读，又能抄写，但是要完全恢复仍是一个漫长的过程；④能够自发地书写并写得正确。

尽管人们的膳食以素食为主，但仍有相当一部分的男人和不少的女人面临中风的危险。在病人血压这么高的情况下——最高超过200mmHg，除非心脏损坏了，否则大脑的某条血管迟早会出现问题。

这些病人成了一个最令我们困惑的问题。

霍乱流行

霍乱流行是去年最突出的事件。霍乱病人不允许进医院治疗，且他们也不能在家中接受恰当的治疗。当出现感染病例时，医院对面的寺庙仁慈地把病人安置在“临终之家”并交由我们照管。然而在太多霍乱病人出现的情况下（在1912年），寺庙容纳不下这么多病人，而理论上肩负着汕头人民健康平安的监督官员竟然说他们无法提供一个地方来治疗这些病人。

心慈人善的米尼拿医生（Dr. Beath）将女医院的一幢楼隔离出来供治疗霍乱病人使用，并允许我们使用部分房间，即使如此，病房仍然不够。

我们的朋友蔡彦士（Tshua Ngan Su）先生过来援助我们（在1912年），在离医院很近的地方为我们提供一个大棚屋。这里有3间木制地板的大病房以及大约50张病床，还有一个护理人员的房间。

在医院两名医院助理（蔡先生和谢先生）和5名“护士”的协助下，我们治疗了大约350位病人，死亡率大约是20%。如果没有医院员工辛勤的工作，是不可能取得这样的成绩的。

有一位霍乱病人到医院的时候，已经由于呕吐流失了大量的体液，大量体液流失使眼球深深地陷入了眼窝，整个身体变得干瘪，血液如此枯竭因而不容易通过血管流动，结果几乎触不到脉搏，全身也变得冰冷。很明显，首先需要补充体液，这很容易做到，我们将4.5到6品脱的盐水直接输入静脉，病人的身体经历了一次急剧的反应，血液循环恢复了，干瘪的身体又鼓起来了，呈现了生命的温度及肤色。

但是到了这个治疗阶段病人还没有脱离危险，他仍然有（通常会发生）再次病危的可能，因此需要静脉注射更多的盐水。另一方面，如果反应过度，病人的体温会升得很高而降不下来，直到病人死亡。防止由于这个原因而死亡的可靠方法就是从病人体温开始上升的时候起就一直保持警惕，并马上采取措施，通过冰敷防止体温升得太高。

我们对麦高恩先生（Mr. Macgowan）的感激之情怎样都道不尽，他每天慷慨地给霍乱医院送来100磅冰块。我们有了充足的冰块供应，从而得以挽救那些因为体温过高而必定死亡的病人。

朋友们对医院的慷慨捐赠

朋友们对医院的资助和以往一样慷慨。

捐款列表显示了我们所收到的款项的捐赠者。如果没有整个汕头社会年复一年地作为坚强后盾，很明显就无法顺利进行工作。

我们也必须对以下的绅士表达热烈的感激之情：感谢蔡彦士和他的朋友为临时的霍乱医院所做的努力。

感谢德记洋行（主要经由亚瑟·麦高恩先生之手）为临时的霍乱医院捐出6 000磅冰块。

感谢汕头自来水公司及开明电灯公司提供免费的水电给霍乱医院，并同意给汕头福音医院每月费用的慷慨折扣。

感谢陈长荣（Tan Chang Yong）先生也向医院供应半价自来水。

感谢庆成兴（Kwang Seng Hong）行捐赠亚洲石油公司的蜡烛两箱。

感谢唐宏祥（Tung Hong Seang）先生（怡和洋行）及陈辑尧（Tan Chhip Ngian）先生（德记洋行）为病人送来大篮橘子作为圣诞礼物。

感谢汕头电话公司为医院免费安装了一部电话，而且免收月租，还从这里将电话线拉到了医生房间。

感谢德记洋行、曬士洋行提供资源这样丰富的布类样本，使怀敦干医生（Dr. Duncan Whyte）能够解决“缝缝补补”的问题。

实际上是中国妇女为医院缝制了这些被套，我们对此表示感谢。

财务形势严峻

尽管我们很感激所有年复一年对医院慷慨捐赠的人们，但是我们还是要提请注意，这些收到的捐款还是不够的，我们需要更多的资金。截至去年年终，账本显示财务赤字为800美元，其中500美元是去年产生的。

赤字上涨的原因：

（1）英镑的汇率降低意味着我们已收到的来自英兰长老会的拨款只有几百美元，英镑拨款总数现在与在战争前是相同的，而当时拨款折算超过一千美元。

（2）受汕头的中国人生活成本的提高的影响，员工的薪水增加，导致我们的支出比去年增加了大约600美元。

（3）最近几年药品、棉花、羊毛制品、软麻布等物品的费用急剧增加。

去年我们共治疗了超过40 000人次，这就意味着要花费很多的钱。我们是非常不愿意向这些贫穷的病人收取任何费用的。怎么能因为病人付不起费用就不去给他们提供简单的必要的治疗呢？但是除非财政状况得到改善，否则一些这样的做法就不可避免了。

X光设备

在这一年，我们等待已久的从英国来的X光设备已经到达，最终安装好并已投入正常运转了。之后它首先向纪万顺（Kee Buan Soon）、老实琴（T. M. King）、萧少南（Siau Siau Lam）先生和为购买这台设备募集捐款的这些绅士朋友们展示，再向对医院捐赠的全体人士展示。同时我们利用这一机会邀请到包括当地官员及商人等400名来宾，一起参观这台设备。事实证明这台X光设备在内科及外科医疗实践方面都有非常宝贵的作用。在外科手术方面，当体查无法发现子弹或玻璃碎片时，用X光设备或许能够看到；当骨折和脱位由于局部肿胀明显而体查不能查到时，用X光设备也能明确诊断；还有误吞的硬币及金属纽扣等等，也能够被清晰地看到。

在内科方面，X光设备能够识别心脏的大小及形状的变化，并适用于肺结核及肺炎等疾病的诊断。通过让病人吞下不透明的药物（如铋和钡），可以看到胃和肠道的大小及形状。

一些皮肤疾病是可以通过X光来治疗的，或许通过这种方法还可以用来预防癌症的复发。

遗憾的是，有些人不愿意相信 X 光检查的好处，他们已经被 X 光可能造成的伤害吓到。为了排解这种不必要的忧虑，我们特意说明：

（1）随着 X 光的使用，放射性疾病（如湿疹、手部溃疡、不育症等）的影响主要发生在从事过 X 光工作的医生和助理身上，而不是发生在病人身上。

（2）我们的 X 光设备的球管由铅或其他无法穿透材料构成的防护层严密屏蔽，绝对没有理由去担心。

传教工作

如果医学传教没有体现人文关怀，报告中所提到的所有努力都是无足轻重的，医院将被证明是名不副实的。

为什么医学传教工作始于汕头呢？①为了帮助缓解不适和治愈中国贫穷病人的疾病。②帮助中国人摒弃愚昧和邪恶鬼神思想（这种思想使他们经常上当受骗），并予以抚慰。③为改变这种错误的思想，认为宇宙的最高统治者与世上任何父母一样，用更温柔、更智慧、更愿意宽恕的爱去爱我们每一个有罪的人。耶稣基督对一个人表现出的最清楚的一种爱就是去帮助和治愈受难的人。

医院的目标就是在实际工作中展现爱，不管有多少其他工作要忙，我们在这方面的工作不能不做好，或者说，这是我们存在的价值。过去的失败会让我们降低目标吗？不会。我们必须敢于去坚持我们的崇高目标，我们必须下决心做好医学传教，以展示上帝的爱为最大的满足。

我们怀着最大的荣幸来记载，医院在引导男男女女进入上帝的王国的过程中起到了重大作用。

1920 年 5 月福音女医院职员表

（略）

汕头女医院统计表

1918—1919

住院病人	1 303
门诊病人	3 032
到病人家中出诊	672
个体病人总数	5 007
就诊总人次（初诊、复诊）	10 775
到病人家中出诊人次	1 271

手术

普通外科	215
眼科	333
妇科	44

产科 ………………………………………………………………… 176
牙科 ………………………………………………………………… 175
氯仿麻醉下手术 …………………………………………………… 260
小手术（不完全统计） …………………………………………… 186

米尼拿（N. H. Beath）
夏理德（F. W. Heyworth）

1918—1919 年度汕头福音女医院之收支表

单位：美元

收入

中国汕头捐款	1 370.60
中国上海捐款	468.00
中国香港捐款	461.13
外国人捐款	125.15
新加坡的小汽船公司付给的医生诊金	450.00
售卖所得	300.12
病房租金	435.80
对学生收费	146.20
来自国内（英国）的拨款	654.69
来自国内（英国）贫穷者基金的款项	154.50
公共捐款分配	649.72
	5 215.91

支出

去年赤字	136.79
火灾保险费	37.50
电费、水费	267.82
药品费用	1 105.13
外科敷料	324.56
修理和杂项费用	1 103.70
工资	753.20
帮助贫穷病人	226.83
兑换损失	116.82
教学仪器等	179.00
印刷和邮资	33.25
结余	931.31
	5 215.91

福音女医院诊金诸君芳名

（略）

福音女医院捐银诸君芳名

（略）

汕头福音医院全年进支总数

（详见上卷第428页，因原文已有翻译，此处不再赘述。）

本院向各善士捐题者

（略）

各善士亲至本院向捐题者

（1918年11月1日—1919年10月31日）

（略）

诊金一览表

（1918年11月1日—1919年10月31日）

（略）

（翻译：陈练意、许思婷　校译：朱文平　审校：胡卫清、余维泉、江建安　中文校正：许党泉、杨柳婷）

1925 年汕头福音医院报告

（1925 年度英兰长老会汕头教会医院和汕头女医院报告
和账务与捐款等列表　电话号码：64）

1925 年 6 月女医院职员

（略）

1924—1925 年汕头女医院统计表（病汇表）

（详见上卷第 458 页，因原文已有翻译，此处不再赘述。）

手术统计表（解剖表）

（详见上卷第 458 页，因原文已有翻译，此处不再赘述。）

1925 年 6 月汕头教会医院职员

（略）

汕头福音医院 1924 年 10 月 1 日至 1925 年 9 月 30 日年度报告

病人统计表（病汇表）

（详见上卷第 459 页，因原文已有翻译，此处不再赘述。）

汕头福音医院 1924 年 10 月 1 日至 1925 年 9 月 30 日年度报告

在过去几年中，汕头的环境不稳定，医院员工，尤其是来爱力医生（Dr. Lyall）的工作压力有增无减。在如此困难的情况下，我们很难发布医院工作和财务状况的常规报告。

我们觉得我们有责任向汕头和其他地方的许多朋友及支持者发布现在这份简明的报告，朋友们可以得知医院工作进展和捐款及其他物资的使用情况。尽管现在处于非常时期，我们以后仍将尽力保持每年发布报告。

在财务方面，我们的报告包含一份统计表，上有台风救灾基金收到的各项捐款的支出情况。

报告还包括 1924 年至 1925 年常规账目。

尽管简短，但这份报告必须提及医院承受的巨大损失——与来爱力医生在总医院长期合作的怀敦干医生（Dr. G. Duncan Whyte）和主管女医院将近 20 年的米尼拿医生（Dr. Nina Beath）的不幸逝世。

怀敦干医生于 1923 年 11 月在香港逝世，作为每个中国人和外国人所尊敬和喜爱的榜样，已在礐石（Kakchieh）的墓地里安息。米尼拿医生 1925 年秋天在伦敦逝世，让人深感痛惜。汕头和教区的许多人都应对这两位为事业献身的医学工作者心存感激。

这几年虽然政局变化，社会动荡，我们庆幸仍能保有汕头人民的信心和美好祝愿，为汕头人民谋福祉的工作得以继续进行。

我们需要保有这种良好的愿望，也需要经济援助措施，让我们能为病人们，特别是为汕头穷困的病人们提供更加有效的服务。

应我主和耶稣之精神，我们对帮助了那些最有需要的灵魂和身体的牧师表达最崇高的敬意。那些打算贬低基督教的人要在这里忏悔，若非耶稣基督和他的教义及范例，就不可能有汕头福音医院为了贫穷受苦的中国人的利益而长期服务的记录。

和以往一样，我们迫切需要经济援助，我们愿意承担医院的发展责任，使工作更为高效。

必须提及的是我们治疗的麻风病病人的增加。几年前来治疗的病人为 12～20 人，此后病人数量一直在稳步增长，直到现在我们每周有 80～90 位病人为接受免费治疗而来。治疗方法为注射疗法，这种方法已被证明对于治疗麻风病是有效的。我们需要你们的帮助，使我们能够开展和改进这项工作，这是非常必要的，这也是最有希望的。

原来中国朋友捐助的 X 光机在台风中损坏严重，必须送去英国维修。最终，根据专家的意见，该设备不能再使用了，我们便从北京购买了一台简单而更先进的成套 X 光设备。设备已安装完毕，由尼尔·斐义礼医生（Dr. Neil Fraser）主管，斐义礼医生在北京协和医学院参加了一期放射学特殊课程的学习。斐义礼医生在逐步开展这一方面的工作，在资金允许的情况下我们将安装更多的设备，从而提高 X 光部门对医院和社会的效能。

我们要感谢汕头自来水公司及开明电力公司一直以来对每月费用的优惠折扣。

同样也要感谢汕头电话公司让我们免费使用电话。

越晏如（A. Wight）

1925 年捐款名单

（略）

汕头教会医院账务

（详见上卷第 468 页，因原文已有翻译，此处不再赘述。）

台风救灾账务（注：收入）

（1922—1925 年）

（略）

台风救灾账务（注：支出）

（1922—1925 年）

单位：大洋

		墨洋	直平银
1922 年 8—9 月	医院清洁	30.31	

1922年10月	更换女医院电灯	134.74	
1923年10月	X光机送伦敦修理	62.21	2.26
1923年12月	助理宿舍修葺	105.67	
1922年和1923年	医院屋顶和其他地方的修葺		13 122.50
	助理宿舍的修葺		20.80
1922年	潮州府医院的修葺		276.00
1924年7月1日	半价更换医院电线		159.00
	医院厨房为病人供应食品		792.80
	杂项开支		59.41
1924年9月5日	X光机送修后返税	109.66	
截至1924年底开支合计		442.59	14 432.77

汕头女医院1925年10月31日年终账务

单位：大洋

收入

上年度结余	42.58
场地捐款	778.00
来自英国的特殊物资捐款	277.24
病人捐款	908.16
私人病房租金	908.20
销售药物等	540.04
学生缴费	97.60
人力车收入	132.05
存款利息	589.14
超支（110英镑）	918.69
合计	5 191.70

支出

薪金与工资	1 557.81
燃料与电费	111.36
食物和牛奶	159.14
药品	1 005.56
维修与装修	304.22
医院必需品	1 003.10
杂项	77.00
兑换损失	3.05
水费	155.57
运费、海关等	99.56
印刷	8.10

贷方余额	707.23
合计	5 191.70

I. E. Brander（审计员）

1926年2月8日

台风救灾账务

单位：大洋

1926年3月15日	结余	4 852.94
	以上金额有一部分使用与X光机有关，剩余部分转入由汕头教会理事会指定授权的一般账户。	
	特殊支出如上	
1925年4月20日	斐义礼医生到北京学习放射学课程旅费	95.00
	其他的旅程开支	35.00
	支付给斐义礼医生的X光机账户	2 000.00
	银行汇票和兑换佣金	77.19
1925年12月21日	X光机房装修	18.55
1926年2月3日	斐义礼医生装配X光机	219.46
		2 445.20
		4 852.94
		-2 445.20
		2 407.74

结余2 407.74美元转入医院一般账户。

除去1923年医院的一般收入，一笔3 000美元的慷慨捐款来自香港和汕头商会的台风救济委员会办公室，选择性地用于一些建筑或若干特殊需求设备的购买。迄今为止，没有合适项目可以在经过论证后使用这笔钱，但现在正考虑将医院的一栋大楼改建为门诊部，在本年度结束前大部分资金将用于该方案。

（翻译：陈练意、朱悦阳　校译：朱文平　审校：胡卫清、余维泉、江建安　中文校正：许党泉、龙欣）

1926—1927 年汕头福音医院报告

（1926—1927 年度英兰长老会汕头教会医院和汕头女医院报告和账务）

1926 年 6 月汕头福音医院职员

（略）

1926 年汕头福音女医院职员

（略）

1927 年 6 月汕头福音医院职员

（略）

1927 年汕头福音女医院职员

（略）

汕头福音医院自 1925 年 10 月至 1926 年 9 月 30 日报告

（详见上卷第 475 页，因原文已有翻译，此处不再赘述。）

1925—1926 年汕头福音女医院报告

（详见上卷第 475 页，因原文已有翻译，此处不再赘述。）

汕头福音医院自 1926 年 10 月至 1927 年 9 月 30 日报告

（详见上卷第 476 页，因原文已有翻译，此处不再赘述。）

1926—1927 年汕头福音女医院报告

（详见上卷第 476 页，因原文已有翻译，此处不再赘述。）

1926—1927 年报告

我们将为朋友们呈现一份包括近两年来最新的福音医院工作记录的报告。

首先，我们怀着感恩的心写这份报告，尽管频繁受到当地状况的干扰，但医院仍然能不间断地开展工作。

无须多言，从医院创建至今，我们一直做着有益于身体及灵魂的工作。日复一日，耶稣的福音和治疗身体的神职人员一直与病人同在，众所周知，医院是双重救赎的地方。

1926年3月，有一件事需要特别提到，那就是来爱力医生（Dr. Alex. Lyall）退休了，他的名字与汕头福音医院连在一起已经长达47年。来爱力医生1879年从苏格兰来到汕头接管教会医院，当时医院在吴威凛博士（Dr. Wm. Gauld）的带领下已经开始走向繁荣。在医院发展的早期有许多困难及偏见要克服，来爱力医生通过他的技术及善意逐渐消除了偏见，并使人们获得了信心。随着时间的流逝，他的名字和威望带来了越来越多的就诊病人，人们心怀感激地记住了他。带着各阶层人士的深深喜爱和赞誉，他离开了汕头，他的名字将永远与汕头福音医院同在。

另一位受人尊敬的员工罗玛鉴医生（Dr. Malcolm Ross）也在1927年退休，汕头许多人都记得这位医生。罗玛鉴医生负责汕尾医院的工作，在那里他有很高的声望，而且他一次又一次他给了汕头福音医院最宝贵的帮助，我们将不会忘记他的经验和技术。

去年夏天，来自福建永春（Yung-chun）的J. H. 拉姆博士（J. H. Lamb）为医院提供了长达两个月的服务，令人感激。

这份报告还包括斐义礼医生（Dr. Fraser）对汕头总医院更为详细的叙述，以及罗希拉医生（Dr. Hera Ross）（华河力夫人）为汕头女医院所作的贡献。所以现在谨让我对中国和国外所有朋友表示诚挚感谢，感谢他们在这两年的时间里给予的各种帮助。另外，除了捐款名单上出现的名字，我们将记下对汕头自来水公司以及开明电力公司的感谢，他们在每个月结账时都给予我们慷慨的折扣。当然还要感谢汕头电话公司让我们免费使用电话。

在上海负责对麻风病病人传教的医学主管亨利·福勒医生（Dr. Henry Fowler）也慷慨地提供了用于治疗麻风病的注射药物。

最后要提醒朋友们，在潮州府和汕尾，教会医院正以同样的方法运行，或正在进行良好的工作，我们希望这些医院得到关注、同情和支持。

越晏如（A. Wight）

医学记录

麻风病

最鼓舞人心的成果是埃塞尔酯类大枫子油和橄榄油的使用。这种药物注射基本无痛，有大量的病人每周定期就诊。一个17岁的女孩走了3英里的路、坐了30英里的船后来到汕头，继续进行治疗。每天平均有60例病例。少数病人来治疗一两次后就停止了复诊，而大部分病人由于看到有人在定期治疗后情况得以改善，因此备受鼓舞而坚持治疗。

霍乱

过去的几年时间里，到医院治疗霍乱的汕头病人数已大幅下降，这归功于大峰寺无私地提供房间作为病人的“临终之家”。如果没有这些地方，医院不可能承担这些霍乱病人的治疗。霍乱暴发一段时间后，公共卫生局开了一所霍乱专科医院，之后我们就很少负责治疗霍乱的工作了。然而，夏天过去后霍乱医院便被关闭了，在疫情进一步发展的大约两个月里，部分员工又参与了这项工作。大约200位病人在医院接受了高渗盐溶液的注射治疗，取得了良好的疗效。

钩虫病

去年在总医院有 1 300 位感染钩虫病的病人接受了四氯化碳治疗，结果证实了四氯化碳的疗效良好。

我们预留的作为医学案例的病人很少离开病房，因此我们有大量的机会对心脏和循环系统、神经系统、呼吸系统和肺部疾病进行研究。

外科手术

在过去的两年时间里，我们治疗了许多枪伤病人，为他们取出子弹及异物。在很短的一段时间内我们的病房没有受伤的士兵，但随后内战的浪潮在短时间内迅速席卷这个地区，每个高峰过后都有不少伤员滞留在医院。有段时间医院的病房已经被住满，在一个临时救助站里，医院派出的外科手术助手治疗了超过 200 名的伤员。

某军事当局试图接管医院，幸运的是，他们并没有成功，我们进行的工作没有受到干扰。

X 光机对于寻找体内子弹、针及其他异物，以及对于许多骨科疾病病人的外科手术案例来说具有非常宝贵的价值。在没有 X 光机的辅助的情况下，骨脓肿及骨疽性坏死、骨折和脱位的手术困难会很大，甚至无法完成。我们万分感激那些促成 X 光机安装的朋友。尽管有个病例不需要 X 光检查，也值得我们注意：一个小男孩来医院就诊，一根金属管嵌入他鼻子一侧的眼内角。探针可以进入这根金属管 2 英寸，金属管可以绕轴心转动，但是轻微的拉力并不能拉动它。使用麻醉后，稍加用力，便取出了一个弹壳。这个男孩因为 6 个月前在玩火药时发生爆炸，弹壳深嵌在他的脸上了。

放射科

过去 X 光机的使用范围局限于拍 X 光片，并不适用于透视及治疗。但是我们认为，与仅用于治疗相比，这台简单的设备能实际应用于更大范围，由此证明这个选择是合理的。不久医院的电力供应将会改善——据悉这将在春节动工——我们希望开始使用 X 光机辅助诊断胸部及腹部的健康状况。与 X 光检查相关的费用是很高的，对于那些付得起费用的病人，拍一张小片的价格是 5 美元，大片的价格是 10 美元。大部分 X 光项目是免费的。由于准确读片需要经验及不断的实践，所有的 X 光片将由医院保存，归档备查。假如病人需要获取一张胶片，则需要另付 5 美元。

如果私人执业医生提出要求，认为 X 光检查对他们的病人有好处，医院可以为此做出安排。

斐义礼（N. D. Fraser）

外科工作

一年割症目录

（详见上卷第 481 页，因原文已有翻译，此处不再赘述。）

财务状况

多年来，医院引以为豪的是，由于部分汕头人的慷慨相助，我们已经做到尽可能免除大部分病人的问诊及治疗费用。近来，需要进行一个小小的改变，就是对于那些有支付能力的病人，我们要求他们支付一些药品及治疗费用。我们还必须强调的是，没有人因为贫穷或没带钱而被拒绝问诊或治疗。

病人需要支付10美分的挂号费，如果每个月都需要到医院问诊或治疗，则需要在每月首次就诊时支付挂号费。病人如果没有带足够的钱也不会被拒之门外，但是需要在下次就诊时带来。这些费用包括问诊、药物及敷料的费用，事实上病人只支付了其中的一小部分。当然，事故和急症不论何时到来都能得到医治，每天都有一名资深的中国医生夜以继日地负责这些病例的治疗。

上午8点半之后来挂号的病人要额外支付40美分，要求立刻看病和下午2点至4点来就诊的病人则需要支付1美元。

一年多前，我们就发现门诊每日从上午9点开始就诊是可行的。这个举措令人满意，防止病人过多导致候诊时间过长。以前，大量的病人在周二和周五前来就诊，现在已分散到每周的6个工作日中去了。

我们再次呼吁汕头的朋友，尤其是曾在医院问诊或接受治疗的人，希望得到你们的慷慨援助。今年开始我们的负债已经超过700美元，另外还要负担沉重的药品及敷料账单。到目前为止，捐款的增长没有跟上薪水及药品费用的增长速度。医院的福利完全依靠所收到的资助，你们慷慨的资助可以减轻医院的经济负担，让我们能够把精力投入到提高为社会服务的效率中。

港汕商会的台风救济委员会为医院捐献的一些专用资金，现在部分被用于重新装修3间外科公共病房，并配备提高疗效所必需的设备，每间病房花费了大约150美元。一间私人病房的墙壁也得以彻底翻修，我们希望不久后能对其余的病房进行装修。

来爱力医生（Dr. Lyall）

前面已经提到，服务医院长达47年之久的来爱力医生退休了。他在英格兰的朋友希望募集资金来表彰其所做的出色工作，作为最合适项目——他们建议重新装修手术室。假如来爱力医生在汕头的朋友希望用一种类似的方式去表达他们的赞赏，没有比提供一间新的手术室更为合适的了。一部分台风救济委员会的资金用于翻修现有的手术室，将小窗更换为大窗，为外科手术提供更好的光线。一间储存室被改建成仪器存放室和消毒室，而在紧急情况下现有手术室可以在治疗事故受害者及脓毒性病例时使用，但我们仍迫切需要另外一间手术室用来做无菌手术。需要提及的是，目前这一需求十分迫切，因为我们几乎每天都要用到现有的手术室。

怀敦干医生（Dr. Duncan Whyte）

同样是为了纪念怀敦干医生，他的朋友在英格兰募集了资金以重新装修实验室。我们的实验室仪器新增了一个恒温箱，并不时购置其他物品。在诊断和治疗许多疾病时，高效的实验室服务能够提供的帮助是不可估量的。洪作樑先生（Mr. Ang Tsak Liang）在安庆的医院技术研究所学习实验室技术长达6个月时间，我们希望随着时间的推移，实验室会被证明越来越有用。怀敦干医生在汕头的许多朋友希望能一同表达感谢，以此为目的的专项捐款将得到相应的使用。

对新大楼的需求

我们还要利用这一机会谈一谈，那就是我们急需选取一块土地并建设新大楼。汕头道路的拓宽及改进正在快速进行，根据这个计划，医院将会失去一幢有 14 间私人病房的大楼。即使这个计划改变得以保留这些建筑，这仍然是最不可取的方位之一，因为窗户正对着宽阔繁忙的大街，噪音和灰尘不利于病人的康复。

我们强调医院保有足够的开放性空间的重要性，这样治疗才可以在尽可能最好的条件下进行。一所医院如果被周围的建筑物所封闭，就会缺乏足够空气和阳光这些基本需求；我们现在的病房就有被包围封闭的危险，因此不适合用作医院病房。此外，医院现有的病房大楼对前来接受治疗的病人数量来说是不够的。结核病人的治疗要求有新鲜的空气和阳光，然而我们医院的病房却无法满足这些要求。医院附近有可以使用的土地；一所最新的医院应该建在理想的环境上，汕头是否已将这片土地预留用作扩建现有建筑？我们希望汕头当局能对这个关系到整个社会福利的问题采取行动。

全体员工

多年来，每当汕头医院人手短缺的时候，越晏如医生屡次放下潮州府的工作来帮助我们；来爱力医生退休后也同意继续负责管理医院一段时间。然而，由于要继续管理潮州府医院，越晏如医生表示他无法长期停留，因此在为斐义礼医生安排了一名新同事后，越晏如医生就会回到潮州医院。对于越晏如医生住在汕头期间所做的宝贵的工作，我们希望表达我们的感激，并对他的离去表示遗憾。

我们要对 Dr. T. C. Pan 的帮助表示感谢。最近他已在汕头开展医疗业务，每天早上他都会安排两个小时为医院做义务工作。他在英国格拉斯哥（Glasgow）学习医学，毕业后又在伦敦、意大利和上海工作，从中获得的技术和知识使医院受益匪浅。

我们还要欢迎贺尔德医生（Dr. Worth）及其夫人的到来，在这篇报告发布之前他们将会到达汕头。又有一名从国内（英国）来的医生成为医院的员工，我们因此能为进一步提高技术水平及拓展医院的工作作打算。

斐义礼（N. D. Fraser）

工作重组

1927 年，我们对医院助手的工作进行了重新调整。男性助手在被雇用的 4 年期间，将要接受医院各个工作部门的实践指导。

在洪先生的指导下，他们要学习使用显微镜对寄生虫感染进行诊断，学习最基本的细菌学及无菌技术，另外还有一般的实验室检查。

李家隆先生（Mr. Li Kia Long）在安庆学习了由医院技术研究所主办的 6 个月的课程后，现负责药房管理，助手们将在这里受到系统的药房工作训练。

在医生和助理的监督下，助手们在病房更换外科敷料，病人们对治疗的指令表示理解并执行。

助手们在 Mr. Tan Sia Chhin 负责管理的手术室里培训，协助所有的手术作业，包括准备手术器械、消毒敷料等手术室常规工作的各个环节。

在这些助手参与医院常规工作变得更有效率后，我们希望能有机会给他们进一步作系统指导，并安排了一门“急诊病人的急救措施”课程。

如果我们没有经过正规培训的护士员工，就不可能训练这些助手去完成所有住院病人所需要的工作，由于他们的协助，我们得以为大量来诊病人提供治疗。

同时，在住院期间会有一个朋友或是家属来帮助照顾病人。

当助手们完成4年的课程后，我们希望一部分人能留下来管理一个部门或从事医院某个部门的工作。如果我们在潮州府及汕尾的医院能够继续运营的话，也会需要我们医院培训的助手。

斐义礼（N. D. Fraser）

医院助理宿舍的重建

列表中的捐款用于重建之前为了拓宽马路而拆掉的两栋楼。由于筹集的资金仍然不足，我们卖掉了一块土地，所得资金和捐款一起用于在剩余的土地上建大楼。现在已经开始施工，我们希望不久后建成。

财务状况表将会择时发布。

斐义礼（N. D. Fraser）

汕头女医院

统计显示了整整两年来女医院的工作。

在我们所治疗的疾病当中，钩虫病是最为普遍的常见病了。我们不仅看到了处于该疾病各个阶段的病人，也看到了大量导致其他病症恶化的病例，其中最显著的或许是沙眼和麻风病。这些疾病极大地降低了病人的抵抗力。牙周类疾病和沙眼在这一地区极为流行，我们必须治疗大量由于忽视沙眼而导致睑内翻的病人。这种情况下，手术几乎全部由张小姐（Miss Chang）及陈小姐（Miss Chen）执行。

结核病的死亡人数很多，令人痛惜的是，许多年轻人患上了晚期肺结核。大量的儿童被确诊患有骨结核及关节结核。今年夏天我们治愈了很多伤寒及痢疾病例，这些病症在去年还是重症病例。有意思的是助产工作方面，大部分都是常见病，这与以往不同。过去人们没有意识到，尽早寻求技术性帮助是明智之举。

不久前医院的外科大楼进行了改建，为病房提供了浴室，且在病房之间新建了一条宽阔的楼梯。Mrs. Ou Pek Thiu 友善地支付了这些改建的资金，并为这次改建筹集了相当慷慨的资金。详细内容将会发布在下一年度的财务报告上。

这些改建完成之后不久，一间外科病房的房顶塌陷了。这是由于一根大的房梁突然断裂了。这些横梁被白蚁啃食且埋于墙内，因此尽管我们定期检查房顶但没有发现这个情况。病人幸运地躲过了伤害，他们在扭曲变形的铁床上被拉出来，注视着横梁、瓦片、水泥堆。人们认为，是神的护佑拯救了他们。修复这里以及其他被发现不安全的屋顶的花费超过1 000 美元。关于这些修复工作的完成，我们必须感谢太古洋行（Messrs. Butterfield and Swire）的格姆雷先生（Mr. Gumley）所给予的权威建议。

我们诚挚地呼吁建设更多的房间及建筑物。我们必须将传染病病人隔离在单独的病房，但有时没有空余的病房。在医院繁忙的时候，甚至没有足够的住处提供给普通病人，他们中很多人来自农村，在汕头没有朋友可以投靠。

在 1926 年的春夏之际，我们很幸运地得到了夏理德医生（Dr. Winifred Heyworth）的援助，她来给医院提供短期的服务。我们非常不希望她离去，不想她由于家庭原因提前回国了。我们也非常感谢泉州的萨克医生（Dr. Thacker)，她因此有段时间不能够待在她的驻地，她给予了我们最需要的帮助。

大部分传道工作是在志愿者的帮助下进行的，我们感谢很多中国及外国的朋友，他们定期用这种方式给予了帮助。每周日下午，我们为在医院的儿童及附近的贫困儿童开办了主日学校。在过去的一年半的时间里，这所学校由佩顿小姐（Miss Paton）管理。

我们希望表达对越晏如医生（Dr. Wight）的感激之情，感谢他在过去几个月里对我们的帮助，我们对他离开汕头深表遗憾。

我们也感谢 Dr. T. C. Pan，他最近在二年级学生的临床教学中给予了宝贵的帮助。

我们现在有 10 位在医院工作的学生助理，他们中的两位将会在今年夏天毕业。现在我们不再招收任何新的医学学生，因为我们希望开设护理及助产课程。

罗希拉（H. Ross）

汕头福音医院全年进支总数

（1925—1926 年）

（详见上卷第 489 页，因原文已有翻译，此处不再赘述。）

旅港潮州八邑商会汕头赈灾团捐款

（略）

叶克斯镜房进支数目

（1925—1926 年）

（略）

汕头福音医院捐款芳名

（1925—1926 年）

（略）

汕头福音医院全年进支总数

（1926—1927 年）

（详见上卷第 493 页，因原文已有翻译，此处不再赘述。）

叶克斯镜房出入数目

（1926—1927 年）

（略）

旅港潮州八邑商会汕头赈灾团捐款

（略）

再建辅理医生新屋住宅诸君捐款芳名

（略）

汕头福音医院捐款芳名

（1926—1927 年）

（略）

汕头福音女医院进支总数

（1926 年 9 月 30 日年终账目）

（详见上卷第 499 页，因原文已有翻译，此处不再赘述。）

汕头福音女医院全年进支总数

（1927 年 9 月 30 日年终账目）

（详见上卷第 500 页，因原文已有翻译，此处不再赘述。）

汕头福音女医院捐款芳名

（1925—1926 年）

（略）

汕头福音女医院捐款芳名

（1926—1927 年）

（略）

（翻译：陈练意、许思婷　校译：朱文平　审校：胡卫清、余维泉、江建安　中文校正：许党泉、龙欣）

1930—1931 年汕头福音医院报告

（汕头教会医院 1930—1931 年报告）

男医院

我们将简单谈谈各个部门以回顾上一年的工作。

常规医疗及外科工作：

很大一部分的常规医疗及外科工作由洪伟勋先生（Mr. Ang Ui Hun）、陈养颐先生（Mr. Tan Iang Hi）与洪作樑先生（Mr. Ang Tsak Liang）先生 3 位医院助理承担。他们总共完成了 838 例手术，其中全麻手术 506 例，眼科手术 230 例。

医院已接诊门诊患者超过 8 000 名，诊疗记录总共有 39 500 人次。

麻风病诊所：

麻风病诊所由洪作樑先生负责。就诊人数保持平稳，令人鼓舞的是，治疗已进一步取得成效。一些病例的病变迹象已全部消失，其他许多病例逐步好转，有望治愈。就诊麻风病人总数是 3 704 人。

目前为止，我们发现无法推进我们的工作计划——发展这一分支的工作及建立一家小型麻风病院，但是我们觉得我们正在做的工作是值得的。我们要感谢教会为麻风病防治工作给我们汇来拨款，也感谢中国教会向每一位麻风病人赠送的圣诞礼物和布道短文。

实验室：

在洪作樑先生和林庭汉先生（Mr. Lim Theng Hang）管理之下，实验室完成了很有价值的工作，已经完成的检测超过 2 300 份。实验室也被用作护士卫生学和细菌学、解剖学和生理学方面的教学展示室和讲堂。

X 光工作：

不幸的是，在今年年中时 X 光机损坏了，更换该设备耗费了数日的时间。这笔花费由部分特殊捐款和特殊专项基金支付。新设备安装后，由于市电厂供电出现问题，致使 X 光工作暂时不能开展。无论如何，我们希望不久后能恢复正常。

福音工作：

教堂服务和病房探望工作一直由医院的牧师和女传教士忠实地进行着。在这一年里，工作人员已经成立了一个委员会来安排奉爱服务，并在患者中增加福音工作。现在汇报任何成效还为时过早，但该委员会良好的工作开端给未来提供了保障。

建筑：

在这一年中，我们已经设法用钢筋混凝土重修阳台、走廊和医院两侧的楼梯。正如我们预计，开展这项工作会困难重重，但是我们也正在享受预期的好处。

财务状况：

本地运营总费用为 30 470 美元，其中 8 510 美元为所得捐款，12 400 美元为私人病房及特殊处理费用。

人事：

我们的事务总管史葛先生（Mr. Scott）由于语言不通度过了艰难的一年，我们期待他能接替我们很大一部分工作的那天到来。暑假期间他参观了许多所教会医院，所收集的数据和经验对于我们计划的推进是非常宝贵的。

关于新医院的诉求：

我们曾希望截至今年年底，我们为新医院募集资金的诉求将会顺利落实，但由于抗洪救灾工作和随后东北的“九一八”事变耗尽了当地商人的资金，我们不得不撤手。我们仍然强烈希望明年可以开展。

最后，我们想说明的是，在中国，战乱对于传教工作来说意味着更多（而非更少）的机遇。我们仍急需医生，我们衷心地欢迎他们，有大量的工作等着他们。

斐义礼（N. D. Fraser）

女医院

常规医疗和外科工作：

尽管存在缺点，医院的工作总体进行得非常好。我们对一整栋有着 50 个床位的大楼进行了爆破，以及拆建和更换原有的木制走廊和楼梯，代之以混凝土，并因此造成了不便。大约 20 名“旅社病人”的住处已经由教堂提供。即便如此，我们的“病床等级”也已经从 11 级下降到 7 级。这一年完成的手术在 2 500 例以上，张博士（Dr. Chang）负责的手术超过 2 000 例。手术包括在全身麻醉下进行的大手术，并完成了将近 300 例产科手术。

护理：

护理系统的引进使治疗效果大大提高，而患者也在很快学着适应这种创新疗法。

福音工作：

这方面在护士长的报告中已充分描述，随着护理的引进，我们现在得以进一步利用这些工作机会表达我们的喜悦之情。

助产与妇科学：

除了儿科的工作以外，妇科和产科成为医院最重要的部门。比起其他的工作，这部分的工作更为中国病人所感激。张博士负责监督我们目前的院外助产工作，有两名助产学生在她的指导下工作。今年接受院外助产的产妇超过 800 例，许多是磋商的性质的，由院外的中医来请教我们。妇科卵巢囊肿切除手术往往比其他任何类型的手术更多。

儿科：

这是我们要做的最重要的，也是最令人愉快的一项工作。旧的儿童病房已被拆除，现在我们把儿童安排在综合医疗病房和外科病房，他们给周围成年人的生活和医院工作人员带去了许多阳光和欢笑。

人事：

张步周博士（Dr. P. C. Chang）工作的勤奋程度一再让人们感到惊讶，她在处理医院运行中的一系列令人不愉快的细节时所展现的工作技巧和耐心，极大减少了外籍员工的不快。

不幸的是，宋玛利小姐（Miss Macpherson）在本该是暑假的时间里接受了一次大手术。她将会为我们感到自豪，因为在短短的一年内，护理工作在汕头已经从一个模糊的梦变成了现实，而且显而易见的，这会被保留下来。

邓慕德小姐（Miss Martin）在语言学习方面做得很好，虽然她没有正式进入医院“内部”，但已经与中国员工成为朋友。我们期待着有一天，她能更好地进行医疗工作，不再为语言所累。

我们期待华莱士夫人（Mrs. Wallace）休假后回归，并且希望她能再次帮助我们，特别是在妇科和助产方面的工作。

最后但也是很重要的，斐义礼医生和佩吉·切兹沃思小姐（Miss Peggy Chesworth）刚刚在佛山医院完婚，我们必须祝贺他们。

贺尔德（Harold R. Worth）

护理报告

今年，当我们开始在汕头实施护理方案时，有很多机遇。这里的东西更先进，因为这是一个港口，而且非常接近香港。地处广东省，其首府——广州——为中国的先行试点地。受过教育的女孩非常愿意到这里来接受护理训练。对于护理工作，我们说：“一切随缘不强求。”因为我们并不担心会缺少人手来执行医院的工作，也没有必要通过增加任何其他方式的培训和学习来粉饰。由于接收了3名新的会说汕头方言的实习生，我们的士气大不相同，从而促使我们在4月有一个良好的开端。

与我同来的5位泉州女孩，两位已在夏天完成培训，其余3位已签约完成培训，培训将依照新教学大纲来进行。为了让两位高年级学生在暑假之前完成培训，她们需要更多的关注。事实上，过去的3个月中，我在汕头的工作正式开始，在这段时间内，我试图全力投入。它让我想起了万圣节的咬苹果游戏——有些问题十分难以捉摸，而且如果缺乏时间和耐心则无法解决。

我不知道你是否想象过一所医院如果没有任何护理服务将会是什么状况。最初的困难之一是患者想带上自己的亲属（他们不相信我们会真的愿意为他们做任何事情），如果他们离家不远的话，有时他们愿意回家去；但更多的时候他们想留下来。他们毫无顾忌地躺在同一张床上，或躺在地板上。如果他们不占用别的床位，尤其是他们为病人所做的我们不希望的事，例如为病人提供其不能食用的食物，或是毫不在乎地在病房内制造一些“愉快的混乱”，我们其实无从担忧，然而这些外人的行事实在不可理喻。尽管如此，因为他们有我们所需之物，所以除非必要之时我们并不会加以阻拦。

重要的是，他们开始意识到这些担心是没有必要的，在我们主要工作开展的第二病房，越来越多的患者并没有携他们的亲属前来，这是令人鼓舞的。

我们已经接管了楼下的一些工作，但那要另当别论。那些病人不需要护理，他们只需要包扎伤口。他们停留在医院是因为他们来自很远的地方，虽然他们是门诊病人，却把医院当作酒店。让人担忧的是，他们走进来，没有经过你的允许就走向一张床，然后当他们认为他们康复了，或者他们自己断定我们不能治愈他们时，他们没有任何示意就消失得无影无踪了。我们设法使主要工作的病房甚至楼下保持一点秩序。当我们提醒自己“本应如此”的时候，我们会在还没有接管的病房的周围散步。

我们开始接管门诊部的一些工作。迄今为止，之前的学生都参与门诊工作，但她们已逐渐离开，很快这里就没有人了。我们希望不久后可以接收新班级的护士，然后我们的工作会越来越令人满意。

星期日下午我们为无法去教堂做礼拜的病人提供一项病房活动服务，一些能行走的病人也会过来，参与的人数逐渐增多。女传教士教患者阅读诗歌，并进行短暂祈祷。另一种方法是将课程用大字写好，挂在整个病房都看得到的地方。每课由几个短句组成，他们很快就熟记于心了。当他们能够复述课程时，会被奖励一张上面印有相同文字的彩色小纸条。当病房里的大多数人都学会了一个课程，我们就换另一个课程。我们只有前六个课程的大表，不停更换病房的患者会一次又一次重复学习这些课程，但停留时间更长的患者能从小纸条中学到更高级的课程。我们的目的是教给他们福音的基本真理，如果他们用足够长的停留时间来学习前六个课程，会打下一个很好的基础。

幸运的是，汕头女孩学厦门话比我学本地方言快得多，所以我们相处得很好。尽管事情进展缓慢，却确实有进展，我们有充分理由期待不久能看到一所好的护士培训学校，每个病房看上去干净整洁，所有的病人都被照顾得很好。在今年年底，邓慕德小姐（Miss Martin）将会和我们一起工作，我们很快会达到所预想的完美水平。

宋玛利（Macpherson）

汕头教会医院统计

1930—1931 年

1. 医疗传教士	2
英国护士	2
业务管理人	1
3. 中国助手	5
4. 中国护士	6
助产学生	1
配药师、服装管理员等	12
6. 7. 住院病人	2 910
8. 9. 门诊病人	11 374
16. 总人数：首次和再次就诊	92 919
18. 手术	1 847
19. 眼部手术	1 495
	3 342
23. 一般麻醉下的手术	735
拔牙（仅女医院）	741
25. 医院床位	272
仅女医院——出诊	501

总探访量	1 306
产科与妇科	274
注射	800

（翻译：朱文平　校译：魏菁　审校：胡卫清、余维泉、江建安　中文校正：许党泉、龙欣）

1932—1933 年汕头福音医院报告

（汕头教会医院 1932 年 10 月—1933 年 9 月报告
史葛　英兰长老会　中国汕头）

这一年来汕头医院的工作有许多值得一提的地方，我们只挑选出 12 个月中最突出的事件来报告。

福音工作： 毫无疑问地，这项工作的质量得到了提高。由长老会任命的牧师比他的许多前任更有“活力”，他可以更有效地组织信息来适应和抓住观众的兴趣。他的努力得到一位盲人客家牧师的支持，而且几乎每天，都有一位汕头人们熟知的自由牧师为他提供免费的帮助。他走进医院，并向在登记处等待问诊的病人传道。他总是随身携带小册子等，并向人们大量派发。女传教士在女病房进行她们的工作。在邓慕德小姐（Miss Martin）的指导下，这些病房的福音传播工作已被协调好。每个星期日，所有患者都会收到一张配文图片，在随后的病房礼拜中会讲述。在每次做礼拜之前，护士会领唱赞美诗，这对教育病人有一定的帮助，尤其是对儿童听和唱的教育。赞美诗限于简单的几首，他们唱功已有进步，许多人会将赞美诗的要义深深印在脑海中并带回家中。另一种较有条理的方法就在墙上悬挂印有日常简单语句的大幅海报。

我们成立了一个由中国员工管理、为全院员工服务的奉爱社团，它有助于增强员工的团结和服务的精神，如果缺乏这种精神，福音传道工作的效率就会降低。

在平安夜，我们在病房放映了一部描述基督生命的电影。令人感动的是，年轻的护士会站在病床边，为病人讲解画面。

我们把与员工一起做祈祷作为一天的开始，我们希望随着时间的推移，员工们能更好地利用机会，为病人传播福音。

护理服务： 我们怀着深深的感激之情汇报这方面工作持续取得的进展。有资历的和正在训练的护士员工现在共 16 人。这一年的重大事件是首批在医院完成学业的 3 名护士的毕业典礼。她们中的两人回到泉州，协助当地护理工作的开展。

这项新服务的效率稳步提高。宋玛利小姐（Miss Macpherson）最早将护理工作引进本院，她勇敢地克服了诸多初始困难（它们的数量惊人），使这项新业务取得了很大的成功，我们怀着喜悦的心情深表谢意。我们对所有她所做和想做的（其中大部分现在已完成）竭诚表示感谢，希望她在国内这个新的服务领域中工作愉快。

麻风病： 今年已经有治疗病例数的记录，许多病例既有意思又鼓舞人心。

我们已经通过其他地方对这个专科感兴趣的医生扩大了工作范围，他们所采取的治疗麻风病的方法与我们这里所采用的方法相同。

斐义礼医生（Dr. Fraser）应邀对治疗麻风病的某些药物的作用做研究，现正在进行这方面的特殊调查。

新医院的计划： 在这一年中，我们有很多夜晚都在对新医院进行讨论和规划，我们希望在能出售现有土地之后将其建成。事实证明这是项有吸引力的工作，它意味着集思广益，我们有理由感恩，事实上我们终于能够制订出为各个有关方面所能接受的初步方案。

随后的土地谈判使该计划需要进行修改。此外，在最终的计划完成之前还需要进行其他的改进和修订。与此同时我们非常欣慰地获知，我们提出新医院的综合“布局”已由英国董事会批准。

改变和改进现有的医院：由于中国普遍的贸易萧条和政治形势的动荡，很明显，要立即出售该土地是无法实现的，所以建立一个全新的医院仍需时间。因此我们的注意力转移到改善现有的建筑设施的可能性上。我们被汕头董事会引荐，随后经英国董事会批准，获得了 1 万美元上限的预算，这使我们备受鼓舞。经过仔细制定的有关改建的账目归于本年度工作报告，但大部分最为紧迫、急需改进的事项的初步想法已在年内提出。简单来说，我们主要决定将一个危险的木、瓦结构的阳台改建成混凝土结构；将两间大的公共病房改成护理病房；为医院护理部门、护理人员搭建新的厨房；改善浴室和厕所用房；将一座旧建筑重建为整个医院的门诊部，这座旧建筑是 54 年前吴威凛博士（Dr. William Gauld）建造新医院时唯一留下的建筑。所有这些计划已进行最仔细的检查。前两个项目，即阳台和两间病房的改建已完成，由此带来的改善令我们十分高兴，剩下的工作正在进行中。

郑博士加盟：另一个重要的决定是在今年邀请郑迁适博士（Dr. C. S. Cheng）加入员工队伍。郑博士毕业于上海圣约翰大学，并在北京协和医科大学做了两年的研究生工作，随后在揭阳美国浸礼会医院就职两年。他是个技术精湛的博士和外科医生，且声名远扬，与其能力相称的是他和善的性格，他将自己的能力与讨人喜欢的性格相结合。显而易见，他是一个虔诚的基督教徒，值得一提的是，他放弃揭阳每月 200 美元的薪水，愿意领我们每月 150 美元的薪水。我们对他的帮助寄予厚望。

他的加入使医院机构需要相当大的改变，工作人员也需要调整。总的来说，令我们相当满意的是，员工正以忠诚和热情投入所有的重建和重组计划中。我们觉得这种遍及医院的精神比近几年进步多了。

财务：由于汕头贸易萧条，加上我们的两个主要收入来源（即病房的租金和中国朋友捐款）显著减少，今年可谓困难重重。我们的员工努力募集常规捐款，尽管大都令人失望。另一方面，部分外国社区的支持十分慷慨，令人鼓舞。我们认为，总体上我们做得很好，在从一个特殊基金借款 1 000 美元后，年终仅有 15 美元的借方余额。

今年我们开始向所有住院病人收取小额的治疗费用，由此我们的收入大量增长。现在进行中的重建工作也会节省一些行政管理费用，尽管部分增加的收入将被郑博士的高额薪水抵消，但我们预计今年年底的财政状况将会改善。

一般情况：在其他方面的发展中，值得一提的是我们参与了中华医学会研究部门承担的一项流行病学研究。这包括向中华医学会提供每一个住院患者和门诊患者的详细记录。尽管这意味着要给我们的医生额外增加很大的工作量，然而一分耕耘，一分收获，我们提供各种病例信息，得到的是对这些病例的分类记录，最主要的好处是对中国不同地区的各种疾病进行了有用的调查。

贺尔德医生（Dr. Worth）6 月回英国，他可以好好休息一下了。

根据一年一度的惯例，我们会向很多在这一年中捐款捐物及在其他方面帮助和鼓励过我们的朋友说声“谢谢”。

同时我们非常清楚，在工作中我们存在很多不足之处，我们所取得的一切应感谢上帝。在一年的时间内我们面临的许多问题太复杂，难以满意地解决，我们原先预期的一些困难却没有出现，还有一些困难在我们的诚意和克服困难的决心面前消失了。道路已经在我们面前铺开，在最需要的时候我们总能得到指引。感谢一切。

史葛（Scott）

（翻译：朱文平　校译：林帆　审校：胡卫清、余维泉、江建安　中文校正：许党泉、龙欣）

1934—1935 年汕头福音医院报告

（汕头教会医院 1934—1935 年报告）

在去年大规模的重建和改建后，今年主要合并了医院的内部机构。相对而言，少有让人明显感兴趣的事件可以报告。

在员工中发生了一些人事变动，员工的健康状况和素质与多年来的状况相比，或许更好了。今年所做的最重要的决定就是邀请郑迁适博士（C. S. Cheng M. D.）留任医院员工，期限为 5 年。在过去的两年里他与我们的合作非常愉快，他已经证明了自己是一位能力很强的内外科医师。此外，尽管事实上以前的经历使他习惯于非常现代化的设备和护理服务，但他表明已调整适应了在现有建筑内的工作困难；在没熟练护理助理的情况下开展工作也表现出他的耐心和机智。我们相信他会证明自己是一名更为有用的员工。

我们已经详细报告了本年度财务状况。我们说过由于存在外债而无法结算，因而感到很失望，但这种失望被深深的感恩所取代。我们在 10 月收到了 250 元的匿名捐款，抵消了今年运营的财务赤字。有迹象表明，汕头经济萧条最严重的时期已经过去。年内最后 6 个月表明，我们的收入有一个稳定的增长，而且今年第一季度的业绩也是令人鼓舞的。因此我们有理由持谨慎的乐观态度。这一进步体现在与前一年相比，今年来诊患者的数量大幅增加。住院病人总数从 1 662 例上升到 1 748 例，同时，门诊病人数从 45 500 例上升到 77 000 例。

今年最后几个月以一种严重而且长时间流行的伤寒疫情为特征。几个月来我们的病房都挤满了这种疾病的患者。

在这一年里福音工作一直被虔诚地继续进行着，更多的跟进工作也已经完成，然而在这个方面我们仍然有很多工作要做。通常所做的大部分工作都没有可见的结果，但我们记录了至少两个在住院期间开启了新的精神世界的患者实例。其中一位患者在去年的报告中已提及，她找到了生命中新的意义和欢乐。今年她回医院，介绍一位她村里需要得到治疗的乡亲。在这几天里她和我们一起，并证明了她自己是一名有效的福音传播者，她从来没有停止将自己在医院的经历告诉其他病人，她的脸上总是带着“有事情发生了”的表情。第二个例子是一位住院长达 18 个月的女孩。她初来医院时感觉枯燥乏味，无精打采，而且不愉快，但她在住院期间学会了阅读圣经和赞美诗集，无精打采和坏脾气逐渐消失了。她离开我们时郑重地向我们表达谢意并感谢在此得到的精神和肉体的改善，她还明确表示要在她家最邻近的教堂加入教会。我们专门给该教堂的牧师发去一封推荐她加入教会的信函。

去年我们开展了肺结核的外科治疗，并进行了一直以来在我们的医院从未开展的其他类型手术，拓展了外科工作范围。这些医院发展的消息通过教区迅速传播，因此我们预计未来的外科工作的范围会更广。

汕头麻风病诊所和去年开业的盐灶（Iam Tsau）乡村诊所继续接诊。病人数量持续保持，然而盐灶的当地人开始对周边地区的麻风病人每周集中就诊表示关注。樟林（Tsng Lim）居民的恐惧和缺乏热情使在当地开第二个乡村诊所的计划搁浅。

需要提到的是，在邓慕德小姐（Miss Martin）休假期间，两个训练有素的中国修女承担护士长的职责。在过去的3个月中，她们向我们证明了她们的能力。

正如我们所讨论的，本报告记录了我们沿着现代化服务道路前进的一些重要进展，很大程度归功于我们的女子学校校长。我们似乎已经到达一个关口，我们进一步的发展不能因为缺乏受过正规教育的护士而延后。在接下来的3个星期，我们期望能接收六七名实习护士，同时随着她们的到来为男性患者开放第一间护理服务病房。在允许开放第二间护理服务的私人病房的情况下，我们可以进一步接收4名护士。

我们还总结出，现在到了将男医院和女医院整合的时候，这将通过合并两间手术室的护理服务来实现。为此，改造方案正在考虑中。

正如我们的许多中国朋友向我们提出的，也与我们的愿望达成一致的，我们另一重要的进展就是提供更多、更好的有足够护理照料的私人病房，以吸引汕头更富有的赞助者。我们可以从他们那获得大量的额外收入；同时，还要扩大我们影响的范围来接受这个类型的患者。我们已经决定采纳这个策略，并对我们的公共病房作一些调整，将护理部门的私人病房从6个增加至12个，此外我们将投入2 000美元为这些特殊病房配备精致的家具、病床及常用仪器。

当所有这些计划实现时，我们将拥有70张配有全面护理服务的病床。在随后的日子里，我们把儿童病房也加入这一数字，在我们的医院场所所允许的最大限度下，使护理照料下的病床达到80张。即便如此，该设施也只是“权宜之计”。无论如何，在年底前拥有80张全面护理服务的病床是这5年来令人鼓舞的发展。在1930年年底，中国最古老、最大的教会医院之一——汕头医院还没有护理服务，我们深深感激现在这条道路已经稳步打开，它为我们带来了改变。此外，我们将拥有一所配有100～110张病床的全新医院，这些病床全都具有现代化的环境和护理服务，这将是快乐的日子，现有的80张病床就像是一颗定心丸。

我们已经与长老会中学的董事会商议，准备为那里的550名学生提供完整和全面的医疗管理和治疗，包括他们在整个学校生活中住院时必要的照料。如果该方案可以投入运行，我们的工作领域将要添加另一项非常重要且有价值的服务。

因此我们对近一年的稳定工作表示感谢，在这期间接受治疗的患者大幅增加，我们期待新的一年会有新的进展和机遇。

史葛（Scott）

（翻译：朱文平　校译：林帆　审校：胡卫清、余维泉、江建安　中文校正：许党泉、龙欣）

1937 年汕头福音医院报告

（英兰长老会汕头教会医院 1937 年年度报告）

过去的一年，医院经历了数个极端的时期。在最初的几个月里，我们开始从过去几年的调整和重组中受益，同时贸易萧条结束，经济状况有所好转，这对医院的运营产生非常有利的影响。我们已经好多年未有这样一个繁荣时期。医院收支平衡，私人病房的患者人数增加，并且愿意支付“护理之家”的费用，我们从而能免费对公共病房的贫困患者进行大量的治疗。除了少数人能够支付昂贵的注射、手术或 X 光检查费用以外，平均来说，有一半的公共病房患者没有支付任何食物和治疗费用，而剩下的一半只支付了七分之一的治疗费用。我们不断收到自发捐款，总之，我们觉得已经渡过困境，无论将会遇到什么困难和问题，我们都能在发展的道路上脚踏实地走下去。

在这良好的发展时期，我们明显感觉到，原先计划在中国社区提前筹集重建医院资金的诉求是合理的，我们也已经开始安排筹集资金购买一台新的 X 光设备和一辆急需的电动救护车。

护理学校的发展在继续推进，政府的规定促使我们根据未来的护理需要，初步考虑与汕尾和五经富合作，建立一所自主管理和拥有大型设备的“护理联校”。这是一项艰巨的任务，需要认真思考和规划。我们已经对华人社区做了初步的咨询，得到了令人鼓舞的回应，这使我们期待能够较快、较顺利地去实施工作。一位著名的中国汕头籍女士接受了调查，当被告知这项任务的规模和难度时，她提出的意见很有启发性：“就让汕头的女士们去做吧。”

私人病房的重建正朝着预期的方向进行，除了富有的中国病人，我们具备为欧洲患者提供医疗和外科手术的条件，并能提供治疗和舒适，因此我们觉得没有必要为此感到羞愧。

1936 年，几乎医院所有的管理部门都被重组，我们由此体会到提高效率和经济效益的好处。

可以毫不夸张地说，去年 7 月，医院的繁荣达到了顶点。

7 月，抗日战争在中国北部暴发。8 月 12 日，日本领事带着所有日本侨民离开汕头。8 月 13 日，上海近郊的战斗开始了。显而易见，这是一场比 5 年前的战争性质更严重的抗争，汕头预计至少会遭受空袭和来自海上的炮击。当地富人很快就开始离开并前往比较安全的地方，而中国当局开始鼓励妇女、儿童和老人离开港口前往内陆的安全地区。防空演习正在继续进行着，一些小街道开始设防。贸易额立即下降，封锁给商品的自由流通增加了进一步阻碍。为了防止资金流出中国，政府宣布暂停贸易，并“冻结”所有的银行存款。我们很快就清楚，即使战争没有波及汕头，医院的财政也将经历一个非常困难的时期。我们的私人病房很快就空了，除了少数私人病房的病人仍能支付费用之外，我们只剩下人数众多的不能支付任何费用的穷困病人了。物价不可避免地开始上涨，尽管政府努力防止有人牟取暴利，生活费用和药物的成本还是大大增加了。

由于附近有被烈性炸弹轰击的危险，我们的建筑并不适合作为医院。哪怕没有直接命中，我们的建筑物也会倒塌。尽管如此，我们希望通过在屋顶画上大旗帜的方式提供识别标志。另外，如里军事目标不在附近，我们应该能够继续运营。不幸的是，中国军方将高角度的相当大口径的防空机枪安装在与医院相邻和对街的建筑物上，我们所有要求拆除这些武器的努力都白费了。在9月的第一周，汕头遭受了一系列的空袭和一次海军的炮击。正如我们所担心的那样，医院的公共病房周围区域的枪支成为袭击的目标。飞行员显然试图仅攻击军事目标，飞行风险相当大，飞得非常低，以确保目标的准确性，他们首先仅用机枪扫射医院旁边的建筑物。袭击并没有停下来，炸弹随之落下，与医院毗邻的消防站被一枚炸弹直接命中，其他的炸弹则落在消防站前面的道路上。医院建筑物摇晃得很厉害，并有一些轻微的损坏。中国员工越来越害怕，威胁说要撤离。医院临时转移到港口对岸的礐石驻扎，我们得以留下三分之一的员工，其余的逃到了内地。由于警察对空袭采取了很好的防护措施，人员伤亡较少，约有10人遇难，20人受伤，伤者都在我们医院接受治疗。

在过去一年里，医院和市政当局及公共卫生部门的关系日益融洽。所有影响城镇的健康和医疗福利的重大事项都会向教会医生咨询。在战争初期，我们成立了一个探讨空袭防护的医生特别委员会。这个委员会代表医院向市政当局提交建议。其中一个建议是，市政当局应该承担照顾伤亡人员的费用，我们医院的伤员救治费用大约25%由市政当局承担。

笔者已被任命为中国预防空袭和紧急医疗措施委员会顾问。

可以看出，在很短的时间内，医院的前景已经从繁荣而满怀希望突然转向飘摇动荡，还有一系列新的问题必须面对和即将遭遇。根据目前的情况，任何重建的想法，以及扩大护士学校都要无限推迟。另一方面，我们必须认识到，人们对医院的需求随时有可能比以往任何时候都大。我们不得不面对这样的事实：试图使用和平时期正常工作的方法，将会在很短的时间内削弱我们的财政；但同时，我们必须随时准备应对大量的人员伤亡，以及在这附近可能发生的地面作战导致的巨大的人员伤亡。我们必须认识到，尽管在进行战争救济工作的时候，有资金和物资可用，并可以很容易获取；然而针对普通民众的运营时，我们无法从私人病房病人那里获得资金，因为大部分人已离开这个地区。我们也不能获得更多的当地捐款，因为无论是通过战争救济捐赠，还是通过增加税收而半强制征收，或是通过购买救国公债的方式获得，每一分钱都将用于填补战争基金。再加上商业萧条，这些战争基金已经成为公众的负担。此外，我们认识到，现阶段必须尽一切努力避免为维持医院的日常运营而呼吁外国使团委员会提供额外的财政援助。而且，我们不能被目前的紧急情况所蒙蔽，更应展望未来，尽管未来也充满着不确定性。我们必须做好准备，在战争结束时能尽快恢复正常公众医院业务，尽可能不给当地民众或英国教会带来沉重的负担。我们意识到，如果日本占领了这里，我们必须尽可能做好准备去满足新政权对我们的严格要求。然后，我们一直面临着一个问题，就是如何减少开支和节约成本，以便在本地没有战事，或有可用的资源时，来年能够继续运作。同时，要做好立刻开展处理大量伤亡者的准备，以及在战争停止的时候随时开始恢复正常的工作的准备。如果可能的话，要做到不把任何额外的负担抛给外国使团委员会。

如果在这里没有发生地面的战争，只有空袭或海军轰炸，这个愿望是能够实现的。正如前面已经指出的，我们的工作人员减少了约三分之二，然而大多数离开的人要么是无偿员工，要么是低收入的工人，这样就有效地节省了一大笔不相称的工资。医院在目前驻扎的临时建筑运营比在我们自己的场地运营要省下许多花销。药物处方实行严格节制，我们已经削减了医院工作中最昂贵的和最不重要的部分——门诊工作。许多病床长时间留空，留给可能出现的伤员；我们已经做好了安排，可以在紧急情况下救治多达150名伤员。

最近在中国南部的一次袭击威胁改变了我们所面临的问题，尽管袭击没有成为现实，但人们普遍认为这早晚是不可避免的。若是如此，我们要比现在做更多的战争准备，我们也正在考虑制订计划来应对这种形势。

战争中的一件事已经清楚地告诉我们，我们必须调整在紧急情况下的行动与想法，使之与中国员工的态度相适应。这个问题在中国各地已经出现了，至少在战争环境中中国员工无法继续工作。如果坚持我们的行动准则，我们的工作将面临完全崩溃，而这正是要维持运营的关键时刻。因此为了能继续运营，我们必须设计出满足中国观念的方法。我们一直试图找到一些方案，可以让我们回到自己的建筑，在那里我们有病房可以去接收更多的紧急病人。我们的中国员工都愿意去，但明确表示，只要遇到麻烦，他们将不会留下来。目前我们无论如何都应考虑采取一些措施，让他们觉得不管发生什么都能留下来。

在今年孟玲医生（Dr. Milne）的休假期间，邵志安医生（Dr. S. L. Strange）第一次从英国来到这里。我们希望孟玲医生有一个悠闲的假期，并重温美好的时光。我们对邵志安医生致以热烈的欢迎，令人沮丧的是他第一次来中国就面临如此艰难的时期，这使他在这里开展工作面临了比原来更多的困难。

史葛先生（Mr. Scott）一休假回来就立刻到汉口帮助J. L. 麦斯威尔医生（Dr. J. L. Mexwell）组织国际红十字会分队了。在这样的时刻失去史葛先生的协助对我们是一个很大的打击，但我们感到自豪的是，在中国各地，即使是最小的医疗传教所，人们也认为只有史葛先生能胜任汉口的工作，报告也表明这项工作他做得非常好。

我们必须提及一个中国员工——郑博士（Dr. Cheng），在繁荣岁月，甚至在最近的动荡时期，他一直是我们的中流砥柱。难能可贵的是，他的机智和智慧帮助我们解决了许多问题。

不可避免，这份报告省略了人们通常发现的诸多细节，而且这一年发生的事因为中国发生的悲剧而蒙上了阴影，对此我们无须致歉。我们试图描绘过去12个月中医院工作真实、相应的画面，希望并祈祷明年我们能汇报更好的消息。

贺尔德（Harold R. Worth）

（翻译：朱文平　校译：林帆　审校：胡卫清、余维泉、江建安　中文校正：许党泉、龙欣）

1939 年汕头福音医院报告

（英兰长老会汕头教会医院 1939 年年度报告）

我们在战争环境中的第二年已经结束，我们能够在报告中说，医院和护士学校仍在运营，并做了很多有用的工作。

1938 年 10 月，广东被占领，我们经历了不安定的几天，海军轰炸了口岸以外的地方，空袭仅限于军事目标，没有造成城里平民伤亡。接下来，情况逐渐稳定下来，频繁的空袭警报和飞机掠过已成为战时的日常，但这里有一段时间没受到进一步的轰炸。

医院工作限于接收病情严重的病人，还有大量的门诊病人。那些患病但自我感觉不太严重的人不愿意来住院，主要是害怕空袭。我们的中国员工进一步减少，战争暴发时我们还有 5 名中国医生，而现在只剩下两名。私人病房的病人少之又少，原因是许多富裕的中国人已经离开城里。

1939 年春天，粤汉铁路段新开通了潮州府和韶州之间的道路运输，卡车队行驶在这些道路上。高运费率让运输服务变得昂贵，但我们收到大量远至湖南北部的内地医院的请求，包括从其他地方采购和运送医疗物资，以及直接从汕头采购或运送。有时采购的医生有自己的卡车，并持有需要在 24 小时内办妥的大批量物资订单；有时我们不得不请求到内陆去的商用货车预留空间。空袭警报每隔几天被拉响，3 月 1 日，汕头的空袭又开始了。

开始有来自内地的流言，大意是不久将进攻汕头。到今年 3 月底，海面上的飞机开始向河里的电船和舢板扫射并投下炸弹。中国当局开始逐步组织市民自愿撤离，愿意撤离的约有 30 000 人，大约占此时市区人口的一半。4 月份空袭放缓，但到 4 月底空袭卷土重来。5 月份我们经历了战争期间最大范围的轰炸。炸弹并未投向人们熟知且避开的常规目标，而是投向了许多新的地方，开始出现伤亡。大多数攻击有俯冲轰炸的特点，飞机显然有明确的目标，但我们却常常很难分辨出被轰炸的区域有哪些军事目标。随后发生的事情使我们确信这些袭击是为了辅助封锁以终止贸易。

在这一系列袭击期间，有一批炸弹被扔在教区，其中 8 枚落在三个方向距医院边界 50 码的地方。作为一项预防措施，我们把最西面普通病房的患者转移到淑德（Sok-Tek）学校的房子里面，这是在早晨两次袭击的间隙快速完成的。医院的工作人员在困难的情况下仍表现得很好。

5 月 7 日星期天，一场自然灾害加重了汕头人已经遭受的苦难。每天早晨，成千上万的人习惯于过海到礐石（Kak Chieh）以躲避可能的空袭，在下午晚些时候回汕头。而在这一天，港内挤满了带着难民返回的舢板，突如其来的风暴席卷了汕头。许多船只倾覆，成千上万的人落入大海。英国驱逐舰和英国商船救了许多人的性命。我们没有统计出确切的死亡人数。

在 6 月份，除了轰炸外，汕头还有大量的空中侦察。6 月 21 日，空袭警报在凌晨

4：45分最后一次响起。上午10：00，一队日本驱逐舰入港。一些小口径舰炮和多管自动高射机关炮进行了射击。12枚炮弹落在我们的教区，一枚炮弹落在医院，在教区有3位难民受轻伤。教区有4间房子被弹片击中，但没有受到严重损坏。飞机在我们头上盘旋了一整天，轰炸城市郊区。这是令人难以忍受而劳累的一天，但医院员工表现得很好。到了晚上，附近才安静了些，直到晚上8点我们看到离医院很近的地方的上空有红色的光，并发现撤退的中国警察放火焚烧了他们在消防站后面的宿舍，那些宿舍紧靠我们医院的病房和手术室。另外还发生了两起火灾，其中一场大火是在汕头其他地方发生的。由于没有自来水供应，没有可用的消防车，所以医院的工作人员竭尽全力地传递水桶灭火，并拆掉了木制的百叶窗，以防止火势蔓延到我们的建筑。许多伤者躺在靠近火灾的急救站，他们被迅速转移到安全的地方。医院的工人都在帮助灭火，而医院的传教人员，包括女士们，都在抬担架运送伤员。幸运的是，在一个小时左右，火灾被扑灭了，医院得救了。

晚上11点钟，我们接到正在撤退的中国当局的一个电话，说疏散平民的道路开放了。我们说服了相当数量的难民踏上这条路。我们不知道有多少人平安地走了出去。有一批人在一个小时后回来，说他们不得不返回，因为中国士兵在黑暗中用机枪向他们开火。在回来的路上，他们遇到了一队日本兵，告诉他们要静静地回家并待在那里，什么都不用怕。

夜很安静。大约凌晨3点，第一支日本兵队伍沿着崎碌路行进，路过医院。天亮后不久，几百名士兵露宿在医院外的道路上。他们显得疲惫但情绪高涨，还把粮票和香烟分给遇到的中国人。一名官员带着一名翻译访问医院并请求送水给他的士兵。他们允许医院的工人出去把伤员运送进来。告示迅速出现，宣布成立新政府，日本和中国清政府的旗帜在各地开始并排出现。

两个月来，我们一直将一个装满开水的大容器放在医院门口。事实证明，它给中国的黄包车车夫和其他人带来了福利，但到目前为止我们可以确定日本士兵没有使用。

除了偶尔发生的机枪射击，一切都保持平静。飞机不断在城里低空飞过，占领行动快速并悄然进行，在城里基本没有引起骚动。事实上，这是因为在汕头被占领之前，一队日本军队就到达汕头北面的庵埠（Am-Pou），迫使中国军队撤出，并避免在汕头附近引起任何激烈的战斗。

我们有大约120位住院患者，几乎都是炸伤和枪伤，其中40%是妇女和儿童。没有电又没有水，井水是咸的，但我们的储罐中有一定量的雨水。井水正在尽快地进行氯化，但其速度太慢，没能避免阿米巴痢疾在患者和工作人员中小规模暴发。痢疾迅速得到了控制。没有其他流行病的发生。

在接下来的几周，医院不断被日本海军和陆军医疗单位访问。他们都渴望获得港口地区的健康状况信息，并问到可能会暴发的流行病。所有的人都非常有礼貌，医院的工作没有受到任何方式的干涉。我们接到了驻汕头的高级医疗官员礼节性的来电，后来整个广东远征军的高级医疗官员访问并参观了医院。他派下属来汕头，间接地转告了高度的赞许，几天之后，他要求我们让他们复制一些自制的设备，特别是手术室灯。

我们最近增加的两台设备大大减少了占领第一周的困难。一是一台冰箱，这是邵志安医生（Dr. Strange）用捐赠给他的资金购买的。二是一台带有小型发电机的便携式X光机，是由英国的救济基金会为中国购买的。这两台设备都是在被占领的几天前收到的，现已证实是非常宝贵的。我们可以在炎热天气下保存大量库存的血浆，并能继续进行X光工作及使用手术室灯做手术。日本军队在一个月内的自用电力供应是有限的。虽然几乎所有其他线路都被切断了，但医院被允许保留其电力供应，前两个月免费，直到供电公司被移交给日本公司运行。然后我们的电线被立即切断，我们向日本公司陈述后，医院的供电立即恢复了。尽管我们自己住的房子还没有获得供电，但医院被确认为是“公共事业”，不仅给予供电，而且没有限制用电量，但还是要支付费用的。

我们很快就获得限量的供水。由于水压低，十分有限，但还是能够满足我们的需要。

食物依然是一个大问题。在为汕头的占领行动做准备时，中国当局给医院供应了大米，可供食用近3个月，使我们度过了这段时期。在此期间，我们不可能购买到我们所需要的大量大米。食品和燃料仍然是我们面临的一个最困难的问题。燃料短缺，大米昂贵。过去的6个月中，生活费用增长了近3倍。我们没有增收患者的费用，那些需要自己解决膳食问题的工作人员仍允许按旧的价格从医院的厨房购买食品。超过半数的住院病人没有支付食物和治疗费用。为了弥补为穷人服务所增加的成本，我们对私人病房增加了一倍的租金。

两年来，我们得到英国驻中国救济基金会的协助，我们一直在积累医疗用品，这种积累已经给我们带来好处。我们没有想到占领后汕头贸易会完全封闭，现在已经发生了，然而我们还能够维持6个月。尽管患者数量比平常多，但医疗用品供应没有大的缺口。一些用品开始出现短缺，但现在可以获得特别许可证进口医疗用品供医院使用。这是一个漫长而疲惫的流程。由于运输船舶不常来这里停靠，货物到达之前许可证可能已过期。

由于工作难找和生活费用上涨，中国的贫困阶层有很多人营养不良，虽然还没有真正的饥荒。营养不良已导致下肢脓毒性溃疡流行。这些和多年前吴威凛博士（Dr. Gauld）在他早期的报告中对困难时期以及营养不良的记述是一样的。只要给患者的食物补充些营养，就会有良好的治疗效果，我们发现最简单的方法是将含鱼肝油的食物配给所有患者。在过去的6个月，我们已经用完两大箱鱼肝油，现在需要更多的鱼肝油。

我们认为营养不良引起的另一个问题是疟疾的流行。疟疾类型主要为间日疟，这种病今年秋天在汕头周边地区流行起来，许多人因此而死亡。人们都知道，中国人通常对疟疾有很高的忍受力，所以他们来求医时往往为时已晚。原本可用一年的奎宁两个月就用完了。

另一个比较小的疫情值得注意，因为到目前为止我们还诊断不了。多年来汕头存在这种病情：病人出现持续低烧，欧洲人尤其易受感染，现已确认病源在汕头。今年欧洲人和中国人都出现大量病患。患者自己的感觉比低烧似乎严重得多，但大多数成人患者不需要卧床。这种症状可能会持续几个月，当寒冷的天气到来时症状就缓解了。年龄小的孩子偶尔呈现出严重的病情，包括高热、谵妄。我们接到的报告称，今年这种发热病人在从厦门到广州的中国沿海一带均有发现，它在沿海地区被俗称为“汕头热”。我们希望最终能够找到这种疾病的病因，但到目前为止没有发现任何有效的治疗方法。

本年度工作的另一个方面就是欧美病人对医院的使用。几乎每段时间我们的私人病房都至少会有一个欧洲的病人。医院因此为外国社区所熟知，我们由此所获得的利益远比所显示的不少经济回报要大得多。

年内，来自教会的非医务人员给予了我们宝贵的帮助，特别是梅乐光小姐和黎节小姐（Misses Muloock and Richards），她们着手做了许多不同的工作，包括从秘书工作到对感染性伤口进行敷料包扎，以及与患者之间沟通的工作。

我们的大部分伤员现在已经离开了医院，从1937年战争开始至今，我们所接收的常规医疗和外科病人第一次接近过去的数量。我们希望情况能迅速得到改善，使这部分工作可以得到恢复和加强。

护士学校得以继续开办，有新护士被录取。学校已不可能完全按我们计划的那样与五经富保持合作，但是只要条件允许，合作将重新开始。目前五经富医院的工作人员肩负着给那些应该回到汕头的护士讲课的重任，在目前的状况下那些护士是不能回汕头的。这意味着在五经富需要教两个（而不是一个）年级的护理课程，而在汕头又要教3年的时间。尽管课程中断，但各类教学仍在进行。

现在，淑德（Sok-Tek）学校的建筑物已移交给医院，它被计划改建成一所护士学校，以适应护理联校计划。在该校毕业的护士可以在五经富和汕尾医院工作（如果她们希望如此），这将使护士学校与汕头医院有较多的联系。汕头医院承担对学校的建筑物进行必要改建的全部费用，使之能够达到这个目的。当护士学校迁新址后，我们期待他们尽快设置独立的预算机构。

医院全年都在进行福音传播工作，包括日常的门诊服务、病房和工作人员的礼拜，以及星期天的病房服务。医院工作人员举办了自己的青年联谊会。

我们与中国教会的关系一年比一年密切。战争这种非正常状态在很大程度上帮助医院提高了声望。令人感动的是，尽管近来仍有许多的困难，周边农村的小教堂纷纷向医院基金捐赠。在非基督教华人社区，医院也享有极好的声誉，这不仅体现在捐款方面，也体现在穷人和富人都来我们这里治疗。

尽管遭遇战争和经济紧缩，我们仍然能够对在用的旧建筑进行必要的维修，使之能继续使用。此外，还粉刷和修饰了部分墙面，使患者生活得更快乐。我们拆除了男医院和女医院之间的隔墙，以改善医院的整体外观。

未来难以预测。不可避免，明年将是困难的一年，某些方面可能出现最困难的局面，我们必须去面对。欧洲战争暴发意味着药品价格立即大幅上涨，生活成本的增加和汕头的贸易限制也加剧了药品价格上涨。在过去的两年中，我们原来计划逐渐提高病床的强度使之达标，现在这项计划不得不推迟，但我们必须努力，尽快地放置更多的配备护理服务的病床。医院的重建计划无限期推迟，我们必须寻求在现有建筑中进行高效运营而无须高昂开销的方法。

C. H. Brangwin医生虽然不与医院有直接联系，但他一直对教会和医院非常友好。我们将以更多的帮助、建言和治疗来回报他。1939年1月他突然去世使我们深有感触。

1939年9月30日年终统计

住院病人：	男病人	596	这些病人中大约60%接受免费治疗和食物。
	女病人	378	
	儿童病人	116	
	合计	1 090	
门诊病人：	首诊	8 507	
	复诊	11 090	
	敷料包扎	14 452	
	眼科	9 477	
	合计	43 526	

伤员：在年内住院患者中，311人因炸弹或机枪子弹受伤，或被倒塌的建筑物压伤。1939年5月，在对汕头的空袭中有58人死亡，160人受伤，其中，当月被送到我们医院的有143人。

1939年1月1日至6月30日的6个月期间，汕头有108次空袭警报，炸弹落在汕头26次。

工作人员：	医生	欧洲	3	护士长	1
		中国	2		
	技师		2		
	助产士		1		
	毕业护士		10		
	培训中的护士		28		
	学生技师		3		

贺尔德（Harold R. Worth）

（翻译：朱文平　校译：许思婷　审校：胡卫清、余维泉、江建安　中文校正：许党泉、龙欣）

1940—1941 年汕头福音医院报告

（英兰长老会汕头教会医院 1940—1941 年年度报告）

敬畏来年，去年年终报告提到“我们希望有实力和机会继续运营”。又一年结束了，我们写到，感谢上帝在我们一年比一年困难的情况下，给予我们力量和继续运营的机会。

6 年前的一份医院报告提到“当建成一所拥有 100 或 110 张护理病床的新医院时，那将是个快乐的日子”。在今年 4 月到 8 月之间我们拥有了 120 张护理病床，不是在“新医院”，而是在翻新的旧医院里，尽管如此我们仍然感到自豪，我们的目标已经达到。不幸的是，由于财政原因，两个新病房在 8 月再次关闭，这将在稍后解释。我们希望下一次的书面报告将能够记述这些病房已重新开放。实际上，由于占领区和非占领区之间的通信中断，最近几个月增加病房的需求已不再迫切。通常我们接收了相当数量的未占领地区的患者，但由于管制仍然有效，他们一直无法前来汕头。

食品和燃料的间断供应让我们感到焦虑，不只是因为成本大幅度上升，也由于难以获得这些物资。今年上半年我们获得购买“官价”大米的许可，价格很便宜，但是我们大部分精力放在获得许可上。不幸的是，后来我们不得不在附近的自由市场购买，成本因此增加了。年内，药品价格上升速度稳定，然而由于英国和美国政府宣布了冻结的规定，平均价格陡涨 70%。

由于药品、食品和燃料成本不断上升，医院的财务运行令人担忧，但我们能够很高兴地报告今年收支平衡，略有结余。在过去的一年里，医院的运营成本已达每天 8 英镑，其中 5 英镑花在食品、燃料上，1 英镑花在药品上。医院的财务状况，就像许多汕头人一样，在很大程度上依赖抽纱制品行业，目前由于冻结的政策而停滞了。近年来，我们收到来自抽纱制品公司的大笔捐款。此外，我们的许多私人病房的病人与抽纱制品行业有关系，许多公共病房病人支付食品和治疗费用的能力取决于这个行业的就业情况。鉴于这种收入来源大幅度减少的可能，我们除了实施其他严格的节俭制度以外，还极不情愿地决定关闭另外两间公共病房。这意味着我们的公共病房床位从 104 张减少到 80 张，这和去年可用的病床数量是一样的。让人自豪的是，我们医院有着不考虑病人的支付能力而进行治疗的传统，在中国很少有教会医院能给予如此高比例的免费治疗。在过去的 6 个月里，我们医院平均每天有 100 名住院病人，其中平均每天有 54 名病人的治疗和膳食是免费的。我们一直都很关注持续提供大量免费治疗的能力，所以在一个星期前收到 15 000 美元的捐款时，我们非常高兴。这笔捐款使我们目前能够暂时保持免费治疗的工作量。这笔非常慷慨的捐款来自上海的一个管理委员会，该委员会正在管理由美国基督教会募捐的资金，除了给医院的资金外，他们已经为汕头地区的救济工作提供了大笔捐赠。

现代的治疗方法开销很大。夏天，有一位老人因为在 10 天前受伤，手部有一个严重感染的伤口而来到医院就诊。病人由于广泛感染致使血管侵蚀，造成严重出血并发破伤风——一种更严重的并发症。痊愈的唯一希望是截肢，还要在术前和术后注射大剂量的抗破伤风血清。10 天后他康复了，可以出院了，我们相当高兴，虽然他失去了左手。血清用去了 10 美元，他住院期间没有能力支付任何治疗和食品的费用。遗憾的是，最终的结果并不总是像这个病例一样美好，尽管治疗费用昂贵，但患者也可能会死亡，我们只能竭尽全力去面对它。

今年我们收到了宝贵的资金和医疗用品捐赠。中华医学会通过其医院基金赠予我们足够一年病床使用的款项，在汕头的 3 位中国朋友每人捐赠了足供一年使用的病床款项。去年 5 月，长老会对医院的礼拜进行观察，并给了医院一笔很可观的资金。我们收到美国红十字会的一份大礼，包括医疗用品和一批奶粉。奶粉使我们能够为营养不良的儿童开设每日免费供应牛奶的诊所，我们高兴地看到，许多孩子的状况已见改善。他们来到我们这里时要么浮肿要么非常瘦弱，而广泛性浮肿是最难治愈的。相对早期的病例，在接受一个好的日常饮食之后结果有了好转，晚期的病例我们也尝试过治疗，但没有任何效果。

在这一年里医院存在的问题之一就是避免同时成为孤儿院。在过去的两年里，有两个女婴被她们的父母遗弃在医院大门口，因为她家缺少食物。去年，由于经济条件日益恶化，这已经成为一种比较普遍的做法。我们曾一度收留了 6 个小女孩，如果当时没有保持密切关注，会有更多孩子留给我们。幸运的是，我们已经找到两个家庭并说服他们把孩子带回去，但仍然有 4 个孩子留在我们这里。通常孩子可能被其他家庭收养，但目前由于贫困和政治前景的不确定性，要找到这样的人非常困难。我们不愿意接收他们，不仅仅是因为喂养和照顾他们的费用问题，还因为如果人们普遍认为我们会接收他们不想要的孩子，那么将带来数量惊人的弃儿。

汕头除了伤寒病之外，没有其他的传染病流行，这是由于日本当局和中国地方政府在霍乱和天花疫苗接种方面做出了积极的努力。不幸的是，在夏季的几个月里，他们没有做出同样的努力去减少大量的伤寒病例。今年有很多病情异常严重的伤寒病例，对于这些重症病例，我们的努力未能避免生命逝去。这个时候对于我们所有人来说是非常难过的，我们的一名护士尽管接受了疫苗接种，但还是因为患上这一严重的传染病而死亡。这一年我们的病人中营养不良的人占很大比例，很多人由于食品不足或食品质量太差而导致体质虚弱，这也是人们犯病比例高的主要原因。

令人振奋的是，年内我们已经启用一个福音传播的工作场所。近年来，我们每天早晨都在男性和女性门诊部进行福音传播，星期天下午的礼拜在不同的病房依次举行，其他病房一些可以行走或搬动的病人会来参加礼拜。汕头教会的成员已经组成了一个福音团，每个月在门诊部履行福音传播工作职责并为两间病房提供服务。除了这些活动，他们还在下午访问病房患者，在许多患者出院回家后到其家中探访。医院福音传播的机会非常多，我们感激汕头教会的成员帮助我们做这项工作。

年内，我们的工作人员发生了一些变动。洪作樑医生（Dr. Ang Tsak-liang）曾在医院忠实服务超过 10 年，并在福音传播工作中成绩突出，现已辞职并接手内地的医疗实践工作。他的位置由已经成为医院的工作人员的张糜西医生（Dr. Moses Chang）接替。2 月，贺尔德医生（Dr. Worth）作为医院院长，在完成艰难的 6 年任期后离开去休假。在任期间，他还不得不担任业务经理。在过去 3 年的战争环境中，令人担忧的困难增加了他的负担。去年1月，郑博士（Dr. Cheng）和我们签订合同，同意在我们医院留任3年以上，令我们所有人感到十分高兴和满足。1933年郑博士成了医院工作人员，这一时期医院的工作很大程度上要归功于他，他不仅是一名医生，他还以睿智的建议，巧妙地化解了许多困难。除了这些行为外，过去两年他还为医院募集了大量的捐款。

不言而喻，来年很可能比过去的一年更困难。但是，回顾走过的路，在这充满机遇的日子里，倘若我们不怀着勇气和希望前进，那我们的信仰确是脆弱不堪的。

统计

1940—1941年

医学传教士		3
外国护士		1
本国医生		2
本国护士		49
助产士/麻醉人员		1
技师		9
牧师/业务经理助理		1
办事员		1
社会工作者		1
住院病人：	男 454 女 628 儿童 255	1 337
门诊患者：	首次就诊人数	20 315
	总就诊人数	78 243
妇产科：	住院分娩	92
	家庭分娩	93
手术		314
实验室	病理学检测	9 733
病床数		95

邵志安（S. L. Strange）

（翻译：朱文平　校译：林帆　审校：胡卫清、余维泉、江建安　中文校正：许党泉、龙欣）

岭东护士学校 1940 年 10 月—1941 年 9 月报告

今年年初，我们的学校中，除了护士长助理，还有 9 名已毕业的护士、42 名在训护士，其中 5 名将要毕业了。我们期待着有足够的毕业生能成为医院各部门的工作人员，并能有一人做私人护士，因为这在汕头富有的中国人中有不断增长的需求。然而，我们百感交集地发现，有 5 个人打算随红十字会去中国西部为国家服务。后来最终只有 3 个人过去了，其余两个人中有一人成为隶属美国浸信会的一家内地医院的工作人员，还有一人现在在上海医生站工作。尽管我们很遗憾失去了她们，但她们为自己和未来毕业的护士铺开了一个更广泛的服务领域，我们为她们感到高兴。顺便说一句，对更多的初级护士来说，她们的离开是一种激励，会促使她们加倍努力学习，从而接替她们工作。

护士学校从开办到今年已经过了十年，我们已经实现接受训练的护士人数突破一百名的目标。

自从与五经富医院联合办学以来，每年的护士调动的行程都很艰难，今年也不例外。这种变动迟来了一个月，因为中国人被限制出入汕头，原因是一些人被发现走私货物到非占领区。

年内有 9 名护士加入我们教会，两人接受了洗礼。其中一人是非基督徒，但当她来到医院时已经是一名听众；另一人的父亲已加入浸信会，而母亲是一名非基督徒。后者承认，她作为一名学生参加培训的时候，曾坦率地表示怀疑，但在培训中她发现了真理。在此之后，她巴不得让她的妹妹也参加培训，在今年 3 月，她做到了。她做礼拜的持续时间很短，因为虽然我们采取常规的预防措施，她还是在 6 月底感染了一种非常严重的伤寒，大约 3 周后去世了。我们都担心她同学的反应，因为她们也是刚参加培训，但有些人听说后表示，正因为她的离世，她们才打算为病人做更多的护理。在那段艰难的日子里，她的妹妹为姐姐感到自豪。当时她是无法和她家人取得联系的，我们很多人都对她抱有好感。

我们的一位毕业生被允许暂时离开，去北京协和医学院护士学校选修护理管理课程。她做这件事是自费的，只有学校选定的候选人是公费的。

1936 年我校在中国护士协会注册，那一年我们的毕业班通过了他们的考评。次年承担中国政府注册任务的全国咨询委员会本应对所有注册学校进行考评，但是 1937 年以后，他们已不可能这样做下去。今年的全国咨询委员会再次开展了这项工作。今年上报注册的时候，我们被告知联合护校不符合他们的规定。关于这件事我们仍然与他们保持联系。在此期间，我们正在进行护士期末考试。要让护士们看到我们决策的明智之处有些困难，但最终她们都答应参加考试。

明年，至今已经与我们在一起将近 10 年的吴修女将于我不在的时候负责护理工作。

我在这份报告的结尾仍须提及，这一年我们已经接管了对男性门诊部技师工作的监督，在几年前这是完全不可能的事。

邓慕德（Maud. L. Martin）

（翻译：朱文平　校译：林帆　审校：胡卫清、余维泉、江建安　中文校正：许党泉、龙欣）

1948 年汕头福音医院报告

（汕头教会医院 1947 年 10 月 1 日至 1948 年 9 月 30 日年度报告）

1946 年 8 月，医院重新运营并开始重建工作，当时只有 33 张病床。回顾过去一年继续开展的重建工作，我们住院病人床位数从 71 张增至 107 张。这一增长很大程度上归功于越来越多已经过培训的有经验的护士员工，以及这一年外界赠予的病床。

我们是在艰难的经济背景下扩大我们的工作规模的。一年应该有两次粮食收成，但在 1947 年，洪水毁掉了第一次粮食收成，而第二次收成因为台风带来的海啸而毁掉，海水淹没了农田。这场洪水使医院积水达两英尺半之深，医院员工拼命与洪水上升的速度赛跑，最终把病人、食物和药物等搬到高处的安全地带。1948 年，干旱使第一次粮食收成歉丰，但我们仍然很庆幸，在我执笔期间，第二次粮食收成看起来有了较好的保障。所有粮食歉收都引发大米价格的攀升，其他商品也随之涨价。我们的病人中大部分是农民，他们遭受了极大的经济损失。与这一地区大米歉收导致的生活消费增长一起发展的还有其他原因导致的通货膨胀现象。一个成年男人一天需要的大米量约有 1. 3 斤，在 1947 年 10 月，其价格是 3 300 元，而在 1948 年 9 月，需要花费 980 000 元购买同样多的粮食。相应的，医院每月的花费也从 139 000 000 元增长到 25 000 000 000 元。幸运的是，我们的收入和外界的馈赠能够应付开销，但在后半年我们的病房租金逐周增加，有时还更频繁。当我们收到钱的时候，最明智的做法是把它们马上花掉，去买一些用品，赶在货币继续贬值之前花完。钱币的大量印发导致员工半个月的工资需要用大麻袋去装。新的货币在 8 月发行，在其后的 6 周物价恢复正常稳定。但从那之后，生活成本增加了 150%，我们担心这种令人沮丧的进程将重新开始。

在这一年里，来自一个内地村庄的警察来到汕头，逮捕我们医院的秘书，并把他扣留在恶劣的环境中长达 5 周。当事方为转移人们对真凶的注意，栽赃指控他为谋杀凶手。通过多方努力他最终才被保释出来。

在这一年里，医疗主管贺尔德医生（Dr. H. R. Worth）的辞职是我们医院的一大损失。他在 1927 年进入我们医院工作，并在 1935 年升为主管。他在担任主管期间，对推动医院的现代化起到很大的作用。一些病房已经实现了现代护理，到 1938 年，所有病人转而由护士照顾，在这之前部分病人是由家人照顾的。岭东护士学校的建立满足了汕头、五经富医院和汕尾医院对护士的需求。他最大的贡献是在 1946 年，在他回到汕头 4 个月后，使家具、医疗设备缺乏且空荡破旧的医院重新运行，并使其拥有了 33 张床位。吴小姐是我们的护士长，她和贺尔德医生一起为医院的重新运营做准备。她最近向前来拜访我们医院的部长和牧师们演讲，谈到在准备重新运营的时候，很多次她觉得，在那么短的时间且各类物资和设备都缺乏的情况下，要快速恢复医院的运营是一件不可能的事。但贺尔德医生充沛的精力和坚定的信仰使这看起来不可能的事情变成了现实。之前的工作报告中提到，在医院重新开业后的前5个月内有大量的病人，没有其他医生的协助，贺尔德医生独自一人工作。我们真诚地感谢贺尔德医生在各方面对我们的引导，也佩服他对未来发展的远见。在这里他作为一名医生的声誉让人称道，他获得了无数病人的感激和称赞，赢得被他所领导的我们的喜爱。

幸运的是，我们也在这一年吸纳了新员工。在1947年底，郑德悦医生（Dr. T. Y. Cheng）加入我们医院，作为一名内科医生承担内科病房的管理。他是郑少怀牧师（Rev. Sheffield Cheng）的兄弟、北京协和医学院的毕业生。在他的照料下，我们这一方面的工作得到加强。我们也欢迎葛乐辅医生（Dr. Joop Graf）（注：荷兰人）的到来。在一年的语言学习后，他减少了医生的工作，开始在部分时间履行作为一名事务主任的职责。我们期待他对医院这方面工作有更加有效的管理。在这一年中，和我们一起工作的实习医生曾宪庭医生（Dr. H. T. Tseng）毕业了，我们也欢迎他成为我们医院的正式员工。

我们再一次记录各方带给我们的各种馈赠，以示感激。我们收到许多来自联合国善后救济总署（UNRRA）捐赠的医疗物资，其中包括50张病床和一台移动X光设备，后者现在已经投入使用。我们十分感激纽约马克苏德进口公司（Macksoud Importing Company of New York）送给我们的配件，尽管不是供给设备，却是设备运行所需要的。我们只能在夜间运行机器，然而不是每个晚上都可以，因为汕头地区电力供应不足，而我们想要发电机的请求至今仍未实现！英国红十字会赠予我们25张病床和非常实用的设备及药品。我们还收到来自英国联合援华基金会（British United Aid to China）的6套包扎用的敷料和一些纯羊毛衣物，其中有些是由英国的教堂捐献的。我们感谢国际救济委员会（International Relief Committee）把捐赠物品运送过来给我们。经文礼品公司（Scripture Gift Mission）给予我们大量中文印刷的圣经，我们得以分发一些给病人。从美华救济团（U. S. A China Relief Mission）那里我们还收到了大米和住院病人的费用支援。其他一些现金的支援包括医院周日从当地教堂收到的钱，另有600英镑来自海外宣道会，还有当地及远方的英国和中国人的捐助。我们很感谢他们的馈赠，这对我们的工作有了极大的帮助。

这所医院总是人满为患，尤其是在夏天。去年每月就诊的新增病人达到1 000人次，每个月有3 400个“复诊病患”，其中52%的人接受免费治疗，29%的人可享受部分免费治疗。我们之前的门诊部不得不拆除，因为战争结束后病房太少不够住，工作也无法正常开展。我们请求美华救济团捐赠等值8 000英镑的资金，帮助我们新建门诊部。令人遗憾的是，有关此事的信函仍在往来沟通的时候，该团却宣布结业。随着医院员工的增加，有可能会进行工作重组。医院门诊开放不限于一周4天，分诊也不再是男性在一楼就诊、女性在另一层就诊而不管他们的抱怨。我们现在根据疾病的特征对门诊进行分类，如内科、外科、妇产科、麻风病科等等。这些门诊现在每周开放6天，病人们很高兴，尽管还是有些首次就诊的病人会在我们休息日过来。孟玲医生（Dr. Milne）开设了产前门诊，来诊者不断增加，越来越多的妇女了解到产前管理的重要性。

在这一年中，住院床位从71张增加到107张，这些增加的床位都安置在公共病房。1月，妇产科病房重新开放，9月，另一间男公共病房也开放了。随着越来越多的妇女到产前门诊就诊，妇产科病房的负担越来越重，但我们也欢迎这些常规以及非常规的病例来我们医院就诊，因为在这一过程中也锻炼了护士的护理能力。在上一年中，我们总共收治了

1 626 名就诊病人，其中 27% 的人饮食和治疗免费，23% 的人是部分免费。在我们医院规模扩大的现阶段，我们给妇女和儿童增加了房间，并计划下一个开设的病房也是儿童病房，以收治更多患病的儿童，他们多数是营养不良，需要在医院进一步观察一段时间。

在这一年中，有 15 间私人病房和 4 间公共病房进行了油漆和粉刷，而有两间病房走廊部分被特别围起来以提供气泵防护（注：防暴风雨）并增加住宿面积。来自苏格兰和爱尔兰的礼物用来装饰我们的一间员工活动室。另外，我们还对建筑进行了多处修补，这在这么老的建筑物中在所难免。我们已经提请修建新的门诊部，但更为迫切的需要是为我们的医生修建住所，因为他们现在住的地方要另作他用。我们无法接收更多的实习生，除非我们能够建一幢新的大楼。我们希望在新的一年能建成新楼。

上一年没有传染病流行，但常常有伤寒。在 1947 这一年，我们接收了 161 例伤寒病人，其中 32 人死亡。20% 的死亡率是很高的，但这些病人很多是发病数周、病情十分严重时才被送到我们这里医治的。上一年我们免费给想要接种的人提供接种伤寒疫苗，我们在市中心也进行了疫苗接种。总的来说，人们并不害怕伤寒，倒是怕霍乱和天花，遇到那两种病他们会立刻过来接种疫苗；但许多年以来死于伤寒的人数远远超过那两种疾病。我们与汕头卫生局合作，在医院和市中心开展天花和霍乱疫苗接种。

在这一年中，有很多病人对福音传播表现出积极反应。我们有充分的理由认为，这些人在接受基督教信仰方面已迈出了决定性的一步。汕头基督教新教堂选拔出来的布道小组成员协助我们拜访住院病人，并在诊所召集门诊病人谈话。很多住院病人表现出对基督教信息的积极反应，并表示他们出院后将与离家最近的教堂保持联系。由此我们得出了这样的结论，我们是最大的福音传播者，我们需要有一个全天的训练有素的牧师作为医院员工，这样能满足患者的各种需要。根据这个结论，关键在于不仅要找到合适的人选，还要安置他和他的家属。我相信这个问题若能被解决，这样的人应该不难找到。

这一年，汕头长老会的牧师和传教士聚集开会，参观了医院。我们对医院工作进行了概述，述说了我们如何满足病人的需求，之后他们进行了提问和讨论。其他参观者包括从军舰上下来的皇家海军医学军官和汕头放假的医学学生，他们在此期间还参观了医院门诊。

在这一年中，我们能继续保持为公共病房的病人提供无限量免费治疗的制度，让每个无能力支付住院费用的病人能住在公共病房。这也是混乱的一年，有许多动乱和幻灭，但也有很多令人高兴和鼓舞人心的事。我们感谢上帝，让我们可以继续扩大我们的事业和工作范围，并保有免费治疗业务。在 1947 年 11 月，有一个老妇人拜访我们医院并捐资一百万元（那时相当于 3. 1 英镑）。70 年前，医院的第一位医生吴威凛医生（Dr. Gauld）为她父亲非常成功地做了眼科手术，她希望借此表达她的感激。回想过去我们奉行的悠久而光荣的传统，激励我们继续奋斗。

邵志安（S. L. Strange）

1947年10月1日至1948年9月30日统计

	1948年	1947年
医学传教士	2	3
外籍护士	0	0
外籍事务主任	1	0
中国医生	4	2
实习生	0	1
取得资格的护士	13	10
护士学生	48	34
药剂师	2	1
实验室技师	1	1
学生技师	7	6
秘书	1	1
医院社工	3	2
饮食服务人员	1	1
女福音传道者	1	1
住院病人：		
私人病房	273	283
公共病房	1 353	971
合计	1 626	1 254
治疗和饮食免费病人	433（27%）	328（26%）
部分付费病人	368（23%）	177（14%）
门诊病人：		（数字涵盖14个月）
首次就诊	11 953	12 646
复诊	23 727	22 972
换药	16 966	27 596
预防接种	914	230
就诊合计	53 569	63 444
免费治疗（包括用药）	27 818（52%）	18 527（29%）

手术：

主要手术	327	250
小手术	265	326
合计	592	576
正常分娩	145	（无可用数据）
非正常分娩	54	（无可用数据）
实验室检查	13 097	14 728
病床：		
公共病房	91	55
私人病房	16	16
合计	107	71

1947年10月至1948年9月手术分析

腹部：

阑尾切除术	9
阑尾脓肿引流术	1
结肠造瘘术	2
创伤性结肠修复术	1
胃溃疡穿孔手术	1
十二指肠溃疡穿孔手术	1
肠胃造口术	1
胃部分切除术（胃癌）	1
肠套叠复位术	4
右结肠肠套叠复位术	1
肠梗阻（粘连）	2
剖腹手术	3
盆腔结肠肠扭转手术	1

腹壁：

股疝手术	2
腹股沟疝手术	15
嵌顿性腹股沟疝手术	5
脐疝破裂手术	1
腹壁枪伤手术	1
腹部枪伤破裂缝合术	2
腹股沟恶性腺体切开术	1
腹股沟纤维瘤切除术	2

直肠：
痔结扎术……6
直肠息肉手术……2
肛瘘手术……2
直肠脱垂手术……1
缺血性直肠窦手术……3
肛门闭锁手术……2
胸外科：
单纯式乳房切除术……2
根治性乳房切除术……1
乳腺纤维腺瘤手术……6
乳腺囊肿手术……1
腋窝孕期水囊瘤手术……3
胸壁乳头状瘤手术……1
腋窝腺体切开术……1
耳鼻喉科：
鼻息肉手术……13
扁桃腺切除术……5
鼻内异物剔除术……5
乳突根治术……1
鼻中隔纤维瘤手术……1
耳朵整形手术……1
眼科：
眼睛切除术……5
眼窝肿瘤 Kronlein's 手术（注：眶外壁减压术）……1
结膜水肿切除术……1
眼睑痣切除术……2
迈博姆氏（Meibomian's）囊肿（注：睑板腺囊肿）手术……3
睑内翻手术（大约）……400
皮肤科：
皮肤移植术……9
皮脂腺囊肿移植切除术……15
烧伤治疗……6
颈部整形手术……1
皮肤伤口缝合手术（仅统计手术室）……11
纤维瘤切除术……11
乳突淋瘤切除术……3

妇产科：

卵巢囊肿手术	32
刮宫术	31
宫颈扩张术	1
子宫全切除术	6
宫颈切除术	1
膀胱阴道瘘修复术	4
宫颈息肉手术	5
阴道—会阴修复术	3
阴道乳头状瘤手术	1
阴道积血手术	3
阴道整形手术	2
治疗性流产（肺结核）	1
异位妊娠手术	4
尿道下裂手术	1

助产术：

正常分娩	145
剖宫产术	3
前置胎盘	8
钳产术	17
臀位产	12
横位先露	5
脸先露	3
子痫	6

头颈部：

颈动脉外结扎术（中等量出血）	1
甲状腺部分切除术	3
腮腺混合瘤手术	1
颌下腺手术	4
颈部多发性囊肿手术	1
鳃裂囊肿手术	1
甲状舌管囊肿手术	1
颈部纤维瘤手术	1
颈部刺伤手术	1
刎颈手术	1
颈部腺体切开术	1
颈部腺体刮除术	1
颌骨骨髓炎手术	12

拔牙 …… 95
下颌骨腺体细胞瘤手术 …… 1
造釉细胞瘤手术 …… 1
纤维龈瘤手术 …… 1
舌纤维瘤手术 …… 1
舌乳头状瘤手术 …… 2
舌下囊肿手术 …… 1
唇裂手术 …… 17
脸颊囊肿手术 …… 1
面部血管瘤手术 …… 1
其他面部肿瘤手术 …… 5

脊柱和背部：

椎板切除术（子弹） …… 2
脊膜膨出手术 …… 1
骶骨皮样瘤手术 …… 1
髂骨骨髓炎手术 …… 1
石膏床（脊椎结核） …… 2

泌尿生殖系统：

包皮环切术 …… 15
鞘膜积液手术 …… 17
血肿手术 …… 1
尿道破裂手术 …… 5
睾丸切除术 …… 1
阴囊切除术（丝虫病） …… 5
阴茎部分切除术（上皮瘤） …… 3
根治性阴茎和阴囊切除术（上皮癌） …… 1
膀胱结石手术 …… 5
尿道结石手术 …… 3
尿道口狭窄手术 …… 1
耻骨上膀胱造瘘术 …… 4
会阴整形手术 …… 1
膀胱探查 …… 2

肢体：

手臂截肢术 …… 4
大腿截肢术 …… 1
赛姆氏（Syme's）截肢术（注：先天性股骨发育不全手术） …… 1
手指截除术 …… 4
异物手术 …… 6

腿炸伤手术 …… 1
股动脉和静脉结扎术（外伤性动脉瘤） …… 1
臂动脉结扎术（中等量出血） …… 1
手臂纤维瘤手术 …… 1
腘窝黏液囊肿手术 …… 1
脚部脂肪瘤手术 …… 2
膝关节滑膜瘤手术 …… 1
腘窝神经纤维瘤手术 …… 1
其他肿瘤手术 …… 3
胫腓骨骨折手术 …… 6
手指复合骨折手术 …… 1
踝关节严重脱位手术 …… 2
畸形足（石膏固定）手术 …… 4
髋关节固定手术 …… 1
股骨内固定术 …… 1
膝关节穿刺术 …… 3
髋关节人字形绷带固定术 …… 1
腓骨骨髓炎手术 …… 1
股骨骨髓炎手术 …… 2
脚趾骨骨髓炎手术 …… 1
输血 …… 28
脓肿引流 …… 31

1947年10月1日至1948年9月30日收入概述

（按中国国内货币计算）

单位：元

医院：

1947年10月1日贷方余额 …… 5 558 164.96
美华救济团（China Relief Mission, U. S. A.） …… 378 000 000
对残疾人的补助（5英镑） …… 179 310 000
E. M. M. S. 邮票局（3英镑） …… 107 550 000
香港发展（Changing）东方展览（21.13美元） …… 47 550 000
香港马修斯（Matthews）捐赠病床（17.70美元） …… 39 750 000
香港布里斯托（Bristow）捐赠病床（19.58美元） …… 44 100 000
香港援助者捐赠病床（23.57美元） …… 53 040 000
香港爱丁堡医学传教士索笛（Socty）（31.92美元） …… 71 520 000
伯肯黑德圣保罗女校助理（3.3美元） …… 113 100 000
中国人捐助 …… 1 101 777 000

外国人捐助 …………………………………………………………………… 2 259 690 000
病人收款 …………………………………………………………………… 52 855 943 300
销售、银行利息和杂项收入 ………………………………………………… 1 079 928 200
护士学校：
利物浦长老会妇女传教协会（W. M. A.）（16 英镑） ……………… 573 690 000
中国人捐助 ………………………………………………………………………… 6 600 000
食堂收入 …………………………………………………………………………… 623 092 000
银行利息和杂项收入 …………………………………………………………… 782 847 500

60 323 346 164. 96

葛乐辅　邵志安

（翻译：许思婷　校译：朱文平　审校：胡卫清、余维泉、江建安　中文校正：许党泉、龙欣）

岭东护士学校 1947 年 10 月 1 日—1948 年 9 月 30 日报告

自两年前重新运营以来，汕头医院能扩大得那么迅速，主要在于护士数量增长加快，而这主要归功于岭东护士学校培养了有专业技能的护士。因此，我们能很高兴现在有 61 名学生和毕业护士，而一年前我们只有 44 名。虽然现在护士的数量是学校有史以来最多的，但在太平洋战争暴发之前，投入使用的床位更多。一是我们现在总共有 48 名学生护士，其中 29 名要么处在试读期，要么才上一年级，所以她们只能承担有限的工作。二是与战争前相比，现在试读生和护士学生上课的时间要比那时多。去年，学校扩大，新增了两个班的护士学生。由于现在医院有一台运行中的 X 光机，我们能够通过 X 光机对所有刚来学习的学生进行肺部透视，这是一个重要的进步。肺结核病人在中国是非常多的，去年，我们有一个学生不幸染上该病。另有两位上一个班级的学生因 X 光透视之后发现有问题而被拒之门外。去年，有 3 名护士学生毕业并加入我们的员工队伍。

我们的护士学生要上 3 年 4 个月的课程，毕业后，成绩优秀的学生有机会接受进一步培训，在那期间她们可以像护士员工一样进行实践。通过前 4 个月的实习培训，她们将被决定是否适合继续进行护理训练。实习期间不用戴护士帽，去年 2 月，我们护士学校首次为优秀的实习生举行戴帽典礼。在讲完这个典礼的重要性后，这 9 名实习生拿着未点燃的蜡烛，排成一排站在讲台上，面向 9 名手拿着点燃的蜡烛的老护士。老护士逐个点燃对应的新护士的蜡烛，然后由校长彭小姐亲自为她们戴上护士帽。典礼最后由医院院长向护士们作简短的致辞。出席典礼的人都认为这是个印象深刻的典礼，但不幸的是第二天早晨我们就接到一个让我们沮丧至极的消息，20 名刚入行一两年的护士举行罢工，并拒绝履行职责。在中国的学校，罢工这种事情并不少见，原因也有很多，而这次罢工的原因是之前的实习生的新制服都都是长袖的，而现在实习护士只有短袖的，天冷了要在外面加一件夹克。最后决定以后所有学生护士的新制服是长袖的，这个班级将是首批获得新制服的。幸好在中国新年假期后病人数量很少，医院的工作像往常一样继续，36 小时后，之前离岗的护士恢复上班。这次事件是去年我们学校的污点，它的影响不容忽视。

在撰写上一份报告时，为了高级护士班的培训能充分展开，我们申请注册护士学校，希望在 1948 年 7 月接受政府的考核评估，但我们的希望落空了。护理培训归教育部门管辖，注册申请也由汕头市教育局于 1948 年 3 月批准并送达广东省教育部门。如果能批准的话，会进入一下流程，但一直到 7 月我们仍未收到任何消息，于是去查询是不是延迟了。在 9 月我们收到广州的来信说，他们没有收到我们的任何申请，所以我们猜测大概是丢失了。与此同时我们被告知政府条例做出了修改，其中有一些我们难以满足的财务规定，所以我们又回到 1947 年以前的状态。这不仅使校长和董事会失望，也使我们的护士感到失望，她们到现在仍然不能接受政府最终的考核。

1948年1月，我们很高兴欢迎来自英国的护士 M. D. E. 西尔弗小姐（Miss M. D. E. Silver）。她在医学传教工作理事会援助护士学校的专门委员会工作。她的到来令人鼓舞，此行是为了了解我们的现状和需要。自从她来访后，我们收到有价值的馈赠，包括加拿大援助中国的16卷制服布料和来自英国红十字会一个大通娃娃和解剖挂图，此外他们还许诺给我们送来一套人体骨骼架和250美元。学校也很感激由利物浦长老会妇女传教协会（Women Missionary Association of Liverpool Presbytery）送来的16英镑的捐款。

在上一份报告中我们提到了 E. W. 肯尼斯小姐（Miss E. W. Kenneth），她在完成语言学习后要开始工作时，由于健康原因而辞职，我们因此遭受了损失。接下来繁重的责任将由彭小姐和医院护士长吴小姐承担。这些责任在过去几年随着护士学校和医院的发展不断增加，我们很感谢她们为医院病床数扩充至超过100张所做出的努力。她们和我们都期待早期任命的一名护士传教士能分担她们的重担。与此同时我们很高兴欢迎卜瑞德夫人（Mrs. Braisted），她在我们五经富医院当护士时叫许道莲小姐（Miss Doreen Hill），在她丈夫前往美国期间，她来我们这里作4个月的护理顾问。

去年令人沮丧，在中国的许多机构，不论是基督教的还是非基督教的，都有这一经历。但去年也是成长的一年，由于病例数增长比较快，护理工作达不到其应有的标准，但我们感谢已取得的成绩，感谢我们的护士凭着勇气与激情，完成了放在她们面前的工作。

统计

	1948年	1947年
毕业护士	13	10
护士学生		
预读生	13	8
一年级	16	13
二年级	13	7
三年级	6	4
四年级	0	2
护士学生合计	34	48

邵志安

（翻译：许思婷　校译：朱文平　审校：胡卫清、余维泉、江建安　中文校正：许党泉、龙欣）

汕头医院的光荣：
治疗方案被采纳作为中国国家标准

斐义礼医师（Dr. Fraser）应邀在由中华医学会麻风病分会所组织的第一次全国会议上发表演讲。在门诊麻风病病人的治疗方案上，根据斐义礼医师提供的数据，会议组织者安排提供了大量图表，以表格和图形的形式展示了不同年龄和性别组的发病率，并在大标题为“汕头福音医院的门诊工作栏目”下展出。斐义礼医师也给出实际的论证。这些引起人们的热点关注。在会议尾声我们很满意地看到我们的治疗经验得到菲律宾麻风疗养院的推荐与采用，会议将其作为在中国的一项治疗标准，并向那些计划开展麻风病治疗的医院进行推荐。在我们去复印时，收到来自中国麻风救济会的来信，信中写道：“很高兴告诉你们，上周我们发出的关于普及宣传麻风病法律的请愿得到了国民政府卫生署的官方回复，国家麻风病会议决议通过该项提议，相关法律正在起草当中，我们也应邀就相关准则提供参考意见。为了尽可能给我们的政府提出最佳建议，现征集贵医院专家的意见。”显然，我们的会议正初显成效。虽然我们目前触及的只是冰山一角，但对于汕头医院所做的开拓性工作及取得的成效我们心怀感激，回顾一年努力的成果我们还是倍感欣慰。

（摘自《1932—1933 年汕头福音医院文件汇编（第二版）》）

（翻译：陈练意　校译：朱文平　审校：胡卫清、余维泉、江建安　中文校正：许党泉、龙欣）

后　记

汕头福音医院是汕头市第二人民医院的前身，始建于1863年，是英兰长老会创办的教会医院。为迎接150周年院庆，并达到存史、资治、教化的目的，从2012年开始，汕头市第二人民医院进行院志编纂，由笔者牵头完成。

历史资料采集是院志编纂的首要环节。在此过程中，山东大学历史文化学院教授、博士生导师胡卫清给予了极大的帮助。胡卫清教授长期从事中国基督教史和潮汕地方史的研究，颇有建树，有多篇著作发表于权威刊物。胡卫清教授向我院提供了大量极有价值且具有权威性的资料，包括汕头福音医院1866年至1948年多个年度的报告、院长工作手记、信件及其他资料。胡教授提供的资料对于研究潮汕甚至中国的西医学发展史，以及宗教史、战争史和潮汕民风民俗等具有很高的史料价值。

胡教授提供的资料多为英文资料，在医院院志编纂过程中，由谢煊、许思婷、汤意芝、刘慧翔、陈练意、陈坚龙、郑瑞年、郑庭凯等进行翻译，由笔者进行校对、整理。由于资料繁多，时间紧迫，对这些英文资料只能择要翻译，以保证院志编纂按时完成。2013年10月，《汕头市第二人民医院院志（1863—2013）》编纂完成并获得好评，但由于对《汕头福音医院年度报告》等珍贵历史资料未作系统翻译而留下遗憾。

2014年4月21日《潮汕文库》大型丛书编委会发布《关于征集珍稀潮汕历史文献资料启事》，征集范围包括“重要的外文潮汕文献及图书”。笔者从2014年6月9日发行的《汕头日报》上看到启事。笔者与编委会联系人江建安和魏影秋两位老师取得联系，两位老师即亲临笔者所在的汕头市第二人民医院，在亲阅资料后认为资料珍贵，符合征集要求。编委会初定《汕头福音医院年度报告》作为丛书的项目之一。

《汕头福音医院年度报告》基本都是英文资料，根据编委会的要求，必须进行系统翻译。笔者欣然接受了任务，组织许思婷、谢煊、陈练意、朱悦阳、林帆、魏菁等有较好英语基础的年轻人进行再次翻译。对于原来尚未翻译的多个年度报告，由笔者本人进行翻译。翻译者对译文互相进行校对，然后统一由笔者进行校译，由胡卫清教授进行审校。

《汕头福音医院年度报告》涉及大量的医疗卫生专业内容，笔者发挥自身具有扎实医疗卫生专业理论功底的优势，对其中内容进行认真校对，使译文能真正体现专业特色。术科部分笔者还请汕头市第二人民医院原副院长、外科专家李光昭主任医师进行校正，确保了相关译文的准确性。

2014年8月19日，笔者作为推荐人向《潮汕文库》大型丛书编委会推荐《汕头福音医院年度报告编译（1866—1948）》项目，提交“〈潮汕文库〉典籍系列第一批典籍整理项目推荐书”。该项目通过《潮汕文库》大型丛书编委会及组委会评审，成为“文库”文献系列第一批启动项目。2015年3月1日，笔者与潮汕历史文化研究中心签订该项目“〈潮汕文库〉大型丛书典籍系列课题立项书”。按立项书计划，项目分为《汕头福音医院年度报告编译（1866—1948）》原文影印件和中文译文两大部分。

2015 年 4 月 29 日，笔者提交了《汕头福音医院年度报告》英文资料（纸质版）和中文译文第一稿（纸质版和电子版），计有年度报告英文版及其中文译文各 30 份，其他出版稿件英文版及其中文译文各 1 份，由潮汕历史文化研究中心进行结项审批。审稿专家认为：该成果达到了课题的设计要求，可以结项。审稿专家也提出了一些修改意见。

根据审稿专家意见，笔者对翻译稿件进行第二次校译，形成中文译文第二稿，第二稿的纸质版和电子版于 2015 年 6 月 8 日交予江建安和余维泉两位老师进行第二次审校，形成中文译文第三稿。为使中文译文更接近中文的表述习惯，根据编辑部的要求，2015 年 6 月 30 日，第三稿交由许党泉老师进行中文校正。编辑部也将报告的英文版编制成影印件。

2015 年 5 月 23 日，笔者向编辑部提交汕头福音医院历史照片共 25 幅（电子版，含注释），作为《汕头福音医院年度报告编译（1866—1948）》的插图。

至此，本书的编译工作全部完成。

本书在编译过程中得到潮汕历史文化研究中心及其《潮汕文库》大型丛书编委会、组委会、编辑部，以及胡卫清、江建安、余维泉、许党泉、李光昭、许思婷、谢煊、陈练意、朱悦阳、林帆、魏菁等同志的大力支持和帮助，得到陈荆怀、魏影秋等同志的指导，也得到曾旭波、黄晓丹、林志达等同志的帮助，在此一并致谢。

由于内容时间跨度大、资料繁多、工作量巨大，加上编译者的水平有限，书中谬误、错漏在所难免，敬请读者赐教、谅解。

编译者：朱文平
2015 年 7 月 16 日